Urban Bodies

Urban Bodies

Communal Health in Late Medieval
English Towns and Cities

Carole Rawcliffe

THE BOYDELL PRESS

First published 2013
The Boydell Press, Woodbridge
Paperback edition 2019

ISBN 978 1 84383 836 4 hardback
ISBN 978 1 78327 381 2 paperback

The Boydell Press is an imprint of Boydell & Brewer Ltd
PO Box 9, Woodbridge, Suffolk IP12 3DF, UK
and of Boydell & Brewer Inc.
668 Mt Hope Avenue, Rochester, NY 14620–2731, USA
website: www.boydellandbrewer.com

A catalogue record for this book is available from the British Library

The publisher has no responsibility for the continued existence
or accuracy of URLs for external or third-party internet websites
referred to in this book, and does not guarantee that any content on
such websites is, or will remain, accurate or appropriate

This publication is printed on acid-free paper

Designed and typeset in Adobe Warnock Pro by
David Roberts, Pershore, Worcestershire

For
Nicholas Amor, Christopher Bonfield,
Isla Fay, Joy Hawkins,
Carole Hill and Ellie Phillips

❧ Contents

⚜ Illustrations

Maps

The author and publishers are grateful to all the institutions and individuals listed for permission to reproduce the materials in which they hold copyright. Every effort has been made to trace the copyright holders; apologies are offered for any omission, and the publishers will be pleased to add any necessary acknowledgement in subsequent editions.

❧ Acknowledgements

Jeremiads about the pressures of academic life are as old as the hills, or at least as John of Salisbury's *Metalogicon* of *c.* 1159, which begins with a disconcertingly familiar apology. 'I had neither the leisure nor energy to enter into any subtle analysis of opinions, much less to polish my style', he complained, adding for good measure that 'administrative concerns' and other unwelcome duties had consumed all his time, 'save that required for eating and sleeping'. I can offer no such excuse, having been the grateful recipient of generous study leave from both the University of East Anglia and the Wellcome Trust for work on the final stages of this book. I am, as ever, indebted to the staff of the UEA and Wellcome Libraries for their assistance, and to those of the British Library, the Warburg Institute, the Institute of Historical Research and of all the other institutions that I have visited during the course of many years' research. To Dr John Alban, the County Archivist, and his colleagues at the Norfolk Record Office, I owe particular thanks for expert help far beyond the call of duty.

I first became interested in the topic of urban health almost three decades ago, at which point I began to accumulate material that might one day form the basis of a full-length study. Since then, so many scholars have shared their findings with me that it is impossible to thank them all. However, especial mention is due to Professor Caroline Barron, Professor James Bolton, Dr Elma Brenner, Professor Martha Carlin, Professor Sandra Cavalli, Dr Paul Cavill, Mr Giles Emery, Professor Guy Geltner, Professor Roberta Gilchrist, Dr Teresa Huguet-Termes, Mr David King, Dr Hannes Kleineke, Professor Maryanne Kowaleski, Dr Keith Lilley, Mrs Elizabeth Rutledge and her husband, Mr Paul Rutledge, Dr Sheila Sweetinburgh, Dr Sethina Watson and Dr Matthew Woodcock, each of whom has been generous with help and information. The former Norfolk County Archaeologist, Mr Brian Ayers, has proffered invaluable advice about medieval urban archaeology in both England and continental Europe, along with a constant stream of references and photographs. I also wish to thank Mr John Allan of the Exeter Archaeology Unit for sending me copies of unpublished reports on the city's medieval water supply. Phillip Judge and Cath D'Alton skilfully interpreted my rather impressionistic drawings to produce the maps.

Among the many other distractions endured by John of Salisbury were 'the interruptions of friends', which proved just as exasperating as the demands made by his employers. Here, too, I have been infinitely more fortunate, not least in the support offered by my colleagues in the School of History at UEA, and especially by Professor John Charmley, whose many acts of kindness deserve an acknowledgements page of their very own. Hospitable as ever, Professor Joel Rosenthal made possible a memorable visit to New York for work on manuscript collections at the time of the 2008 presidential elections. I am particularly indebted to Dr Linda Clark (who cast her keen editorial eye over each one of the following chapters as it appeared), Ms Elizabeth Danbury and Ms Heather Creaton-Brooke both for their constant encouragement and their cheerful accommodation of my interest in diseased paupers, cesspits and drains. I have profited greatly from the expertise of Professor John Henderson, whose work on public health in Tuscany has prompted so many interesting and illuminating discussions. Nor should any list of debts incurred omit Mr Peter Martin and Master Basil Pug.

It has once again been a pleasure to collaborate with Ms Caroline Palmer and her associates at the Boydell Press, and to thank their reader, Professor Peregrine Horden, for his characteristically insightful and constructive comments. Dr David Roberts copy-edited the final text with meticulous attention to detail.

This book is dedicated to six former research students who have explored medieval sickness and health with me since I arrived at UEA two decades ago. Without their generosity and enthusiasm it would not have been written. Particular thanks are due to Dr Nicholas Amor for allowing me to use his databases of material from Ipswich leet courts and to Dr Isla Fay for commenting on several draft chapters, which have been greatly improved as a result of her perceptive suggestions. But each will recognise in the following pages his or her individual contribution to what is, in so many respects, a work of collaboration.

Carole Rawcliffe
Norwich, September 2012

❧ Abbreviations

BAR	British Archaeological Reports
BHM	*Bulletin of the History of Medicine*
BL	British Library
BTD	A. F. Leach, ed., *Beverley Town Documents*, Selden Society 14 (London, 1900)
CBA	Council of British Archaeology
CCA	Chester City Archives (Cheshire and Chester Archives and Local Studies Centre)
CCR	*Calendar of Close Rolls, 1277–1509*, 63 vols (London, 1892–1963)
CCRCL	R. R. Sharpe, ed., *Calendar of Coroners' Rolls of the City of London, 1300–1378* (London, 1913)
CEMCRL	A. H. Thomas, ed., *Calendar of the Early Mayor's Court Rolls of the City of London, 1298–1307* (Cambridge, 1924)
CIMisc	*Calendar of Inquisitions Miscellaneous, 1219–1485*, 8 vols (London, 1916–2003)
CLB	R. R. Sharpe, ed., *Calendar of Letter-Books Preserved among the Archives of the Corporation of the City of London, 1275–1498*, 11 vols, A–L (London, 1899–1912)
Coventry Leet Book	M. Dormer Harris, ed., *The Coventry Leet Book, 1420–1555*, 4 parts, EETS o.s. 134, 135, 138, 146 (London, 1907–13)
CPMRL	A. H. Thomas, ed., *Calendars of Plea and Memoranda Rolls Preserved among the Archives of the Corporation of the City of London, 1298–1482*, 6 vols (Cambridge, 1926–61)
CPR	*Calendar of Patent Rolls, 1216–1509*, 54 vols (London, 1894–1916)
CS	Camden Society
CSPVenice	R. Brown, ed., *Calendar of State Papers and Manuscripts Relating to English Affairs, Existing in the Archives and Collections of Venice, 1202–1554*, 5 vols (London, 1864–73)
CUHB1	D. M. Palliser, ed., *The Cambridge Urban History of Britain*, vol. 1: *600–1540* (Cambridge, 2000)
CWCHL	R. R. Sharpe, ed., *Calendar of Wills Proved and Enrolled in the Court of Husting of London, 1258–1668*, 2 vols (London, 1889–90)
DRO	Devon Record Office, Exeter
EAA	East Anglian Archaeology
EconHR	*Economic History Review*
EETS	Early English Text Society
EHD	*English Historical Documents*
EHR	*English Historical Review*
e.s.	extra series
HMC	*Historical Manuscripts Commission*
JHM	*Journal of the History of Medicine*
KLBA	King's Lynn Borough Archives
LAN	H. M. Chew and W. Kellaway, eds, *The London Assize of Nuisance, 1301–1431*, LRS 10 (London, 1973)
LPFD	J. S. Brewer *et al.*, eds, *Calendar of Letters and Papers Foreign and Domestic, Henry VIII*, 21 vols, and *Addenda*, 2 vols (London, 1862–1932)

LRBB	F. B. Bickley, ed., *The Little Red Book of Bristol*, 2 vols (Bristol, 1900)
LRS	London Record Society
MCO	H. E. Salter, ed., *Munimenta civitatis Oxonie*, Oxford Historical Society 71 (Oxford, 1920)
MGL	H. T. Riley, ed., *Munimenta Gildhallae Londoniensis* , 3 vols RS 12 (London, 1859–62)
NA	*Norfolk Archaeology*
NRO	Norfolk Record Office
n.s.	new series
OPT	Bartholomaeus Anglicus, *On the Properties of Things: John Trevisa's Translation of Bartholomaeus Anglicus' De Proprietatis Rerum*, ed. M. C. Seymour, 3 vols (Oxford, 1975–88)
o.s.	original series
P&P	*Past and Present*
PL	N. Davis, ed., *Paston Letters and Papers of the Fifteenth Century*, 2 vols (Oxford, 1971–6)
PROME	C. Given-Wilson *et al.*, eds, *The Parliament Rolls of Medieval England, 1275–1504*, 16 vols (Woodbridge, 2005)
RBC	R. Britnell, ed., *Records of the Borough of Crossgate, Durham, 1312–1531*, Surtees Society 212 (Woodbridge, 2008)
RBL	Bateson, M., ed., *Records of the Borough of Leicester*, vols 1 and 2 (London, 1899–1901)
RBN	C. A. Markham and J. C. Cox, eds, *Records of the Borough of Northampton*, 2 vols (Northampton, 1898)
RCN	W. Hudson and J. C. Tingey, eds, *Records of the City of Norwich*, 2 vols (Norwich, 1906–10)
RP	J. Strachey, ed., *Rotuli Parliamentorum*, 6 vols (London, 1783–1832)
RPBC	W. G. Benham, ed., *The Red Paper Book of Colchester* (Colchester, 1902)
RS	Rolls Series
SCH	*Studies in Church History*
SR	A. Luders *et al.*, eds, *Statutes of the Realm*, 11 vols (London, 1810–28)
SROI	Suffolk Record Office, Ipswich
s.s.	supplementary series
TLMAS	*Transactions of the London and Middlesex Archaeological Society*
TNA	The National Archives, Kew (formerly Public Record Office)
TRHS	*Transactions of the Royal Historical Society*
VCH	*Victoria County History*
YASRS	Yorkshire Archaeological Society Record Series
YCO	M. Prestwich, ed., *York Civic Ordinances, 1301*, Borthwick Paper 49 (1976)
YCR	A. Raine, ed., *York Civic Records*, vols 1–4, YASRS 98, 103, 106, 108 (Wakefield, 1939–45)
YMB	*York Memorandum Book*, vols 1 and 2 ed. M. Sellars, Surtees Society 120, 125 (Durham, 1912, 1915); vol. 3 ed. J. W. Percy, Surtees Society 186 (Gateshead 1973)

✒ Introduction

Of hygiene in the whole of this period there is little that can be said.[1]

From a twenty-first-century perspective, the towns and cities of medieval England seem surprisingly small in terms of their size and population density. Although the nation became far more urbanised between the twelfth and late thirteenth centuries, as trade flourished and the birth rate rose, approximately four-fifths of all Englishmen, women and children continued to pursue a rural or semi-rural existence.[2] This state of affairs remained virtually unchanged until the 1500s: allowing for the widespread contraction occasioned by successive outbreaks of plague and other epidemics from 1348 onwards, urban and suburban communities still accounted for roughly the same proportion of the overall population.[3] Only London, which boasted as many as 80,000 inhabitants before the Black Death, stood comparison with the great cities of continental Europe, such as Bruges, Paris or Florence.[4] By contrast, recent estimates suggest that, of the 690 or so communities which merit the name of town (and there is invariably a grey area that shades into sizeable villages and hamlets), the great majority comprised far fewer than 2,000 souls, and a mere sixteen ever exceeded the 10,000 mark.[5]

Even so, despite their modest size, these towns and cities have consistently punched above their weight, both in terms of the political, legal, economic, social and cultural influence that they exercised during the later Middle Ages, and in the attention paid to them by successive generations of historians since the nineteenth century. Almost every conceivable aspect of life within the walls, from civic display and ceremony to the minutiae of the rental market, has been subject to meticulous study, and sometimes heated debate – none more lively and protracted than the still contested question of 'urban decline'. Did English towns really succumb to lengthy periods of economic hardship and 'sore decay' after the Black Death? Or has the phenomenon been greatly exaggerated? However, one crucial topic of

---

[1] S. G. Blaxland Stubbs and E. W. Bligh, *Sixty Centuries of Health and Physic: The Progress of Ideas from Primitive Magic to Modern Medicine* (London, 1931), p. 106.

[2] R. H. Britnell, *The Commercialisation of English Society, 1000–1500* (Cambridge, 1993), p. 167.

[3] R. H. Britnell, 'Town Life', in R. Horrox and W. M. Ormrod, eds, *A Social History of England, 1200–1500* (Cambridge, 2006), p. 145. Some historians believe that the proportion may have risen slightly: A. Dyer, '"Urban Decline" in England, 1377–1525', in T. R. Slater, ed., *Towns in Decline, AD 100–1600* (Aldershot, 2000), pp. 266–88.

[4] C. Barron, 'London, 1300–1540', *CUHB1*, p. 396. It was four times larger than Norwich, then England's second city in terms of population, but the number of inhabitants may have fallen to 60,000 by 1348 as a result of the early fourteenth-century famines: B. Sloane, *The Black Death in London* (Stroud, 2011), p. 15.

[5] Britnell, 'Town Life', p. 145. Christopher Dyer identifies 667 communities with populations of between about 300 and 2,000, noting that very few towns in the North and West, including Carlisle, rose above this size: C. Dyer, 'Small Towns, 1270–1540', *CUHB1*, pp. 505–6. By contrast, only twenty-four towns were larger: J. Kermode, 'The Greater Towns, 1300–1540', *CUHB1*, pp. 442–3.

obvious relevance to this issue, and a host of others, has been largely ignored by historians, who have yet convincingly to address the ways in which members of these communities sought *collectively* to protect themselves from sickness, debility and disease in a period notable for the looming spectre of *mors improvisa* (sudden death).[6] Nor has the consuming interest shown by scholars in relations between central and local authority extended to an evaluation of the crown's role in protecting the urban environment and encouraging its subjects to do likewise. As the first chapter of this book reveals, a significant number of publications dealing with specific aspects of communal health, such as waste disposal, water supply and medical regulation, has appeared since the 1930s. To them may be added a few studies of the sanitary measures adopted in London and in a handful of provincial cities. Nonetheless, there has so far been no attempt to develop this material into anything approaching a national survey, along the lines pursued in France by Jean-Pierre Leguay,[7] nor to set it within the wider context of rising literacy rates and growing familiarity with ideas about human physiology that had previously been confined to a narrow academic elite.[8]

This state of indifference is all the more striking in view of the vulnerability of late medieval town dwellers to that lethal combination of endemic and epidemic disease known to historians of later periods as 'the urban penalty'.[9] As Richard Britnell observes, the dramatic, often capricious, effect of pestilence and other vicissitudes (such as fire, coastal erosion and loss of trade) is strikingly apparent from a comparison of the taxable wealth of English towns in 1334 and 1524. Just as today, in the case of school league tables or Michelin-starred restaurants, there were clear 'winners' and 'losers', whose dramatic reversals and recoveries underscored 'the shortnes and unstablenes of this lyf'.[10] Reading rose from fortieth to twelfth place, and Exeter (the great success story of the period) from twenty-eighth to sixth. York, on the other hand, fell from third to eleventh place, while the once-prosperous Yarmouth plummeted from seventh to twentieth.[11] Yet not even the most economically buoyant communities escaped unscathed, especially as plague mutated during the fifteenth century into a more specifically

---

[6] For example, S. Sheard and H. Power, eds, *Body and City: Histories of Urban Public Health* (Aldershot, 2000), moves from the early European Middle Ages to early modern France, without mentioning English health provision before 1847.

[7] J.-P. Leguay, *La Rue au Moyen Âge* (Rennes, 1984); *La Pollution au Moyen Âge* (Paris, 1999); and *L'Eau dans la ville au Moyen Âge* (Rennes, 2002).

[8] D. Jørgensen '"All Good Rule of the Citee": Sanitation and Civic Government in England, 1400–1600', *Journal of Urban History* 36 (2010), pp. 300–15, for instance, ignores the effect that epidemics and contemporary ideas about them might have had on schemes devised by the rulers of Coventry and Norwich. In contrast, see Isla Fay's forthcoming study: *Health and the City: Environment and Politics in Norwich, 1200–1600* (York, forthcoming).

[9] See, for example, G. Kearns, 'The Urban Penalty and the Population History of England', in A. Brändström and L. Tedebrand, eds, *Society, Health and Population during the Demographic Transition* (Stockholm, 1988), pp. 213–36.

[10] R. Horrox, 'Introduction', in R. Horrox, ed., *Fifteenth-Century Attitudes: Perceptions of Society in Late Medieval England* (Cambridge, 1994), p. 3.

[11] Britnell, 'Town Life', pp. 145, 150.

urban and local, rather than a national, phenomenon. However much scholars may disagree about its long-term consequences, the close relationship between these 'continuing and ubiquitous' epidemics and stagnating levels of population is now widely recognised, if still perhaps not fully understood.[12] So too is the impact of high mortality rates upon the art, literature and religious practices of the period. That the citizens who gazed in trepidation upon the vivid imagery of the Dance of Death in the painted cemetery cloister of St Paul's, London, or in the stained glass of St Andrew's, Norwich (plate 1), may have sought to postpone their own confrontation with the Grim Reaper by ameliorating the conditions in which they lived can seem, nonetheless, a leap of the imagination too far.[13] On a more positive note, the extent to which clean streets, salubrious market places and well-maintained hospitals constituted a source of communal pride, projecting a conscious image of success, independence and civic virtue, is still not as widely appreciated as it might be.

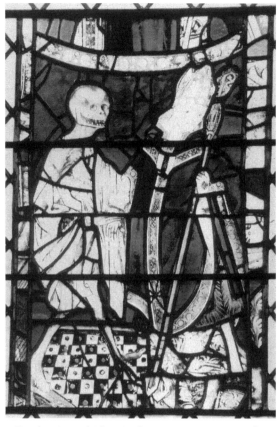

1 Death seizes a bishop in the one surviving image from an early sixteenth-century series of up to thirty-three stained glass panels depicting the Dance of Death in St Andrew's parish church, Norwich.

A number of factors explain our tendency to belittle medieval approaches to health and hygiene, not least being the long shadow cast by a *cadre* of influential Victorian sanitary reformers and polemicists whose commitment to the ideal of scientific progress made them contemptuous of a society so different from their own. It is instructive to contrast the tenacity of these assumptions with

---

[12] M. Bailey, 'Demographic Decline in Late Medieval England: Some Thoughts on Recent Research', *EconHR*, 2nd series 49 (1996), pp. 1–19, on p. 1.

[13] C. Platt, *King Death: The Black Death and its Aftermath in Late-Medieval England* (London, 1996), chaps 9 and 10, discusses this type of imagery, as, more recently, do P. Berger, 'Mice, Arrows and Tumours: Medieval Plague Iconography North of the Alps', in F. Mormando and T. Worcester, eds, *Piety and the Plague from Byzantium to the Baroque* (Kirksville, MO, 2007), pp. 23–63; E. Gertsman, 'Visualising Death: Medieval Plagues and the Macabre', in *ibid.*, pp. 64–89; and J. Aberth, *From the Brink of the Apocalypse: Confronting Famine, War, Plague, and Death in the Later Middle Ages*, 2nd edn (London, 2010), pp. 214–70.

the fate of other, equally trenchant nineteenth-century opinions about the later medieval period, such as those voiced in the fields of political and constitutional history by scholars fixated upon the development – and innate superiority – of parliamentary institutions. The comprehensive reassessment of aristocratic activities and aspirations that has taken place over the last seventy years certainly bears little relationship to Charles Plummer's damning indictment of 1875. His celebrated introduction to Sir John Fortescue's tract on *The Governance of England* depicts a world brutalised by

> that pseudo-chivalry, which, under a garb of external splendour and a factitious code of honour, failed to conceal its ingrained lust and cruelty, and its reckless contempt for the rights and feelings of all who were not admitted within the charmed circle; and it saw the beginning of that bastard feudalism, which, in place of the primitive relation of a lord to his tenants, surrounded a great man with a horde of retainers, who wore his livery and fought his battles ... so that by a sort of ignoble caricature of the feudal system the whole structure of society from the apex to the base was knit together in a hierarchy of corruption.[14]

Delivered shortly afterwards, Bishop William Stubbs's verdict upon the fifteenth century as an 'age of obscurity and disturbance', memorable for 'little else than the details of foreign wars and domestic struggles', proved rather more enduring, at least in its conviction that the political classes lacked any coherent ideology for the conduct of 'public life' beyond the pursuit of personal interest, however enlightened.[15] Not until the late 1980s did it appear that a 'new constitutional history' of Lancastrian England might be envisaged in terms of 'common principles and structures' which transcended the baronage's preoccupation with the networks and connections through which they exercised power.[16] Significantly, many of these 'common principles' derived from current ideas about the working of human and political bodies, and proved just as attractive to the rulers of English towns and cities.

The contention that civic authorities and other members of the mercantile elite espoused a growing commitment to matters of *communal* welfare, over and above the specific needs of their own families and households, is one of the main themes of this book. Frequently self-serving, and all too often hampered by lack of money and technological resources, their efforts nonetheless constituted a pragmatic response to contemporary beliefs about the spread of disease, which was designed to improve the quotidian lot of their fellow men and women. Can we justifiably describe these various initiatives in terms of a coherent agenda for the betterment of public health? And, if so, how might we define it? George Rosen's checklist, presented at the start of his pioneering *History of Public Health*, which traced developments from Ancient Greece to the 1940s, constitutes a useful point of departure. Measures for 'the control of transmissible disease, the control and

---

[14] C. Plummer, 'Introduction', in Sir John Fortescue, *The Governance of England*, ed. C. Plummer (Oxford, 1875), pp. 15, 25.

[15] W. Stubbs, *The Constitutional History of England*, vol. 3 (Oxford, 1878), pp. 2, 4.

[16] J. Watts, *Henry VI and the Politics of Kingship* (Cambridge, 1996), pp. 1–9, 363.

improvement of the physical environment (sanitation), the provision of water and food of good quality and in sufficient supply, the provision of medical care, and the relief of disability and destitution' were widely adapted in most medieval English towns, and form the basis of five of the following chapters.[17] Many of them will seem surprisingly familiar to a modern reader whose weekly visit to the supermarket is marked by the careful scrutiny of 'sell by' dates and a nagging anxiety over rising levels of traffic pollution. He or she may, indeed, reflect enviously upon the number of public lavatories situated along busy medieval thoroughfares, or the twice-weekly refuse collections instituted (but perhaps not always carried out) by the more zealous authorities.

However, this sense of recognition can be deceptive. Few leading burgesses would have questioned society's obligation 'to protect, promote and restore the people's health',[18] although their choice of remedy might be influenced as much by the Bible and Church Fathers as it was by the work of Hippocrates or Galen. Underlying such ostensibly 'progressive' innovations as the supply of fresh piped water and the construction of purpose-built slaughterhouses lay a very different understanding of sickness from our own, and a religious imperative that gave the most practical of regulations a moral dimension. As the editors of a recent collection of essays on medieval domesticity remind us, 'the boundaries between the sacred and the profane, the spiritual and the secular, appear porous, even illusory'.[19] Today's medical historians are sometimes as dismissive of these ideas as their Victorian predecessors, ignoring the context in which they developed and the impact which they had upon so many aspects of urban life. We are, for example, faced from the outset with a more fluid and wide-ranging concept of what actually constituted *public* health.[20] Alfons Labisch's insistence that it should be 'situated in differently structured dimensions in a qualitatively different way compared to individual health' would have puzzled a medieval magistrate, who made few distinctions between the working of the civic body and the complex network of veins, arteries, nerves, spirits and organs encased within his own mortal flesh.[21] *He* inhabited a world in which such personal vices as gluttony, sexual promiscuity and the reluctance to work seemed to threaten the wellbeing of entire communities like a toxic miasma, weakening their resistance to disease

[17] G. Rosen, *A History of Public Health* (New York, 1958; rev. edn, Baltimore, 1993), p. 1.

[18] This definition appears in a text-book for today's health professionals, who are, incidentally, informed that 'the Middle Ages marked a dark period in the history of public health', notable only for pestilence and the crusades: M. L. Fleming and E. Parker, *Introduction to Public Health*, 2nd edn (Sydney, 2012), pp. 7, 29.

[19] P. J. P. Goldberg and M. Kowaleski, 'Introduction', in P. J. P. Goldberg and M. Kowaleski, eds, *Medieval Domesticity: Home, Housing and Household in Medieval England* (Cambridge, 2008), p. 12.

[20] A point succinctly made by G. Geltner, 'Public Health and the Pre-Modern City: A Research Agenda', *History Compass* 10.3 (2012), pp. 231–45, on pp. 231–2. I am indebted to Professor Geltner for allowing me to read this article before publication.

[21] A. Labisch, 'History of Public Health: History in Public Health Looking Back and Looking Forward', *Social History of Medicine*, xi (1998), pp. 1–13, on pp. 9–10.

and even inviting divine retribution. The drains, cesspits and 'political statutes' so beloved by earlier generations of scholars are, in short, just one part of our story.[22]

This book covers a time span of just under three centuries, between c. 1250 and c. 1530, during which English towns and cities experienced the cataclysmic impact of rapid population growth, followed by famine and repeated outbreaks of pestilence. By investigating attitudes to public health over such a lengthy period, it is possible to establish a clear sense of the extent to which fear of plague, and subsequently of the pox and sweating sickness, proved both an impetus and an opportunity for environmental improvement. Research on urban communities in France, Italy and Spain suggests that many of the measures deployed from 1348 to combat epidemics were, in fact, in place before then. As Chapter 1 reveals, the English experience, at least in London and the leading provincial centres, seems to have been little different. It was, after all, during the later thirteenth century that medical theories about the communication and prevention of disease (theories first developed by the Ancient Greeks and later refined by Muslim scholars) began to gain greater currency, initially in Latin texts and then in abridged and simplified English versions. These ideas and their influence upon an increasingly well-informed urban elite are examined in greater detail at appropriate points in the following chapters, notably with regard to the ways in which they may have shaped approaches to the management of the communal body, its environment, its supply of food and water and the provision of care for its sick and incapacitated members.

The popularity of advice literature which so obviously derived from pagan sources owed much to its ready acceptance by the medieval Church, whose teachings exerted a powerful influence upon all aspects of urban life. Changing attitudes to collective health and welfare clearly reflect many of the developments in popular piety and devotional practice discernable between 1250 and the Dissolution of the Monasteries. The desire for personal commemoration, increasingly apparent among the merchant class from the thirteenth century onwards, prompted significant investment in public utilities. Activity increased after the Black Death, when the purchase of paradise was routinely transacted through the hard currency of bricks, mortar, lead pipes, paving stones and emergency grain supplies. A telling reappraisal of what constituted a 'comfortable work' meant that by the fifteenth century many testators were more interested in schemes that would ameliorate the lives of their fellow citizens than they were in traditional forms of pious provision. But at the same time a conviction that, whatever its immediate terrestrial causes, plague was God's judgement upon sinners encouraged, if it did not directly provoke, a growing concern with the *moral* health of the individual burgess or citizen. His or her propensity for fornication, idleness and gambling in low dives became as urgent a problem as the removal of festering dung heaps and stagnant ponds.

The dramatic fall in urban populations apparent by the later fourteenth century was not an unmitigated disaster. With better and cheaper food to eat, greatly improved lodgings and more opportunities for employment, those members of

---

[22] For a summary of general developments in the historiography of public health, see D. Porter, *Health, Civilisation and the State* (London, 1999), pp. 1–4.

the urban proletariat who survived successive epidemics appear to have enjoyed a considerably higher standard of living than their predecessors. Despite the sanitary nuisance posed by abandoned tenements and garbage-strewn wasteland, towns were generally easier to keep clean and free of rubbish; markets could be more effectively regulated, and populations adequately fed, save in the worst of shortages. Artisans and tradesmen began to acquire washing equipment and to express an interest in matters of domestic hygiene. Less fortunate were the hospitals and *leprosaria* which succumbed in considerable numbers to a combination of economic hardship and chronic mismanagement from the early fourteenth century onwards. By adopting a longer perspective, we can trace the shifts in institutional support for the sick and debilitated poor, as townsmen and women began to exercise far tighter control over foundations which they endowed and ran themselves for the benefit of deserving cases. Even more than the hospitals that they replaced, the new almshouses that sprang up across England conveyed a powerful moral and political message designed to serve an agenda set by the ruling elite.

Being in many respects a preliminary sortie into uncharted territory, this study does not claim to offer a comprehensive analysis of every aspect of late medieval public health, much less a full coverage of English towns. The focus rests almost exclusively on lay rather than ecclesiastical responses, with a particular emphasis upon the role played by central government, urban authorities, craft guilds (whose involvement in sanitary policing has been consistently underestimated) and ordinary householders in the collective battle against privation and disease. Inevitably, given the quantity of published primary sources and the even greater profusion of unedited manuscript material that has survived in both local and national archives, a selective approach has proved essential. Having worked for several years on various aspects of health provision in Norwich and other East Anglian towns, I have naturally drawn on this research, supplemented by a close analysis of the King's Lynn Hall Books, which constitute as valuable a resource as the better-known volumes from Bristol, Coventry, Southampton and York, also featured here. Care has been taken to examine smaller towns as well as large, the impoverished (Carlisle) as well as the successful (Exeter), and to achieve a correspondingly wide geographical span – from Chester on the Welsh March to Hull on the North Sea coast. Since the level of autonomy enjoyed by citizens and burgesses could have a significant impact upon the nature and extent of urban improvements, seigniorial boroughs, such as Wells and Salisbury, merit consideration alongside more independent self-governing communities. Although it was in so many ways *sui generis*, London makes frequent appearances, in part because provincial magistrates used it as 'a mirror and example' upon which to base their own endeavours.[23] Its early history of sanitary legislation and concern for the cleanliness of the environment furnishes us with more than enough evidence to question entrenched assumptions about the 'primitive' nature of late medieval health provision in general, and of the benighted state of English cities in particular.

The genesis of these pervasive ideas among the 'sanitarians' of Victorian Britain is explored at the start of Chapter 1, which provides an overview of the

---

[23] Sloane, *Black Death in London*, p. 18.

relevant historiography to date. A more systematic and sensitive analysis of the available sources, including archaeological evidence, suggests that few established orthodoxies can pass unchallenged. Indeed, a comparison between the health measures instituted in English and Italian cities both before and after the Black Death confirms that the conventional view of England's particular 'backwardness' needs revision. The final part of the chapter questions another widespread supposition, no less tenacious, that whatever limited initiatives were eventually adopted must have been imposed from above, by the crown, upon a resistant and ignorant populace. Equipped with a basic level of medical knowledge, if only by virtue of their manifold legal responsibilities, the *mediocres*, or 'middling' citizens, of fourteenth- and fifteenth-century England were far from indifferent to matters of public health.

Chapter 2 reveals that the Church's emphasis upon the intimate connection between spiritual and physical health was reinforced by long-established medical theories regarding human physiology. The heavy burden of chronic and epidemic disease shouldered by urban populations, especially during 'the golden age of bacteria' that followed the Black Death, more than justified such beliefs, and framed official responses to a raft of sanitary issues.[24] Having considered the psychological as well as the physical impact of repeated outbreaks of pestilence on the residents of English towns and cities, we explore the ways in which ideas about the working of the body politic may have influenced expectations of how magistrates should react. They were, for instance, urged to lead by virtuous example, exercising a duty of care towards the more vulnerable parts of this living and breathing organism. Alongside these exhortations of mutual support and comfort ran a more brutal attitude that demanded the excision of corrupt members before they infected the rest. Recourse to spiritual prophylaxis, in the form of 'celestial helpers', civic processions and religious imagery formed an important weapon in the authorities' armoury. Yet, in the final resort, they were responsible for diverting the arrows of divine wrath by eliminating sources of moral pollution. For this reason, attempts to curtail the potentially lethal effects of prostitution and the proliferation of idle beggars ranked alongside the more seemingly 'conventional' sanitary measures discussed in the rest of this book.

Chapter 3, which concentrates upon the physical environment, begins by examining late medieval attempts to explain the rapid spread of pestilence in somatic terms. Since polluted air and, to a lesser extent, disgusting sights such as rotting carcasses and overflowing latrines had long been recognised as principal vectors of disease, the elimination of nuisances likely to breed miasmas and offend spectators became a priority. Already common by the mid-fourteenth century, ordinances for the removal of the intimidating quantities of garbage, dung and other detritus that accumulated in urban thoroughfares and markets increased exponentially after the Black Death. Archaeological research suggests that programmes for street paving, refuse collection and the construction of

---

[24] The phrase was coined by Sylvia Thrupp, 'The Problem of Replacement Rates in the Late Medieval English Population', *EconHR*, 2nd series 18 (1965–6), pp. 101–19, on p. 118.

public and private cesspits had a significant impact upon standards of hygiene in some towns, although the financial and logistic challenges faced by magistrates remained daunting. The regulation of butchery and the disposal of butchers' waste proved no less troublesome, especially as the demand for meat was rising steadily throughout our period. Even more truculent than their owners, butchers' dogs posed another threat to life and limb, along with the pigs that roamed at large like sturdy beggars, spreading disease and even attacking children. And what was to be done about the cattle, sheep, horses and carts that jostled for space in congested thoroughfares? From attempts to control the filth and chaos generated by animals, we turn to the atmospheric pollution caused by lime-burning, brick-making and other dangerous industrial activities, which invariably involved noise as well as smoke. The close proximity of industrial and domestic premises meant that fire posed a constant risk, and we conclude with an assessment of the measures taken to protect populations against one of the greatest hazards of urban life.

Because stagnant water was regarded as another prime source of the noxious vapours that spread infection, urban magistrates went to great lengths to maintain drains, wells, gutters and canals in public places. Having noted their commitment to the upkeep of these common utilities, Chapter 4 explores the extent of individual liability for keeping watercourses clean: householders who caused obstructions or allowed their own property to become flooded faced heavy fines, and were frequently required to contribute towards the general cost of repairs and improvements. As we shall see, members of the civic elite heeded medical advice about the importance of providing fresh, uncontaminated water for human consumption. Piped water was freely available in many towns, the heavy expenditure involved being often shared with religious houses and supported by donations from wealthy philanthropists. Zoning was widespread by the thirteenth century, but commercial interests still made it difficult to prevent the pollution of rivers and streams by butchers, brewers, cloth workers and tanners. Nevertheless, the authorities did their best to ensure that ordinary men and women had controlled access to wells and conduits. Their concerns bring us back to the symbolic aspects of public health, since water, in particular, carried powerful religious connotations. Navigable rivers – the arteries of the civic body – were essential for commercial health, while the association of cleanliness with godliness meant that donors were particularly drawn towards schemes that promised so many spiritual benefits.

Like the provision of drink for the thirsty, feeding the poor ranked as one of the comfortable works that Christ had urged His followers to perform if they hoped to escape the flames of hell. Chapter 5 deals with food, 'the first instrument of medicine', upon which the survival of both the urban and the human body depended. Anxious lest their readers should become more vulnerable to infection by adopting an unsuitable diet, the authors of medieval *regimina* warned against the dangers of consuming unseasonable or contaminated food. The very real prospect of popular unrest, as well as disease, made magistrates particularly sensitive to issues surrounding the quality, availability and pricing of essential commodities, as well as the conditions in which they were sold. A raft of legislation aimed to protect the consumer from potentially lethal practices on the part of butchers, cooks (the most notorious and persistent offenders), bakers, fishmongers and other victuallers. Brewers, innkeepers and taverners were also required to take basic sanitary precautions and to refrain from adulterating their wares. In practice, quality control was exercised through the medium of local courts and craft guilds, which had a vested interest in ensuring that their members retained public confidence. The rulers of many English towns turned their attention to the crowded and insanitary state of market places well before the first outbreak of plague. Where possible, they provided designated sites with adequate drains and facilities for waste disposal; sometimes markets were even paved and covered. The task of supervisory officials was more than simply hygienic: they had to enforce statute law regarding the uniformity of weights and measures, regularly inspect the ale and bread on sale and ensure that traders did not exploit the poor or deny them cheaper food. Price-fixing, cornering the market in vital foodstuffs and similar commercial abuses constituted an assault upon the most vulnerable members of the urban body (as well as Christ's representatives on earth), and could be punished accordingly.

What happened to these people when they became too sick, disabled or aged to work? The final chapter deals with the medical services and hospital provision available in English towns and cities. In contrast to Continental practice, neither magistrates nor guilds retained salaried physicians and surgeons to serve the public, with the result that they had either to pay for their own treatment or hope that it might be offered *gratis* on a charitable basis. We start by investigating attempts at reform, which came nearest to fruition in London, but failed because of political circumstances and professional rivalry. Not surprisingly, given the risks involved, civic authorities took a firmer stand when ensuring that practitioners should possess appropriate levels of education, training and skill. As in the case of the victualling trades, supervision was chiefly exercised through the medium of craft guilds, including the London Grocers, who oversaw the quality and price of all the drugs imported into England and sold locally by apothecaries. Incompetence, profiteering and quackery were punishable at law, both in central and local courts. The sick poor rarely had such redress, and it is far harder to trace the informal networks of support upon which they customarily relied. However, the changing pattern of institutional care offers a more revealing insight into responses to poverty, as well as the wider political and religious aspirations of the men and women who provided it. Having noted the ubiquity of hospitals and almshouses in the spiritual and physical topography of English towns, the second part of this chapter investigates the variable fortunes of *leprosaria*, open ward or 'common' hospitals and almshouses during the three centuries before the Dissolution. Once again, we return to the preoccupation with spiritual health and salvation – as well as more immediate issues of discipline and order – that prompted so many of the initiatives described in preceding chapters.

Much of the evidence used in this book derives from the plethora of regulations and decrees issued by urban magistrates, sometimes at the behest of central government or in accordance with the vernacular advice literature in their possession. The dangers of assuming that practice obediently followed precept are well enough known, yet worth reiterating. 'Fixated on what was recommended rather than on what people actually did', historians all too often forget that 'earthier behaviours' tend to defy the most stringent of injunctions, which may well reflect mounting desperation rather than success.[25] On the other hand, pronouncements of this kind provide us with a very clear idea of what members of the ruling elite (and a growing number of the 'middling sort') *believed* to be important, and of how seriously they regarded the threat posed by particular nuisances. The close connection between specific epidemics and the sudden bouts of intensive regulatory and administrative activity apparent throughout the fifteenth century speaks volumes, irrespective of whatever improvements may actually have been achieved on the ground. Although any conclusions on the latter score must remain more impressionistic, we are fortunate that the survival of so much medieval infrastructure, along with other material remains, can often shed light upon the success or failure of particular ventures. The copious records generated by late medieval English courts likewise provide a fascinating insight into the mechanics of law enforcement as magistrates struggled to translate legislation into action.

In this context, a word about the relative value of the fines imposed for the various offences and nuisances proscribed by urban authorities will prove useful. Although the latter sometimes had recourse to the pillory and other humiliating physical punishments, as well as imprisonment and the threat of expulsion, financial deterrents were most commonly employed. In 1459 the Norwich Assembly introduced a typical penalty of 6s. 8d. for fly-tipping, in an attempt to keep the River Wensum free of 'mukke and fylth'; at current local rates that represented twenty days' work by a mason and twenty-six by a thatcher, and was by most reckonings a substantial sum. Repeat offenders stood to forfeit two or three times this amount.[26] From the standpoint of the working man or woman, even the routine amercements of 4d. or 6d., payable by householders who allowed their drains to overflow or who left stinking garbage in the street, were far from negligible. Exemplary fines, like the £5 or more faced by suspect lepers who refused to remove themselves to the suburbs, were designed to convey the enormity of their transgression and to secure prompt compliance. In most instances, miscreants were simply threatened with forfeiture should they fail to amend their ways, while in others a draconian fine might well be substantially reduced once a suitably abject apology had been tendered before the court. Recidivism was all too common and on many occasions the authorities resigned themselves to taxing what they could not effectively prohibit. Their widespread reliance upon the salutary effects of peer pressure and public shame nonetheless suggests that a sense of communal responsibility, or active membership of the urban body, may not have been quite as unusual as some historians suppose.

---

[25] V. Gatrell, *City of Laughter: Sex and Satire in Eighteenth-Century London* (London, 2007), p. 17.

[26] NRO, NCR, 16D/1, Assembly Proceedings, 1434–1491, fol. 44r; NCR, 24/A, Great Hospital Accounts for Norwich Properties, 1415–1460, account for 1460–61.

❧ Chapter 1
Less Mud-Slinging and More Facts

CART DRIVER: Bring out your dead!

We follow the cart through a wretched, impoverished, plague-ridden village. A few starved mongrels run about in the mud scavenging. In the open doorway of one house perhaps we just glimpse a pair of legs dangling from the ceiling. In another doorway an OLD WOMAN *is beating a cat against a wall rather like one does with a mat. The cart passes round a dead donkey or cow in the mud ...*

   They turn ... suddenly all in the village fall to their knees, touching forelocks, etc. ARTHUR *and* PATSY *ride into shot, slightly noses in the air, they ride through without acknowledging anybody. After they pass the* LARGE MAN TURNS TO THE CART DRIVER.

LARGE MAN: Who's that then?

CART DRIVER (*grudgingly*): I dunno, must be a king.

LARGE MAN: Why?

CART DRIVER: He hasn't got shit all over him.

Monty Python and the Holy Grail (1974)[1]

FROM the searing intensity of Ingmar Bergman's *Seventh Seal* to the surreal humour of Monty Python, the Middle Ages invariably emerge smeared with excrement and littered with garbage. Yet, however fanciful they may appear, few cinematic representations of this seemingly benighted period can rival the truly dismal picture of urban life presented by the scholars and sanitary campaigners of Victorian England. Thus, for example, in *The Coming of the Friars*, a book of essays composed in 1890 for the popular market, the antiquary Augustus Jessopp observed that:

> The sediment of the town population in the Middle Ages was a dense slough of stagnant misery, squalor, famine, loathsome disease and dull despair, such as the worst slums of London, Liverpool or Paris know nothing of ... What greatly added to the dreary wretchedness of the lower order in the towns was the fact that the ever-increasing throngs of beggars, outlaws and ruffian runaways were simply left to fend for themselves. The civil authorities took no account of them as they quietly rotted and died ...[2]

Five years later, the physician, Sir George Newman, cited this passage as evidence of the foetid conditions in which leprosy was bound to flourish, adding further embellishments of his own about the grim business of survival in a society which 'knew little of decency, cleanliness and order' and was chiefly characterised by its

---

[1] J. Cleese *et al.*, *Monty Python and the Holy Grail: The Screenplay* (London, 2002), pp. 3, 5.

[2] A. Jessopp, *The Coming of the Friars and other Historic Essays* (London, 1890), p. 6.

'total neglect of all hygienic or sanitary laws'.[3] That both men should have formed such a depressing view of the later medieval city and the apparent indifference of its magistrates to matters of public health is entirely understandable. They were, after all, products of a culture which basked in 'the revealing light of science', and tended as a result to disparage those unfortunates who had 'aforetime walked in darkness'.[4] As the reformer Benjamin Ward Richardson observed not long before, it was only during his own lifetime that 'the actual effect of civilisation, so fragmentary and so overshadowed by barbarism', had been brought to bear upon 'the work of sanitary progress'.[5]

We should remember, too, that Jessopp and his contemporaries had witnessed at first hand the impact upon English towns and cities of unfettered industrialisation, population growth and devastating epidemics caused by widespread malnutrition and chronic overcrowding. It is surely no coincidence that the Norwich of Jessopp's boyhood ranked as one of the most insalubrious provincial cities in England, with an infant mortality rate almost as high as those of Manchester, Leeds and Liverpool.[6] The appalling state of the slum housing around the River Wensum was vividly described in December 1849 as part of a campaign for sanitary reform mounted by *The Morning Chronicle*. In words that were to be replicated almost verbatim by Jessopp in a medieval context, the author noted that 'the ground is constantly damp and moist, while heaps of filth and rubbish, open bins and privies, decaying vegetable and other matters, are constantly contaminating, by their offensive *malaria*, the unwholesome atmosphere in which the wretched inhabitants live'.[7] Despite the many approving references to its clean, well-paved streets, sophisticated water supply and fresh air made by seventeenth-century visitors, there was a growing consensus that Norwich must always have been filthy.[8]

This presumption was reinforced by an excoriating report of 1851 commissioned by the Board of Health on the 'infamously bad' sanitary conditions which still blighted the city. As a good Victorian progressive, William Lee, the superintending

---

[3] G. Newman, *On the History of the Decline and Final Extinction of Leprosy as an Endemic Disease in the British Isles* (London, 1895), pp. 70–9.

[4] The sanitary reformer Sir William Collins, cited by L. G. Stevenson, 'Science Down the Drain', *BHM* 29 (1955), pp. 1–26, on p. 22. For a striking example of this optimistic view of human progress, see C. F. H. Marx and R. Willis, *On the Decrease of Disease Effected by the Progress of Civilization* (London, 1844). In France, 'progressivists', such as François Guizot (d. 1874), adopted a similar stance: A. Guillerme, *The Age of Water: The Urban Environment in the North of France*, AD *800–1800* (College Station, TX, 1988), p. 96.

[5] B. W. Richardson, *Hygeia: A City of Health* (London, 1876), p. 14.

[6] A. Armstrong, 'Population, 1700–1950', in C. Rawcliffe and R. Wilson, eds, *Norwich since 1550* (London, 2004), pp. 252–3, 535 n. 31.

[7] 'Letter XVI: The Rural Districts: Norfolk, Suffolk and Essex', *The Morning Chronicle*, 12 December 1849, cited by J. F. Pound, 'Poverty and Public Health in Norwich, 1845–1880', in C. Barringer, ed., *Norwich in the Nineteenth Century* (Norwich, 1984), p. 48.

[8] C. Rawcliffe, 'Introduction', in C. Rawcliffe and R. Wilson, eds, *Medieval Norwich* (London, 2004), pp. xxiv–xxv.

inspector, was determined to provide some sense of perspective, and began with a graphic account of 'the ravages of disease in former times'. Drawing on his own experience, he assumed that even larger 'accumulations of offensive organic matter' must then have littered the streets and river banks, generating the toxic fumes of pestilence. Since he rammed home the point by citing grossly inflated mortality figures sustained in Norwich during the first seven months of 1348 alone (57,374, 'besides religious and beggars'), we can readily appreciate why Jessopp came to adopt such a pessimistic tone.[9] Significantly, in its lengthy catalogue of nineteenth-century shortcomings, Lee's report drew particular attention to the absence of any public measures for the removal of refuse or the repair of the rudimentary sewerage system, to the flooding caused by stagnant waste in open drains, and to the proliferation of noisome slaughterhouses, all of which had been subject to stringent regulation during the later Middle Ages.[10] That the city might ever have been cleaner or that the corporation might once have played a more active role in the struggle to protect the health of its inhabitants nonetheless seemed unimaginable to right-thinking 'sanitarians'. As chronicled in the chapter headings of student text-books, progress from 'the dark ages of public health' *via* 'the great sanitary awakening' to a 'golden age of bacteriology' represented the inexorable advance of science in the face of irrationality and superstition.[11] This was precisely the type of facile generalisation that the medical historian Lynn Thorndike called into question as much for its arrogance as its ignorance of primary sources. In a groundbreaking article of 1928 he urged his readers to avoid 'regarding as a lineal heritage from the Middle Ages the bad new conditions which actually resulted from the industrial revolution of the eighteenth and nineteenth centuries, and the negligence of early modern medicine'.[12]

On the rare occasions that it was commented upon by nineteenth-century historians, evidence of the fight against urban pollution waged by medieval communities generally elicited a patronising response. H. T. Riley's reaction to complaints made by the residents of Hythe about a range of unpleasant nuisances

---

[9] W. Lee, *Report to the General Board of Health on a Preliminary Inquiry into the Sewerage, Drainage and Supply of Water, and the Sanitary Conditions of the Inhabitants of the City of Norwich* (London, 1851), pp. 21–2. Lee appears to have derived this astonishing figure from the recently calendared 'Mayor's Book of Norwich': G. Johnson, ed., 'Chronological Memoranda Touching the City of Norwich', *NA* 1 (1847), pp. 140–66, on p. 141. According to his calculations, barely one in seven residents would have survived. In fact, when the Black Death struck the city in 1349 (not 1348), the population had probably fallen well below the 25,000 mark estimated for the early 1330s: see p. 65 below.

[10] Lee, *Report to the General Board of Health*, pp. 49–61. For earlier criticisms, see also *Second Report of the Royal Commission for Inquiring into the State of Large Towns and Populous Districts* (London, 1845), appendix: 'Norwich'.

[11] C.-E. A. Winslow, *The Evolution and Significance of the Modern Public Health Campaign* (New Haven, CT, 1923). See also V. Smith, *Clean: A History of Personal Hygiene and Purity* (Oxford, 2007), pp. 309–10.

[12] L. Thorndike, 'Sanitation, Baths, and Street Cleaning in the Middle Ages and Renaissance', *Speculum* 3 (1928), pp. 192–203, on p. 193. His appeal for 'less mud-slinging and more facts' (p. 203), provides the title for this chapter.

exemplifies this combination of distaste and condescension. Unlike most of the scholars assigned by the Royal Commission on Historical Manuscripts to catalogue municipal archives, Riley did at least address this topic in his report of 1874 on the town's records. Yet the 'few extracts' which he reproduced from a longer list of presentments about blocked drains and the dumping of waste clearly offended his sensibilities. The town struck him 'as being in a state of such utter filth and squalor, that we are not all surprised to learn from the Release by Henry the Fifth … that the place was devastated by pestilence in this reign'.[13] It certainly did not occur to him that, in accordance with current medical advice, the jurors of Hythe might have been trying to *avoid* any further epidemics by reporting such unacceptable activities as the butchering of pigs ('skaldynge de hogges') near a public highway.[14] But Riley did at least acknowledge that some effort, however basic, was being made to improve the environment, an assumption shared by few of his contemporaries.[15]

Two examples from a wide range of eminently quotable material will here suffice to illustrate the stance adopted by Victorian sanitarians, notably in talks and pamphlets designed to generate popular support for their cause. Others appear at the start of subsequent chapters of this book. In an influential series of lectures delivered in 1861, the Edinburgh physician W. T. Gairdner bemoaned the complete dearth of health provision in British medieval towns, where, he maintained,

> all the first wants of humanity were utterly neglected or left to chance, and to the imperfect legislation of civic authorities, limited mostly to deciding disputed cases; there was no drainage; masses of filth lay piled about the streets; water was everywhere procured from wells or from rivers, and was often of bad quality; food was frequently salted, long kept, half putrid, and not rarely at famine prices, or not to be procured at any price.[16]

Another pioneer, the clergyman and author Charles Kingsley, reassured a crowded and largely female audience in 1869 that he would not 'disgust' them with statistical information about the striking incidence of disease and mortality in nineteenth-century Britain. However, he did expand upon the 'more rational and

---

[13] HMC, *Fourth Report*, Royal Commission on Historical Manuscripts 3 (London, 1874), p. 431. As the editor of the impressive three-volume *Munimenta Gildhallae Londoniensis* (RS 12, 1859–62), and of the substantial collection *Memorials of London and London Life in the XIIIth, XIVth and XVth Centuries* (London, 1868), Riley was by then well aware of the numerous sanitary regulations already adopted in the capital.

[14] C. Rawcliffe, 'The Concept of Health in Medieval Society', in S. Cavaciocchi, ed., *Le interazioni fra economia e ambiente biologico nell'Europa preindustriale. Secc. XIII–XVIII* (Florence, 2010), pp. 317–34.

[15] The compilers of a series of extracts from the late medieval Basingstoke court rolls constitute one notable exception, remarking with evident surprise that 'the sanitary arrangements are of a more extended character than might be expected'. They went on to list a comprehensive range of measures designed to keep the town clean: F. J. Baigent and J. E. Millard, *A History of the Town and Manor of Basingstoke* (Basingstoke and London, 1889), p. 246.

[16] W. T. Gairdner, *Public Health in Relation to Air and Water* (Edinburgh, 1862) p. 11.

cleanly habits of life' that nevertheless distinguished Victorian society from what had gone before:

> Knowing something, as I happen to do, of the social state and of the health of the Middle and Elizabethan Ages, I have no hesitation in saying that the average of disease and death was far greater than it is now. Epidemics of many kinds, typhus, ague, plague – all diseases which were caused more or less by bad air – devastated this land and Europe in those days with a horrible intensity, to which even the choleras of our times are mild. The back streets, the hospitals, the gaols, the barracks, the camps – every place in which any large number of persons congregated, were so many nests of pestilence, engendered by uncleanliness, which defiled alike the water which was drunk and the air which was breathed.[17]

Despite their obvious appeal, such views were hard to reconcile with the archival evidence that was already beginning to attract more systematic historical scrutiny.[18] When compiling his 1915 edition of court cases relating to medieval public works, C. T. Flower reported a dramatic increase in litigation over the upkeep of drains and watercourses during the second half of the fourteenth century, accompanied by the introduction of more streamlined procedures for recording disputes. 'It is impossible to avoid connecting these developments with the Great Pestilence of 1348–9', he remarked, conceding that 'even in that period of *unscientific medicine* (my italics) it would be apparent that stagnant sewers and ditches were bad from a sanitary point of view, and the necessity for providing adequate remedies would be brought home by the visitation of the plague'.[19] Flower was one of the first English scholars to note the unambiguous connection

---

[17] C. Kingsley, *Sanitary and Social Lectures and Essays* (London, 1889), pp. 61–2.

[18] The years between 1882 and 1915 witnessed the publication of such important sources for urban history as: M. Bateson, ed., *Records of the Borough of Leicester*, vols 1 and 2 (London, 1899, 1901); W. G. Benham, ed., *The Red Paper Book of Colchester* (Colchester, 1902); F. B. Bickley, ed., *The Little Red Book of Bristol*, 2 vols (Bristol, 1900); M. Dormer Harris, ed., *The Coventry Leet Book, 1420–1555*, 4 parts, EETS o.s., 134, 135, 138, 146 (London, 1907–13); W. Hudson, ed., *Leet Jurisdiction in the City of Norwich during the Thirteenth and Fourteenth Centuries*, Selden Society 5 (London, 1892); W. Hudson and J. C. Tingey, eds, *Records of the City of Norwich*, 2 vols (Norwich, 1906–10); A. F. Leach, ed., *Beverley Town Documents*, Selden Society 14 (London, 1900); C. A. Markham and J. C. Cox, eds, *Records of the Borough of Northampton*, 2 vols (Northampton, 1898); C. H. Mayo and A. W. Gould, eds, *The Municipal Records of the Borough of Dorchester, Dorset* (Exeter, 1908); M. Sellars, ed., *York Memorandum Book*, vols 1 and 2, Surtees Society 120, 125 (Durham, 1912, 1915); R. R. Sharpe, ed., *Calendar of Letter-Books Preserved among the Archives of the Corporation of the City of London, 1275–1498*, 11 vols, A–L (London, 1899–1912); W. H. Stevenson, ed., *Records of the Borough of Nottingham*, vols 1–3 (London, 1882–5); W. H. Stevenson, ed., *Calendar of the Records of the Corporation of Gloucester* (Gloucester, 1893); P. Studer, ed., *The Oak Book of Southampton of c. AD 1300*, 3 vols, Southampton Record Society 10, 11 (Southampton, 1910, 1911).

[19] C. T. Flower, ed., *Public Works in Medieval Law*, vol. 1, Selden Society 32 (London, 1915), p. xxviii.

between outbreaks of epidemic disease and the more stringent enforcement of health measures, a connection clearly evident in the surviving records of towns such as Ipswich, King's Lynn and Yarmouth.

The next part of this chapter considers the extent to which twentieth- and twenty-first-century historians and archaeologists have overturned entrenched assumptions about 'the triumphant emancipation of modern society from the primitive bondage of ignorance' (1.1).[20] Research into the regulatory procedures adopted by Italian cities both before and after the Black Death has contributed in no small measure to this process of revision, while at the same time fostering a widespread belief that medieval England remained, at best, a remote backwater, untroubled by any impetus for change (1.2). We move on to discover how far the surviving evidence actually supports this viewpoint (1.3), before turning to the vexed question of agency. Was sanitary reform simply a matter of royal decree, supported perhaps by a small but unrepresentative urban elite (1.4)? Or did legal and administrative developments foster a broader consensus, not least among the 'middling sort' who played such an important part in urban policing (1.5)? The final section examines the spread of medical ideas and information in a society that was increasingly receptive to advice about the preservation of health (1.6).

1.1 The Victorian legacy

The equation between medieval urban life and unrelieved squalor came automatically to many writers, especially when they were describing conditions in the capital. In 1925, for example, Dorothy George drew attention to an emergent sensibility during the later eighteenth century, as London finally shed the unprepossessing image immortalised by Fielding and Hogarth. So great, she concludes, was the scale of the transformation that 'its dirt and insecurity' seemed 'no longer worthy of a mediæval town'.[21] However, in less than a decade a major contribution to the rehabilitation of the fourteenth-century City had been made by the historian E. L. Sabine, whose three seminal articles on butchery, sanitation and street cleaning in late medieval London appeared in the American journal *Speculum* between 1933 and 1937.[22] Although he did not explore the underlying medical beliefs that drove members of the elite to embark upon their campaign, his meticulously documented survey of their efforts to safeguard the health and environment of Londoners is notable for its emphasis upon the importance of historical context. In particular, his caveat about the dangers of 'hasty generalization, gleaned from a cursory sampling of data' – with its inevitable focus upon the worst and most offensive cases of 'sickening nuisance' – still bears repetition:

> It does not indicate anything as to changes and developments in ... regulation and practice ... It does not point out times when insanitary

[20] Porter, *Health, Civilisation and the State*, p. 3.

[21] M. D. George, *London Life in the XVIIIth Century* (London, 1925), p. 10.

[22] E. L. Sabine, 'Butchering in Mediaeval London', *Speculum* 8 (1933), pp. 335–53; 'Latrines and Cesspools of Mediaeval London', *Speculum* 9 (1934), pp. 303–21; 'City Cleaning in Mediaeval London', *Speculum* 12 (1937), pp. 19–43.

conditions were especially acute, or, at any rate, especially criticised; nor does it seek to link up such times with their specific underlying causes. Indeed, such a generalization leads to a grave misapprehension and unjust depreciation of the zealous civic spirit often active in mediaeval London for the improvement of sanitary conditions.[23]

Independently of these developments, in 1939 G. T. Salusbury-Jones produced a short study of *Street Life in Medieval England* that was intended 'to serve as a signpost to stores of facts which although known to specialists have remained largely outside the knowledge of the general reader'.[24] Despite its modest aspirations, this little book is no less remarkable for its use of primary source material and its stress upon the need 'to look further back than the industrial revolution for profit and enlightenment'.[25] *Inter alia*, Salusbury-Jones dealt with the repair and cleaning of the streets, the regulation of traffic and other potential hazards, improvements to the water supply and attempts to protect the consumer in a number of provincial towns. His findings were evidently unknown to George Rosen, whose *History of Public Health*, first published in 1958, has little to say about pre-Reformation England. Even so, his praise for the 'rational system of public hygiene' that developed in continental Europe during the Middle Ages sets his work apart from 'the grand narrative of progress' presented by so many writers of his generation.[26]

Recent work by historians such as Mark Jenner, Derek Keene and Margaret Pelling offers a salutary reminder that the history of public health cannot be envisaged in terms of a slow but unwavering march towards the shining citadel of mains drainage.[27] The banner first raised by Sabine has been carried forward by Caroline Barron, whose study of *London in the Later Middle Ages* (2004) provides a comprehensive account of the measures taken by ordinary citizens, as well as members of the ruling elite, to maintain communal wellbeing and provide care for the sick.[28] Writing from a literary and cultural perspective, Susan Signe Morrison,

---

[23] Sabine, 'Butchering in Mediaeval London', pp. 335–6.

[24] G. T. Salusbury-Jones, *Street Life in Medieval England* (Oxford, 1939; repr. 1948), p. 3.

[25] Salusbury-Jones, *Street Life in Medieval England*, pp. 8–9.

[26] Rosen, *History of Public Health*, chap. 3; Porter, *Health, Civilisation and the State*, pp. 1, 80.

[27] See, respectively, M. S. R. Jenner, 'Underground, Overground: Pollution and Place in Urban History', *Journal of Urban History* 24 (1997), pp. 97–110; M. S. R. Jenner, 'Civilisation and Deodorization? Smell in Early Modern English Culture', in P. Burke, B. Harrison and P. Slack, eds, *Civil Histories: Essays Presented to Sir Keith Thomas* (Oxford, 2000), pp. 127–44; D. Keene, 'Rubbish in Medieval Towns', in A. R. Hall and H. K. Kenward, eds, *Environmental Archaeology in the Urban Context*, CBA research report 43 (London, 1982), pp. 26–30; D. Keene, 'Issues of Water in Medieval London to *c.* 1300', *Urban History* 28 (2001), pp. 161–79; M. Pelling, 'Health and Sanitation to 1750', in Rawcliffe and Wilson, *Norwich since 1550*, chap. 5.

[28] C. Barron, *London in the Later Middle Ages: Government and People, 1200–1500* (Oxford, 2004), chaps 10 and 11.

Paul Strohm and other scholars of late medieval English poetry have likewise campaigned against 'stereotypes of the Middle Ages as a foul, foetid and filthy period', pointing out with some justice that only 'unusual and extraordinary' cases of urban pollution tend to feature in the documentary record.[29] Signe Morrison, in particular, mounts a robust (and entertaining) assault on our desire to infantilise and denigrate the past 'as a site of waste, rubbish and excrement'.[30]

While accepting that, in many respects, the medieval and early modern urban population remained powerless in the face of epidemic disease, overcrowding and pollution, each of these authors has demonstrated that a sustained and inherently rational effort *was* made to minimise perceived risks to survival. But Jenner's warning that 'historians have too often depicted the inhabitants of pre-industrial cities as wallowing cheerfully in grime' often goes unheeded, and what, for want of a better phrase, we may call the 'Victorian' view of medieval and early modern urban standards of hygiene lingers on in some of the best current scholarship.[31] Thus, for example, in her richly detailed and evocative *Hubbub* (tellingly subtitled *Filth, Noise and Stench in England, 1600–1770*), Emily Cockayne argues that, before the later eighteenth century, town-dwellers had little sense of the threat posed by poor sanitation and even less interest in issues of public health. Yet if 'a lack of genuine concern about pollution and contamination (in food, water and the environment)' did, indeed, characterise much of the early modern period, the same cannot be said of the preceding centuries.[32]

[Nor is it helpful to evaluate whatever sanitary measures may have been promulgated in medieval and early modern towns by the exacting standards of modern technology and biomedicine, rather than contextualising them within the cultural, medical and religious *milieux* of the time.] Inevitably, the concerns expressed by fourteenth- and fifteenth-century men and women seem very different from our own, not least because of the symbiotic relationship that bound concepts of individual and collective health so closely to religious belief. As we shall see in the next chapter, there seemed little point in cleaning streets or constructing piped water systems without first removing the lethal miasmas of idleness and vice. While dismissing such attitudes as inherently 'superstitious', advocates of medical materialism are also inclined to belittle pragmatic responses

---

[29] S. Signe Morrison, *Excrement in the Late Middle Ages: Sacred Filth and Chaucer's Fecopoetics* (New York, 2008), p. 61; P. Strohm, 'Sovereignty and Sewage', in L. H. Cooper and A. Denny-Brown, eds, *Lydgate Matters: Poetry and Material Culture in the Fifteenth Century* (New York, 2007), pp. 57–70. See also D. N. DeVries, 'And Away Go Troubles Down the Drain: Late Medieval London and the Poetics of Urban Renewal', *Exemplaria* 8 (1996), pp. 401–18.

[30] Signe Morrison, *Excrement in the Late Middle Ages*, pp. 134–8.

[31] Jenner, 'Underground, Overground: Pollution and Place in Urban History', p. 101. See also, M. S. R. Jenner, 'Follow your Nose? Smell, Smelling, and their Histories', *American Historical Review* 116 (2011), pp. 335–51, on pp. 339–40.

[32] E. Cockayne, *Hubbub: Filth, Noise and Stench in England, 1600–1770* (New Haven, CT, 2007), p. 244, and also pp. 156, 245. For a different viewpoint, see A. Wear, *Knowledge and Practice in Early Modern English Medicine, 1550–1680* (Cambridge, 2000), chap. 4.

to disease in a society that lacked the complex infrastructures characteristic of the modern city. Yet a society without mains drainage or any knowledge of germ theory can still devise coherent strategies for the preservation of health, as is apparent from the numerous vernacular advice manuals that found a ready market among the educated urban elite.[33] The temptation to dismiss or denigrate these ideas nonetheless remains hard to resist. Norman Pounds's belief that 'the casual attitude of medieval people towards matters of cleanliness and sanitation can be excused by their ignorance of the nature of infection and the reality of pathogens' epitomises a common, but misleading, presumption that such an ostensibly backward society nursed few aspirations with regard to the quality of the urban environment. As both the medical literature and the sanitary regulations of the period confirm, Pounds's strictures about the collective 'failure to associate morbidity with filth', and to recognise the dangers of contaminated food, find scant support in the historical record, although they continue to surface in surveys of civic life.[34]

From this perspective it is, indeed, easy to assume the worst. Asserting that 'in Medieval Europe, virtually everyone was infested with blood-sucking parasites and their homes were colonized by equally infested mice and rats', the microbiologist Dorothy Crawford rivals Jessopp in her portrayal of a society choking in its own effluvia:

> ... As the population expanded and small communities grew into towns the situation got steadily worse. With *no facilities for waste disposal* [my italics] everything was thrown out into the narrow lanes that ran between the dwellings so that these dark, dank conduits became quagmires of mud, human and animal excreta and garbage, most of which ended up in the rivers that served as the water supply. In these unhygienic surroundings it is no wonder that microbes flourished ... poor ventilation and overcrowding made life easy for airborne microbes; *non-existent sanitation* [my italics] meant that gut pathogens had easy access to food and water; and lack of personal hygiene allowed vectors like fleas and lice to prosper.[35]

For most medieval town-dwellers the defining feature of any urban body was its ability to care for those members of the workforce who could no longer support themselves because of age or sickness. The availability of reasonably priced and well-regulated medical services was a high priority in major centres of population, while all but the smallest communities could boast at least one hospital or almshouse for the deserving poor, as well, perhaps, as a refuge for lepers and the victims of other 'intolerable' diseases.[36] By and large, however, neither practitioners

---

[33] C. A. Bonfield considers these topics in depth: 'The *Regimen Sanitatis* and its Dissemination in England, *c.* 1348–1550' (PhD thesis, University of East Anglia, 2006).

[34] N. Pounds, *The Medieval City* (Westport, CT, 2005), pp. 68, 141.

[35] D. H. Crawford, *Deadly Companions: How Microbes Shaped Our History* (Oxford, 2007), p. 82. I am grateful to Dr Isla Fay for this reference.

[36] See Chapter 6 below.

nor institutions have fared well at the hands of urban historians, who are reluctant to tread 'the long and weary road' away from medical positivism.[37]

For example, reflecting upon the 'squalid and insanitary conditions' endured by the inhabitants of sixteenth-century York, one distinguished scholar refers disparagingly to the 'rudimentary' and 'especially inadequate' levels of medical provision that must have prevailed in a city without many university-trained physicians.[38] The impressive roster of barbers, barber-surgeons and apothecaries listed in the local records, not to mention the empirics, herbalists and midwives whose services were more affordable, merit little in the way of serious consideration, since from a modern perspective they do not rank as qualified professionals.[39] The level of medical expertise on offer in an age without antibiotics, blood transfusion and effective anaesthesia may all too readily be deemed 'lamentable', but such a bleak assessment brings us no nearer to an understanding of contemporary attitudes and expectations.[40] Books aimed at today's popular market are even less inclined to contextualise attitudes to sickness and health, on occasion outdoing the Victorians in their condescension. To dismiss medieval medicine as 'a bizarre mixture of arcane ritual, cult religion, domestic invention and a freakshow' does scant justice to the complexity and sophistication of many of the ideas about the preservation of health discussed in the following pages.[41]

Historians are not the only culprits in this respect. The belief that medieval cities constituted a haphazard jumble of overcrowded and dirty streets that had evolved unplanned from 'the pack donkey's way' was fostered in the 1920s by the influential Swiss architect Le Corbusier.[42] His frequently quoted remarks about the 'heedlessness, looseness, lack of concentration and animality' of these congested spaces, whose layout condemned them to 'sickness and death', have prompted the historical geographer Keith Lilley to stress the importance of challenging such *ex cathedra* pronouncements, and, above all, of recognising that our 'imaginings' may bear little relation to the documentary or topographical record.[43] Just as attempts by urban magistrates to 'modernise' and improve the layout of towns have often been ignored because they so rarely

[37] M. Pelling, *Medical Conflicts in Early Modern London: Patronage, Physicians and Irregular Practitioners, 1550–1640* (Oxford, 2003), p. 8.

[38] D. M. Palliser, 'Civic Mentality and the Government of Tudor York', in J. Barry, ed., *The Tudor and Stuart Town: A Reader in English Urban History, 1530–1688* (London, 1990), pp. 215–24. However, Professor Palliser does acknowledge that the council was 'far from complacent' in matters of public health: p. 223.

[39] For a survey of some available options, see P. Stell, *Medical Practice in Medieval York*, Borthwick Paper 90 (York, 1996).

[40] J. M. Theilmann, 'The Regulation of Public Health in Late Medieval England', in J. L. Gillespie, ed., *The Age of Richard II* (Stroud, 1997), p. 216.

[41] I. Mortimer, *The Time Traveller's Guide to Medieval England* (London, 2008), p. 190.

[42] Le Corbusier, *The City of Tomorrow and its Planning*, trans F. Etchells (London, 1947), pp. 13–14.

[43] K. D. Lilley, *Urban Life in the Middle Ages, 1000–1450* (Basingstoke, 2002), pp. 18–21.

conform to our own ideas of formal planning,[44] so too the apparently piecemeal nature of many of the public works undertaken in medieval England has led us to underestimate the level of communal activity involved. The cumulative effects of epidemic disease and intermittent recession made it difficult, even in a prosperous city such as Exeter, to complete ambitious projects without proceeding in fits and starts as funding became available. Fortunately, in this particular case, sufficient archaeological and archival evidence has survived for us to appreciate the enterprise and expenditure involved in conveying a piped water system through lofty stone-lined subterranean passages (see plate 15).[45]

Archaeology can often provide a valuable supplement, and sometimes a much-needed corrective, to the written sources upon which medical historians customarily rely.[46] Recent excavations in Norwich on the site of the Franciscan friary about which Jessopp wrote so disparagingly have uncovered an extensive but almost entirely undocumented system of waste and water management whose sophistication was matched by its effectiveness.[47] Monastic water systems are rightly celebrated, but it would be mistaken to assume that, until the fourteenth century at least, major engineering projects of this kind were undertaken only by religious houses or the crown. A lack of archival evidence certainly cannot be equated with inactivity. For example, we know that by the mid-twelfth century, man-made canals conveyed essential supplies of fresh water some distance across country and through the middle of Sandwich, but our information comes entirely from archaeological and topographical sources.[48] By then, too, some of the natural streams, or 'cockeys', that provided Norwich with its principal source of clean water had been diverted or merged so as better to support the needs of the residents.[49]

It is, on the other hand, all too apparent that practice did not always accord with precept. Edward III's orders of 1336 for the removal of noisome refuse from the castle ditch at Newcastle upon Tyne seem to have been ignored by the mayor and bailiffs, who made no significant attempt to address the problem, either because

[44] Lilley, *Urban Life in the Middle Ages*, p. 168.

[45] See section 4.1 below.

[46] For stimulating explorations of the value and limitations of archaeological evidence in the study of urban health, see I. H. H. Fay, 'Health and Disease in Medieval and Tudor Norwich' (PhD thesis, University of East Anglia, 2007), pp. 23–30; and I. H. H. Fay, 'English Hygiene', in M. Carver and K. Klapste, eds, *The Archaeology of Medieval Europe: Twelfth to Sixteenth Centuries* AD (Aarhus, 2011), pp. 136–9.

[47] See pp. 176–7 below.

[48] The project was almost certainly executed by the lay community, possibly with advice from the monks of Christ Church priory, Canterbury, who were skilled in hydraulics: H. Clarke *et al.*, *Sandwich: A Study of the Town and Port from its Origins to 1600* (Oxford, 2010), p. 37.

[49] For example, water from the 'Dalymond Dyke' was diverted into a second, probably man-made, cockey to serve new settlements on the north of the River Wensum: J. Kirkpatrick, *The Streets and Lanes of the City of Norwich*, ed. W. Hudson (Norwich, 1889), pp. 88, 102.

of the cost or the inconvenience of losing such a convenient rubbish dump.[50] Even in London, fly-tipping was ubiquitous and hard to control. There can be little doubt that the vociferous complaints about the 'dung and other nuisances' that constantly clogged the Walbrook stream owed little to exaggeration (the authorities eventually decided to cover it over).[51] The hyperbole so often employed in parliamentary petitions for tax relief was certainly unnecessary in the case of Carlisle, where the combined impact of endemic warfare and pestilence (among animals as well as humans) is vividly apparent from the archaeological record. The striking absence of any major civic projects, such as the introduction of piped water or adequate street paving, is hardly surprising in a community that was so often subject to arson as well as epidemics. Indeed, the lack of spatial barriers between domestic and industrial activities of the sort that were elsewhere confined to the outer suburbs, and the presence of unduly large numbers of livestock within the walls, furnish eloquent testimony to the sanitary problems of living under constant threat of siege.[52]

Not all such findings are as clear-cut or easy to interpret. The discovery of thick deposits of earth and rubbish between successive layers of paving in Winchester's medieval thoroughfares led Derek Keene to conclude that 'in wet weather most streets and lanes would have been at least ankle deep in refuse'.[53] Yet in both England and Scandinavia rubbish was often used deliberately to level uneven road surfaces before new paving was laid. Had this common practice been followed in Winchester, the city might well have been far cleaner than hitherto supposed.[54] The study of waste management constitutes one of the major advances in medieval urban archaeology over the last few decades, confirming both the ingenuity and pragmatism of ruling elites in the face of a potentially intractable problem. As we shall see in Chapter 3, many European cities deployed vast quantities of garbage in reclamation schemes that transformed the landscape; among them, London constitutes a notable, but far from unusual, example.[55]

---

[50] *CCR, 1333–1337*, p. 697; B. Harbottle and M. Ellison, 'An Excavation in the Castle Ditch, Newcastle upon Tyne, 1974–6', *Archaeologia Aeliana*, 5th series 9 (1981), pp. 75–250, on pp. 85–93. In the sixteenth century the ditch became an officially supervised civic dump.

[51] J. Drummond-Murray and J. Liddle, 'Medieval Industry in the Walbrook Valley', *London Archaeologist* 10.4 (2003), 87–94; see section 4.3 below.

[52] M. Brennand and K. J. Stringer, *The Making of Carlisle: From Romans to Railways*, Cumberland and Westmorland Antiquarian and Archaeological Society e.s. 35 (Kendal, 2011), pp. 125–6, 131–2.

[53] Keene, 'Rubbish in Medieval Towns', p. 28.

[54] D. Jørgensen, 'Co-operative Sanitation: Managing Streets and Gutters in Late Medieval England', *Technology and Culture* 49 (2008), pp. 547–67, on p. 560. Since stone paving was often taken up and re-used elsewhere before new surfaces were laid, the quality of excavated roads can often appear much worse than was actually the case: C. A. Martin, 'Transport for London, 1250–1550' (PhD thesis, Royal Holloway University of London, 2008), pp. 96–7, 101–2.

[55] J. Schofield, *London, 1100–1600: The Archaeology of a Capital City* (Sheffield, 2011), pp. 34–7.

Archaeological discoveries about urban infrastructure are making it increasingly apparent that schemes for environmental improvement may have had a significant impact upon collective health. For example, work undertaken in Southampton during the 1950s and 1960s demonstrated that more stringent building regulations and compulsory measures for waste disposal (both prompted by the growing fear of polluted air), correlate with evidence of rising standards of cleanliness on the ground (see plates 8 and 16).[56] More recently, in 2004, a pioneering volume of comparative essays assembled by Manfred Gläser surveyed the provision of such vital utilities as piped water, cobbled streets, hospitals and facilities for removing refuse in thirty-nine 'Hanseatic' towns, including London, Norwich, Hull and York. Together the contributors paint a convincing picture of the ways in which these communities sought to achieve a better and more salubrious quality of life.[57] As one author tellingly observes, 'we like to imagine medieval streets as public rubbish tips and latrines, along which people trudged through drifts of stinking garbage', whereas in reality it was a matter of collective pride that major thoroughfares, at least, should appear attractive and welcoming to visitors.[58]

In this respect, it is easy to be seduced by Italian authors such as Leonardo Bruni, whose panegyric to the unique virtues of Florence, composed in 1402, tends to overshadow the less polished tributes paid by northern Europeans to the towns and cities in which they lived.[59] 'It seems to me that Florence is so clean and neat that no other city could be cleaner', he boasted, in a passage which frequently finds its way into histories of the Renaissance:

> Surely this city is unique and singular in all the world because you will find here nothing that is disgusting to the eye, offensive to the nose, or filthy under foot. The great diligence of its inhabitants ensures and provides that all filth is removed from the streets, so you see only what brings pleasure and joy to the senses ... such unparalleled cleanliness must be incredible to those who have never seen Florence, for we who live here are amazed daily and will never take for granted this fine quality ... Moreover, however big a rainstorm, it cannot prevent you walking through the city with dry feet since almost before it falls the rainwater is taken away by appropriately placed gutters.[60]

Recent studies focussing upon the reality behind the rhetoric suggest that fifteenth-century Florentines were, in general, far from scrupulous about the dumping of waste in public places and that, as a result, their sanitary provisions left much to

---

[56] See section 3.4 below.

[57] M. Gläser, ed., *Lübecker Kolloquium zur Stadtarchäologie im Hanseraum IV: Die Infrastruktur* (Lübeck, 2004).

[58] G. Westholm, 'Sanitary Infrastructure in Mediæval Visby', in Gläser, *Lübecker Kolloquium*, p. 491.

[59] A point made by D. Keene, 'The Medieval Urban Environment in Documentary Records', *Archives* 16 (1983), pp. 137–44, on p. 137.

[60] B. G. Khol and R. G. Witt, eds, *The Early Republic: Italian Humanists on Government and Society* (Manchester, 1978), p. 138.

be desired.[61] Nor, despite some remarkable feats of hydraulic engineering, were other late medieval Italian cities necessarily as clean as is often supposed. For instance, although subterranean aqueducts brought fresh water into the centre of Siena from the thirteenth century onwards, there was no comparable system for sewage disposal, which depended upon the open channels to be found in all major urban thoroughfares. Allowing for the obvious bias of a writer who came from Florence, Leon Battista Alberti's conviction that Siena was 'filthy and offensively vaporous' because it lacked proper drainage may well have rung true. Certainly, by 1450 the residents were conscious that the slaughtering of cattle in the mercantile centre was not only 'inappropriate to decorum' but also offensive to visitors and a significant health hazard.[62] The decision to provide designated slaughterhouses well away from 'showplace areas' had already been taken in London well over a century earlier, thereby placing it among those 'well governed' cities which the Sienese sought to emulate.[63] Such considerations, however, have rarely carried much weight with the historians who maintain that medieval England lagged slowly and painfully behind the rest of Europe, and most notably Italy, in matters of public health.

1.2 In the shadow of Italy

The great nineteenth-century public buildings of cities such as Bradford, Birmingham, Glasgow, Leeds and Manchester still bear witness to the English love affair with Italy, as newly successful northern capitalists sought to project themselves as latter day Medici.[64] Being so firmly wedded to the ideals of Empire, Victorian progressives felt a similar affinity with the Romans, whose achievements in the fields of hygiene and urban planning appeared to cast the limitations of their medieval successors into even sharper relief. The surgeon and reformer Sir John Simon spoke for many when reflecting that during 'the ten dark centuries,

---

[61] D. Biow, *The Culture of Cleanliness in Renaissance Italy* (Ithaca, NY, 2006), pp. 83–94; J. Henderson, 'Public Health, Pollution and the Problem of Waste Disposal in Early Modern Tuscany', in Cavaciocchi, *Interazioni fra economia e ambiente biologico*, pp. 374–5. Although he considered its political system to be unhealthy, the Venetian Marco Foscari (d. 1551) felt that Florence was, indeed, 'neat and clean' in comparison to his native city, where as late as 1529 disembarking visitors encountered butchers' stalls and effluvia from public latrines: Biow, *Culture of Cleanliness*, pp. 76–82. For a perceptive examination of the discrepancy between Italian civic propaganda and 'the very real limits and inefficiencies of early modern health controls', see J. Wheeler, 'Stench in Sixteenth-Century Venice', in A. Cowan and J. Steward, eds, *The City and the Senses: Urban Culture since 1500* (Aldershot, 2007), pp. 25–38.

[62] M. Kucher, 'The Use of Water and Its Regulation in Medieval Siena', *Journal of Urban History* 31 (2005), pp. 504–36; F. Nevola, *Siena: Constructing the Renaissance City* (New Haven, CT, 2007), pp. 22–4, 93, 97–8.

[63] Sabine, 'Butchering in Mediaeval London', pp. 335–6. As early as 1301–2, local juries had complained when butchers' waste was deposited in public places: pp. 339–40.

[64] T. Hunt, *Building Jerusalem: The Rise and Fall of the Victorian City* (London, 2004), chaps 5 and 6.

by which the age of Attila and Genseric was separated from the auroral epoch of Gutenberg and Columbus ... the proportion of thought vouchsafed to sanitary ordinances and constructions remained everywhere at the lowest level'.[65] Indeed, the Roman city still constitutes a benchmark against which the fifteenth-century urban experience seems at best inadequate. Such is the view of the archaeologist Peter Addyman, who concludes that, despite the evidence of a steady 'amelioration in sanitary conditions', late medieval York was still only 'slowly beginning to climb back to something like' the levels of cleanliness evident in Roman times.[66]

Setting aside the validity of such comparisons, it is interesting to note that historians of the Ancient world are now far less inclined to regard the Roman city as a paradigm of environmental health, although the jury is still out on the amount of filth through which residents had to wade. The streets of Pompeii were undoubtedly far less salubrious than modern tourists tend to imagine, not least because they functioned as refuse tips and drainage channels for the elimination of decaying rubbish and water in wet weather.[67] In a celebrated article on 'Slums, Sanitation and Mortality in the Roman World', Alex Scobie effectively shattered many cherished illusions by comparing the 'overcrowded and squalid' housing, minimal drainage, substandard food, contaminated water and high levels of violent crime endured by most town-dwellers with the conditions described in 1842 by the reformer Edwin Chadwick, in his famous *Report on the Sanitary Condition of the Labouring Population of Great Britain*.[68]

The attention focussed by historians of medieval medicine upon southern Europe also tends, implicitly, to portray English towns and cities in a bleak light, if only because they so rarely figure in any discussion of incipient attempts to improve urban health. In his exploration of 'the increasing concern for the physical environment' apparent 'all around the Mediterranean' in the decades before the Black Death, Jon Arrizabalaga highlighted the fact that, as early as 1330, the people of Barcelona protested about the corrupt air (*fetores*) emanating from noisome sewers.[69] Yet it would be possible to cite many similar complaints voiced in English towns and cities from the latter half of the thirteenth century, few of which have

[65] J. Simon, *English Sanitary Institutions Reviewed in their Course of Development* (London, 1890), p. 35. Following his lead, C.-E. A. Winslow described the public health measures of the Romans as 'transitory gleams of intelligence to be quenched in the intellectual darkness of medieval Europe': *Evolution and Significance of the Modern Public Health Campaign*, p. 4.

[66] P. V. Addyman, 'The Archaeology of Public Health at York, England', *World Archaeology* 21 (1989), pp. 244–64, on p. 257.

[67] M. Beard, *Pompeii: The Life of a Roman Town* (London, 2008), pp. 55–7.

[68] A. Scobie, 'Slums, Sanitation and Mortality in the Roman World', *Klio* 68 (1986), pp. 399–433, especially p. 417. Greek and Roman medical authorities commented on the unhealthy nature of towns, which they attributed, *inter alia*, to the effects of poor diet and pollution: V. Nutton, 'Medical Thoughts on Urban Pollution', in V. M. Hope and E. Marshall, eds, *Death and Disease in the Ancient City* (London, 2000), pp. 65–73.

[69] J. Arrizabalaga, 'Facing the Black Death: Perceptions and Reactions of University Medical Practitioners', in J. Arrizabalaga *et al.*, eds, *Practical Medicine from Salerno to the Black Death* (Cambridge, 1994), p. 276.

attracted much attention from scholars. By the same token, although, in theory at least, Italian communes adopted a more systematic approach to the regulation of public nuisances, the widespread assumption that English magistrates showed no interest in such matters is hard to sustain in the face of so much documentary and archaeological evidence of prolonged activity. On the contrary, claims that an awareness of the environmental benefits of 'municipal law and policies' spread slowly across Europe to England from northern Italy take little account of the chronology of sanitary measures either imposed from above by the English crown or instigated at a local level by the residents themselves.[70] It is easy to overlook the fact that London's piped water system, begun during the 1230s, was one of the very first ventures of its kind documented in any medieval western city.[71]

Bye-laws for the disposal of waste, the regulation of food markets and the control of industrial pollution adopted in cities such as Bergamo and Bologna from the late 1250s onwards have, in particular, been described as the first stirrings of 'communitywide responsibility' on the part of European magistrates, providing a model which eventually crossed the English Channel centuries later.[72] Yet already by the 1270s the mayor and aldermen of London were taking similar steps, not least for the election at ward level of officials with specific responsibility for keeping the streets free of dung and other unpleasant nuisances.[73] Comprehensive assizes promulgated between 1276 and 1278 codified long-established civic customs, which, *inter alia*, determined both the price and quality of bread and ale, the dietary staples of the urban proletariat; insisted upon the removal of rubbish, manure and stray pigs from public thoroughfares; controlled civic markets; consigned lepers and brothels to the suburbs; and prohibited street cleaning when it rained, lest the attendant mess cause 'a nuisance to the neighbours'.[74] Not coincidentally, this process was accompanied by a number of administrative innovations, whereby 'traditional' practices, which had hitherto often been passed on by word of mouth from one generation to the next, were written down and rationalised.[75]

Many initiatives came from above, especially in the reign of Edward I, whose efforts to impose a centralised legal and administrative system upon the nation

---

[70] R. E. Zupko and R. A. Laures, *Straws in the Wind: Medieval Urban Environmental Law* (Boulder, CO, 1996), p. 114.

[71] Schofield, *London, 1100–1600*, pp. 30–1.

[72] Zupko and Laures, *Straws in the Wind*, p. 114.

[73] *CLB*, A, p. 183. As was frequently the case, both the officials and their superiors, the aldermen, could be fined for failing to perform their duties. It is interesting to compare early thirteenth-century Italian building regulations (such as those adopted in 1216 in Milan) with London ordinances of a similar date: F. Bocchi, 'Regulation of the Urban Environment by the Italian Communes from the Twelfth to the Fourteenth Century', *Bulletin of the John Rylands Library* 72 (1990), pp. 63–78, on pp. 63–6; see section 3.4 below.

[74] *CLB*, A, pp. 215–20.

[75] G. A. Williams, *Medieval London: From Commune to Capital* (London, 1963), p. 248. For the early documentation of urban customs, see M. T. Clanchy, *From Memory to Written Record: England, 1066–1307* (Oxford, 1993), p. 96; J. Campbell, 'Power and Authority, 600–1300', *CUHB1*, p. 61.

made him impatient of the 'juridical peculiarity' and 'contentiousness' of cities such as Lincoln and London.[76] His intervention in the capital, first through the mayor and then directly through the appointment of a royal warden in 1285, had a dramatic impact upon standards of policing, not least with regard to the enforcement of existing measures relating to hygiene, food standards and the organisation of the City's numerous markets.[77] By the close of the century Edward had turned his attention to York, which became the *de facto* capital of England while he was at war against the Scots. Reports were not encouraging. Alarmed lest he and his men might succumb to disease before they even reached the border, he wrote sternly to the authorities in 1298 complaining that:

> The air is so corrupted and infected by the pigsties ... and by the swine feeding and frequently wandering about ... and by dung and dunghills and many other foul things placed in the streets and lanes, that great repugnance overtakes the king's ministers staying in that town and others there dwelling and passing through, the advantage of more wholesome air is impeded, the state of men is grievously injured, and other unbearable inconveniences and many other injuries are known to proceed from such corruption ... to the peril of their lives, and to the manifest shame and reproach of the bailiffs and other the inhabitants of that town.[78]

Ordinances devised three years later by the royal council and the rulers of York reveal continuing anxiety about the state of the streets, along with additional concerns regarding the availability of fresh, reasonably priced food, the quality of the drugs sold by apothecaries and the competence of medical practitioners. As well as insisting once again upon the removal of stray animals, and demanding regular inspections for cleanliness, they decreed that:

> No one is to put out excrement or other filth or animal manure in the city, nor shall canvas or linen be placed in the drains. Tree trunks and other timbers are to be removed. Ordure is to be carried away and the gutters and drains cleaned. There shall be four public latrines in the four quarters of the city. The people of each trade shall ... remain in a specific place, so that no degrading business or unsuitable trade is carried out among those who sell food for humans.[79]

A close study of late medieval urban records reveals that most English towns readily absorbed this message, even though they were not always able to act upon it. The fact that so many Continental cities appear more 'advanced' can generally be explained in terms of their relative size and prosperity; the amelioration of public services in England was more often hampered by shortage of money than

---

[76] Williams, *Medieval London*, pp. 250–51.

[77] Further ordinances, which reinforced the 1276–8 Assizes and have been described as 'the manifesto of a model regime', were drawn up in 1285: Williams, *Medieval London*, p. 255; *MGL*, I.280–97.

[78] *CCR, 1296–1302*, p. 218; reproduced in H. Rothwell, ed., *EHD*, vol. 3: *1189–1327* (London, 1975), pp. 854–5.

[79] *YCO*, p. 17.

by lack of knowledge or commitment on the part of local magistrates. During the mid-fifteenth century, for example, the urban economy as a whole succumbed to 'an extraordinary range of powerful depressive forces', with inevitable consequences for building programmes and utilities.[80] The once bustling common quay of Ipswich, which in 1344 had been leased out by the authorities at £17 a year, was at this time worth less than £3, being littered with rubbish and the filth of unauthorised pigsties. Only during the economic upturn of the 1470s was it possible to contemplate essential cleansing and repairs, which were funded by a combination of public subscription and the money raised from an influx of newly admitted freemen.[81] As we have seen, even the affluent merchants of Exeter had to stagger investment in their impressive new piped water system, while similar works in towns such as King's Lynn and Hull became largely dependent upon donations from wealthy residents. Significantly, though, none of these projects was mentioned by Richard Holt in the rather apologetic survey of English medieval water technology that he produced for a collection of comparative essays in 2000. Indeed, beyond reflecting upon the alleged failure of 'indifferent' English magistrates to ape their Italian peers, he effectively ignored their efforts.[82]

It is also worth noting that approaches to record keeping and preservation varied considerably from place to place. Italian cities such as Venice maintained detailed registers of sanitary decrees and ordinances as they were promulgated, whereas most English towns and cities adopted a less structured approach. Notwithstanding the shift during the late thirteenth century to the formalisation of custom, and the compilation of two substantial volumes of documents for civic use, memory continued to play a major part in the government of London.[83] The production of the *Liber albus* (White Book), which lists many 'ancient' regulations for the avoidance of environmental problems, was undertaken at the late date of 1419 because 'all the aged, most experienced and most discreet' aldermen had been 'carried off at the same instant, as it were, by pestilence', with the result that 'younger persons who have succeeded them in the government of the City, have on various occasions been often at a loss from the very want of written information; the result of which has repeatedly been disputes and perplexity among them as

[80] J. Hatcher, 'The Great Slump of the Mid-Fifteenth Century', in J. Hatcher and R. Britnell, eds, *Progress and Problems in Medieval England* (Cambridge, 1996), pp. 237–72, quotation on p. 240. See also M. Kowaleski, *Local Markets and Regional Trade in Medieval Exeter* (Cambridge, 1995), p. 90.

[81] N. R. Amor, *Late Medieval Ipswich: Trade and Industry* (Woodbridge, 2011), pp. 133, 186.

[82] See section 4.1 below.

[83] One 'miscellaneous collection' of customs, along with other legal material relating to civic government, appeared between 1311 and 1319 in the volume now known as *Liber Horn*. A slightly earlier custumal, the *Liber legum regum antiquorum*, or *Greater Liber Horn*, was dismembered in the seventeenth century: J. Catto, 'Andrew Horn: Law and History in Fourteenth-Century England', in R. H. C. Davis and J. M. Wallace-Hadrill, eds, *The Writing of History in the Middle Ages* (Oxford, 1981), pp. 371–2, 376–8.

to the decisions which they should give'.[84] The search for reliable precedents was hardly helped by the practice, common among English magistrates and their clerks, of keeping archival material relating to their administrative duties at home and even allowing people to borrow items of particular interest.[85] As a result, many documents were either lost, stolen or not 'duly ordered whiche for the more partye have rested in billes and skroules some tyme in one mannes handes and kepyng and some tyme in another'.[86]

1.3 The Black Death and its aftermath

On the face of things, the contrast between England and the Continent can seem even sharper after 1348, as successive outbreaks of plague prompted very different responses.[87] The failure of English towns to introduce specific measures, such as quarantine and the establishment of isolation hospitals, for the containment of epidemics has been widely regarded either as evidence of passive resignation in the face of divine will or as further proof of collective incapacity and ignorance.[88] Even today, we can still hear echoes of W. T. Gairdner's assertion that:

> the fear of contagion amounted to a frenzy, absorbing all the energies that ought to have been devoted to the removal of the local causes of epidemic disease … The disease itself was supposed to be simply a visitation of God, inscrutable, intangible, unassailable, borne on the wings of the wind, having no relation to diet, drink, habitation, or, indeed, any purely physical cause.[89]

---

[84] H. T. Riley, ed., *Liber albus: The White Book of the City of London* (London, 1861), p. 3. Disputes in Lincoln in 1393 between members of the elite and those of lower status were blamed upon 'verbal traditions (*oracula*) not founded on the solid basis of clear conscience': *CPR, 1391–1396*, pp. 355–6; S. H. Rigby, 'Urban "Oligarchy" in Late Medieval England', in J. A. F. Thomson, ed., *Towns and Townspeople in the Fifteenth Century* (Gloucester, 1988), pp. 65–6.

[85] The problem appears to have been particularly bad in London, although this may simply be because we know more about it. In 1537 'stringent regulations' were introduced to prevent the clerks of the mayor's court from keeping books and calendars at home for reference. Already by then one of the Letter Books had 'been longe myssyng', to be recovered three years later: *CLB*, A, pp. ii–iv.

[86] D. Harrington and P. Hyde, eds, *The Early Town Books of Faversham, c. 1215–1581* (Chippenham, 2008), pp. 98–9. The first town book was compiled between 1382 and 1405, probably in circumstances similar to those leading to the creation of London's *Liber Albus*.

[87] Porter's brief survey of medieval responses to plague is, for example, solely concerned with Italy: *Health, Civilisation and the State*, pp. 34–7.

[88] J. P. Pickett observes that in fifteenth-century England 'the idea of fighting a disease on a wide scale was just beginning', and that Italy was 'unusual in taking civic action' to combat plague: 'A Translation of the "Canutus" Plague Treatise', in L. M. Matheson, ed., *Popular and Practical Science of Medieval England* (East Lansing, MI, 1994), pp. 263–81, on p. 265.

[89] Gairdner, *Public Health*, p. 12. See also Charles Kingsley's remarks quoted at the start of Chapter 3 below.

There was certainly no sustained attempt by urban magistrates to promulgate sanitary regulations during the Black Death of 1348–50, at least so far as we can tell from the surviving sources. As Richard Britnell observes, local authorities 'took little initiative in coping with the crisis, partly because there was nothing they could do and partly because the problem was not recognized as one of their responsibilities'.[90] In extreme cases, the crown itself stepped in to ensure that basic standards of hygiene could be maintained, most notably in London. It was thanks to the foresight of Bishop Stratford, a couple of royal servants and some influential but anonymous Londoners that three cemeteries were established on the outskirts of the City in East and West Smithfield for the emergency burial of plague victims. Their methodical layout has led one archaeologist to detect the work of an official body 'concerned with public health' which functioned throughout the epidemic, but, if so, its impact was limited.[91] When street cleaning operations ground to a halt as plague intensified its grip in early April 1349, Edward III ordered the mayor and aldermen:

> to cause the human *feces* and other filth lying in the streets and lanes of that city and its suburbs to be removed with all speed to places far distant ... and to cause the city and suburbs to be cleansed from all odour and to be kept clean *as it used to be in the time of preceding mayors* [my italics], so that no greater cause of mortality may arise from such smells, as the king has learned how the city and suburbs, which are under the mayor's care and rule, are so foul by the filth thrown out of the houses both by day and by night into the streets and lanes where there is a common passage of men that the air is infected, the city poisoned to the danger of men passing, especially in the mortality by the contagious sickness which increases daily.[92]

A more proactive stance was taken in Italy, where from the very outset in 1348 some communes, such as Florence, Genoa, Pisa, Pistoia and Venice, mobilised committees and tried their utmost to curb the spread of infection both within the walls and from outside. In keeping with contemporary ideas about the transmission of disease by miasmatic or corrupt air, they restricted personal mobility, placed embargoes on the transport of cloth, ordered the destruction of infected bedding, regulated the burial of the dead, curbed industrial pollution and

---

[90] R. Britnell, 'The Black Death in English Towns', *Urban History* 21 (1994), pp. 195–210, on p. 203.

[91] D. Hawkins, 'The Black Death and the New London Cemeteries of 1348', *Antiquity* 64 (1990), pp. 637–42. For a detailed description of these cemeteries and the burials in them, which suggest that there was both 'some centralised pattern of corporate or civic management of the dead not recorded in documents', and 'an organised collection system', see Sloane, *Black Death in London*, pp. 41, 46–8, 52–5, 90–103; quotations on pp. 96 and 100, respectively.

[92] *CCR, 1349–1354*, pp. 65–6. In late August 1357 Edward again complained about the lamentable state of the river bank and streets, where piles of filth were generating 'fumes and other abominable stenches'. He reiterated the fact that 'in the times of our forefathers and our own' the city and suburbs 'were wont to be cleansed from dung, laystalls, and other filth, and ... to be protected from the corruption arising therefrom': Riley, *Memorials of London*, pp. 295–6; *CLB*, G, p. 92.

augmented existing arrangements for cleaning streets and sewers. In Florence and Perugia, magistrates even commissioned autopsies in order to gain a better understanding of the problem.[93]

Once it became clear that outbreaks of plague would recur at regular intervals, more sophisticated procedures were developed. In Milan at the turn of the fourteenth century, for instance, rigid exclusion zones were enforced and extramural plague hospitals set up for the reception of victims. Inevitably, as these regulations became more complex, semi-permanent bodies were needed to implement them. Health boards soon became ubiquitous throughout Italy, especially during the fifteenth century, when urban epidemics were characterised by their increasing virulence and frequency.[94] First instigated in 1377 by the rulers of the Adriatic port of Ragusa (now Dubrovnik), quarantine took longer to gain widespread acceptance on the Italian mainland, although prohibitions on travel were common.[95] The fact that the English government did not contemplate its first 'slight and tentative' steps in this direction for the best part of 150 years has inevitably prompted unfavourable comparisons with continental Europe.[96] Even so, although some foreigners may well have feared visiting such an apparently 'benighted, backward country' as England, we should be wary of equating the lack of a centralised policy for segregating the afflicted with more general passivity on the part of the governing elite.[97]

On the contrary, despite their apparent failure to institute emergency measures once plague struck, the rulers of English towns and cities were well aware of the environmental hazards which bred the miasmas of disease, and launched vigorous (if sometimes belated) campaigns to eliminate them. One has only to observe the efforts made during the fourteenth and fifteenth centuries to restrict the

[93] J. Henderson, 'The Black Death in Florence: Medical and Communal Responses', in S. Bassett, ed., *Death in Towns: Urban Responses to the Dying and the Dead, 100–1600* (Leicester, 1992), pp. 136–50; K. Park, *Doctors and Medicine in Renaissance Florence* (Princeton, NJ, 1985), p. 4; R. J. Palmer, 'The Control of Plague in Venice and Northern Italy' (PhD thesis, University of Kent at Canterbury, 1978), pp. 18–23.

[94] Palmer, 'Control of Plague', pp. 33–47; C. M. Cipolla, *Miasmas and Disease: Public Health and the Environment in the Pre-Industrial Age* (London, 1992), p. 15; A. Carmichael, 'Plague Legislation in the Italian Renaissance', *BHM* 57 (1983), pp. 508–25.

[95] A. Carmichael, *Plague and the Poor in Renaissance Florence* (Cambridge, 1986), pp. 110–16. It was initially adopted only in Mantua and Milan, which were ruled by tyrants. The foundation of a plague hospital often served the interests of political propaganda and one-upmanship rather than helping the sick. As John Henderson points out, Florence's first *lazarreto* took thirty years to build (1464–94) and accommodated only twenty-eight patients: *The Renaissance Hospital: Healing the Body and Healing the Soul* (New Haven, CT, 2006), p. 94.

[96] R. S. Gottfried, *The Black Death: Natural and Human Disaster in Medieval Europe* (London, 1983), p. 122, dates the arrival of 'public health' in north-European cities to the sixteenth century, as Italian practices spread across the continent.

[97] P. Slack, *The Impact of Plague in Tudor and Stuart England* (London, 1985), pp. 201–3. Quarantine was first attempted in London on the orders of Cardinal Wolsey in 1518, almost certainly in consultation with his celebrated physician, Thomas Linacre, who had studied in Padua: see section 6.1 below.

movement of lepers because of their presumed infectiousness to recognise that segregation had already become commonplace in urban society.[98] It is, indeed, the local records rather than those of central government that furnish evidence of pre-emptive action. During the 'great pestilence' of 1467, for example, the rulers of Rochester ordered each of the borsholders, or local headmen, 'every night diligently [to] search within their several boroughs for all new comers and such as may prove infectious persons whereby the city may be in danger of infection by the plague or any other noisome disease'.[99] The names of any suspects were to be reported immediately to the mayor and aldermen so that the necessary steps could be taken for their expulsion. In Durham, by contrast, residents were threatened with heavy fines by the borough courts should they receive visitors from areas where pestilence had already broken out.[100] *Ad hoc* measures, such as the decision to hold Hereford's market some distance outside the walls during the Black Death, the burning of straw from the beds of plague victims, recorded in the Book of Fines kept by the mayor of Southampton in 1501–2, and the removal of butchers' stalls from an infected parish in Shrewsbury sixteen years later, confirm that some communities were unexpectedly proactive.[101]

Although it has so often been regarded as a benchmark of medical progress, quarantine (along with a policy of compulsory isolation in plague hospitals) may have been less successful during the pre-modern period than once supposed. Not only was it socially divisive, commercially disruptive and hard to enforce, but there are good reasons to question its efficacy: even in cities where it appears to have encountered less resistance, plague deaths per head of population were not significantly lower than elsewhere.[102] Moreover, it is important to

[98] C. Rawcliffe, *Leprosy in Medieval England* (Woodbridge, 2006), chap. 6.

[99] F. F. Smith, *A History of Rochester* (London, 1928), pp. 164–5. For details of the 1467 epidemic see Appendix below. In March 1498 the Edinburgh authorities refused to admit persons or goods from areas afflicted with 'this contagious infirmity of pestilence' under pain of death, while anyone who received a suspect was threatened with forfeiture and banishment. An embargo was subsequently placed on the import of English cloth, lest it carry infection: J. D. Marwick, ed., *Extracts from the Records of the Burgh of Edinburgh, 1403–1528* (Edinburgh, 1869), pp. 72, 74.

[100] M. Bonney, *Lordship and the Urban Community: Durham and its Overlords, 1250–1540* (Cambridge, 1990), pp. 223–4.

[101] W. J. Dohar, *The Black Death and Pastoral Leadership: The Diocese of Hereford in the Fourteenth Century* (Philadelphia, 1995), p. 39; C. Butler, ed., *The Book of Fines: The Annual Accounts of the Mayor of Southampton*, vol. 1: *1488–1540*, Southampton Record Society 41 (Southampton, 2008), p. 57; B. Champion, *Everyday Life in Tudor Shrewsbury* (Shrewsbury, 1994), p. 27.

[102] A point made by John Henderson in his unpublished inaugural lecture, 'Death in Florence: Plague, Public Health and the Poor in Early Modern Italy', delivered at Birkbeck College, London, in May 2011. Many of the factors militating against the use of quarantine in the Ancient world still obtained in the later Middle Ages, being compounded by Christian sensibilities with regard to the care of the sick: V. Nutton, 'Did the Greeks Have a Word for It? Contagion and Contagion Theory in Classical Antiquity', in L. I. Conrad and D. Wujastyk, eds, *Contagion: Perspectives from Pre-Modern Societies* (Aldershot, 2000), pp. 154–62. For the economic hardship caused by quarantine, see K. W. Bowers, 'Balancing Industrial

recognise that frenetic legislative activity does not always produce an effective and prompt response on the ground, while an apparent reluctance to innovate cannot necessarily be regarded as 'evidence of apathy'. Health-conscious Italian communes like Bologna had already introduced such comprehensive sanitary regulations over the previous century that it was simply a matter of enforcing them more strictly in plague time, rather than devising new ones.[103] Close analysis likewise reveals that most of the *ordinamenta* issued in Pistoia and Florence during pestilences drew heavily upon existing precedents, to which were added a few supplementary prohibitions upon the entry of people and goods from infected places.[104]

The rulers of English cities also opted to rely upon tried and tested sanitary measures, while simultaneously tightening up the machinery for waste removal and the regulation of insalubrious activities, often through the medium of local ward-moots or craft guilds, which were responsible for policing their own members. Thus, despite the fact that medieval London never possessed anything resembling a board of health or sanitary committee on the Milanese or Venetian model, an analysis of the memoranda entered chronologically from 1276 in the City's Letter Books reveals a four-fold rise in the number of orders for cleaning the streets in the second half of the fourteenth century, and a corresponding increase in the size of the fines imposed for infractions.[105] A similar trawl through the late medieval Hall Books of King's Lynn indicates that between 1431 and 1519 steps for scouring and repairing watercourses were taken on average every two years, either 'at the common cost' or by householders under threat of heavy financial penalties.[106] Being frequently hidden among a mass of other official business, orders of this kind rarely receive much in the way of systematic study. Our preoccupation with novelty and innovation may also explain their general neglect, since historians of public health and medicine are notoriously prone to seek out whatever seems 'progressive and evolutionary' at the expense of less dramatic or traditional practices.[107]

Late medieval English towns and cities were undoubtedly far more salubrious than most Victorian authors and their intellectual heirs would have us believe, but it is certainly not the intention here to depict them as bastions of health and cleanliness. From a highly sanitised twenty-first-century perspective, they would have seemed dirty, noisome and profoundly *un*healthy places: an opinion that

and Communal Needs: Plague and Public Health in Early Modern Seville', *BHM* 81 (2007), pp. 335–58, pp. 341, 343.

[103] S. K. Wray, *Communities and Crisis: Bologna during the Black Death* (Leiden, 2009), p. 151.

[104] Palmer, 'Control of Plague', pp. 21–2; Henderson, 'Black Death in Florence', p. 143.

[105] Sabine, 'City Cleaning in Mediaeval London', p. 28.

[106] See section 4.1 below.

[107] R. W. McConchie, *Lexicography and Physicke: The Record of Sixteenth-Century English Medical Terminology* (Oxford, 1997), p. 4. A similar focus upon 'breakthroughs in theory and therapeutics' explains the comparative neglect of vernacular health advice: M. Solomon, *Fictions of Well-Being: Sickly Readers and Vernacular Medical Writing in Late Medieval and Early Modern Spain* (Philadelphia, 2010), p. 3.

some of their fourteenth- and fifteenth-century inhabitants clearly shared, at least when they were campaigning for better utilities. Despite the earnest intentions of magistrates, food might be contaminated and water polluted, while the threat of plague and other lethal epidemics was never far away. Inscribed into the urban landscape, the names of streets and watercourses bear eloquent testimony to the limitations of medieval technologies for waste disposal and drainage. The stream known as 'Shytebrok' on the outskirts of Exeter, 'Shitebourne lane' in both London and Oxford, and the pungent 'Shite lane' in Bristol leave little to the imagination.[108] Other, less immediately apparent, sanitary problems are reflected in names such as Drummer (Drusemere) Street in Cambridge, and Lothmere in Norwich, both of which were once notable for the pools of stagnant mud and refuse that accumulated there.[109] Even so, as we will see in the following chapters, strenuous and consistent efforts *were* made to rectify all these problems, often involving the investment of large sums of money and considerable human endeavour. As we gain a greater understanding of the ways in which communities sought to arm themselves in the battle against disease, the image of abject passivity that took shape in the aftermath of the Industrial Revolution may, at last, be replaced by something more positive. *truly Communal ?*

[The extent to which schemes for environmental improvement were, in fact, truly *communal* or simply imposed from above by the crown with the support of a well-educated urban elite nonetheless remains an important question,] since one of the principal caveats about the effectiveness of medieval sanitary measures hinges upon the striking level of collaboration required to implement them.[110] The threat of draconian fines, imprisonment or even of humiliation in the pillory is unlikely to have won more than grudging support for measures whose long-term success depended upon the voluntary compliance of individual tradesmen and householders. It has been argued that the civic ordinances compiled by the royal council and rulers of London in the late thirteenth century resulted in 'the massive reinforcement of the executive arm and the *bludgeoning of the public* [my italics] into a sense of responsibility'.[111] Was it really necessary to dragoon the lesser orders in this way, or can we detect a far wider consensus with regard to the threat posed by specific nuisances, such as industrial pollution and fly-tipping? The rest of this chapter will examine some initiatives for change, both from above and below, as we attempt to discover how far ordinary citizens may have come to appreciate the benefits of tighter regulation and collective action.

---

[108] DRO, ED/MAG/62, 76, 168; E. Elkwall, *Street-Names of the City of London* (Oxford, 1954), p. 155; A. H. Smith, *The Place-Names of Oxfordshire*, vol. 1 (Cambridge, 1953), p. 43; *LRBB*, I.7.

[109] P. H. Reaney, *The Place-Names of Cambridgeshire and the Isle of Ely* (Cambridge, 1943), p. 45; K. I. Sandred and B. Lindström, *The Place Names of Norfolk*, vol. 1 (Nottingham, 1989), p. 131. The aptly named 'Niedham Slothe' in Norwich was likewise 'a deep miry place ... made by the conflux of the Water of several Kennels (gutters) before the Streets were paved with Stone': Kirkpatrick, *Streets and Lanes*, pp. 14–15.

[110] Jørgensen, 'Co-operative Sanitation', p. 566.

[111] Williams, *Medieval London*, pp. 255–6.

1.4 The impetus from above

The apparent frequency with which exasperated English monarchs criticised the insanitary habits of their subjects seems to confirm that most urban communities remained cheerfully resigned to the squalor that surrounded them. As we shall see in Chapter 5, early attempts to regulate the quality and pricing of basic foodstuffs owed much to royal initiatives. On many other occasions, though, the crown chose to act at the behest of aggrieved third parties who took exception to the behaviour of their feckless neighbours. During the late thirteenth and early fourteenth century, for example, the rulers of Oxford were repeatedly ordered to prohibit a variety of practices deemed unacceptable, if not overtly dangerous, by staff and students at the university. A royal writ of 1293 censured the townspeople for keeping pigs in their tenements and clogging the streets with dung, 'by which the air is infected and corrupted to the grave damage and danger of loss of life of both clergy and laity living in the said town and others gathering there'.[112] Six months later the mayor and bailiffs were hauled before the king's justices because they had taken so long to clean up the town, and were ordered to do so without further delay. This humiliating experience was evidently soon forgotten, since in both 1301 and 1305 the university authorities protested volubly about the parlous state of the pavements, made worse by heaps of filth and garbage which not only provoked 'horror abhominabilis' in the viewer, but were poisoning the air and taking a serious toll upon the health of residents and visitors alike.[113]

Once again, King Edward demanded immediate compliance, this time under threat of an unspecified but serious punishment. He also acted upon a more particular grievance with regard to the melting of tallow in public places, the unbearable stench of which reputedly occasioned 'illness and debility' among those who inhaled it.[114] Five years later Oxford's butchers were singled out for causing 'so great a corruption' when slaughtering their beasts 'that many people, according to the scholars of the aforementioned university, are made gravely sick ... and some die'.[115] Fraught relations between town and gown inevitably lent colour, if not a touch of melodrama, to these complaints, but the underlying sense of anxiety was real enough. Given that several of these scholars were interested in medicine, and might well have been familiarising themselves with the lengthy section on contaminated air to be found in Avicenna's newly available *Canon of Medicine*,

---

[112] *MCO*, p. 293. For additional complaints about the pollution of the water supply used by brewers and bakers, see section 5.5 below.

[113] *CCR, 1296–1302*, p. 484; *MCO*, pp. 10–11. For the impact upon the body of disgusting sights and smells, see section 3.1 below.

[114] *MCO*, p. 13. Tallow, which was principally used for making candles and soap, came from rendered animal fat, which had to be boiled. Its production was notoriously unpleasant, resulting in the type of miasma that was increasingly associated with disease. When Queen Elizabeth visited Norwich in the summer of 1578, the 'trying' or testing of tallow was prohibited throughout her stay, while any butchers who failed to remove their waste promptly and effectively were threatened with imprisonment: NRO, NCR, 16D/3, Assembly Proceedings, 1553–1583, fols 270v–271r. I am grateful to Dr Matthew Woodcock for this reference.

[115] *MCO*, pp. 13–14.

it is easy to see why they should have been so exercised about environmental hazards.[116] The onset of plague clearly intensified their fears: among the various concessions extracted from the mayor and burgesses by the University in its royal charter of 1355 was an undertaking that they would implement whatever sanitary measures the chancellor might require, or risk the appalling prospect of excommunication.[117]

Not coincidentally, a similar charter awarded almost a century earlier, in 1268, 'for the peace and tranquillity, as also for the utility of the scholars of Cambridge' was notable for its requirement that the town should be

> cleansed of dung and filth and be kept clean, and that the conduits be opened as of old they used to be and kept open, in order that filth may flow away through them … and that obstacles impeding their passage be removed; and especially that the great ditch of the town be cleansed: for the observing of which things there shall be ordained two of the more lawful burgesses in every street, sworn before the mayor and bailiffs, the chancellor and masters being invited to this if they wish to come.[118]

Here, too, questions of hygiene remained contentious. In both 1320 and 1330 the Cambridge university authorities petitioned parliament about the sanitary shortcomings of the burgesses, reporting with shocked disapproval that they had not only failed to pave the streets as required, but had also diverted royal grants made specifically for this purpose to other uses. Since, by all accounts, the pavement had previously been well maintained, it looks as if a decade of famine and exceptionally bad weather rather than outright corruption or negligence had taken its toll on the urban infrastructure.[119] At all events, while insisting that the residents should address the problem at once and render proper accounts for whatever sums had already been collected, the king seemed happy to provide more financial support for essential improvements.[120]

Central government took a close and continuing interest in the upkeep of major urban thoroughfares, as much for the protection of commerce as the avoidance of injury and disease. They were, indeed, crown property and thus, almost without exception, subject to royal jurisdiction.[121] Occasionally, local magistrates would

[116] O. Cameron Gruner, ed., *A Treatise on the Canon of Medicine of Avicenna* (London, 1930), pp. 185–203, 444–5. Further complaints about environmental pollution were made in 1311 and 1339: *MCO*, p. 18; H. E. Salter, ed., *Mediaeval Archives of the University of Oxford*, vol. 1, Oxford Historical Society 70 (Oxford, 1920), pp. 136–8; *CCR, 1337–1339*, pp. 634–5.

[117] C. H. Lawrence, 'The University in State and Church', in J. I. Catto, ed., *The History of the University of Oxford*, vol. 1: *The Early Oxford Schools* (Oxford, 1984), p. 138.

[118] *CPR, 1266–1272*, p. 196. It is, however, apparent that the colleges were just as culpable where the disposal of waste was concerned: R. Williams, 'The Plague in Cambridge', *Medical History* 1 (1957), pp. 51–64, on p. 54.

[119] *RP*, I.381; *RP*, II.48.

[120] *CPR, 1317–1321*, p. 542; *CPR, 1330–1334*, pp. 75, 285, 570.

[121] As Martin explains, the interests of crown and people rarely diverged in practice, especially in London, where unusually from 1444 the citizens enjoyed sole ownership of the streets and 'common soil': 'Transport for London', pp. 159–63.

be instructed to force householders to pay for repairs themselves, as was the case in Lincoln in 1286, when 'the better sort' were ordered to shoulder most of the burden in order that the poor might be spared.[122] The impact of two devastating outbreaks of plague on the city had by 1365 accelerated an ongoing process of decline, which could no longer be ignored. Condemning a 'default of good rule' on the part of the elite, Edward III observed that trade was bound to suffer since 'merchants on account of the deep mud and the dung and filth thrown in the streets and lanes, and other loathsome things lying about and heaped up there, come but seldom and thereby the evil name of [the inhabitants] and the city grows worse'.[123] Perhaps because of the hardship experienced by so many residents, his requirement that they should be 'charged and, if need be, compelled by grievous methods' to pave the streets in front of their dwellings failed in its objective, and in 1371 further powers of distraint were accorded to the authorities so that they could pay workmen to do the job instead.[124]

However, direct intervention of this kind was comparatively rare and almost always arose in exceptional circumstances, often associated with pestilence. A classic case occurred in Norwich during the aftermath of the Black Death, when King Edward commanded the citizens to remove the garbage and filth that had recently accumulated in the streets and to lay adequate paving without delay.[125] In general, the crown was *responding* to petitions from members of the urban elite who actively sought to initiate civic projects, or from local interest groups, among whom the universities of Oxford and Cambridge were predictably the most vocal. As we shall see in Chapter 3, it made far more sense to contract the upkeep of pavements and gutters to trained craftsmen than to rely upon the good will and expertise of individual householders. Moreover, by allowing municipal authorities to raise levies for this purpose the government was able to encourage activity at a local level, offering a carrot before it began to brandish a stick. Grants of pavage, which bestowed the right to impose tolls on specific commodities, such as firewood, salt, corn or iron goods, at the point of entry, were certainly in great demand.[126] Some, such as an award made to the residents of Shrewsbury in 1276 for paving their new marketplace, were intended to assist in the execution of a royal mandate (occasioned in this instance because of 'the filth and mud' that

---

[122] *CPR, 1281–1292*, p. 260.

[123] *CPR, 1364–1367*, p. 89.

[124] *CPR, 1370–1374*, p. 47; J. M. F. Hill, *Medieval Lincoln* (Cambridge, 1948), pp. 253–4.

[125] *CPR, 1350–1354*, pp. 283–4. The streets of London were also in a bad state at this time: *CLB*, E, p. 116.

[126] For a detailed list of the commodities upon which pavage might be levied, and the rates charged, see the 'chartor for a petie custome' granted by Edward I to the city of Exeter: John Vowell, *alias* Hooker, *Description of the Citie of Excester*, vol. 3, Devon and Cornwall Record Society o.s. 14 (Exeter, 1919), pp. 540–3; and similar awards from Edward III and Henry VI to the burgesses of Gloucester: Stevenson, *Records of the Corporation of Gloucester*, pp. 50–1, 57–9. Unlike other towns and cities, London did not require a royal licence and levied tolls from at least 1304: Martin, 'Transport for London', pp. 125–6.

had hitherto deterred visitors), but most were requested by, or on behalf of, the communities themselves.[127]

Between 1268 and 1308 alone the crown made at least fifty-nine awards of pavage to thirty-four towns and cities for periods of up to seven years.[128] Renewal was common, leading in some instances to abuses of a kind practised at Beverley in Yorkshire. Having benefited from a regular series of grants from 1249 onwards, the burgesses came to regard pavage as a supplementary source of income that could be used to make good any shortfall in revenue and spent accordingly.[129] At least the town was 'sufficiently paved' well before the late fourteenth century, but elsewhere the money might be siphoned off into other projects, or even embezzled, before a single flagstone had been laid. By way of deterrent, royal commissioners would be instructed to audit the accounts of collectors, especially when allegations of malfeasance had already been made. The most flagrant cases were, of course, impossible to conceal, as the half-completed paving in Derby, the filthy streets of Worcester, the impassable highway through Southwark and the above-mentioned problems in Cambridge and Lincoln so clearly reveal.[130] Yet, for all its limitations, the system does appear to have promoted an awareness of the importance of collective responsibility that repeated outbreaks of plague served to intensify. By the fifteenth century, magistrates had grown acutely conscious of the corrosive effects of 'foule, noyous and uneasy' streets upon commercial and physical health. And it was they who took the first steps to rectify the situation by petitioning parliament for the right to exact contributions for this purpose.[131]

As Edward III reminded the citizens of London in 1357, clean streets were as much a matter of 'honour and decency' as of hygiene, reflecting the good order of the community and, by implication, the prestige of the crown itself.[132] Not surprisingly, the prospect of a royal visit, when the urban body had to appear at its most fragrant and respectful, proved a particular spur to action.[133] Perhaps

[127] *CPR, 1272–1281*, p. 129.

[128] *CPR, 1266–1272*, p. 228; *CPR, 1272–1281*, pp. 103, 129, 281, 311; *CPR, 1281–1292*, pp. 79, 111, 163, 165, 168, 172, 175, 221, 228, 336, 358, 391, 447; *CPR, 1292–1301*, pp. 13, 22, 24, 59, 144, 358, 408, 514, 576, 581; *CPR, 1301–1307*, pp. 48, 52, 69, 71, 267, 318, 360–1, 374, 396, 463 *(bis)*, 495, 498; *CPR, 1307–1313*, pp. 15 *(bis)*, 33, 73, 76, 90, 92, 96, 120, 173, 194, 416, 430, 440–1, 553, 572, 710–11.

[129] Before the 1430s the town raised between £20 and £30 a year in pavage, spending about half the sum on other purposes: J. K. Allison, ed., *VCH York: East Riding*, vol. 6 (Oxford, 1989), p. 31.

[130] *CPR, 1281–1292*, pp. 223–4; *CPR, 1313–1317*, p. 236; M. Carlin, *Medieval Southwark* (London, 1996), pp. 233–4; Hill, *Medieval Lincoln*, pp. 253–4; see n. 119 above.

[131] Jørgensen, 'Co-operative Sanitation', pp. 554–7; see section 3.3 below.

[132] Riley, *Memorials of London*, pp. 295–6; *CLB*, G, p. 92; Strohm, 'Sovereignty and Sewage', p. 6. Royal writs demanding the more effective enforcement of measures for the removal of waste from London and Westminster, originally adopted during the Winchester parliament of 1393, stressed that they had been devised *'for the credit of the city'* (my italics) as well as the elimination of polluted air: *CCR, 1392–1396*, p. 133.

[133] As in 1274, when the butchers and fishmongers of Cheapside in London were obliged to move their stalls before Edward I processed through the City on his

because they had already been reprimanded over the filthy and congested state of the River Wensum, the rulers of Norwich embarked upon a comprehensive programme of environmental improvements during the late 1460s, while awaiting news of the impending arrival of the Yorkist court.[134] Even if they could not be eliminated altogether, disagreeable nuisances could at the very least be temporarily removed, as was the 'dongehll' at the water gate of Southampton, which was carted away by order of the mayor in 1513 just before Henry VIII embarked for France.[135] Contemporary sensibilities demanded that even in death a monarch should be transported through freshly swept streets. Preparations for the funeral procession of Henry V, whose remains were brought from France to St Paul's cathedral in 1422, involved clearing dirt from the major thoroughfares of Southwark and London, in part because 'the more sufficient persons of the whole city' were to escort the hearse on foot.[136] Since King Henry's father had previously ordered the bailiffs of Southwark to enforce the law against the dumping of dung and offal in ditches, watercourses and other prohibited places much more strictly, we may assume that such an exercise was far from cosmetic.[137]

The statute in question had been passed by the Cambridge parliament of 1388, as a delayed response to complaints by prominent Londoners about the health hazards arising from the wholesale disposal of butchers' waste along the banks of the Thames.[138] Parliament customarily met at Westminster and was therefore alert to such potential dangers, but, as we shall see in the next chapter, it had sometimes to assemble elsewhere, especially during times of war or epidemics. These provincial meetings tended to inspire an even greater 'flurry of local cleansing activity', albeit not always without a sharp reminder from above.[139] In October 1332, for example, the mayor and bailiffs of York were warned that:

> The king, detesting the abominable smell abounding in the said city more than any other city of the realm from dung and manure and other filth and dirt wherewith the streets and lanes are filled and obstructed, and wishing to provide for the health of the inhabitants and of those coming to the present parliament, orders them to cause all the streets and lanes of the city to be cleansed from such filth before St Andrew [30 November] next, and to be kept clean.[140]

---

return from France: H. T. Riley, ed., *Chronicles of the Mayors and Sheriffs of London* (London, 1863), p. 173; see section 5.7 below.

[134] See section 4.5 below.

[135] Butler, *Book of Fines*, p. 82. The extramural rubbish tips which marked the approaches to most English towns were a perpetual source of anxiety on such occasions. Preparations for Queen Elizabeth's visit to Norwich in 1578 involved the removal of the massive and noisome 'muckhill' outside Brazen Gate, near her point of entry: NRO, NCR, 16D/3, Assembly Proceedings, 1553–1583, fol. 271r.

[136] *CLB*, K, p. 2.

[137] *CCR, 1402–1405*, p. 5.

[138] See sections 3.5 and 4.3 below.

[139] Keene, 'Rubbish in Medieval Towns', p. 28.

[140] *CCR, 1330–1333*, p. 610.

Had the citizens so quickly forgotten Edward I's efforts to eliminate these very same problems? Or was his grandson, whose entourage also included Continental physicians abreast with the very latest theories concerning the preservation of health, even more sensitive about such matters? Was it really necessary to warn the chancellor of Cambridge university to prepare for the arrival of the Lords and Commons in 1388 by clearing the streets of 'all swine, and all dirt, dung, filth and trunks and branches of trees'?[141] There was by this point no lack of rules and regulations for the guidance of urban communities; and, indeed, most already possessed at least some of the legal and administrative structures necessary for the implementation of sanitary measures at a local level.

1.5 Customary law and the machinery of local government

As we have already seen in the case of London's *Liber albus*, long-established civic and borough customs were being formalised into 'digests of borough law' (generally known as custumals) throughout the later Middle Ages.[142] We will encounter many specific ordinances relating to public health in subsequent chapters of this book, but it is worth noting here how widespread they were. Six of the thirty-two bye-laws inscribed in 1414 in the imposing book of memoranda known as the Dorchester 'Domesday' deal with sanitary problems. Indeed, the very first three concern the disposal of dead animals, the weekly removal of garbage from the market and the protection of food outlets from contamination. Further measures addressed such common nuisances as stray dogs, wandering pigs and the blockage of gutters in public thoroughfares.[143] That a far smaller town such as Dunstable should pay so much attention to the wellbeing of its residents is perhaps unsurprising given the fact that the regulations recorded in about 1221 had been devised in consultation with the prior, who was lord of the borough, and, as was so often the case, drew their inspiration from London.[144] Even so, the prohibition of obstructive dung-heaps and pigsties and of the abandonment of butchers' waste in streets or markets, the careful monitoring of bread and ale prices and the elimination of potential fire hazards confirm that vigilance on this score was not confined to the larger and more prosperous self-governing urban bodies.[145]

The machinery for addressing individual as well as collective problems was

[141] C. H. Cooper, ed., *Annals of Cambridge*, vol. 1 (Cambridge, 1842), p. 133.

[142] For an introduction and a list of sources by place, see M. Bateson, ed., *Borough Customs*, vol. 1, Selden Society 18 (1904; repr. 1972), pp. xv–lvi. For the burgeoning of this 'literate civic self-awareness', see Rigby, 'Urban "Oligarchy"', p. 62,

[143] Mayo and Gould, *Records of the Borough of Dorchester*, pp. 104–12.

[144] For the extent to which London's customs were adopted elsewhere, see pp. 108, 135, 137, 144, 152, 170, 203, 211, 218, 252–3, 261, 272, 276 below. Most urban elites appear to have had access to information about them by the later fifteenth century, if not long before. In 1447, for example, the 'usages and privileges' of Exeter were recorded in a 'black roll', and soon after the city acquired a 'booke' describing those of London. Both roll and book were passed on from mayor to mayor: J. W. Schopp, ed., *The Anglo-Norman Custumal of Exeter* (Oxford, 1925), p. 14; DRO, ECA, book 51, Commonplace Book of John Hooker, fol. 324r.

[145] W. Page, ed., *VCH Bedford*, vol. 3 (London, 1912; repr. 1972), pp. 360–1.

also developing apace. Although legal historians tend to date the emergence of a discrete body of law concerning 'nuisance affecting the senses' to the Tudor period, its origins are, in fact, far earlier.[146] From at least the 1270s, Londoners were expected to abide by a series of building regulations relating to the construction of walls, drains, cesspits, windows and pavements, which were subsequently enforced by means of a specially constituted assize.[147] Elsewhere, in towns such as Bury St Edmunds (by 1327), Ipswich (by 1291) and Northampton (by 1190), borough custom provided residents with a (theoretically) prompt and accessible means of obtaining redress should their homes or neighbourhoods be threatened by overflowing drains, noisome privies, dangerous working practices and the like.[148] The Norwich custumal of *c.* 1306 refers to a similar procedure whereby aggrieved neighbours could set in train an inquiry by 'sworn men', following which the authorities were empowered to discipline any offenders, force them to pay appropriate damages and, most important, deal effectively with the source of contention.[149]

At the same time, registers of writs, which constituted an essential guide to the principles and application of the English common law, began to include a growing body of material relating to unacceptable activities and structures that damaged private property or threatened the health of the occupants.[150] By the fifteenth century, these legal formularies also contained copies of royal directives on the subject of communal health, not simply for the benefit of government clerks, but for magistrates and other prominent citizens who might themselves wish to initiate proceedings. Based upon late medieval models, the collection assembled in 1534 by Sir Anthony Fitzherbert described the form of writ to be sued out of Chancery 'if the ways be straightned, or the allies or lanes in any town, city or borough corporate be filled with filth or dung or such things by which means infection may increase'.[151] Significantly, he chose to cite one of the crown's tersely worded missives to the mayor and bailiffs of Oxford.

However, not all urban communities were at liberty to adopt and enforce health measures as they saw fit. The confirmation of borough status by royal charter formalised and defined a town's capacity for self-government, notably in cases where the ruling elite answered directly to the crown rather than to an ecclesiastical or aristocratic overlord.[152] From 1345 onwards (when Coventry's growing importance as a centre of cloth production was formally recognised by

---

[146] J. H. Baker, *An Introduction to English Legal History*, 2nd edn (London, 1979), pp. 357–60. However, the law relating to nuisance was more clearly defined after 1550: Robert Monson, *A Briefe Declaration for What manner of Speciall Nusance concerning dwelling Houses, a man may have his remedy by Assize* (London, 1639), p. 1.

[147] *LAN*, pp. ix–xxx.

[148] Bateson, *Borough Customs*, pp. 245, 249, 250.

[149] *RCN*, I.152.

[150] E. de Haas and G. D. G. Hall, eds, *Early Registers of Writs*, Selden Society 87 (London, 1970), pp. 370–1.

[151] Anthony Fitzherbert, *The New Natura Brevium* (London, 1677), pp. 410–11.

[152] Britnell, 'Town Life', pp. 154–5.

Edward III), the legal doctrine of incorporation allowed some towns to assume a 'fictitious personality' and thus, crucially, to acquire property. Several of England's larger provincial centres, beginning with Bristol (1373), York (1396), Newcastle-upon-Tyne (1400) and Norwich (1404), secured additional privileges through the award of county status, which further augmented the independent authority of their magistrates.[153] In principle, it was far easier to effect environmental improvements in incorporated towns and cities, largely because rates could be levied and land purchased for the construction and upkeep of whatever utilities seemed necessary, including almshouses and hospitals. Moreover, along with fiscal autonomy went a formidable range of judicial and disciplinary powers exercised principally through the medium of local courts. Given a reasonable degree of consensus, the most hazardous and unpleasant activities would be targeted at street level through the imposition of fines and other deterrents, among which public opinion proved a significant force.[154]

Seigniorial boroughs remained under the immediate jurisdiction of a monastic lord (as at Bury St Edmunds, Cirencester, St Albans and Reading), a bishop or archbishop (Beverley, Lynn, Salisbury and Wells) or a member of the baronage (Chester, Leicester, Richmond and Warwick), although the residents might still enjoy a considerable amount of freedom to manage their own affairs.[155] In Wells, for example, the bishop permitted the community to appoint 'shambles keepers', who supervised the slaughtering of animals and inspected their meat, and also four officials with responsibility for ensuring the cleanliness of the streets.[156] Moreover, as we shall see in Chapter 4, Bishop Beckington gave generous support to the residents when they embarked on a costly project for the introduction of piped water.[157] Monastic overlords, too, were likely to look sympathetically upon schemes of this kind and could often provide valuable technical expertise as well. Unity of purpose was harder to achieve in places such as Southwark, where five different and sometimes competing jurisdictions overlapped.[158] Durham, which

---

[153] M. Weinbaum, *The Incorporation of Boroughs* (Manchester, 1937), pp. 2–3; C. Liddy, *War, Politics and Finance in Late Medieval English Towns* (Woodbridge, 2005), chap. 5; S. H. Rigby and E. Ewan, 'Government, Power and Authority, 1300–1540', *CUHB1*, pp. 298–9; C. Platt, *The English Medieval Town* (London, 1976), chap. 5.

[154] Britnell, 'Town Life', p. 157.

[155] R. H. Hilton, *English and French Towns in Feudal Society* (Cambridge, 1992), p. 48.

[156] D. G. Shaw, *The Creation of a Community: The City of Wells in the Middle Ages* (Oxford, 1993), p. 132, and chap. 4 in general. Notwithstanding their sometimes fraught relationship with their overlord, the bishop, the residents of Salisbury also enjoyed a relatively free hand with regard to the regulation of nuisances, repairs and improvements to the urban infrastructure, and the enforcement of food standards: D. R. Carr, 'From Pollution to Prostitution: Supervising the Citizens of Fifteenth-Century Salisbury', *Southern History* 19 (1997), pp. 24–41; D. R. Carr, ed., *The First General Entry Book of the City of Salisbury, 1387–1452*, Wiltshire Record Society 54 (Trowbridge, 2001), pp. xxvii–xxix.

[157] See section 4.6 below.

[158] Carlin, *Medieval Southwark*, chap. 4. However, as Hilton points out, most towns and cities 'were riddled with feudal jurisdictions' that were exempt from regulation: *English and French Towns*, p. 48.

comprised four separate boroughs, certainly had neither an overreaching sense of community, nor a unified approach to issues of public health. There was, for instance, no consistent attempt to reduce the risk of fire by restricting building materials to stone and tile, as happened so often in places where magistrates could unilaterally forbid the use of thatch, wood and straw. Only the bishop's borough possessed a market and an independent piped water supply, which was installed in 1450.[159]

Such diversity was matched by corresponding variations in the opportunities available to residents for involvement in the business of local government. Small towns without a franchise might well be run by the lord's bailiff or steward rather than elected officials, sometimes because there were too few available candidates, but also because of a desire to curtail any nascent signs of independence.[160] Notwithstanding his obvious concerns about the sanitary condition of the borough, the prior of Dunstable was reluctant to relinquish any of his judicial authority to the residents. Although they could present negligent butchers and fishmongers who sold contaminated food and report disagreeable nuisances in the local courts, it was the prior who devised the bye-laws and his officers who enforced them, not always as effectively as the burgesses might have wished.[161] Yet, however many liberties a town or city might possess, only a small proportion of its inhabitants ever rose to occupy high office and thus to make meaningful decisions that would affect the health and welfare of the entire body politic. With a few notable exceptions, women played no formal role in urban government, which was, in practice, increasingly dominated by members of a narrow, often self-perpetuating mercantile oligarchy.[162]

This was in part because the number of male householders admitted to the freedom (which bestowed the right to vote in local elections in return for the payment of rates and taxes) might be surprisingly small. In Exeter during the 1370s, for example, only about four per cent of adult males became freemen, of whom just one quarter made up the ruling elite.[163] In York, by contrast, the entry rate was nearer half, although here, too, a coterie of wealthy merchants tended to dominate civic life. The aldermen of fifteenth-century Norwich, where on average fewer than forty new freemen were enrolled every year, have recently been described as an 'aristocracy' of mercers, grocers and drapers, whose power was reinforced by a tight network of familial as well as commercial relationships.[164] Affluent, literate

---

[159] Bonney, *Lordship and the Urban Community*, pp. 33–4, 41–9, 219–23.

[160] Britnell, 'Town Life', p. 156.

[161] Page, *VCH Bedford*, III.357–8, 360; *CCR, 1364–1368*, p. 304.

[162] Rigby and Ewan, 'Government, Power and Authority', pp. 300–1, 306–11; Rigby, 'Urban "Oligarchy"', pp. 62–86; Platt, *English Medieval Town*, pp. 118–24.

[163] Britnell, 'Town Life', p. 158. Lorraine Attreed suggests a slightly higher level of involvement, of about 6 per cent: *The King's Towns: Identity and Survival in Late Medieval English Boroughs* (New York, 2001), p. 22.

[164] R. Frost, 'The Urban Elite', in Rawcliffe and Wilson, *Medieval Norwich*, pp. 235–53, notably p. 243. Their hold on power was based upon a disproportionate share of the city's wealth. Returns to the 1525 subsidy reveal that 60 per cent of taxable goods and property lay in the hands of 6 per cent of the population. Indeed, whereas 29 individuals were then taxed on possessions worth over £100, at least

and well informed about developments in other English and Continental cities, such individuals were clearly disposed to take an interest in matters of public health, often digging deep into their own pockets to provide the necessary funding for improved amenities. In light of much of the evidence considered above, it is tempting to assume that they were swimming against a tide of ignorance and indifference. But there is copious evidence to suggest that a desire for cleaner and more salubrious living conditions was not confined to the upper echelons of urban society, especially once fear of plague brought home the potential dangers lurking in every wayside rubbish dump or flyblown joint of meat.

1.6 The response from below

Historians disagree over the extent to which ordinary men and women actually cared about their living conditions, or whether, as Anthony Wohl argues for the nineteenth century, 'the majority, it seems, accepted filth and smell as parts of their world, as unremarkable and unnoticeable, perhaps, as peeling paint or smog-laden air'.[165] Such assumptions can be dangerous as well as patronising, irrespective of the period in question. As the sanitary reformer, Charles Cochrane, observed in 1849, 'poor people are not absolutely fond of wallowing in filth'. It was then (and almost certainly with his assistance) that spokesmen from one of the most deprived areas in London addressed a celebrated letter to *The Times*. 'We live in muck and filthe', they protested, 'we aint got no priviz, no dust bins, no drains or suer [sewer] in the hole place ... the stench of the Gully-hole is disgustin. We all suffer, and numbers are ill ... we are livin like piggs, and it aint faire we soulde be so ill-treated.'[166] The briefest glance at the complaints made by local juries, largely drawn from members of the artisan class, reveals that such sentiments had hardly changed over the previous four hundred years.[167] In 1415, for example, residents of the area near the ebb gate at the north end of London Bridge fired a barrage of 'loud expostulations' at the mayor and aldermen, because

> the blood from the raw flesh slaughtered by the butchers of Estchepe [East Cheap], and the water in which fish, both fresh and salt, was washed daily, and all the other kinds of filth that had been thrown out of the houses of all sorts of persons, situate to the north of them, into the kennels [gutters] of the said city, usually made their way into a certain gutter, called 'the Swolne', at the end of the said bridge ... until at last the said course has become choked up; and then, by reason of some works lately begun by Thomas Fauconer, the then mayor, was turned out of its course to discharge itself

one third of the residents were too poor to contribute: J. F. Pound, 'The Social and Trade Structure of Norwich, 1525–1575', *P&P* 34 (1966), pp. 49–69.

[165] A. S. Wohl, *Endangered Lives: Public Health in Victorian Britain* (London, 1983), p. 77.

[166] J. Winter, 'The "Agitator of the Metropolis": Charles Cochrane and Early-Victorian Street Reform', *London Journal* 14 (1989), pp. 29–42, on p. 38.

[167] As D. R. Carr points out, 'dwellers in cities had sensibilities seldom attributed to medieval people': 'Controlling the Butchers in Late Medieval English Towns', *The Historian* 70 (2008), pp. 450–61, on p. 460.

and fall [into the Thames] at the gate of Ebgate aforesaid, to the very great nuisance of the neighbours.[168]

Given that the 'works' in question were designed to *facilitate* effective waste disposal into the river, and in fact proved to be only a temporary, if deeply unpleasant, nuisance, it would appear that medieval Londoners responded just as quickly and forcefully to the threat of any 'horrible, corrupt and infected atmosphere', as their Victorian descendants. Even in small provincial towns, officials could face public censure for failing to maintain communally acceptable standards of cleanliness. The people of Basingstoke were so critical of their bailiffs' failure to remove heaps of filth from the marketplace that in 1511 they had them fined for negligence and bound over under sureties of 6s. 8d. to address the problem forthwith.[169]

The implementation of sanitary regulations and the presentment of infractions at this level depended heavily upon that group of relatively prosperous and communally minded householders known in the early modern period as 'the middling sort' or 'honest men'. The role of these solid, politically conservative figures in enforcing the more repressive aspects of Tudor social policy went hand in hand with a less contentious and long-established involvement in the lower echelons of local government and in matters of environmental health.[170] From a comparatively early date men of this stamp had access to a useful store of legal and medical knowledge and were increasingly likely to have mastered the ability to read, if not necessarily to write, in English.[171] Some became minor office holders, acting as tax collectors, constables, gate keepers and surveyors of public works and markets.[172] Almost all served as jurors and capital pledges in local courts, where they were responsible, among other things, for presenting a wide variety of sanitary offences, from the pollution of water supplies to the sale of substandard

[168] Riley, *Memorials of London*, p. 616.

[169] Baigent and Maillard, *History of the Town and Manor of Basingstoke*, p. 316.

[170] See, for example, A. Wood, '"A Littull Worde ys Tresson": Loyalty, Denunciation and Popular Politics in Tudor England', *Journal of British Studies* 58 (2009), pp. 837–47; A. R. De Windt, 'Local Government in a Small Town: A Medieval Leet Jury and its Constituents', *Albion* 23 (1991), pp. 627–54, on p. 628.

[171] Rawcliffe, *Leprosy in Medieval England*, pp. 192–3. Estimates of literacy levels in late medieval England vary widely, but it seems likely that at least a quarter of the urban male population, and perhaps far more, could read: P. Pahata and I. Taavitsainen, 'Vernacularistaion of Scientific and Medical Writing in its Sociohistorical Context', in I. Taavitsainen and P. Pahata, eds, *Medical and Scientific Writing in Late Medieval English* (Cambridge, 2004), pp. 15–16. Certainly, by 1469 the ability to read and write in English was a prerequisite of admission to apprenticeship in many London and provincial guilds. An earlier 'surge in literacy' may have occurred between the 1380s and 1410, when the number of artisans working in book production in London alone almost trebled: M.-R. McLaren, 'Reading, Writing and Recording: Literacy and the London Chronicles in the Fifteenth Century', in M. Davies and A. Prescott, eds, *London and the Kingdom: Essays in Honour of Caroline M. Barron* (Donington, 2008), pp. 347, 350.

[172] The hitherto neglected role of these men is explored by S. Sagui, 'Mid-Level Officials in Fifteenth-Century Norwich', *The Fifteenth Century* 12 (2013), pp. 101–21.

or contaminated food. They were empowered to fine petty offenders and demand remedial action, while more serious cases would be referred to a higher authority.

The urban custumals which so often itemise the various types of antisocial behaviour likely to attract attention would sometimes be read aloud in open court for the guidance of the assembled jurors.[173] The latter might also work from a short checklist of specific misdemeanours and 'common annoyances' that had to be reported, adding complaints of their own as circumstances required. A few such documents have survived, demonstrating, once again, a lively interest in matters of communal health. The *inquisitiones wardemotarum* copied into London's *Liber albus* reveal that an ongoing campaign was being fought at neighbourhood level against dirty and impassable streets, dung-heaps, the keeping of domestic animals, fire hazards, overpriced and substandard food and lepers who frequented public places.[174] In most cases, however, we are obliged to deduce from the number and frequency of presentments made by juries what precisely these lists may have contained and where the court's priorities lay.[175] In Ipswich during the early 1470s, for example, the town's four leet courts launched an unprecedented assault on sanitary offences relating to stray pigs, the dumping of dung in ponds, ditches and other prohibited places, and the failure to clean 'noxious' drains. In 1471, the year of 'the most vnyuersall dethe' in living memory, between a quarter and a third of all presentments related to such offences; and in 1472 over a third. Another 'blitz' occurred in 1479, when pestilence again struck East Anglia. People were clearly responding to the need for greater vigilance.[176]

By the closing years of the fourteenth century, if not long before, the threat posed by miasmatic air was understood at all but the lowest levels of society.

---

[173] An abridged version of civic regulations was read aloud in London ward moots from at least 1311, and from the middle of the century each mayor began his term in office by arranging for *communes proclamaciones* to be made through the streets, alerting the populace to the measures which he deemed especially important. In 1357, for example, John Stodeye 'presented himself as a genuine Mr Clean': F. Rexroth, *Deviance and Power in Late Medieval London* (Cambridge, 2007), p. 124; *CPMRL, 1413–1437*, pp. xxvi–xxvii. During the late fifteenth century, the rulers of Worcester likewise sought to remedy what they regarded as an alarming level of ignorance about local bye-laws by having both new and old ones read to the residents every year: T. Smith, L. T. Smith and L. Brentano, eds, *English Gilds*, EETS o.s. 40 (London, 1892), p. 402.

[174] *MGL*, I.337–8. Every London alderman had to make sure that these articles were enforced in his ward. In 1343, for example, each was ordered 'to see that the streets were properly kept and that rubbish and dung were removed, under pain of imprisonment of the serjeants' who were responsible for policing the system: *CPMRL, 1323–1364*, p. 156.

[175] F. J. C. Hearnshaw, *Leet Jurisdiction in England* (London, 1908), pp. 43–71.

[176] SROI, C/2/8/1/13, 14; C/2/10/1/7; see sections 3.2 and 3.6 below. For details of these epidemics, see Appendix. The same phenomenon, accompanied by growing popular awareness of health issues, is documented by A. Kinzelbach, 'Infection, Contagion, and Public Health in Late Medieval and Early Modern German Imperial Towns', *Journal of the History of Medicine and Allied Sciences* 62 (2006), pp. 369–89, on p. 376.

And besides protecting the community from any potential sources of airborne corruption, jurors had to demonstrate more specialist medical expertise. As Faye Getz observes, 'the ability of the layperson to make medical decisions was in fact the rule rather than the exception'.[177] Ordinary citizens might be called upon to assist local coroners in determining how and why someone had died and to pronounce in cases involving claims of physical incapacity, insanity, pregnancy, injury, rape or impotence. In thirteenth-century Norwich, for instance, coroners' juries expressed opinions with regard to the effects of atmospheric pollution, the mental health of suicides, the debility of vagrants and the probable onset of septicaemia in untreated wounds.[178] It was, moreover, often necessary to establish whether or not officials were too sick, disabled or senile to discharge their duties. In contrast to continental Europe, where suspect lepers were increasingly subject to a formal examination, or *judicium*, by trained physicians and surgeons, in England the decision to segregate them from the community was taken by laymen. Despite the complaints sometimes voiced by qualified practitioners, many of these 'amateurs' appear to have acquired considerable diagnostic expertise. A panel of twelve leading burgesses, or jurats, 'with knowledge of the disease' was elected specifically to determine cases of leprosy in King's Lynn in 1376; and it was generally assumed that the 'discreet and law-worthy men' who presented suspects elsewhere would be sufficiently familiar with the challenging range of symptoms to reach an informed decision.[179]

How could one acquire this type of information? The later Middle Ages witnessed a growing demand for accessible advice manuals that would enable men and women to avoid serious illness without recourse to costly professional care or the blandishments of quacks and charlatans.[180] Increasingly seen as a work of charity, the abridgement and translation into English of medical and surgical texts, plague tracts and guides to healthy living may initially have been undertaken at the behest of practitioners who had little or no Latin, but soon catered for a far wider audience.[181] Not all the intended beneficiaries of this self-help literature

[177] F. Getz, *Medicine in the English Middle Ages* (Princeton, NJ, 1998), p. 75; Rawcliffe, *Leprosy in Medieval England*, p. 167.

[178] NRO, NCR, 8A/1–2; R. F. Hunnisett, *The Medieval Coroner* (Cambridge, 1961), chap. 2.

[179] Rawcliffe, *Leprosy in Medieval England*, pp. 192–3.

[180] The most comprehensive studies of the development and transmission of this literature in continental Europe may be found in P. Gil-Sotres, 'Els regimina sanitatis', in Arnald de Villanova, *Arnaldi de Villanova opera medica omnia*, vol. 10.1: *Regimen sanitatis ad regem Aragonum*, ed. L. García-Ballester and M. R. McVaugh (Barcelona, 1996), pp. 25–105; M. Nicoud, *Les Régimes de santé au moyen âge*, 2 vols (Rome, 2007); and Solomon, *Fictions of Well-Being*. For England, see Bonfield, '*Regimen Sanitatis* and its Dissemination', pp. 24–36.

[181] S. Cohn, *The Black Death Transformed: Disease and Culture in Early Renaissance Europe* (London, 2001), chap. 9; P. Murray Jones, 'Medical Books before the Invention of Printing', in A. Besson, ed., *Thornton's Medical Books, Libraries and Collectors*, 3rd edn (London, 1990), pp. 10–16; P. Murray Jones, 'Information and Science', in Horrox, *Fifteenth-Century Attitudes*, pp. 97–111; P. Murray Jones, 'Medicine and Science', in L. Hellinga and J. B. Trapp, eds, *The Cambridge History*

were themselves able to read; those who could commonly acted as 'interpreters' by transmitting and explaining the contents to others – a task greatly facilitated by the fact that many *regimina* were written in verse.[182] As the fifteenth century drew to a close, vernacular texts began to appear quickly in response to specific epidemics, reflecting both the level of demand and the conviction that they served a useful purpose. Thus, for example, at least three separate translations of the well-known 'Canutus' plague tract were produced in 1485 to combat the spread of the sweating sickness, perhaps on the orders of Henry VII himself.[183] Within three years of its publication in 1497 Gaspar Torella's *Tractatus* on the French pox had also been partially translated so that English readers would be better equipped to deal with this terrifying new disease.[184] The burgeoning new print culture accelerated this process.

It is, of course, one thing to own, or even study, a health manual and quite another to act upon its recommendations, as the rapidly escalating levels of obesity in twenty-first-century Britain clearly demonstrate. Yet some advice found a receptive readership. In late October 1479 John Paston II reassured his mother that he had survived a devastating outbreak of pestilence in London, 'whereoff the first iiij dayes I was in suche feere off the syknesse, and also fownde my chambre and stuffe nott so clene as I demyd, which troblyd me soore'.[185] Members of the gentry and civic elite had grown extremely particular about such matters. In accordance with the guidance offered in *regimina* and plague tracts, and no doubt also in order to ape the manners of the nobility, they placed a high premium upon personal and domestic hygiene.[186] Popular verses of Arab origin, reputedly composed for an English king by the physicians of Salerno, stressed the importance of washing the hands and face, combing the hair, rinsing the eyes and cleaning the teeth every morning on rising. A light, well-ventilated home, free from noxious

of the Book in Britain, vol. 3: *1400–1557* (Cambridge, 1999), pp. 433–48; F. M. Getz, 'Charity, Translation and the Language of Medical Learning in Medieval England', *BHM* 64 (1990), pp. 1–15; G. Keiser, 'Scientific, Medical and Utilitarian Prose', in A. S. G. Edwards, ed., *A Companion to Middle English Prose* (Cambridge, 2004), pp. 231–47.

[182] P. Strohm, 'Writing and Reading', in Horrox and Ormrod, *Social History of England*, p. 466; Kinzelbach, 'Infection, Contagion, and Public Health', pp. 380–3.

[183] G. R. Keiser, 'Two Medieval Plague Treatises and their Afterlife in Early Modern England', *JHM* 58 (2003), pp. 292–324, on pp. 318–19.

[184] BL, MS Sloane 398, fols 147r–153r; E. L. Zimmermann, 'An Early English Manuscript on Syphilis', *Bulletin of the Institute of the History of Medicine* 5 (1937), pp. 461–82.

[185] *PL*, I.515. For the Pastons as owners of medical literature, see C. Jones, 'Discourse Communities and Medical Texts', in Taavitsainen and Pahata, *Medical and Scientific Writing*, p. 33.

[186] For the cleanliness of domestic space , see D. Shaw, 'The Construction of the Private in Medieval London', *Journal of Medieval and Early Modern Studies* 26 (1996), pp. 447–66. However, Shaw's contention that Londoners were reconciled to 'sensory assaults' and 'physical aggravation' outside the home (p. 448) runs contrary to much of the evidence presented in this book.

odours, dirt, stagnant water and other health hazards, was deemed equally beneficial.[187]

In the early 1390s, the anonymous Ménagier de Paris composed a guide to successful housekeeping for his young bride. No English equivalent survives, but it seems unlikely that the English bourgeoisie were any less attached to their creature comforts. Not only was the assiduous chatelaine expected to wage war against all manner of vermin, but also to ensure that her husband was constantly supplied with hot water for washing, freshly laundered linen and spotless bed sheets. It is interesting to note that the daily dusting and sweeping of public rooms was seen as much in terms of 'estate' as of hygiene, since dirt reflected badly upon anyone with aspirations to gentility.[188] Affluent Londoners invested in basins, ewers, tubs, fixed *lavatoria* (which empted directly into gutters), soap and sponges, while some possessed their own bathing facilities.[189] Testamentary evidence from the port of Ipswich suggests that the growing demand for washing utensils was not confined to a few wealthy merchants, but had, by the later fifteenth century, spread down the social hierarchy to embrace 'the middling sort' as well.[190] Although they survive in far smaller numbers, inventories are even more revealing about rising standards of cleanliness. The goods of a moderately successful Winchester fuller appraised by the courts in 1433 included a basin, ewer and other items designed for care of the person; the hundred or so probate inventories surviving from the late medieval diocese of York also contain numerous references of this kind. Not surprisingly, the well-connected York MP Robert Talkan (d. 1415) kept washing equipment in both his hall and chamber, but within a few decades even a humble city shoemaker could lay claim to some towels and basins.[191]

[187] Sir John Harington, *The School of Salernum: Regimen sanitatis salernitanum* (London, 1922), pp. 76, 87. A short fifteenth-century vernacular tract, allegedly based on a regimen sent to Queen Isabella, promised its English readers that they would 'neuer neden leche crafte' if they took these precautions: Wellcome Institute Library, Western MS 408, fol. 13v.

[188] E. Power, ed., *The Goodman of Paris* (London, 1928), pp. 15, 173–6, 211. For the enduring connections between cleanliness, refinement and status, see R. Cox, 'Dishing the Dirt', in R. Cox *et al.*, *Dirt: The Filthy Reality of Everyday Life* (London, 2011), p. 47; and K. Ashenburg, *Clean: An Unsanitised History of Washing* (London, 2007), chap. 3.

[189] S. L. Thrupp, *The Merchant Class of Medieval London* (Ann Arbor, MI, 1962), pp. 138–9.

[190] N. Amor, 'The Trade and Industry of Late Medieval Ipswich' (PhD thesis, University of East Anglia, 2009), p. 63. Advice literature recommending that servants in great households should clean their nails and wash their hands before and after eating undoubtedly made an impression lower down the social hierarchy: F. J. Furnivall, ed., *The Babees Book*, EETS o.s. 32 (London, 1868), pp. 22, 29, 309; C. Woolgar, *The Senses in Late Medieval England* (New Haven, CT, 2006), pp. 132–5.

[191] Keene, 'Medieval Urban Environment', p. 44; P. Stell and L. Hampson, eds, *Probate Inventories of the York Diocese, 1350–1500* (York, 2006), pp. 72–6, 305–6, and *passim*. Despite the poor sanitary provision in Carlisle, many of the more affluent residents still possessed basins and ewers for washing: H. Summerson, *Medieval*

The conviction that medieval people rarely, if ever, washed either their bodies or their clothing has proved almost as tenacious as assumptions about the filth of the towns and cities in which they lived.[192] However, recent scholarship has revealed a society which enthusiastically embraced the pleasures and rituals of grooming and bathing.[193] Although, as we shall see, even the most reputable public bath-houses fell out of favour during epidemics, great emphasis was placed in elite circles upon keeping one's person – especially the hands and face – scrupulously clean, while also changing one's underwear as frequently as possible. This was not simply a matter of aesthetics or even status. An English translation of the *Hortus sanitatis* (Garden of Health) of 1491 warned that lice were generated 'out of the filthi and onclene skyne', adding that the best way to avoid them was 'to wasche the[e] oftentimes and to chaunge often tymes clene lynen'.[194] Since medical opinion made a direct connection between dirty clothes, insanitary habits and skin disease, it is hardly surprising that negligent employers who obliged their apprentices to work and sleep in squalid, vermin-ridden conditions could face imprisonment.[195] The preoccupation, apparent in both health manuals and remedy collections, with the elimination of 'stynkynge brethe that comyth out of the stomake' and with 'stynkyng teth' likewise reflects the deep-seated anxiety felt

Carlisle: The City and the Borders from the Late Eleventh to the Mid-Sixteenth Century, 2 vols, Cumberland and Westmorland Antiquarian and Archaeological Society e.s. 25 (Kendal, 1993), I.372.

[192] Rawcliffe, *Leprosy in Medieval England*, pp. 226–7.

[193] Smith, *Clean: An Unsanitised History of Washing*, chap. 6. While recognising the popularity of bathing, G. Vigarello underplays the importance accorded to the wearing of clean linen in the later Middle Ages: *Concepts of Cleanliness: Changing Attitudes in France since the Middle Ages* (Cambridge, 1988), pp. 48–54. For a different view, see C. Rawcliffe, 'A Marginal Occupation? The Medieval Laundress and Her Work', *Gender and History* 21 (2009), pp. 147–69. Vigarello's assertion that washing the hands and face was a question of morality and decency *rather* than health (pp. 46–8) is also debatable in light of the emphasis placed upon it in *regimina*. Washing the hands after meals was, for example, believed to benefit the eyes as well as maintaining personal hygiene: R. Loewe, 'Handwashing and the Eyesight in the *Regimen sanitatis*', *BHM* 30 (1956), pp. 100–8.

[194] N. Hudson, ed., *Hortus sanitatis* (London, 1954), p. 65. Far from tolerating lice, 'nyttes' and fleas, medieval men and women devoted considerable energy both to the elimination of vermin and to removing the sweat and grime from which they apparently sprang. However, ingredients such as mercury, aloes, arsenic and lead monoxide, which were employed against body lice, are likely to have produced unpleasant side-effects (for use of these ingredients, see BL, MS Harley 2390, fol. 150r; MS Sloane 73, fol. 31r; MS Sloane 213, fol. 155v; MS Sloane 983, fols 72v–73r; Wellcome Institute Library, Western MS 408, fol. 49v). I am most grateful to Professor Martha Carlin for these references and others in n. 196 below. See also W. R. Dawson, ed., *A Leechbook, or Collection of Medical Recipes of the Fifteenth Century* (London, 1934), pp. 132–5, 278–9 (fleas and lice), 200–1 (nits).

[195] In 1492, for instance, a merchant tailor was 'committed to warde' for his 'ungodeley dealyng' in forcing an apprentice to live 'foule shirtyd above his midyll and full of vermin, etc': M. Davies, ed., *The Merchant Taylors' Company of London: Court Minutes, 1486–1493* (Stamford, 2000), p. 198.

about any source of corrupt air and its potential impact upon the body. Clearly, too, there was a growing sense that appearances mattered; if the human form was a gift from God, it should be preserved for as long as possible in the divine image.[196]

Other factors besides fear of plague and an attendant desire to eliminate miasmatic infections explain the interest shown by late medieval urban communities in matters of public health. Royal intervention (especially during the reigns of Edward I and Edward III) was a powerful spur to action, as well as a remarkably effective means of alerting people to the hazards in their midst.[197] The development of administrative and legal mechanisms for the enforcement of a growing corpus of customary law enabled neighbours, as well as magistrates, to take steps against potentially dangerous nuisances and reckless behaviour, with the result that responsibility for the actual implementation of sanitary measures frequently lay with those who suffered most from environmental pollution and the sale of substandard goods. At the same time, the enfranchisement and incorporation of boroughs made it possible to secure long-term funding for more ambitious public works and amenities through the acquisition of property. As we shall see in the next chapter, the dramatic fall in urban populations during the second half of the fourteenth century may have caused a raft of social, economic and political problems, but it at least eased the chronic overcrowding and food shortages that had hitherto blighted the lives of so many men, women and children. Indeed, it was during the aftermath of the Black Death that standards of living among the urban workforce began steadily to rise, permitting a modestly successful artisan to invest in the goods and services deemed beneficial to health by his social superiors.

Less apparent to a modern reader, but of paramount importance to the thoughtful citizen, was a widespread conviction that the urban body functioned organically in exactly the same way as that of the individual baker, butcher or apothecary who sold his wares in the local market. It followed logically from this assumption that the health, prosperity and *moral rectitude* of each resident could affect the wellbeing – and perhaps even the survival – of the whole, which was no less vulnerable to the malign effects of bad air and physical indulgence.[198] In short, the public and the personal merged seamlessly in one simple physiological metaphor. As the Tudor polemicist Thomas Starkey (d. 1538) explained: every 'cyte or towne hathe hys commyn wele & most perfayt state, when fyrst the multytude of pepul and polytyke body ys helthy beutyful & strong … then plentuously nuryschyd wyth abundance of al thyngys necessary … and so thyrdly lyve togyddur

---

[196] See, for example, BL, MS Harley 2378, fols 39v–40r; MS Harley 2390, fol. 150r; MS Sloane 122, fols 55v–56r; MS Sloane 983, fols 6r, 76r; Dawson, *Leechbook*, pp. 190–1, 280–1, 333. For the growing preoccupation with cleanliness and aesthetics in European towns, see L. Demaitre, 'Skin and the City: Cosmetic Medicine as an Urban Concern', in F. E. Glaze and B. K. Nance, eds, *Between Text and Patient: The Medical Enterprise in Medieval and Early-Modern Europe*, Micrologus' Library 39 (Florence, 2011), pp. 97–120.

[197] See section 3.1 below.

[198] G. Rosser, 'Urban Culture and the Church, 1300–1540', *CUHB1*, pp. 340–1.

in cyvyle ordur ... ychone lovyng other as partys of one body'.[199] In practice this superficially inclusive concept was fraught with difficulties, not least the problem of dealing with any diseased limbs or organs that threatened to contaminate the rest.

---

[199] Thomas Starkey, *A Dialogue between Pole and Lupset*, ed. T. F. Mayer, CS 4th series 37 (London, 1989), p. 38.

Chapter 2
Urban Bodies and Urban Souls

Those who study the physical sciences, and bring them to bear upon the health of Man, tell us that if the noxious particles that rise from vitiated air were palpable to the sight, we should see them lowering in a dense black cloud above such haunts, and rolling slowly on to corrupt the better portions of a town. But if the moral pestilence that rises with them, and in the eternal laws of outraged Nature, is inseparable from them, could be made discernable too, how terrible the revelation! Then should we see depravity, impiety, drunkenness, theft, murder, and a long train of nameless sins against the natural affections and repulsions of mankind, overhanging the devoted spots, and creeping on, to blight the innocent and spread contagion among the pure.

Charles Dickens, Dombey and Son (1846)[1]

This chapter begins with a tale of two priests, each of whom was censured by his parishioners and neighbours for conduct that seemed to threaten their wellbeing as much as his own. The first, John Leche, a Yarmouth chaplain, faced charges of incest, adultery and brothel-keeping, committed 'to the great detriment' of the entire community. The fines of 20s. and 18s. 4d. which he paid in 1440–1 ranked among the heaviest imposed by the local courts during the fifteenth century, being on a par with the penalties faced by incorrigible prostitutes and lepers who persistently refused to live beyond the walls. They clearly reflected the 'insult, affray [and] rebellion in great disturbance of the people' of which he was deemed guilty.[2] Even more heinous were the offences reputedly committed by John Scarle, the parson of St Leonard's church, Aldgate, as reported to the mayor and aldermen of London two decades earlier. According to his indignant congregation, he was

> a commyn putour [pimp or fornicator] of his owne parischens alle wey duryng, and a baratour [brawler], and a scolde, and a perilous rebaude [ribald] of his tunge and a discurer of confessioun of the whiche women that wole not assent to his lecherie, the whiche is *gret dissese* [my italics] to alle the parisshe. Item, we endite the same parsoun … for by cause that he presentit hym self a surgeoun & a visicioun [physician] to disseive the peopl with is false connynge, that he scheuithe unto the peopl, by the whiche craft he hathe slayn many a man.[3]

---

[1] Charles Dickens, *Dombey and Son* (Harmondsworth, 1985), p. 738.

[2] NRO, Y/C4/149, rot. 19r–v. Assertions in one local chronicle, now lost, that no Yarmouth cleric had ever been publicly detected in a 'fleshly sin' were demonstrably wide of the mark, as a brief perusal of the leet rolls reveals: P. Rutledge, 'Thomas Damet and the Historiography of Great Yarmouth', *NA* 33 (1965), pp. 119–30, on p. 129 n. 58.

[3] *CPMRL, 1413–1437*, p. 127. For the role of London ward moots in policing sexual misbehaviour, see S. McSheffrey, *Marriage, Sex and Civic Culture in Late Medieval London* (Philadelphia, 2006), pp. 144, 158–61.

In the eyes of their contemporaries both men appeared to undermine public health as well as decency. A twenty-first-century reader would undoubtedly agree that, if true, Scarle's misguided attempts to practise medicine and surgery without proper training must have put vulnerable people at risk. He or she might also regard the pair as grossly negligent, not only setting a poor example to their congregations but also as potential vectors of sexually transmitted diseases. However, fears that their lack of restraint might itself spread through the urban body like cancer, even unleashing the catastrophic forces of pestilence, are likely to strike such a reader as at best misplaced and at worst as the product of ignorance and superstition. Why should courts that customarily dealt with insanitary nuisances such as blocked drains, fly-tipping and the sale of contaminated food regard questions of clerical morality as a legitimate cause for concern?

In order to answer this question and, indeed, to provide an appropriate context in which to evaluate the various initiatives considered in the rest of this book, it is first necessary to outline the basic tenets of human physiology as understood by the late medieval medical profession and a steadily growing proportion of the educated laity. Since, as we shall see in later sections of this chapter, towns, cities and entire nations were believed to function – and malfunction – as bodies writ large, such an exercise will also help to explain how the analogy became so pervasive. Reverence for a system of belief that in some cases had already endured for over a millennium ensured the survival of ideas whose continuing appeal lay as much in their coherence and logic as in their universal applicability. The Ancient Greeks, along with the Muslim scholars who organised and developed much of their work, believed that the preservation of health hinged upon comprehensive, but essentially simple, holistic principles. Because each individual represented a microcosm of the universe, he or she appeared to share the same component parts and obey exactly the same natural laws. Just as the cosmos had been created out of earth, water, fire and air, and became seriously disturbed if one of these four elements predominated, so the human body could only work effectively if its levels of coolness, moisture, heat and aridity remained in a state of equilibrium.

The complexion of each individual was determined by a combination of four 'interactive qualities', or humours, which under ideal circumstances were balanced so that none grew too weak or too powerful. As originally defined in Classical times, the melancholic humour was cold, dry and earthy; the phlegmatic chilly and wet, like water; the choleric as hot and dry as fire; and the sanguine warm, moist and airy. Each was the product of an ongoing culinary process, having been generated in the liver from partially cooked food conveyed from the oven of the stomach.[4] When all was going well, the bulk of this mixture would be converted into blood, while the residual matter became phlegm (potential blood). The foam on top was transformed into choler, or yellow bile, and the sediment at the bottom into black bile, which was melancholic. Reserves of choler and black bile were stored, respectively, in the gall bladder and spleen, the rest being transported with the blood and phlegm along the *vena cava* into the venous system, and thence

---

[4] P. Brain, ed., *Galen on Bloodletting* (Cambridge, 1986), pp. 5–10; N. Siraisi, *Medieval and Early Renaissance Medicine* (Chicago, 1990), pp. 97–100.

as nourishment to the vital organs, limbs and extremities. In a healthy body any surplus humoral matter would be expelled in the urine, sweat, mucus and faeces before it could do too much damage.[5] The overproduction of any humour might trigger serious illness, although choler and black bile seemed the most dangerous because of their capacity to promote anger, paranoia and depression, as well as to cause terminal diseases, such as cancer and leprosy.[6]

Being unaware of the circulation of the blood, medieval physicians believed that the veins, arteries and nerves functioned as quasi-independent networks, akin to irrigation canals.[7] The venous blood, with its potent mixture of humours, or natural spirits, nurtured the entire body, enabling it to grow and reproduce. Some of this blood was diverted to the heart, the source of natural heat and thus of life itself, where it appeared to pass through a filter from the right ventricle to the left before mixing with air from the lungs. Thus transformed into light and frothy *pneuma*, or vital spirits, it travelled along the arteries, carrying warmth and life to the rest of the body, any noxious vapours generated in the process being immediately exhaled in order to eliminate poison. The vital spirits destined for the brain underwent a further process of refinement on their journey through a filter (the *rete mirabile*) at the top of the spine, which allegedly turned arterial blood into superior matter known as animal spirits. Once invigorated by air from the nostrils, these spirits not only served to activate the entire nervous system but also to animate thought and thus directly to control the 'inward wits' or powers of reason.[8] Mind and body consequently enjoyed a symbiotic relationship which depended upon the smooth working of this complicated, finely tuned physiological system. An imbalance in the humours or the inhalation of corrupt air threatened to create a vortex of mental and physical instability, which might prove impossible to rectify. Excessive choler would, for instance, stoke the fires of wrath, suffusing the body with heat, seriously weakening the heart, perverting the judgement and endangering the immortal soul through deadly sin.

As we have already seen, a specific genre of medical literature, known as the *regimen sanitatis*, or guide to health, developed in the later medieval West to provide advice for those who were understandably anxious about falling ill. Drawing heavily upon the work of Galen (d. 216) and other eminent Greek and Muslim physicians, the authors argued that, through the careful manipulation of six *res non naturales*, or external agencies, it should be possible to preserve a reasonable state of equilibrium and thus to remain well.[9] Composed initially in

---

[5] E. Grant, ed., *A Source Book in Medieval Sciences* (Cambridge, MA, 1974), pp. 705–15.

[6] Rawcliffe, *Leprosy in Medieval England*, pp. 64–72.

[7] Brain, *Galen on Bloodletting*, p. 156; G. K. Paster, 'Nervous Tensions: Networks of Blood and Spirit in the Early Modern Body', in D. Hillman and C. Mazzio, eds, *The Body in Parts: Fantasies of Corporeality in Early Modern Europe* (London, 1997), pp. 112–16.

[8] R. E. Harvey, *The Inward Wits: Psychological Theory in the Middle Ages and Renaissance* (London, 1975), pp. 2–28.

[9] P. Gil-Sotres, 'The Regimens of Health', in M. D. Grmek, ed., *Western Medical Thought from Antiquity to the Middle Ages* (Cambridge, MA, 1998), pp. 296–300;

Latin for affluent individuals and medical students, these manuals explained how careful attention to such factors as diet, rest, exercise, sexual activity, the environment and psychological stress could help to maintain the humoral balance and keep disease at bay. In accordance with the needs of a popular audience, the use of rhyming couplets became widespread, most notably in a poem known as the *Regimen sanitatis Salernitanum*, over 100 versions of which proliferated across Europe. A fifteenth-century commonplace book compiled by an anonymous London citizen contains a short metrical digest of this work entitled 'the wisdom of physicians', together with a longer prose regimen largely concerned with exercise and diet.[10] Although they have been dismissed as the work of 'obscure physicians of no particular renown', texts of this type are of particular interest to historians of public health, since they supplied much of the information that underpinned the sanitary measures adopted by urban magistrates.[11]

The zeal with which the medieval Church embraced the message of the *regimen sanitatis* accounts in no small measure for its dissemination across the social spectrum, not simply in texts but also through the powerful medium of the pulpit and confessional. The absorption of rules originally devised by pagan Greeks and Muslims for the preservation of physical health into the mainstream of Christian life casts a fascinating light upon medieval attitudes to the body. Both regular and secular clergy were increasingly exposed to, and influenced by, medical literature, such as the *Pantegni* of Al-Majusi (Haly Abbas), which drew a clear connection between rational thought, morally acceptable behaviour and the preservation of humoral balance.[12] Perfection on this score had, it seemed, been realised only in paradise, where Adam and Eve had been vouchsafed the prospect of eternal life and health – or at least extreme longevity. However, following their expulsion from the Garden of Eden they and all their descendants had become trapped in a vicious circle of transgression and humoral instability, each of which exacerbated the other.[13] Although the *Regimen* could never promise a return to paradise, it did offer a means of delaying this process of decline by following the Aristotelian principles of temperance and moderation. Notwithstanding its pagan antecedents, its emphasis on the physical damage likely to be caused by sinful and self-indulgent behaviour proved immensely attractive to clerical propagandists, who enthusiastically endorsed Galen's strictures on the importance of sexual continence and dietary restraint in preserving health.[14] His acerbic remarks on the futility of treating 'immoderate winebibbers and gluttons' who accumulated 'a mass of crude humours through intemperate living' resonated through the ages.[15]

L. J. Rather, 'The Six Things Non-Natural: A Note on the Origins and Fate of a Doctrine and a Phrase', *Clio Medica* 3 (1968), pp. 337–47.

[10] BL, MS Egerton 1995, fols 77v–81v.

[11] Gil-Sotres, 'Regimens of Health', p. 301.

[12] Al-Majusi, *Liber pantegni* (Lyon, 1515), 'Theorica' book 4, caps 19–20, fol. 17v; Harvey, *Inward Wits*, p. 14.

[13] J. Ziegler, 'Medicine and Immortality in Terrestrial Paradise', in P. Biller and J. Ziegler, eds, *Religion and Medicine in the Middle Ages* (York, 2000), pp. 201–42.

[14] C. Rawcliffe, *Medicine and Society in Later Medieval England* (Stroud, 1995), p. 30.

[15] Brain, *Galen on Bloodletting*, p. 3.

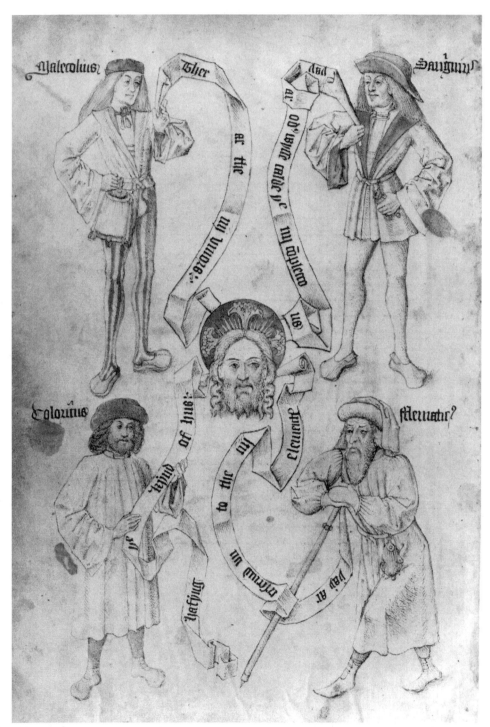

2 The four humoral types or temperaments personified in the late fifteenth-century guild book of the York Barber Surgeons, Christ alone, in the centre, being possessed of perfect balance. The images would have been used as an *aide memoire*, especially for teaching apprentices.

Significantly, an elegant depiction of the four humoral types in the late fifteenth-century guild book kept by York's barber surgeons centres upon Christ as the platonic form of *homo temperatus* (plate 2).

Secular rulers and magistrates were equally susceptible to the force of these arguments, which, as we shall see, were as applicable to them as to the people they governed. John Evelyn's (d. 1706) contention that men and women who enjoyed the benefits of pure, clean air and well-calibrated humours would be less prone to rebellion than others boasted long antecedents.[16] Fear that excess of any kind would generate all manner of social and economic ills had long found expression in the language of the *Regimen*. Writing in 1433, the canonist Nicholas of Cusa stressed that a monarch's principal task was to act as a good physician in order to avoid such dangers:

> whether because the melancholy which is abundant avarice has produced various diseases in the body – usury, fraud, deceit, theft, pillage and all these ways in which great wealth is acquired without labour through some deceptive artifice ... or if he sees the body grow feverish because of choleric wars, dissension and division, or swell up with sanguine pomposity, luxury, banqueting and the like, or become morose because of a temperament which is phlegmatic concerning virtuous efforts both to gain a livelihood and to protect the fatherland.[17]

Both individual *and* communal health were increasingly seen as desirable goals to be actively pursued, since they not only constituted the bedrock upon which profit and prosperity depended, but were necessary preconditions for the development of a just, orderly and God-fearing society.[18] Many writers and preachers, such as the eloquent Benedictine Robert Rypon (d. 1419), drew close analogies between the human and the urban body in this specific regard. Comparing the organs of sense perception to 'the town gates, through which the populace enters and goes', he observed that, in a well-regulated community (or healthy body) the residents, who constituted the flesh and blood, would be governed jointly by the intellect and the will, which in turn would cheerfully obey the commands of God as manifest through the sovereign powers of reason.[19]

Unfortunately though, as everyone knew, life after the Fall was fraught with the perils of misbehaviour and insubordination. Indeed, in the words of one twelfth-century homilist, the human body more often merited comparison with a town

[16] John Evelyn, *Fumifugium: Or, the Inconvenience of the Aer and Smoak of London Dissipated* (London, 1661), p. 1.

[17] Nicholas of Cusa, *The Catholic Concordance*, ed. and trans. P. E. Sigmund (Cambridge, 1995), p. 321.

[18] As Sir Thomas More explains in his *Utopia*, ed. and trans. R. M. Adams (New York, 1975), p. 49.

[19] G. R. Owst, *Literature and Pulpit in Medieval England* (Oxford, 1996), pp. 29–30. See also F. Choay, 'La Ville et le domaine bâti comme corps dans les textes des architectes-théoriciens de la première Renaissance italienne', *Nouvelle Revue de psychanalyse* 9 (1974), pp. 239–51, on p. 246. For the Classical derivation of these ideas: K. D. Lilley, *City and Cosmos: The Medieval World in Urban Form* (London, 2009), pp. 140–1.

because 'many sins and foul lusts dwell therein, just like people in a burgh. And in it the carnal appetites reign, just like a lord in his city, and in it the carnal will rules, like an alderman in his burgh.'[20] The consequences of wanton behaviour, as exemplified by the conduct of the two lecherous priests discussed at the start of this chapter, therefore came to be viewed in collective as well as personal terms, especially from the mid-fourteenth century, when epidemic disease concentrated the minds of English magistrates upon any potential sources of moral or physical infection. Their concern was two-fold: on the one hand, epidemics in general were widely regarded as wholesale acts of retribution upon a sinful populace, while on the other men and women whose reckless lifestyle had already put their own health at risk would be less able to resist the toxic effects of pestilential air. Since, once infected, a single individual might contaminate an entire community, the way that citizens comported themselves was clearly of pressing importance.[21]

By this date, more precisely targeted advice literature, based upon the format of the *regimen sanitatis*, had begun to proliferate across western Europe, offering guidance on such topics as care of the elderly, pregnancy, long-distance travel and bringing up children.[22] The outbreaks of plague that occurred at regular intervals after the Black Death gave rise to the most popular type of specialist manual, the *concilium contra pestilentiam*. Significantly, one of the very first, by the Catalan physician Jacme d'Agramont, was composed in the vernacular in April 1348 for 'the common and public utility' of the people of Lerida. It provided a brief regimen for protection against the miasmatic vapours that were already regarded as a primary terrestrial cause of the disease. But Jacme was, nonetheless, anxious to stress that, 'if corruption or putrefaction of the air is due to our sins or faults, the remedies of the medical art are useless', and urged his readers to repent, confess and do penance for their misdeeds.[23] Many other *concilia* followed, mostly in Latin, warning their readers against a raft of morally and physically risky activities, including heavy drinking and sex, which would render the body vulnerable to external corruption. The avoidance of anxiety, especially when occasioned by a guilty conscience, was also deemed highly desirable.[24]

Although, so far as we know, no English physician produced an original plague tract, some Continental offerings, most notably that composed by John of Burgundy in 1365, lent themselves readily to translation and, in an abridged format, were often copied into domestic remedy collections and commonplace

---

[20] R. Morris, ed., *Old English Homilies of the Twelfth Century*, EETS o.s. 53 (London, 1873), p. 55; and section 5.5 below.

[21] P. Horden, 'Ritual and Public Health in the Early Medieval City', in Sheard and Power, *Body and City*, p. 21.

[22] Rawcliffe, 'Concept of Health', pp. 327–8.

[23] Jacme d'Agramont, *Regiment de preservació de pestilència*, ed. J. Veny (Lerida, 1998); Arrizabalaga, 'Facing the Black Death', pp. 251, 272. For a partial translation, see J. Aberth, ed., *The Black Death: The Great Mortality of 1348–1350* (Boston, 2005), pp. 51–5.

[24] Arrizabalaga, 'Facing the Black Death', pp. 237–88. See also Cohn, *Black Death Transformed*, pp. 233–8.

books.[25] When the Dominican friar and medical practitioner Thomas Multon translated and reorganised the longer version of John's treatise for a lay readership, probably during the epidemic of 1479, he explained his motives in a preface. It was, he felt, the duty of every Christian to assist those 'in grete perell or likely to fall in grete myscheues', especially as there was such a demand for accessible vernacular literature. For this reason, he deemed it a work of charity to 'gader this trety and sette it in Englissh that euery man, both lerned and lewde, may the better vnderstond hit and do thereafter, and to be his owne phisicien in tyme of nede ayenst the venym and the malice of the pestilence'.[26] Multon's work subsequently eclipsed the original in popularity, achieving wide circulation in print during the next century. This was largely because of some very personal interpolations on the close relationship between the natural and supernatural causes of plague, which Multon added to John of Burgundy's more empirical text. As both a friar and a physician, he readily accepted that divine will could create the precise conditions in which pestilence would strike those whose disobedience to the teachings of the Church had already poisoned their bodies with 'venemes and corrupt humours'.[27] Citing biblical precedents for the many occasions on which God had chastised his people with plague, he exhorted his readers to 'putte away the syn thorgh verry sorowe and contricioun', before embarking upon the specifically medical precautions and remedies that followed.[28]

The extent to which urban magistrates may have sought to implement the more pragmatic recommendations about food, water and environmental health set out in these manuals will be explored in the rest of this book. Yet few measures, however ostensibly mundane, were free from wider spiritual considerations, if only because cleanliness was increasingly regarded as a manifestation of civic virtue, while dirt and disease prompted associations with sin.[29] Given the intimate relationship between humoral balance, order and self-discipline, the possibility that physical health might be achieved *without* a moral dimension would have seemed remote, as much on physiological as religious grounds. Even so, as we saw in the previous chapter, a tendency to ignore the underlying sophistication of this holistic approach still continues to dog the study of medieval responses to epidemic disease, especially when such apparently 'unscientific' or 'superstitious' attitudes are judged by the criteria of modern laboratory-based biomedicine. For example, the widespread belief that temperance, piety and charity would offer protection against pestilence, which finds expression in many plague *concilia*,

---

[25] R. Horrox, ed., *The Black Death* (Manchester, 1995), pp. 184–93. At least thirty-four manuscripts of the shorter version survive in English: Keiser, 'Two Medieval Plague Treatises', p. 299. For vernacular plague tracts in general, see G. Keiser, ed., *A Manual of the Writings in Middle English, 1050–1500*, vol. 10: *Works of Science and Information* (New Haven, CT, 1998), pp. 3662–7, 3853–60; Pickett, 'Translation of the "Canutus" Plague Treatise', pp. 263–82.

[26] BL, MS Sloane 3489, fol. 44r. For the charitable imperative to disseminate medical knowledge, see Getz, 'Charity, Translation and the Language of Medical Learning', pp. 1–15.

[27] BL, MS Sloane 3489, fol. 45v; Keiser, 'Two Medieval Plague Treatises', pp. 292–324.

[28] BL, MS Sloane 3489, fol. 44v.

[29] See sections 3.1 and 4.6 below.

has been disparaged by some historians as an unfortunate aberration from an otherwise 'rational' attempt to combat the spread of disease in ways that a microbiologist might deem effective.[30] Yet, to the reflective medieval or early modern citizen, it seemed self-evident that unrestrained or 'rebellious' conduct would invite disaster. The reckless abuse of 'meat and drink, of sleep and watching, of labour and ease, of fullness and emptiness, of the passions of the mind, and of the immoderate use of lechery' led inevitably to gluttony, sloth, avarice, anger, envy and lust, each of which not only destabilised the body's intricate network of natural, vital and animal spirits, but was also likely to prompt far more dramatic displays of divine displeasure.[31]

That such fears seemed eminently justified will be apparent from the next part of this chapter, which examines the ubiquity of both endemic and epidemic disease (2.1) and the impact of plague upon late medieval urban populations (2.2). It was against this background of recurrent and often devastating epidemics that established ideas about political and civic bodies underwent further development, most notably with regard to concepts of mutual obligation and civic responsibility. The Church's emphasis upon charity and compassion, which drew upon the Galenic theory that healthy members would assist those prone to weakness or infection, inspired a striking variety of public works and environmental improvements. On the other hand, magistrates needed little persuasion when there was a call for more drastic surgical procedures designed to eliminate undesirables (2.3). Indeed, although recourse to the saints and other apotropaic rituals remained an important weapon in the civic armoury (2.4), the need for direct action assumed increasing urgency. The influence of medical as well as religious and political ideas upon office holders who attempted to regulate the behaviour of their fellow citizens is further explored in two final sections dealing specifically with responses to the idle or unproductive poor (2.5) and to prostitution (2.6). The rulers of English towns devoted considerable time and effort to the management of these problems, which were perceived in terms of both moral and environmental health. Not coincidentally, their efforts intensified from the 1460s onwards, when a series of particularly virulent epidemics, including sweating sickness and the Great Pox, as well as plague, took a heavy toll on many English cities.

2.1 Endemic and epidemic disease

Medieval urban populations shouldered a heavy burden of sickness, notably in periods of growth, when overcrowding and food shortages exacerbated an already formidable roster of potentially fatal or chronically debilitating conditions.[32] Although it was by far the most dramatic and feared, leprosy was only one of many endemic diseases, such as scurvy, trachoma and a raft of enteric disorders, that are today associated with the Developing World rather than the British Isles.

[30] R. S. Gottfried, for example, observes in this context that 'for every step forward, there is the inevitable step back': *Epidemic Disease in Fifteenth Century England* (Brunswick, NJ, 1978), p. 69.

[31] Slack, *Impact of Plague*, pp. 28–9.

[32] C. Roberts and M. Cox, *Health and Disease in Britain* (Stroud, 2003), chap. 5.

Already on the decline by the closing years of the thirteenth century, when, not coincidentally, standards of diagnosis became far more precise, leprosy generated such complex responses in both ecclesiastical and secular society that historians have tended to focus upon it to the exclusion of more common but less well-documented diseases.[33] Yet these other diseases claimed the overwhelming number of fatalities, either directly or through a steady process of attrition. Where areas of settlement abutted on marshland and slow moving stretches of water, malaria (then known as ague) flourished, attacking the bloodstreams of men, women and children who were often already weakened by a chronic lack of protein and essential vitamins and minerals.[34] Evidence of progressive anaemia is, for instance, apparent in a significant proportion of skeletal remains from twelfth- to fourteenth-century urban cemeteries (plate 3).[35] Although unlikely to prove terminal, a serious deficiency in iron and vitamin B12 would undermine the body's resistance to pathogens, and increase the risks faced by women in childbirth.[36] Even so, the impact of both malaria and tuberculosis on the townspeople of medieval Europe has still to be satisfactorily explored, in part because, unlike leprosy, the former leaves no trace upon the human skeleton, while the latter is detectable in only a small percentage of cases.[37] Infection rates must have remained high, since increased consumption of meat and milk, evident from the mid-fourteenth century onwards, spread bovine tuberculosis among the human population, giving rise to a range of severe gastrointestinal symptoms, fevers, lassitude and weight

[33] See, for example, L. Demaitre, *Leprosy in Pre-Modern Medicine: A Disease of the Whole Body* (Baltimore, 2007); Rawcliffe, *Leprosy in Medieval England*; and F. O. Touati, *Maladie et société au moyen âge* (Paris, 1998).

[34] For the neglect of malaria in the study of medieval urban health, see P. Horden, 'Disease, Dragons and Saints: The Management of Epidemics in the Dark Ages', in T. Ranger and P. Slack, eds, *Epidemics and Ideas: Essays on the Historical Perception of Pestilence* (Cambridge, 1992), pp. 45–76. M. J. Dobson assesses the impact of the disease in the seventeenth century, in *Contours of Death and Disease in Early Modern England* (Cambridge, 1997), pp. 287–350.

[35] Previously attributed to iron deficiency (Roberts and Cox, *Health and Disease*, pp. 234–5), skeletal damage to the orbital roof and cranial vault has recently been linked to a shortage of vitamin B12: R. Gilchrist, *Medieval Life: Archaeology and the Life Course* (Woodbridge, 2012), p. 51.

[36] K. L. Pearson, 'Nutrition and the Early-Medieval Diet', *Speculum* 72 (1997), pp. 1–32; V. Bullough and C. Campbell, 'Female Longevity and Diet in the Middle Ages', *Speculum* 55 (1980), pp. 317–25. Since malaria attacks red blood cells, it would have caused particular damage in anaemic populations.

[37] Roberts and Cox, *Health and Disease*, pp. 230–2. Strikingly, thirty of the 384 individuals whose remains were excavated from the cemetery of the leper hospital of Saints James and Mary Magdalen, Chichester, had apparently contracted tuberculosis, while seventy showed obvious signs of leprosy. Given that leprosy is far more likely to affect the skeleton, there is a very real possibility that more patients were tubercular than leprous: J. Magilton *et al.*, '*Lepers Outside the Gate*': *Excavations at the Cemetery of the Hospital of St James and St Mary Magdalen, Chichester, 1986–87 and 1993*, CBA research report 158 (London, 2008), pp. 218–23, 265–7.

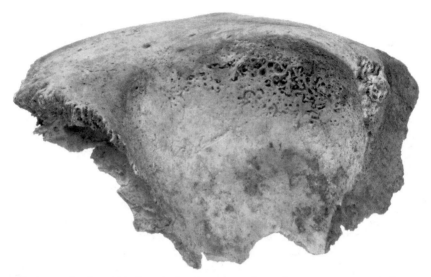

3 Evidence of *cribra orbitalia*, which recent research attributes to a protracted shortage of vitamin B12, in skeletal remains from late medieval London

loss.[38] The cramped and unhygienic living conditions endured by the urban poor, particularly during the century before the Black Death, had already provided an ideal breeding ground for the more lethal pulmonary strain of TB (then termed *phthisis*), which travels rapidly by droplet infection through coughing and spitting.

The effects of famines and food shortages, which occurred at regular intervals throughout the later Middle Ages, were especially severe during periods of high population density, when the land was under pressure and malnutrition was rife. Given the high death rates usual in towns, notably among children, a steady level of immigration from the countryside was essential to maintain economic productivity.[39] However, during the second half of the thirteenth century the influx of casual labourers into English cities began to cause serious problems,

[38] Keith Manchester's supposition that leprosy declined in late medieval England as townspeople who had contracted bovine tuberculosis developed immunity to it is based on some dubious assumptions about rates of urban growth, but does highlight the scale of the problem: 'Tuberculosis and Leprosy in Antiquity: An Interpretation', *Medical History* 28 (1984), pp. 162–73.

[39] Gilchrist, *Medieval Life*, pp. 48–53; M. Lewis, *Urbanisation and Child Health in Medieval and Post Medieval England*, BAR British series 339 (Oxford, 2002). Reliable infant mortality rates can rarely be extrapolated from skeletal evidence (our principal source of information about the health of the urban poor), largely because the remains of children tend to survive in smaller numbers. Evidence from a medieval cemetery in one of the most deprived areas of York suggests a rate of up to 50 per cent among infants: J. D. Dawes and J. R. Magilton, *The Archaeology of York*, vol. 12.1: *The Cemetery of St Helen-on-the-Walls, Aldwark*, (London, 1980), p. 63. The rate in some parts of post-Conquest Norwich was even higher: A. Stirland, 'The Human Bones', in B. Ayers, ed., *Excavations within the North-East Bailey of Norwich Castle, 1979*, EAA 28 (Norwich, 1985), pp. 49–50. B. A. Hanawalt maintains that in late medieval London, too, the death rate among

apparent not only from the rapidly escalating demand for institutional relief but also from attempts by the ruling elite to stem the tide of indigents who lacked any apparent means of support.[40] To contemporaries, the body politic must have appeared swollen with an excess of malignant humours. Norwich's response to these testing circumstances can be documented in unusual detail, thanks to the survival of a remarkable combination of documentary and archaeological evidence. In the early fourteenth century the city was already stretched to capacity. Then the years between 1315 and 1322 were blighted by a run of disastrous famines and cattle plagues that prompted desperate agricultural workers from the East Anglian hinterland to migrate into towns. The population of Norwich rose from about 17,000 in 1311 to as many as 25,000 in 1333, many of the immigrants being men and women whose predicament rendered them especially vulnerable to the ravages of epidemic disease.[41] The city lacked the resources to cope with this unprecedented situation. Most newcomers found cheap accommodation in existing buildings, where rooms were sublet by tenants, or in rows of multi-storey cottages erected speculatively in gardens or on marginal land. Being neither as permanent nor as robust as the timber framed dwellings occupied by the poor of York, these clay-walled buildings lacked damp-courses and cooking facilities, and made scant provision for effective waste disposal.[42] By the 1330s (at which point population levels almost certainly began to decline) a lethal combination of overcrowding, dirt, vermin and parasites must have created optimum conditions for the spread of diseases such as pulmonary tuberculosis, dysentery, diphtheria, typhus and eventually plague among men and women whose formative years had all too often been defined by sickness and hunger.[43] The close proximity of domestic animals, which then constituted a major urban nuisance, added a cocktail of zoonotic diseases to this insalubrious mix.[44]

children remained disproportionately high: *Growing Up in Medieval London: The Experience of Childhood in History* (Oxford, 1993), pp. 23–4, 56–62.

[40] C. Rawcliffe, *Medicine for the Soul: The Life, Death and Resurrection of a Medieval English Hospital* (Stroud, 1999), pp. 13–15.

[41] E. Rutledge, 'Immigration and Population Growth in Early Fourteenth-Century Norwich: Evidence from the Tithing Roll', *Urban History Yearbook* 15 (1988), pp. 15–30, on pp. 25–7. For the background to these natural disasters, see B. F. Harvey, 'Introduction: The 'Crisis' of the Early Fourteenth Century', in B. M. S. Campbell, ed., *Before the Black Death: Studies in the 'Crisis' of the Early Fourteenth Century* (Manchester, 1991), pp. 1–24.

[42] E. Rutledge, 'Landlords and Tenants: Housing and the Rented Property Market in Early Fourteenth-Century Norwich', *Urban History* 22 (1995), pp. 1–24, on pp. 12–14; M. Atkin, 'Medieval Clay-Walled Building in Norwich', *NA* 41 (1991), pp. 171–85. For the 'wretched living conditions' of the city's poor, see Summerson, *Medieval Carlisle*, I.371.

[43] For the 'synergistic package' that bound famine to chronic as well as epidemic disease, see Aberth, *From the Brink of the Apocalypse*, pp. 7–42, especially p. 41.

[44] See section 3.6 below. Both archaeological and documentary sources testify to the ubiquity of parasitic infections, which medieval men and women believed to be the product of humoral imbalance. See, for example, J. Greig, 'The Investigation of a Medieval Barrel-Latrine from Worcester', *Journal of Archaeological Science*

Notwithstanding the fact that standards of living improved appreciably for those who survived successive outbreaks of plague and other epidemics, the long fifteenth century has been memorably described as a 'golden age of bacteria', when the young, in particular, fell victim to a variety of infectious and contagious diseases.[45] Even though between 30 and 40 per cent of the population of England and Wales appears to have perished during the Black Death of 1348–50, some historians believe that the nation as a whole might have staged a convincing recovery from the cataclysmic disaster, and even perhaps have emerged leaner and fitter as a result. We can, however, only speculate on this point, since a series of late fourteenth-century epidemics not only brought incipient regeneration to a standstill, but also inflicted deeper and more lasting damage.[46] Regarded by contemporaries as a children's plague, the outbreak of 1361–2 effectively sabotaged any return to normality, as did those of 1368–9, 1374–5 and 1378–9, which also tended to strike individuals with the least immunity, and thus to cull the next generation of productive adults.[47] How did English towns and cities fare under these repeated blows?

It is notoriously difficult to determine the cumulative impact of pestilence on urban populations with any degree of accuracy, since comparative evidence from *before* as well as after the Black Death and subsequent epidemics is sparse and often problematic. Nor is it possible to establish the extent to which other factors, such as changing levels of fertility or the migration of men and women in search of better opportunities, may have affected whatever rough estimates are available.[48] A general tendency to underestimate the size of towns before 1348 has prompted a corresponding readiness to dismiss as excessive the high levels of mortality recorded by chroniclers and antiquaries. Yet some places did experience catastrophic losses during the Black Death, which, according to Richard Britnell, had such traumatic consequences for many communities as to constitute 'a turning point in urban history'.[49] Even before 1361, therefore, the prospect of resurgence hung in the balance. London, by far the largest and most prosperous of English cities, boasted an impressive tally of 80,000 or more inhabitants at the start of

---

8 (1981), pp. 265–82, on pp. 272, 274–5; and C. de Rouffignac, 'Parasite Remains from Excavations at St Mary Spital, London', Museum of London report 102 (1992). Remedy collections furnish many receipts for the elimination of intestinal worms (Dawson, *Leechbook*, p. 202; T. Hunt, ed., *Popular Medicine in Thirteenth-Century England* (Woodbridge, 1994), pp. 90–1; BL, MS Harley 2390, fols 146r, 151r; MS Sloane 983, fols 8r, 72v), while the physician Gilbertus Anglicus devoted an entire chapter of his *Compendium medicinae* (*c.* 1250) to 'worms in the gut' (F. M. Getz, ed., *Healing and Society in Medieval England* (Madison, WI, 1991), pp. 202, 204, 207–11).

[45] Thrupp, 'The Problem of Replacement Rates', p. 118.

[46] J. L. Bolton, '"The World Upside Down": Plague as an Agent of Economic and Social Change', in W. M. Ormrod and P. G. Lindley, eds, *The Black Death in England* (Stamford, 1996), pp. 26–7; Platt, *King Death*, chap. 1.

[47] See Appendix for details of these and subsequent outbreaks.

[48] For the debate on this point see Bolton, 'World Upside Down', pp. 70–7; and Bailey, 'Demographic Decline', pp. 1–19.

[49] Britnell, 'Black Death in English Towns', pp. 195–200.

the fourteenth century, and just half that number in 1400, although its economic fortunes suffered far less than such a striking decline might suggest.[50] Norwich appears to have sustained even heavier losses, with two-thirds of its residents either dying or leaving between the 1330s and 1370s, yet it still managed to weather the storm because of a well-timed shift to cloth production.[51] The picture was much bleaker in the Lincolnshire ports of Grimsby and Boston: between 1377 and the sixteenth century, their populations fell by 40 and 50 per cent respectively, partly as a result of commercial problems that inhibited economic regeneration, making it impossible to attract the 'new blood' without which plague-hit communities could not recover.[52] The vital importance of maintaining replacement rates in this way is clearly apparent in Colchester, which emerged from the first wave of epidemics relatively unscathed, but entered a long period of decline during the fifteenth century because, like many other towns, it could no longer recruit enough outsiders to compensate for sustained periods of high mortality.[53]

There is a general consensus that, after the serial pandemics of the second half of the fourteenth century, plague became less of a national threat and more of an urban phenomenon as its geographical range decreased.[54] This tendency, which started gradually in the 1370s, struck the chronicler Thomas Walsingham, whose description of the devastating impact of the 1407 pestilence on London is accompanied by a paraphrase of Ovid to the effect that city walls offer no protection against the 'furnace blasts of death' borne on southerly winds.[55] It was, indeed, then that the 'masters and doctors of Oxford' sent the mayor a 'letter', or *concilium*, on the best means of avoiding plague, perhaps at his request and evidently to widespread civic approval.[56] The localised – but still lethal – nature of most epidemics became especially apparent towards the close of the fifteenth century, when the population as a whole, which had for so long remained stagnant,

---

[50] Barron, *London in the Later Middle Ages*, p. 45. For a vivid account of the impact of the 1348–9 epidemic on the City, see Sloane, *Black Death in London*, chaps 2 and 3.

[51] C. Rawcliffe, 'Sickness and Health', in Rawcliffe and Wilson, *Medieval Norwich*, pp. 317–18.

[52] S. H. Rigby, *Medieval Grimsby: Growth and Decline* (Hull, 1993), pp. 126–33; S. H. Rigby, '"Sore Decay" and "Fair Dwellings": Boston and Urban Decline in the Later Middle Ages', *Midland History* 10 (1985), pp. 47–61, on pp. 54–5; Platt, *King Death*, pp. 19–20.

[53] R. H. Britnell, *Growth and Decline in Colchester, 1300–1525* (Cambridge, 1986), pp. 1–6, 159–60, 201–5.

[54] Bolton, 'World Upside Down', p. 32; J. M. W. Bean, 'Plague, Population and Economic Decline in England during the Later Middle Ages', *EconHR*, 2nd series 15 (1963), pp. 423–37, on p. 430; J. Hatcher, 'Mortality in the Fifteenth Century: Some New Evidence', *EconHR*, 2nd series 39 (1986), pp. 19–38, on p. 36.

[55] Thomas Walsingham, *Historia Anglicana*, ed. H. T. Riley, 2 vols, RS 28.1 (London, 1863–4), II.276. For further details of this epidemic, see Appendix; for the source of the verse, see Ovid, *Metamorphoses*, ed. A. D. Melville (Oxford, 1986), pp. 160–2.

[56] BL, MS Sloane 3285, fols 68r–70r. This Latin text was based on John of Burgundy's popular advice manual: D. W. Singer and A. Anderson, *Catalogue of Latin and Vernacular Plague Texts in Great Britain and Eire in Manuscripts Written before the Sixteenth Century* (London, 1950), pp. 27–8.

began to rise, and 'the grip of persistently high mortality' to slacken.[57] Although, as we shall see, few thought of questioning the belief that pestilence was, ultimately, an act of God, regular, occasionally annual, outbreaks of infectious disease had by then become the norm in major commercial centres, such as Norwich, York and, of course, London. The wealth of documentary sources for the capital (which inevitably attracted the attention of travellers from abroad, as well as the government at home) makes it possible to compile a particularly full, although still probably incomplete, list of epidemics in the London area: there were at least twenty-four between 1400 and 1530, in addition to around thirteen national, or at least very widespread, outbreaks during which London was almost always affected.[58] Although less is known about the provinces, serious visitations did find their way into the historical record, such as those which swept through Coventry and Lincoln in 1446–7, Norwich in 1465, and York in 1493, and which brought trade to a standstill in Chester in 1517.[59] In Paul Slack's words, plague had become 'less an autonomous factor, a *deus ex machina* occasionally imposing its will on towns from outside, than ... an integral and in the end familiar part of urban life'.[60]

However, familiarity did not make the advent of pestilence any less alarming. The virulent 'mortalities' of the later fourteenth century were so vividly etched in the collective memory that each fresh outbreak, however minor, must have appeared *potentially* devastating, prompting many to heed medical advice and flee at the first signs of trouble.[61] Nor, indeed, were national or regional epidemics ever such infrequent events as to render these fears unfounded or to mitigate the 'condition of nervous strain' in which entire communities lived.[62] In some places, such as Norwich, King's Lynn and Yarmouth, it was customary by the sixteenth century to display 'tabelles' in prominent places recording the death rate in previous visitations, perhaps sometimes embroidering the evidence for greater effect.[63] Reminders of this kind were hardly necessary in a town like Coventry,

[57] Bailey, 'Demographic Decline', p. 16.

[58] See Appendix. Given the unreliable dating and provenance of some of the chronicle evidence, it can be surprisingly hard to define a 'widespread' epidemic, and I have erred on the side of caution, counting the years 1399–1400, 1407, 1438–9, 1458–9, ?1463, 1467, 1471, 1479, 1485, 1499–1500, 1517, 1518 and 1521 only. Additional outbreaks in London and/or Westminster occurred in 1426–7, 1433, 1434, 1437, 1442–3, 1445, 1449, 1450, 1457, 1464, 1478, 1487, 1490–1, 1504–5, 1511, 1513, 1514, 1515, 1520, 1525, 1526, 1528, 1529 and 1530. Localised plagues affected most major European cities, of which Venice furnishes a striking example. In 1423 the senate noted that outbreaks were occurring almost annually, and, indeed, eighty-eight such 'pestilences' are recorded during the fifteenth century: Palmer, 'Control of Plague', pp. 49–50.

[59] See Appendix.

[60] Slack, *Impact of Plague*, pp. 111–12.

[61] For flight as the best prophylactic, see Horrox, *Black Death*, p. 176; Arrizabalaga, 'Facing the Black Death', p. 274.

[62] Platt, *English Medieval Town*, p. 101.

[63] Slack, *Impact of Plague*, p. 54; John Leland, *Itinerary*, ed. L. T. Smith, 5 vols (London, 1907–10), IV.122; Rutledge, 'Thomas Damet', pp. 124–5. I am grateful to Paul Rutledge for this last reference.

where the 'malignant presence' of infectious disease during the second and third decades of the sixteenth century exacerbated an irreversible process of decline.[64] Even economically successful communities suffered badly. An analysis of death rates at Christ Church priory, Canterbury, between 1395 and 1505 casts valuable light upon the experience of this busy market town, where the monks and their servants interacted freely with their urban neighbours and were exposed to the same risks. It appears that in both the monastic and lay communities a crisis in mortality occurred on average at least once every four years. Significantly, although epidemics were rather less frequent after 1457, they grew more serious, reflecting the vulnerability of young immigrants from the rural hinterland to new pathogens. Expressed in crude terms, during the second half of the fifteenth century (when life expectancy began to fall dramatically), a recently professed monk of twenty, and by inference a migrant worker of a similar age, would have been fortunate to survive for another decade.[65]

Lack of comparative evidence makes it unsafe to generalise on the basis of these statistics, but they were clearly not exceptional. Having successfully weathered a decline in population of about 40 per cent during the third quarter of the fourteenth century, Westminster succumbed in about 1410 to a second period of sustained high mortality, which this time led to protracted contraction and recession. And although fertility levels rose and immigration increased after 1470, the death rate remained 'frighteningly high'. As in Canterbury, data from monastic archives confirms that among the neighbouring Benedictines life expectancy was also falling at an appreciable rate, most notably between 1485 and 1505. By this date the town, which shared with Southwark the dubious accolade of being the most congested in the kingdom, had become a veritable 'death trap' for newcomers.[66]

The urban landscape furnished equally painful and unavoidable reminders of mortality, particularly in the number of tenements, shops and even entire streets left vacant and dilapidated, sometimes for long periods. Semi-rural areas, which had been developed in periods of growth and prosperity, were allowed to revert to empty plots and gardens, a phenomenon clearly apparent in Gloucester,

---

[64] C. Phythian-Adams, *Desolation of a City: Coventry and the Urban Crisis of the Late Middle Ages* (Cambridge, 1979), pp. 52–4.

[65] Hatcher, 'Mortality in the Fifteenth Century', pp. 31–6. P. Nightingale questions this supposition on the ground that infectious diseases, especially tuberculosis, would spread more rapidly in monastic dormitories: 'Some New Evidence of Crises and Trends of Mortality in Late Medieval England', *P&P* 187 (2005), pp. 33–68, on pp. 59–60. However, young migrants almost certainly shared living and working space too.

[66] G. Rosser, *Medieval Westminster, 1200–1540* (Oxford, 1989), pp. 170–1, 177–80; Nightingale, 'Some New Evidence of Crises and Trends of Mortality', p. 58; B. Harvey, *Living and Dying in England, 1100–1540: The Monastic Experience* (Oxford, 1993), pp. 127–9. Harvey's findings are strikingly similar to Hatcher's: between 1390 and 1459 one year in nine might be considered 'bad', an average rising to one in five over the next seventy years (p. 124). This was not solely a southern phenomenon: J. Hatcher, A. J. Piper and D. Stone, 'Monastic Mortality: Durham Priory, 1395–1529', *EconHR*, 2nd series 59 (2006), pp. 667–87.

Wallingford and Wells.[67] In some towns churches were abandoned as it became necessary to merge dwindling congregations. In Norwich, the number of parish churches shrank from well over fifty in the early fourteenth century to forty-six by 1520; St Matthew's, an early casualty of the 1349 epidemic, allegedly became a ruin within a couple of decades.[68] In Winchester the decline was even more striking, the number of churches falling by nineteen (about one third) in the second half of the fourteenth century alone. Although it might be argued that Winchester, like Norwich, was oversupplied with places of worship, this phenomenon testifies eloquently to the effects of plague. Further contraction, occasioned by a slump in the weaving and fulling trades, led to more closures, as well as the depressing spectacle of unoccupied dwellings and streets that had lain almost completely derelict since the great epidemics of 1349 and 1361.[69]

Ambitious building plans conceived in more prosperous times were jettisoned by some beleaguered and demoralised communities. An elegant extension to St Margaret's church, Yarmouth, whose great size and lofty interior testified to the port's erstwhile reputation as a 'forte ville de guerre', stopped abruptly in 1349, leaving the foundations for the new west front to moulder in the grass.[70] A similar project at Winchester cathedral, along with plans for the erection of two new towers, was likewise abruptly shelved.[71] In the north-west, work on Chester castle and a major project for rebuilding the Dee bridge in stone also ground to a halt, the locals being obliged for many years to cross the river by ferry.[72] As the lively and continuing debate about the extent of late medieval urban decline reveals, not all communities suffered permanent damage, and some staged a convincing recovery. But, to a greater or lesser extent, plague inflicted deep and lasting scars upon the collective psyche of them all.

Despite its economic resilience, Norwich, whose population fell by about two-thirds between the 1330s and the early 1370s, had good reason to dread the return of pestilence.[73] We can certainly understand why here, as elsewhere,

[67] B. Dobson, 'Urban Decline in Late Medieval England', *TRHS*, 5th series 27 (1977), pp. 1–22, on p. 11; J. Roskell, L. Clark and C. Rawcliffe, eds, *The Commons, 1386–1421*, 4 vols (Stroud, 1992), I.270, 408; Shaw, *Creation of a Community*, pp. 47–54.

[68] Rawcliffe, *Medicine for the Soul*, p. 16. Bowing to the inevitable, in 1365 the bishop of Ely agreed to a merger between the Cambridge parishes of St Giles, which had experienced a dramatic slump in population, and All Saints, whose parishioners were 'for the most part dead of pestilence': HMC, *Sixth Report*, Royal Commission on Historical Manuscripts 5 (London, 1877), appendix, p. 299.

[69] D. Keene, *Survey of Medieval Winchester*, 2 vols (Oxford, 1985), I.93–4, 97–8, 116–17, 145–6, 367–8. By 1439 Wallingford had lost almost two-thirds (seven) of its churches and was seriously depopulated: D. M. Palliser, 'Urban Decay Revisited', in Thomson, *Towns and Townspeople*, pp. 10–11. (Nonetheless, Palliser urges caution in the use of such evidence.)

[70] N. Pevsner and B. Wilson, *The Buildings of England: Norfolk*, vol. 1, 2nd edn (London, 1997), pp. 494–8.

[71] Gottfried, *Black Death: Natural and Human Disaster*, p. 63. For problems in Hereford, see Dohar, *Black Death and Pastoral Leadership*, pp. 38–9.

[72] J. Laughton, *Life in a Late Medieval City: Chester, 1275–1520* (Oxford, 2008), p. 25.

[73] Rawcliffe, 'Sickness and Health', pp. 317–18.

subsequent generations were inclined to exaggerate the effects of the first epidemic, and why the implausible figure of over 57,000 deaths (for the year 1348) heads the list of memorabilia recorded in the Mayor's Book, which was begun as a civic chronicle during the plague year of 1526.[74] It was at this time that Robert Jannys, the richest member of the ruling elite, commissioned a window in the guildhall reminding his fellow magistrates of the imminence of death and importance of good works. As described by the antiquary Francis Blomefield (d. 1752), the glass painting, now lost, depicted 'a man in his winding sheet, sitting in order to be shot dead with arrows', with Death at his shoulder, ready to carry him away.[75] Both before and after the Reformation, preachers often described plague as a *bellum Dei contra homines*, or a war waged by a vengeful deity who kept his quiver 'full of these arrows, full of the pestilence of fevers, and dropsies and consumptions, and all manner of diseases'.[76] The accompanying verse offered a more explicit warning to those assembled below:

> For all, welth, worship and prosperite
> Ferce Death ys cum, and [ar]rested me,
> For Jannys praise God, I pray you all,
> Whose acts do remayne a memoriall.[77]

In order to leave the type of 'memoriall' about which Jannys was so proud, members of the ruling elite were expected both to invest their time and energy in promoting schemes for civic improvement, and to give generously to such works from their own coffers. We will return to the obligations of office later; at this point it is important to establish how far the threat of epidemic disease, and of the testing economic and social problems likely to accompany even temporary periods of dislocation, may have fostered a particular awareness of the *moral* as well as the physical health of the urban body.

2.2 The consequences of plague

Claims of hardship and decline constitute a recurrent theme in petitions for relief addressed to the crown by the rulers of English towns and cities during the late fourteenth and fifteenth centuries. Notwithstanding the fact that magistrates routinely dramatised their collective predicament in order to secure a reduction in farms or taxes, it is clear that epidemic disease ranked as one of the principal

---

[74] Johnson, 'Chronological Memoranda', p. 141. Hudson and Tingey suggest that this figure relates to Norfolk as a whole (*RCN*, II.cxx–xxi), but William Lee accepted it uncritically in his 1851 report to the Board of Health: see p. 14 above.

[75] F. Blomefield, *An Essay towards a Topographical History of the County of Norfolk*, 11 vols (London, 1805–10), IV.229. The image was later reproduced in a series of portraits of Norwich worthies: Rawcliffe and Wilson, *Medieval Norwich*, plate 21.

[76] Edward Lawrence, *Christs Power over Bodily Diseases* (London, 1672), p. 25; J. B. Friedman, '"He Hath a Thousand Slain in this Pestilence": The Iconography of the Plague in the Late Middle Ages', in F. X. Newman, ed., *Social Unrest in the Late Middle Ages* (London, 1985), pp. 75–112; Berger, 'Mice, Arrows and Tumours', pp. 23–63.

[77] Blomefield, *Topographical History of the County of Norfolk*, IV.229.

reasons advanced for assistance.[78] As early as 1357, the burgesses of Newcastle alleged that the combined impact of warfare and plague had caused wholesale impoverishment; and in 1380 they reported that over 6,000 residents had died in a more recent outbreak. Since the entire population cannot have been much higher than 4,800 in 1377, we should allow for the hyperbole characteristic of such appeals, although the assertion that a third of the town stood 'wasted and uninhabited because of pestilence' seems more credible. The burgesses' woes were compounded by the heavy cost of maintaining their defences against the Scots, which, at the best of times, proved a constant drain on resources.[79]

Contending not only with the *rabie Scotorum*, whose constant raiding parties caused as much damage as full scale campaigns, but also the debilitating economic consequences of protracted sheep murrain, the people of Carlisle had already sunk into 'a state of complete demoralisation' before plague struck.[80] As the wording of royal letters patent of 1345 reveals, conditions within the city had deteriorated so badly that an epidemic of some kind seemed inevitable. 'The air is so corrupted and tainted by dung and manure heaps and much other filth put in the streets and lanes', ran the complaint, 'that the men dwelling there and coming to the city for its defence are stricken with a dreadful horror'.[81] Since, when it arrived, the Black Death followed 'sixty years of almost unremitting calamity', the city's depressed state during the 1350s and for decades afterwards is easy to understand. Warfare and food shortages may well have claimed almost as many victims as successive outbreaks of plague, and certainly made the community more vulnerable to infection.[82]

Elsewhere, the additional burdens imposed by the resumption of the Hundred Years' War inhibited what might otherwise have been a steady process of recovery.[83] The effects of coastal raids and heavy taxes, along with a crisis in mortality, led the residents of Truro to petition parliament for relief in about 1378, and to renew their efforts at intervals over the next fifty years.[84] Similar complaints were voiced by the burgesses of Southampton in 1380, of Sandwich in 1385 and of Ilchester

---

[78] Palliser, 'Urban Decay', pp. 4–7, considers the 'suspicious features' of many such petitions, while accepting the 'frequent and devastating' impact of epidemics on towns.

[79] TNA, SC8/129/6428, 130/6453, 223/11117; *CPR, 1370–1374*, p. 326; *CPR, 1377–1381*, p. 150; Roskell, Clark and Rawcliffe, *Commons, 1386–1421*, I.549; A. F. Butcher, 'Rent, Population and Economic Change in Late-Medieval Newcastle', *Northern History* 14 (1978), pp. 67–77, on p. 74.

[80] Summerson, *Medieval Carlisle*, I.272, and chap. 4 generally. For the archaeological evidence of depression, see section 1.1 above.

[81] *CPR, 1343–45*, pp. 507–8

[82] Summerson, *Medieval Carlisle*, I.281, 299–30. At least the city's vital role in the defence of the border guaranteed a level of royal investment in its military infrastructure, which stimulated the economy (pp. 319–25).

[83] For the economic and political effects of the war effort on a civic community, see C. D. Liddy, 'Urban Conflict in Late Fourteenth-Century England: The Case of York in 1380–1', *EHR* 118 (2003), pp. 1–32.

[84] TNA, SC8/23/1119; SC8/23/1121; SC8/27/1372, SC8/76/3767; *CCR, 1377–1381*, pp. 54–5; *RP*, III.638–9; *CPR, 1408–1413*, p. 215.

in 1407.[85] The destruction of the quay in heavy storms rather than by warfare was advanced as a contributory cause of poverty by the rulers of Scarborough in the early 1360s; and in Hythe a disastrous fire at the start of the fifteenth century likewise exacerbated the devastation already caused by plague.[86] During the 1460s the Yarmouth authorities itemised the causes of the port's steep decline since its glory days in the early fourteenth century, which ranged from the insupportable cost of harbour works and defences to steadily diminishing catches of herring. Worst of all, however, was the long-term effect of depopulation through pestilence, an estimated 7,000 people having expired in 1349 alone 'by the grete visitacion off all myghty God'. It was, they maintained, for this reason more than any other that a once flourishing port 'replenysshed with people' could now claim fewer than 2,000 residents.[87]

The bitter conflict between 'rich' and 'poor' burgesses that contributed in no small measure to Yarmouth's woes during the later fourteenth century also sprang from these demographic upheavals.[88] Medieval urban communities were notoriously prone to unrest and factionalism, their vulnerability on this score in part explaining why so much importance was placed upon the ideal of corporeal unity by members of the governing elite.[89] Like plague, with which it was so closely connected, dysfunction within the body politic seemed an inevitable consequence of human concupiscence. Recalling the earth tremors and pestilence that followed the Peasants' Revolt of 1381, one versifier observed:

> The rysyng of the comuynes in londe,
> The pestilens, and the eorthe-qwake,
> Theose threo thinges, I understonde,

[85] TNA, SC8/142/7088; *CPR, 1377–1381*, p. 448 (Southampton); *CCR, 1381–1385*, pp. 519–20 (Sandwich); *RP*, III.619 (Ilchester).

[86] TNA, SC8/250/12465; SC8/259/12941. The impact of flooding from the late thirteenth century onwards remains to be studied in an urban context, although, as John Schofield points out, it could have serious consequences: Schofield, *London, 1100–1600*, pp. 216–17. In 1423, for example, the residents of Sutton in Lincolnshire petitioned the Duchy of Lancaster for a rent rebate because of the combined impact of devastating floods and 'grete pestilence', which had caused a mass exodus of residents: see Appendix.

[87] P. Rutledge, 'A Fifteenth-Century Yarmouth Petition', *Great Yarmouth District Archaeological Society* 56 (1976), unpaginated; A. Saul, 'English Towns in the Late Middle Ages: The Case of Yarmouth', *Journal of Medieval History* 8 (1982), pp. 75–88. Recent research suggests that this figure, although high, may not be inconceivable: Britnell, 'Black Death in English Towns', p. 200. It was reiterated in a second petition of 1502: NRO, Y/C18/1, fol. 32r–v.

[88] The dispute came to a head in the Parliament of 1376, when 'the great men of the town' were denounced by 'the poor commoners', and thirty-five of their number bound over to keep the peace: *RP*, II.352; *CCR, 1374–1377*, p. 470. Not surprisingly, the homes of some wealthy merchants were plundered during the Peasants' Revolt five years later: B. Dobson, ed., *The Peasants' Revolt of 1381*, 2nd edn (London, 1983), p. 32; William Worcestre, *Itineraries*, ed. J. H. Harvey (Oxford, 1969), pp. 182–3.

[89] C. R. Friedrichs, *The Early Modern City, 1450–1750* (London, 1995), p. 275.

> Beoth tokenes the grete vengaunce and wrake
> That schulde falle for synnes sake.[90]

Matters looked very different from the perspective of the disaffected *mediocres*, or 'middling sort', who resented the concentration of wealth and authority in the hands of narrow and apparently self-serving oligarchs. During the 1430s, for example, Winchelsea was split by 'great diversion and disagreement' as the commons fought to obtain a voice in the election of borough officials. As frequently happened, a compromise was eventually reached through the creation of an enlarged council on which these lesser ranking burgesses could serve, thereby holding their superiors to account.[91] Similar measures were adopted in Norwich, albeit after a longer struggle. The crown's mounting exasperation with the citizens, who were 'hevyly voysed for lak of good and vertuous governaunce' at various points between the 1370s and 1450s, reveals how fragile consensus might be, not only between the rulers and the ruled but also within the fractious ranks of the mercantile elite.[92] The indignation of the *prudeshommes* (dignitaries) of the city when faced in 1414 with demands for a role in government from individuals *de le pluis meindre reputation* (of a lower station) smacks of class interest; yet in 1424 they were taken to task for bickering among themselves, and in the following decade were obliged to surrender their powers to a royal warden, so divisive had their internecine rivalries become.[93]

It would be simplistic to blame these and comparable problems elsewhere in England entirely upon plague, but their genesis can often be traced back to the loss of experienced office holders during the Black Death and subsequent epidemics. This not only caused short-term administrative difficulties as posts fell vacant and replacements could not be found, but also necessitated the promotion of untried 'new men' ignorant or contemptuous of existing practices.[94] Late medieval surgeons might draw a heartening analogy between the reception of outsiders into a city and the body's natural propensity to heal itself after being wounded, but in practice reactions could prove far less harmonious.[95] In 1361, for example, royal letters patent criticised 'the grievous debates and dissensions' that had broken out in Shrewsbury following an influx of ambitious newcomers after the Black Death. True to type, the latter were allegedly plotting to wrest control of the rule

---

[90] T. Wright, ed., *Political Poems and Songs*, 2 vols, RS 14 (London, 1859), I.252.

[91] Roskell, Clark and Rawcliffe, *Commons, 1386–1421*, I.766; BL, MS Cotton Julius B IV, fols 58r–59r.

[92] P. Maddern, 'Order and Disorder', in Rawcliffe and Wilson, *Medieval Norwich*, p. 190.

[93] *RCN*, I.67–108, 273–5; *CPR, 1429–1436*, pp. 29–32; *CPR, 1436–1441*, pp. 76, 123.

[94] Britnell, 'Black Death in English Towns', pp. 205, 208. The loss of eighteen London aldermen in 1348–9 meant that survivors, such as the financier Adam Fraunceys, could rapidly achieve the highest office without significant prior experience: Sloane, *Black Death in London*, pp. 120–1. For the lack of written precedents to guide these *parvenus*, see section 1.2 above.

[95] R. Sennett, *Flesh and Stone: The Body and the City in Western Civilization* (London, 1994), p. 168.

(*regimen*) of the town and overturn established custom.[96] Shrewsbury was already by this date in decline, and thus especially susceptible to internal divisions. Its problems were far from unusual, though, being replicated in other urban centres, such as Lincoln, where the sudden loss of collective memory vested in a generation of magistrates led to protracted conflict over the interpretation of customs and liberties. As a result of pressure exerted from Westminster, the *potentiores* were obliged to accept a degree of popular involvement in the business of government, although the lesser citizens failed in their attempt to control the mayoral elections and thus return one of their own candidates. Significantly, in this instance as in so many others, the solution deemed 'pleasing to God' and most beneficial to the community reinforced existing social hierarchies.[97]

Less dramatic, but equally harmful, was the contraction of credit networks during plague time because entrepreneurs were reluctant to risk lending money, or even to venture into once busy commercial centres. In such a difficult economic climate the effect of adverse competition and lost markets on towns already weakened by pestilence could prove corrosive.[98] Illicit trading in extramural 'kyrkmarkethes' was cited as a particular grievance by the burgesses of Appleby, not least because unscrupulous individuals were able to corner the market in essential goods and push up prices.[99] At Huntingdon, on the other hand, merchants protested that trade had grown so sluggish that they were being taxed on non-existent profits.[100] Like the two pans in a pair of scales, Wells declined as Bristol rose, since the surrounding countryside could not furnish enough people to repopulate both places.[101] Already disheartened by the removal of the valuable Wool Staple in the early fourteenth century, the beleaguered people of Lincoln also lacked the resilience to cope with successive epidemics. Having sought a reduction in the fee farm in 1399 and 1402 because of the effects of disease 'and other insupportable burdens', they secured an exemption from parliamentary taxation in 1447 on account of the most recent outbreak of plague. Over three decades later, in Richard III's reign, they were still blaming 'the grete mortalite that hathe bene here by pestelance and othere sekenez' for the 'dececes, desolacions, and lakke of inhabitantez' which made recovery such a distant prospect.[102] Inevitably, the attendant fall in revenues and proliferation of wasteland and abandoned housing inhibited any attempts at environmental improvement, however desirable.

---

[96] *CPR, 1358–1362*, p. 539; H. Owen and J. B. Blakeway, *A History of Shrewsbury*, 2 vols (London, 1825), I.167–72.

[97] Hill, *Medieval Lincoln*, pp. 260–1.

[98] Nightingale, 'Some New Evidence of Crises and Trends of Mortality', pp. 37–9.

[99] TNA, SC8/90/4470; *CPR, 1377–1381*, pp. 520, 565–6. Similar problems regarding the dislocation of local trade were experienced in Chester: Laughton, *Life in a Late Medieval City*, p. 25.

[100] TNA, SC8/269/13419; *CPR, 1361–1364*, p. 417.

[101] Shaw, *Creation of a Community*, pp. 58–63.

[102] *RP*, III.438, 447, 503; HMC, *Fourteenth Report*, appendix 8: *The manuscripts of Lincoln, Bury St. Edmund's, and Great Grimsby corporations; and of the deans and chapters of Worcester and Lichfield*, Royal Commission on Historical Manuscripts 37 (London, 1895), pp. 10–11, 263–5.

A peremptory letter from Edward III in 1365, drawing attention to the filthy state of the streets, highlights the predicament of magistrates who could not afford the paving and other sanitary measures vital for regenerating the city's economic centre and, indeed, protecting its residents against plague.[103]

Even without such contributory factors as war, factionalism and commercial difficulties, the temporary suspension of trade and the routine business of government occasioned by an exodus of leading citizens during epidemics could prove extremely disruptive. Although, as we shall see, senior officials were expected to remain in post at such times, the temptation to flee, 'like deserters from an army', was often overwhelming.[104] Facing an order from Henry VII in 1493 to place the city on a defensive footing against the Scots, the rulers of York protested that they simply could not mobilise sufficient reserves. They claimed that the city had been left 'in miserable ruyne and decaye and of veray litill power of people', in part because of deaths from 'the lamentable plage of pestilence', but largely as a result of the gentry's reluctance to remain in their town houses while the threat of infection persisted.[105] The king reacted harshly to this dereliction of duty, but there can be little doubt that flight was the preferred option for anyone of means, including the royal family.

In a letter of September 1471 that casts an interesting light on contemporary assumptions about the susceptibility of urban populations to epidemic disease, Sir John Paston warned his brother of the need to protect their younger siblings at the first hint of trouble:

> I praye yow scende me worde iff any off owre frendys or well-wyllerys be dede, fore I feer that ther is grete deth in Norwyche and in other borowghe townese in Norffolk; for I ensure yow it is the most vnyuersall dethe that euyre I wyst in Ingelonde, for by my trowthe I kan not her by pylgrymes that passe the contré, ner noon other man that rydethe er gothe any contré, that *any borow town in Ingelonde* [my italics] is free from that sykenesse ... Wherffor, for Goddysake, late my moodre take heed to my yonge brytheryn, that ... iff ther be any off that syklnesse ded or enffecte in Norwyche, for Goddes sake lete hyre sende them to som frende off hyrse in-to the contré.[106]

Not even the affluent and well connected could be sure of reaching safety, as another member of the Paston clan discovered when finding himself trapped in the plague-ridden city in the autumn of 1479.[107] Hoping to escape the arrows of pestilence, such people generally left for their country estates as soon as an epidemic struck. According to the merchant Richard Cely, the flight of affluent citizens from the pestiferous confines of London 'into the contre for fere of the sekenese' had begun by early May of that year, although he opted to remain behind for as long as possible in order to pursue his business interests.[108]

[103] See section 1.4 above.

[104] Horden, 'Ritual and Public Health', p. 24.

[105] *YCR*, II.102.

[106] *PL*, I.440–1.

[107] *PL*, I.616.

[108] A. Hanham, ed., *The Cely Letters, 1472–1488*, EETS o.s. 273 (Oxford, 1975), p. 48.

During the fifteenth and sixteenth centuries, fear of plague sometimes led to the suspension of legal business at Westminster, as well as the prorogation of parliament, which might in extreme cases decamp to a more salubrious venue. So great was the apprehension generally felt about 'the unhealthiness of the air' in the City that the threat of pestilence may well have served as a useful pretext for the removal of the contentious 1450 parliament to Leicester, a stronghold of the court party.[109] Universities, too, were prone to serious upheavals during epidemics, since it was recognised that disease would sweep like wildfire through the scholars' badly ventilated dormitories and cramped lodgings. As the records of both Oxford and Cambridge attest, the start or finish of term was often postponed so that they could leave for the safety of the surrounding countryside – a practice which the antiquary Anthony à Wood (d. 1695) considered inimical to the cultivation of good manners and morality, as well as learning.[110] It was, perhaps, to avoid these unfortunate contingencies that in 1505 Lady Margaret Beaufort bequeathed her manor house at Malton to Christ's College, Cambridge, 'soo that the maister and scolers may resort thidder, and there to tarry in tyme of contagiouse siknes'.[111] Left behind to face the onslaught of disease, as well as the interruption of food supplies and loss of trade, the less affluent residents of English towns had further reason to resent the conduct of those placed in authority above them.

In this respect, as in so many others relating to the welfare of the urban body, precept and practice were not always at one. Plague tracts and *regimina* recognised an obligation on the part of the ruling elite to work selflessly for the common good through the implementation of projects and policies that would improve the living conditions of residents, as well as adopting whatever short-term measures might prove necessary to halt the spread of specific epidemics.[112] However critical they may have been of the behaviour of individual magistrates, few ordinary burgesses sought to question the general assumption that 'the more worthy, more powerful, more good and true, more discreet, more influential and more sufficient' members of the community would be better qualified for this task.[113] Their acceptance was, however, conditional upon the latter's readiness to 'do right to every person or persons, as well as to poor as to rich', an optimistic expectation that was formally enshrined in the oaths of office taken by the mayors of towns such as Grimsby

---

[109] *RP*, V.172; Bean, 'Plague, Population and Economic Decline', p. 427. In the previous year the king had been obliged to flee in earnest from the corrupt air of the City and Westminster: see Appendix.

[110] Anthony à Wood, *The History and Antiquities of the University of Oxford*, 2 vols (Oxford, 1792), I.651, 658. He nonetheless conceded that 'the lying of many scholars in one room or dormitory ... occasioned nasty air and smells, and consequently diseases' (pp. 596–7). More recently scholars have questioned these assumptions, arguing that the University probably suffered less than the town: T. A. R. Evans, 'The Number, Origins and Careers of Scholars', in J. I. Catto and R. Evans, eds, *The History of the University of Oxford*, vol. 2: *Late Medieval Oxford* (Oxford, 1992), pp. 489–94.

[111] Cooper, *Annals of Cambridge*, p. 275.

[112] Arrizabalaga, 'Facing the Black Death', p. 269.

[113] Hill, *Medieval Lincoln*, p. 279.

and Bristol.[114] Moreover, as members of the same 'bodye corporate', the lesser limbs and organs could lay reasonable claim to a degree of involvement in the decisions made and ratified by the head.[115] How else was such a complex organism to survive?

2.3 The working of the civic body

In keeping with Classical tradition, medieval society was envisaged in organic terms, the ideal community being like a healthy body, which was temperate in its complexion, and in which each part performed its allotted role smoothly, without friction, in the service of the whole.[116] The various limbs and organs did not, of course, rank equally in stature or importance, although the actual 'order of parts' could vary considerably according to the perspective adopted by a particular author. Just as the state recognised a tripartite hierarchy, dominated by prelates, royalty and aristocracy, so the brain, heart and liver generally appeared superior to other less 'spiritual' or 'noble' organs.[117] The sensitive and vulnerable nature of the eyes, as well as their elevated position, likewise set them far above the sturdy and hard-working feet, which were often compared to peasants or artisans (plate 4).[118] Conversely, as we shall see in Chapters 4 and 5, a scale of values predicated on economic productivity rather than social class would inevitably privilege the 'principal' components of the alimentary system, since it was here that the nourishment essential for survival was processed ready for distribution throughout the rest of the body. Both brain and stomach might therefore enjoy the same status, albeit under rather different circumstances. Whereas princes or magistrates were usually regarded as the head or heart of the body politic, a seemingly incongruous comparison with the 'stomake and bowels' made perfect sense in a fiscal context. From the *Policraticus* of John of Salisbury (1159) to a speech drafted by Bishop John Russell for delivery to Richard III's first parliament, the body's dependence upon a regular food supply and the organs that transformed it into life-giving blood and *pneuma* could be employed both to justify the need for equitable taxation and to condemn the dangers of rampant acquisitiveness.[119]

[114] Rigby, 'Urban "Oligarchy"', p. 64.

[115] *YMB*, II.246.

[116] See, for example, L. Barkan, *Nature's Work of Art: The Human Body in the Image of the World* (New Haven, CT, 1975), chap. 2; D. G. Hale, *The Body Politic: A Political Metaphor in Renaissance English Literature* (The Hague, 1971), chaps 2 and 3; M. James, 'Ritual, Drama and Social Body in the Later Middle Ages', *P&P* 98 (1983), pp. 3–29, on pp. 6–9.

[117] Society was traditionally divided into those who fought, those who laboured and those who prayed: P. E. Dutton, '*Illvstre civitatis et popvli exemplvm*: Plato's *Timaevs* and the Transmission from Calcidius to the End of the Twelfth Century of a Tripartite Scheme of Society', *Mediaeval Studies* 45 (1983), pp. 79–119.

[118] M. C. Pouchelle, *The Body and Surgery in the Middle Ages*, trans. R. Morris (Oxford, 1990), p. 119.

[119] John of Salisbury, *Policraticus: Of the Frivolities of Courtiers and the Footprints of Philosophers*, ed. and trans. C. J. Nederman (Cambridge, 1990), pp. 135–6; S. B. Chrimes, *English Constitutional Ideas in the Fifteenth Century* (Cambridge, 1936),

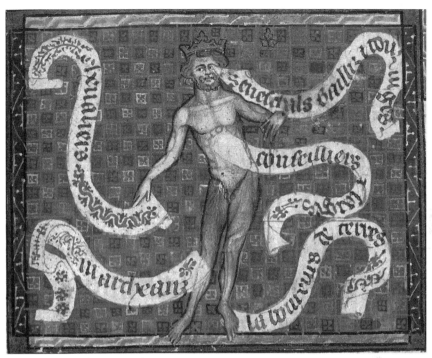

4 In this personification of the body politic from a mid-fourteenth-century French advice manual for princes, merchants (*marcheanz*) who travel the world are the legs, while the labouring classes (*laboureurs*) are the feet which support everyone else.

What anatomical function did the urban workforce perform? Following Plato, early commentators, in particular, took a disdainful view of rude mechanicals, stressing their potential for extravagance and waste, if not worse. John of Salisbury's teacher, William of Conches, for instance, equated 'confectioners, cobblers, skinners and other craftsmen' with the kidneys because, like them, they stimulated greed. An anonymous twelfth-century author drew an even less flattering comparison, noting that 'on the margins of the city live the workers, that is the tradesmen and other servile people, who always desire to acquire things, just as in man lust dwells in the nether quarters'.[120] Demonstrably unfit to govern because of their distance from the citadel of reason, practitioners of crafts and trades had to be kept firmly under control lest they inspired covetousness in others. However, such harsh attitudes were bound to soften, not least because a sustained period of urban growth, together with the rapid development of medical theory and professional education in the West, prompted a more sophisticated use of anatomical imagery.[121] As a result, the correlation between specific parts of the body and particular individuals or social groups became far less prescriptive,

p. 175. See also J. Le Goff, 'Head or Heart? The Political Use of Body Metaphors in the Middle Ages', in M. Feher, R. Naddaff and N. Tazi, eds, *Fragments for a History of the Human Body*, part 3 (New York, 1989), pp. 13–26.

[120] Dutton, 'Tripartite Scheme of Society', pp. 91–2, 95–6 n. 63.

[121] See, for example, Nicholas of Cusa, *Catholic Concordance*, pp. 320–1.

furnishing preachers and poets, as well as political theorists, with a fruitful supply of largely positive metaphors.

Not surprisingly, as the manufacturing and commercial classes acquired greater economic and political influence, their position in the hierarchy of parts began to improve. Although Bishop Brinton of Rochester (d. 1389) compared 'merchants and worthy artisans' with the left hand, thereby underscoring their inferiority to the knights on the right, his belief that 'citizens and burgesses' constituted the heart was telling.[122] As the seat of the vital spirits, this supremely 'spiritual' organ bestowed warmth and life upon the rest of the body, and, according to some authorities, was even home to the soul itself.[123] And if the aldermen of Exeter, London, Norwich or York were unfamiliar with these more recondite flights of corporeal fancy, they would almost certainly have been able to quote vernacular verses which acknowledged the essential role of entrepreneurs and artisans in supporting the commonwealth:

> I likne the thies [thighs], flesch and bon,
> That beren the body quantite,
> To marchaundes, in perile ride and gon,
> Bryngen wynnyng, gold and fee,
> Make highe houses of lym and ston,
> Mayntene burgh, toun and cyte,
> Welthe and worschip in here won,
> And good houshold in gret plente.
> Manys leggis, likne y may
> To all craftes that worche with handes,
> For al the body beren thay,
> As a tre that bereth wandes [branches].[124]

As kingdoms in miniature, cities constituted a very superior type of body, at least according to Thomas Aquinas (d. 1274), who shared Aristotle's belief that, of all the various communities created by man, the city was the most perfect, being 'ordered to the satisfaction of the needs of human life'.[125] His turn of phrase was apt, since *order* was, indeed, the key to prosperity and survival. St Augustine's conviction that 'the peace of the body and soul is the duly *ordered* life and health of a living creature' reflected his gloomy view of mankind's inherent predisposition to sin and need for the structured discipline that only firm municipal government could provide.[126] Written after the sack of Rome in 410, his *De civitate Dei* set

[122] Owst, *Literature and Pulpit*, p. 587.

[123] In the words of Nicholas of Cusa, 'the more immediately accessible seat of the soul is the purest blood contained at the centre of the heart': *Catholic Concordance*, pp. 318–9.

[124] J. Kail, ed., *Twenty-Six Political and Other Poems*, EETS o.s. 124 (London, 1904), p. 66.

[125] C. J. Nederman and K. Langdon Forhan, eds, *Medieval Political Theory: A Reader: The Quest for the Body Politic, 1100–1400* (London, 1993), p. 137.

[126] St Augustine, *Concerning the City of God against the Pagans*, ed. and trans. H. Bettenson (London, 1984), book 19, cap. 13.

a template for the guidance of urban authorities that endured for well over a millennium. In it he explained that, although all the children of Eve were condemned by their inherent corruption, disobedience and selfishness to inhabit an imperfect, disease-ridden, earthly city, the truly virtuous might eventually ascend to the New Jerusalem through divine grace. It was, therefore, the first duty of the ruling elite to facilitate the process of transition from the terrestrial to the celestial city by stamping out evil and leading the populace in the health-giving ways of God.[127] Among the various temporal benefits to ensue from this painstaking spiritual journey would be the creation of a peaceful and salubrious environment, as well, implicitly, as a population whose members toiled obediently together for the benefit of all.

Henry VII deemed it necessary to reiterate this point when instructing the mayor of Northampton to remove any 'vacabunde rioturs or vngodly disposed personnes' from the town without delay. A well-governed community, he tartly observed, 'furst and principally pleaseth God, establissheth parfite reste and tranquillite, noresshech and encreaseth love [and] causith plente and habundance ... the vniuersall wele always inhauncyng and flouryng'.[128] Beleaguered magistrates needed few reminders on this score. Well aware that the urban body could not escape 'much greefe of inflammation, where anie lest part is out of ioint, or not duelie [duly] set in his owne naturall place',[129] they instituted a plethora of regulations that embraced home, workshop and guild, as well as the more public aspects of urban life.[130] As the recorder of Nottingham maintained in 1512, any disturbance of the established social hierarchy could easily unleash chaos. 'If ye shalle suffer the commens to rule and folowe ther apetite and desire', he warned, the ensuing upheavals would inevitably subvert 'alle good and politike order and rule', leading eventually 'to the distruccion of the towne'.[131] It could be only a matter of time before plague and other marks of divine disapproval followed. Yet, as he and his contemporaries clearly recognised, discipline alone was not enough to instil a sense of responsibility into potentially rebellious members of the body politic.

One of John of Salisbury's most innovative – and enduring – contributions to the literature on this topic was his imaginative leap from the concept of a static and essentially elitist hierarchy of parts to a more fluid system that reflected contemporary ideas about the complexities of human physiology.[132] With its emphasis upon the need for mutual cooperation between each separate component of an interconnected network of nerves, arteries, veins, limbs and

[127] St Augustine, *City of God*, book 8, cap. 24. Ordinances produced in Grimsby in 1498 for the regulation of public utilities were dedicated to Christ, the Virgin and 'all the holy citizens of heaven': Rigby, 'Urban "Oligarchy"', p. 67.

[128] C. A. Markham, ed., *The Liber custumarum* (Northampton, 1895), p. 6.

[129] Sir John Cheeke, 'The Hurt of Sedition', in *Holinshed's Chronicles of England Scotland and Ireland*, vol. 3 (London, 1808), p. 1003.

[130] Maddern, 'Order and Disorder', pp. 189–212.

[131] Stevenson, *Records of the Borough of Nottingham*, III.341.

[132] C. J. Nederman, 'The Physiological Significance of the Organic Metaphor in John of Salisbury's *Policraticus*', *History of Political Thought* 8 (1987), pp. 211–23.

organs, his analysis stressed the need for *collaboration* as well as order. This sense of reciprocity emerges clearly in an explanatory letter sent by him, along with a copy of the *Policraticus*, to a friend:

> ∴. thus it is that in the human body the members serve each other, and the offices of each are allotted for the benefit of all. There are less of some and more of others according to the size of the body, but all of them are united to serve the body's health; they differ in their effects, but, if you consider the health of the body, they are all working for the same end. Not all of them are equal, but the inferiors serve their superiors. The foot which moves in the mire does not aspire to the dignity of the head; but the head on the other hand does not, because it is erect to heaven, despise the foot for plodding in the mud.[133]

From John's perspective, it was not enough simply to accept one's allotted place in society and obey the rules; for a community to function at optimum capacity and avoid the ravages of disease its various members were bound to assist each other. And although everyone had a role to play, the heaviest burden inevitably fell upon the ruling elite, or *potentiores*, whose position in relation to the *mediocres* and *inferiores* mirrored precisely that of the head in relation to the chest and feet.[134]

This point was further developed by the Florentine Brunetto Latini (d. 1294), who urged magistrates to govern by example, thereby fostering what might quite literally be termed an *esprit de corps*. They were also encouraged to cultivate the Aristotelian virtues of temperance and moderation, again as a model to others. In his influential *Livres dou tresor*, which was composed for the guidance of the civic authorities, he maintained that:

> ... just as a good doctor looks into the nature of man to keep him in health and to give him medicine against illnesses, so too must man and the rulers of cities be vigilant and strive to bring profit to the citizens and maintain the happiness which belongs to intellective souls, and admonish them to do works of virtue, because their end is felicity.[135]

A number of Brunetto's 'prescriptions for good government' were reproduced, with significant emendations, by the fishmonger Andrew Horn (d. 1328) in his collection of civic ordinances now known as the *Liber custumarum* of London. He

---

[133] John of Salisbury, *The Letters of John of Salisbury*, vol. 1: *The Early Letters, 1153–1161*, ed. W. J. Millor, H. E. Butler and C. N. L. Brooke (London, 1955), p. 181; Nederman, 'Physiological Significance of the Organic Metaphor', p. 216. For the deployment of such concepts in both a medical and personal context, see Pouchelle, *Body and Surgery*, pp. 114–16.

[134] It was, he argued, the responsibility of the elite to ensure that the feet of the body politic were properly shod, since 'the health of the whole republic will only be secure and splendid if the superior members devote themselves to the inferiors': Nederman and Langdon Forhan, *Medieval Political Theory*, p. 43.

[135] Brunetto Latini, *Li Livres dou tresor*, ed. P. Barrette and S. Baldwin (New York, 1993), p. 149. For the trope of prince or magistrate as physician, see J. L. G. Picherit, *La Métaphore pathologique et thérapeutique à la fin du moyen âge* (Tübingen, 1994), pp. 18–21.

chose his material carefully, demonstrating a predictable interest in the qualities desirable in both the governor (in this instance the mayor) and the governed.[136] His very first extract applies the traditional metaphor of the social body directly to this specific urban *milieu*:

> .... the mayor or the governor is, as it were, the chief among the citizens, and everybody wants to have a healthy head, because when the head is unsound all the members fall ill; and for this reason above all else they must study to have such a governor who will lead them to a good end, according to right and according to reason and justice.[137]

As the physician and head of the urban body, a magistrate had to be robust, in both a moral and physical sense, possessing the energy and vigour to implement whatever remedies his patient might require.[138] Bemoaning the failure to complete a programme for cleaning the ditches and repairing the walls of London on schedule in 1477, one chronicler observed that the new mayor 'applyed it not so sore as his predecessour did. Wherfore it had not so good expedicion as it myght haue had; and also he was a syklew [sickly] man, ffeble and weke, wherfore he had not his mynde so fresshely, nothir myght not apply it so well.' He also noted, tellingly, that enterprises begun by one official might have less appeal to his successors, 'for then they thynk the worship therof is ascrybed vnto the ffynder and to the begynner, and not to th'ender; which causeth many good werkes and actes to be put owte of mynd, which is full great pyte.'[139]

Effective leadership certainly demanded a strong personal presence, and could not be properly exercised *in absentia*. Like medical practitioners, who were expected to tend the sick during epidemics (notwithstanding innumerable examples to the contrary), members of the urban elite were called upon to demonstrate their devotion to duty in such testing times.[140] John Warde had good reason to regard his election as mayor of London in late September 1485 with dismay, since the sweating sickness was then cutting a swathe through the City, and

---

[136] Catto, 'Andrew Horn', pp. 387–90. See also, S. Reynolds, 'Medieval Urban History and the History of Political Thought', *Urban History Yearbook* (1982), pp. 14–23, on p. 22; Lilley, *City and Cosmos*, pp. 135–7.

[137] *MGL*, II.i.16–25, on pp. 16–17. See also John of Salisbury, *Policraticus*, pp. 129–31.

[138] Some medical authorities maintained that the physical health of the practitioner was crucial, enabling him to cleanse the air through the purity of his own exhalations. Conversely, if his humours were unbalanced or corrupt he would harm his patients, however skilled he might be: P. Diepgen and J. Ruska, eds, *Quellen und Studien zur Geschichte der Naturwissenschaften und der Medizin*, vol. 5 (Berlin, 1936), pp. 71–2. I am grateful to Maaike van der Lugt for this reference. Surgeons, too, were expected to 'be of a complexioun weel proporciound and ... temperat': Lanfrank of Milan, *Lanfrank's 'Science of Cirurgie'*, ed. R. von Fleishhacker, EETS o.s. 102 (London, 1894), p. 8.

[139] C. L. Kingsford, ed., *Chronicles of London* (Oxford, 1905; repr. Stroud, 1977), pp. 187–8.

[140] The debate about the morality of flight, which so preoccupied sixteenth-century divines, had begun before 1500, it being widely agreed that magistrates and clergy should remain out of duty and conscience: Slack, *Impact of Plague*, pp. 41–4.

had killed his two predecessors in less than a week. While still an alderman he had been threatened with a massive fine of £500 for refusing to leave his Hertfordshire estates and shoulder his full responsibilities, which he now reluctantly agreed to do.[141] Although some members of York's ruling elite proved equally craven at this time by heading for the countryside, they atoned for their derelictions later. During the following decade, in which the city experienced almost annual outbreaks of epidemic disease, two mayors and a sheriff died in office, along with an unusually high proportion of otherwise healthy councillors.[142]

As we shall see in later chapters of this book, such men often continued to fulfil their obligations well beyond the grave by leaving testamentary bequests for public works of the sort advocated by John Jannys. Mindful of the Christian imperative that the rich should succour and assist the poor, magistrates were, moreover, often called upon to contribute personally through loans or donations to schemes for urban development, such as the provision of subsidised food, the laying of drains and the introduction of piped water. More often than not, a persuasive combination of personal vanity, altruism, civic pride and fear of the Last Judgement made coercion unnecessary. In an encomium of the building works undertaken by two leading burgesses in 1373–4, the author of The Red Paper Book of Colchester pays tribute to the strong sense of community that inspired such conspicuous generosity. He was probably familiar with Brunetto's influential *Tresor*, as this passage describing the embellishment of the moot hall shows:

> Just as the head is the substance of the body of every living soul, so this hall is the head and honour of the whole community of Colchester. Take notice, then, of the things which have been done and described previously, the acts of William Reyne and John Clerk this year, and how, towards the end of the same year, they caused the triple seats, benches, and other things visible in public to the eyes of men in the same hall to be ornamented; and how they are mindful of the health [*salutis*] of their souls; and of the welfare [*salubris*] of the whole community of Colchester.[143]

Their desire to achieve redemption in the next life and the health of others on earth also led the two philanthropists to fund extensive improvements to the adjacent gaol, whose inmates had hitherto been confined in unacceptably squalid conditions. The physical care of prisoners became a matter of growing concern during this period, and their spiritual welfare was certainly not neglected either.[144] Thus, for example, the executors of Richard Brown and Ralph Segrym, former aldermen of Norwich, gave £200 in 1472 to fund a priest who would celebrate

[141] *CLB*, L, p. v; Thrupp, *Merchant Class of Medieval London*, p. 227.

[142] *YCR*, I.118; D. M. Palliser, 'Epidemics in Tudor York', *Northern History* 8 (1973), pp. 45–63, on p. 47. The reluctance of some individuals to take up office was almost certainly due to fear of contagion, as well as resistance to the financial demands made upon senior magistrates. However, the extent of the problem has been questioned by J. I. Kermode, 'Urban Decline? The Flight from Office in Late-Medieval York', *EconHR*, 2nd series 35 (1982), pp. 179–98.

[143] *RPBC*, pp. 10–11. For the background to this outpouring of civic pride, see Britnell, *Growth and Decline in Colchester*, pp. 120–5.

[144] See section 4.6 below.

mass daily in the chapel of St Barbara next to the Guildhall 'for the relief and comfort of the prisoners and others incarcerated there', hearing their confessions as appropriate. Significantly, he was also to pray for the salvation of the donors, the mayor and commonalty of the city and another alderman who had endowed and furnished the chapel for the benefit of the prisoners.[145]

Terror at the prospect of *mors improvisa* undoubtedly served to loosen the purse strings of prominent citizens, who nonetheless came increasingly to recognise that good deeds alone, however meritorious, would not suffice. Since sin exercised such a corrosive effect upon urban as well as human bodies, the concept of civic health increasingly came to embrace the moral purity of individual magistrates, as well as their commitment to public works. Even passive collusion in improper behaviour merited censure. From 1417 onwards 'aldermen and substantial commoners' of London who leased their property to men or women of debauched life stood to forfeit whatever rents changed hands, since they were effectively living off immoral earnings.[146] The same Coventry leet court that passed orders in 1429 against the dumping of waste in the town ditch and 'common water', decreed that any sergeant or other official 'taken in adultery' should be immediately discharged.[147] In 1454 the scope of this ruling was broadened to penalise each and every municipal employee who appeared 'vicious of his body', and further reinforced by the threat of exclusion from the prayers and offerings of the community – a draconian punishment with devastating spiritual repercussions. Clearly determined to pay more than lip service to such lofty ideals, the authorities then undertook to sack the town gaoler if he continued his adulterous relationship with the wife of one Thomas White.[148] The drive for moral rearmament continued, notably in the radical programme of reforms launched in 1492 whereby any former officer, councillor or mayor who persistently committed adultery, fornication or usury faced the dual prospect of a permanent ban upon future involvement in civic government and of being 'vtterly … estraunged from all goode companye'. Significantly, this particular measure followed immediately after a ban upon the construction of pigsties within the walls, thereby providing at a stroke for the spiritual as well as the physical health of the population.[149]

Although their long history of sympathy for, if not active espousal of, lollard beliefs made the leading burgesses of Coventry especially keen on this type of prescriptive agenda, they were far from unusual in their insistence upon high standards of behaviour on the part of the ruling elite.[150] In 1439, for example, 'the

[145] NRO, NCR, 24B/25; Rawcliffe, *Medicine for the Soul*, pp. 156–7.

[146] *CLB*, I, p. 178; Riley, *Memorials of London*, pp. 649–50. The connection between morality, 'respectable masculinity' and reputation is considered at length in McSheffrey, *Marriage, Sex and Civic Culture*, part 2.

[147] *Coventry Leet Book*, I.119–20.

[148] *Coventry Leet Book*, II.279–80.

[149] *Coventry Leet Book*, II.344. For a fuller discussion of these reforms, see P. J. P. Goldberg, 'Coventry's "Lollard" Programme of 1492 and the Making of Utopia', in R. Horrox and S. Rees-Jones, eds, *Pragmatic Utopias: Ideals and Communities, 1200–1630* (Cambridge, 2001), pp. 97–116.

[150] Maddern, 'Order and Disorder', pp. 205–12.

commonalty of the City' begged the mayor and aldermen of London to challenge the episcopal confirmation of John Sevenoaks as prior of Holy Trinity, Aldgate, and *ex officio* alderman of Portsoken ward. Their opposition hinged upon the fact that such a notoriously dissolute prelate would bring the *lay* community – which implicitly comported itself with greater decorum – into disrepute. Quite possibly as a result of this scandal and almost certainly in response to the devastating pestilences of the 1430s, a second petition drew attention to 'the detestable synne [of] lecherie' then spreading unchecked throughout the capital, 'in displeasance of almyghti God' and in defiance of existing ordinances.[151] The staunchly and exuberantly orthodox rulers of late medieval Norwich were equally intolerant of improper conduct. New regulations promulgated in 1452 for the religious guild of St George, to which all leading civic officials belonged, insisted that any member who lost either his citizenship or post because of misbehaviour would be expelled from its ranks. By the same token, any brother facing ejection from the guild would automatically be disenfranchised and stripped of his office, 'as a forsworne man and as a man shamed and repreved and renne in the peyne of infamie'.[152] In this way the guild became a highly effective mechanism for disciplining the elite, whose behaviour was closely and constantly monitored.

Late medieval beliefs about human physiology underscored the biblical message that the various limbs and organs of 'Chrystes mistycall body' were joined 'by faythe and charyte' in a union of common sympathy and mutual support.[153] In the words of the encyclopaedist Bartholomaeus Anglicus (d. *c.* 1250): 'the membres beth so isette togedres that, for the byndynge and knettinge togedres, eueryche hath compaciencs [compassion] of othir'. Through selfless generosity, the healthier parts would assist those that were 'sike and sore', drawing 'the matere of the euel' away from the afflicted area and thereby facilitating recovery. There were, however, strict limits to collective altruism. As Bartholomaeus went on to explain, 'if a membre is irooted [rotten] othir deed [dead] it is greuous to itself and to al the body; and therfore is none othir remedye but kutte it of[f] that he destroye not and corrumpe al the body'.[154] Had he lived a century later, he might have added that the removal of contaminated blood by a phlebotomist was a recognised prophylactic against the plague.[155] The implications for urban health were obvious, imposing a duty of care upon the richer and more successful residents, while condemning the intransigent, unruly or criminal of all classes to exclusion or worse:

[151] *CLB*, K, p. 230. See Appendix for details of this epidemic.

[152] B. R. McRee, 'Religious Guilds and Civic Order: The Case of Norwich in the Late Middle Ages', *Speculum* 67 (1992), pp. 69–97, on pp. 92–3. It is interesting to note that, although one Salisbury alderman successfully defended himself against charges of fornication in 1415, he was still 'excused' from holding office: Carr, 'From Pollution to Prostitution', p. 36.

[153] F. R. Salter, ed., *Some Early Tracts on Poor Relief* (London, 1926), p. 41. The reference is to the words of St Paul: 1 Corinthians 12:12–26.

[154] *OPT*, I.166, 168.

[155] Phlebotomy was, significantly, accorded priority in the plague *concilium* sent by 'the masters and doctors' of Oxford to the mayor of London in 1407: BL, MS Sloane 3285, fols 68v–69r. See also Aberth, *From the Brink of the Apocalypse*, pp. 101–4.

> The body, with its various members,
> Together makes a man; and similarly
> The mayor, along with other men,
> Makes up a city. And, by analogy,
> Whereas for his own preservation a person
> Will deliberately cut off his hand
> If it becomes diseased
> And threatens his entire body with death,
> Lest he himself should perish,
> That same individual ought likewise
> To amputate the wicked burgess without compunction,
> Rather than corrupt an entire town with evil.
> God says, 'if a man's hand, or foot,
> Or eye offends him he must always destroy it –
> And deal in the same way with sinners.
> For whoever is contaminated by vice
> Can never earn joy in heaven.'
> It therefore follows that,
> When a citizen rejects the law
> And pursues a life of crime,
> It were best that he were hung or drowned,
> Rather than that he should lead the people astray,
> And thereby divide the city.[156]

Despite their reluctance to employ the agonising and potentially fatal remedies of 'fire and knife' before all other viable alternatives had failed, medieval surgeons recognised that amputation or cauterisation with a hot iron might prove unavoidable.[157] Not surprisingly, the analogy between strong government and aggressive surgery exercised a compelling appeal, being employed, for example, by Henry VIII during the Pilgrimage of Grace in 1536, when he pronounced himself ready to 'cut away all those corrupt members that with wholesome medicines will not be recovered and brought to perfect health'.[158] The excision of 'a rotten and festered member' before it infected the rest of the body was, indeed, widely regarded as an act of *charity* or 'virtuous cruelty', which safeguarded 'them that be good and harmless'.[159] At their most extreme, such procedures would result in the prominent display of the severed heads and dismembered bodies of executed

---

[156] John Gower, *Mirour de l'omme*, in *The Complete Works*, ed. G. C. Macaulay, vol. 1 (Oxford, 1899), p. 292. The biblical quotation is a paraphrase of Matthew 18:8–9.

[157] John of Salisbury, *Policraticus*, pp. 49–50. For a discussion of 'the corrective and punitive aspects' of this analogy, see T. Shogimen, 'Treating the Body Politic: The Medical Metaphor of Political Rule in Late Medieval Europe and Tokugawa Japan', *The Review of Politics* 70 (2008), pp. 77–104.

[158] W. R. D. Jones, *The Tudor Commonwealth, 1529–1559* (London, 1970), p. 16. See also Hale, *Body Politic*, pp. 51–2, 57–9.

[159] J. Griffiths, ed., *The Two Books of Homilies Appointed to be Read in Churches*, 2 vols (Oxford, 1859), I.71–2. The Lancastrian propagandist Sir John Fortescue (d. 1479), who frequently deployed anatomical imagery, made a similar

criminals over the gates of towns and cities as a salutary warning to others.[160] But, as the rulers of Coventry and Norwich recognised, there were other, less brutal ways of eliminating undesirables. As we shall see, prostitutes were often relegated to the urban periphery, along with the practitioners of other insalubrious activities, while lepers were physically (but not spiritually) obliged to dwell 'outside the camp'. It is interesting to note that either banishment or the suspension of trading rights and privileges was often regarded as an appropriate punishment for repeated breaches of local sanitary regulations, especially those involving the sale of substandard food. The fourteenth-century customs of Ipswich, for example, threatened cooks who persistently sold 'vitayles corrupt and disconvenable to mannys body' with permanent expulsion from their craft.[161] The elderly, too, could be cast adrift. At the end of life, improvident paupers who appeared to have brought destitution upon themselves through intemperate behaviour were deemed ineligible for support from guild or community.[162]

Like conscientious surgeons, the rulers of English towns sought to heal any wounds, lesions or inflammations in the body politic at an early stage with soothing poultices and other emollients. Mechanisms for the rapid settlement of quarrels before they escalated into serious confrontations or prompted outside intervention developed at a variety of levels, from informal negotiation to legally binding awards by official arbitrators and umpires.[163] Craft guilds and religious fraternities went to great lengths to 'make an ende and unyte and love betwyne partyes', punishing disputants who refused to seek or accept private arbitration.[164] The Tailors of Lincoln threatened to expel anyone who proved obdurate on this score, clearly fearing the contagious miasma of disunity.[165] At a higher level, urban magistrates regarded their peace-keeping role as a crucial means of upholding law and order, as well as preserving commercial health. The importance of easy access to facilities for the mediation of 'compleyntes and varyaunces' is apparent from a memorandum, composed in about 1480, regarding the duties of the mayor of Bristol. Except on Saturdays and feast days he, the sheriff and various other officials were to be available at regular times 'to sett parties in rest and ease by theire advertisement, compromesse or otherwise'. These daily audiences were

comparison: Sir John Fortescue, *De natura legis naturae*, ed. T. Clermont (London, 1869), p. 216.

[160] Phythian-Adams, *Desolation of a City*, p. 177.

[161] T. Twiss, ed., *The Black Book of the Admiralty*, 4 vols, RS 55 (London, 1871–6), II.146–7.

[162] See sections 6.5 and 6.9 below.

[163] E. Powell, 'Arbitration and the Law in England in the Late Middle Ages', *TRHS*, 5th series 33 (1983), pp. 49–67; C. Rawcliffe, '"That Kindliness Should be Cherished More and Discord Driven Out": The Settlement of Commercial Disputes by Arbitration in Later Medieval England', in J. Kermode, ed., *Enterprise and Individuals in Fifteenth-Century England* (Stroud, 1991), pp. 99–117.

[164] H. F. Westlake, *The Parish Guilds of Medieval England* (London, 1919), pp. 71–3.

[165] Smith, Smith and Brentano, *English Gilds*, p. 183. The confraternity of Garlickhythe, London, which was founded 'to noriche more loue' between its members, also ejected those who refused arbitration (p. 4).

regarded as 'the grettyst preseruacion of peas and gode rule to be hadde within the toune and shire of Bristowe that can be ymagened, for yf it wer anywhiles discontynewid there wolde right sone growe grete inconvenyence amongst th'enhabitauntez of the same, which God forbede'.[166] Once again, stiff penalties upheld procedures that in theory (if not always in practice) had been designed to offer prompt and impartial arbitration. From 1477, partly in order to prevent factionalism, any member of Leicester's ruling elite who failed to submit internal disputes to the adjudication of the mayor and masters of the dominant Corpus Christi guild faced the indignity of ejection as a troublemaker from the aldermanic bench.[167]

Here, as in other towns and cities, the Church's emphasis upon the necessity for unity and concord within the Christian body provided powerful support for the forces of mediation. Not by coincidence, the 'Composition' of 1415, which ended a decade of 'dissensions, trauerses, variaunces and discordes' over the implementation of Norwich's royal charter, was effected 'though love of kynde' on St Valentine's day. The pious expectation that 'poore and ryche' would henceforward remain '*oon in herte*, loue and charite, neuermore fro this tyme forth to ben disseuered' was inevitably doomed to disappointment.[168] Yet throughout England the importance of corporate solidarity was underscored by a constant round of religious observance that punctuated urban life from dawn to dusk, instilling a sense of order into the community.[169] At the same time, these rituals offered the devout a degree of protection against suffering and sickness that no human agent, however zealous, could ever bestow.

2.4 Spiritual prophylaxis

That a wide range of devotional practices, from pilgrimage to the deployment of prayers, amulets and other sacred artefacts, could actually restore or safeguard physical health seemed beyond question during the later Middle Ages, notwithstanding the scepticism voiced by heretics and some empirically minded members of the medical profession.[170] As the symbol of Christ's readiness to taste the bitter medicine of suffering and death, crosses in particular were deemed to possess spectacular therapeutic and prophylactic powers. Frequently employed during the making and application of medicinal preparations, the sign of the cross also sustained women in childbirth, sufferers of ague and those facing surgery. Images of crucifixes and, appropriately, of the five wounds of Christ were to be

---

[166] Smith, Smith and Brentano, *English Gilds*, p. 426; Richard Ricart, *The Maire of Bristowe Is Kalendar*, ed. L. T. Smith, CS n.s. 5 (London, 1872), pp. 84–5.

[167] *RBL*, II.299.

[168] However, the administrative structures then put in place did survive until the 1830s: *RCN*, I.94. See also B. R. McRee, 'Peacemaking and its Limits in Late Medieval Norwich', *EHR* 109 (1994), pp. 831–66.

[169] C. Phythian-Adams, 'Ceremony and the Citizen: The Communal Year at Coventry, 1450–1550', in P. Clark and P. Slack, eds, *Crisis and Order in English Towns, 1500–1700* (London, 1972), p. 61.

[170] Rawcliffe, *Medicine and Society*, p. 95.

found on birth girdles and amulets, including engraved metal plates (*laminae*) which could be placed on or near wounds to facilitate healing.[171] Crosses and holy water together promised to dispel pestilential air as effectively as they drove out devils in rites of exorcism.[172] Not surprisingly, prayers, such as the 'Crux Christi' which had allegedly been sent by the pope to Charlemagne to guard against sudden death, were enthusiastically copied, recited and later printed in plague time. The 'Reproaches' intoned by penitents during the ceremony of creeping to the cross on Good Friday were likewise adopted as 'a good prayer ayenste the pestilence', no doubt on the assumption that heartfelt repentance would deflect the flail of divine wrath.[173] Of particular interest in the present context is the behaviour of the Scottish raiding parties who invaded in England in 1379, hoping to capitalise upon the demoralisation caused by an outbreak of pestilence in the north. On learning that the epidemic 'had come to pass through the special grace of God', to deter sinners and to test the faith of the pious, they allegedly began each day by signing themselves with the cross, 'as though blessing themselves', and enlisting the help of their patron saints. According to Thomas Walsingham, who scathingly observed that the elect would welcome death as a release from earthly tribulation, they believed this ritual to be infallible.[174]

It followed axiomatically that such potent assistance might extend to whole communities, as well as individuals. Representations in stone, timber and paint of the principal instrument of Christ's passion proliferated in English towns and cities, not only in the form of boundary and market crosses, which were often tall and imposing structures (see plate 22), but also in the physical layout of the urban landscape itself. During the mid-fifteenth century, the features most commonly used to mark the 'bounds and metes' of York were crosses, no fewer than eight in stone and wood, often with specific names, being itemised in the civic records, along with a number of ecclesiastical buildings.[175] Coventry, too, was surrounded by chapels, crosses, friaries and churches which, according to Charles Phythian-Adams, denoted sacred points of transit, or spiritual bridges, in the liminal area between town and country. They also offered protection in the ongoing battle against pestilence. One of these chapels was dedicated to the two celebrated dragon-slayers St George and St Margaret, who, along with their fire-breathing adversaries, occupied a prominent place in the civic ceremonies of

---

[171] Hunt, *Popular Medicine*, pp. 84, 87–90, 92, 94–9; Glasgow University Library Special Collections, MS Hunter 117 (T.5.19) fol. 36v; C. Rawcliffe, 'Women, Childbirth and Religion in Later Medieval England', in D. Wood, ed., *Women and Religion in Medieval England* (Oxford, 2003), pp. 108–9; S. Page, *Magic in Medieval Manuscripts* (London, 2005), pp. 29–30.

[172] K. Thomas, *Religion and the Decline of Magic* (Harmondsworth, 1984), p. 32.

[173] E. Duffy, *The Stripping of the Altars: Traditional Religion in England, c. 1400–c. 1580* (New Haven, CT, 1992), pp. 271, 273. For the deployment of crosses as plague talismans and in the administration of remedies, see Wellcome Institute Library, Western MS 404, fol. 32v; BL, Add. MS 6716, fol. 98r; Aberth, *From the Brink of the Apocalypse*, pp. 112–13.

[174] Walsingham, *Historia Anglicana*, I.409–11.

[175] *YMB*, III.131–2, 230–1.

other towns and cities, such as Norwich and Westminster. This suggests that the long-standing association between dragons and epidemics probably continued well into the sixteenth century.[176] It certainly featured in more overtly religious rituals. The Rogationtide processions or 'Cross days' staged before Ascension every year throughout England are now chiefly remembered for the processional crosses and banners carried around the boundaries of towns and villages from one wayside cross to another, cleansing the air and scattering the latent forces of evil. Crucial to the proceedings was another flag bearing an image of a dragon, whose long tail was severed on the final day to symbolise the rout of malignant spirits, circulating 'above in the eyer as thyke as motes in the sonne'.[177] The miasmas of pestilence, too, would surely have been put to flight, if only, alas, for a short while.

Robert Ricart's highly stylised map of Bristol, which appears in the calendar he produced in about 1480 for the mayor, William Spencer, depicts a cruciform street plan, dominated by a tall and elaborately carved high cross in the very centre (plate 5). Although he intended to convey some notion of Bristol's early development, rather than to provide accurate topographical detail of the fifteenth-century city, there is good reason to believe that his drawing of the cross was reasonably accurate.[178] Standing almost forty feet high, with niches containing effigies of English kings and queens, this striking landmark was a source of considerable civic pride. It was painted and gilded at a cost of £20 in 1491, and appears to have been better maintained than the city's three other principal crosses, which by 1525 were beginning to show signs of age.[179] However, Ricart almost certainly wished to do more than simply provide a striking illustration for his chronicle of 'this worshipfull towne off Bristut', since his plan, with its circular walls and four imposing gates at the end of each principal thoroughfare, bears a close resemblance to medieval images of the celestial Jerusalem. In other words, the physical layout of streets, gates, walls and buildings assumed a symbolic meaning, becoming a 'map of Christian belief' that served to link the earthly and the heavenly cities, as so eloquently described by St Augustine.[180] When extolling the powerful

[176] Horden, 'Disease, Dragons and Saints', pp. 45–76; Phythian-Adams, *Desolation of a City*, pp. 176–7; Rosser, *Medieval Westminster*, pp. 272–3. Maddern argues that, in Norwich, these processions symbolised the restoration of order after rebellion: 'Order and Disorder', pp. 208–9. Even so, dragons were more commonly associated with pestiferous exhalations, and Norwich's was not only charged with 'gonne powder' so that it could spit flame, but actually reappeared in civic pageants in 1467, a plague year, after a temporary absence caused by factionalism: B. R. McRee, 'Unity or Division? The Social Meaning of Guild Ceremony in Urban Communities', in B. A. Hanawalt and K. L. Reyerson, eds, *City and Spectacle in Medieval Europe* (Minneapolis, 1994), pp. 200, 206 n. 34.

[177] Duffy, *Stripping of the Altars*, pp. 279–80.

[178] R. A. Skelton and P. D. A. Harvey, *Local Maps and Plans from Medieval England* (Oxford, 1986), pp. 309–16.

[179] Ricart, *Maire of Bristowe Is Kalendar*, pp. x–xi, 48, 51.

[180] K. D. Lilley, 'Cities of God? Medieval Urban Forms and their Christian Symbolism', *Transactions of the Institute of British Geographers*, n.s. 29 (2004), pp. 296–313; Lilley, *City and Cosmos*, chap. 1.

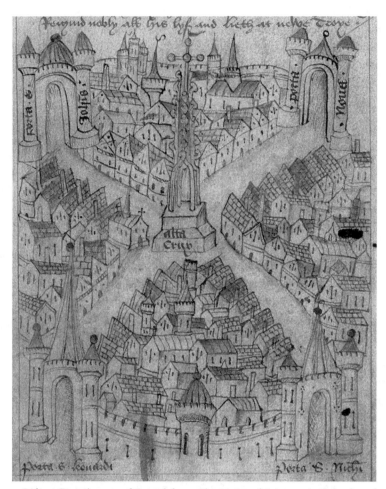

5 Robert Ricart's map of Bristol from *The Maire of Bristowe is Kalendar* of
c. 1480 focuses upon the high cross (*alta crux*) and the cruciform layout of the
streets, reflecting its similarity to the celestial Jerusalem.

protection bestowed upon Chester by virtue of an almost identical street plan, the
Benedictine monk Lucianus (*fl.* 1195) had explicitly likened its four city gates to
the evangelists and its overall layout to that of the City of God. Under the command of Christ, who stood watch over the marketplace, the 'holy guardians' of
these gates, St Michael, St John the Baptist, St Peter and St Werburgh, defended
the residents against the forces of evil. As their patron saint, Werburgh proved a
doughty champion, repaying their trust in times of crisis. When a devastating fire
swept the city in 1180, they invoked her name and, by placing her shrine in the
street, managed to halt the blaze.[181] Celebrated for the healing miracles that she

---

[181] Lucianus of Chester, *Liber Luciani de laude Cestrie*, ed. M. V. Taylor, Lancashire
and Cheshire Record Society 64 (London, 1912), pp. 46–57. For a fuller discussion
of the genre, see J. K. Hyde, 'Medieval Descriptions of Cities', *Bulletin of the John
Rylands Library* 48 (1965–6), pp. 308–40.

worked for the God-fearing residents, Werburgh also turned her wrath upon their enemies, inflicting all manner of horrific afflictions from palsy to blindness, insanity and leprosy upon those who had the temerity to defy her.[182]

Lucianus was writing at the end of the twelfth century, but reliance upon the support of celestial reinforcements lost none of its appeal with the passage of time. The first and most dramatic response to the arrival of plague in Hereford in 1349 was the resumption of work on St Thomas Cantilupe's new shrine, followed by the ceremonial translation of his remains. Convinced that he would 'calm the tumult of the times, drive out the dread infection and lift from them the burden of pestilence', the citizens pinned their hopes upon his intercessionary powers.[183] Statues, as well as relics, could channel these powers. In his will of 1463, John Baret, one of the richest and most ostentatiously pious merchants of Bury St Edmunds, left a generous bequest for rebuilding the town's most dilapidated gate, which was to be 'maad of my coost with fre stoon and bryk, archyd and embatelyd, substancyally to endure'. Above the archway was to be placed 'an ymage of oure lady, sittyng or stondyng, in an howsyng of free stoon, and rememberaunce of me besyde'. While commemorating his bounty through a potent and very public association with the mother of Christ, Baret was simultaneously beautifying the town and strengthening both its physical and spiritual defences.[184] It is tempting to assume that he would have known the prayer for assistance during epidemics addressed to the Virgin Mary by his acquaintance and near neighbour, the Bury monk John Lydgate:

> On vs synneres thi mercy lat doun shyne,
> Off infect heires oppresse al there vttraunce,
> Vs to infect that thei haue no puissaunce;
> From theire batail be thou oure cheef deffennce,
> That theire malis to vs do no grevaunce,
> Off infectynge or strok of pestilence.[185]

A couple of decades later, John Elys of Colchester made similar arrangements for the construction of images of Saints Helen, Margaret and John the Baptist to stand upon the town's east gate, thereby placing his fellow residents under their three-fold protection.[186] Of particular interest in this context is the custom

[182] Henry Bradshaw, *The Life of Saint Werburge of Chester*, ed. C. Horstmann, EETS o.s. 88 (London, 1887), p. 166.

[183] Dohar, *Black Death and Pastoral Leadership*, pp. 59–61. Edward III himself attended the ceremony, no doubt hoping that Cantilupe would save the nation as well as the city.

[184] S. Tymms, ed., *Wills and Inventories from the Registers of the Commissary of Bury St. Edmund's*, CS 49 (London, 1850), p. 37.

[185] John Lydgate, *The Minor Poems of John Lydgate*, ed. H. N. MacCracken, 2 vols, EETS e.s. 107, o.s. 192 (London, 1911, 1934; vol. 2 repr. 1961), I.296. For Baret's association with the elderly Lydgate, see M. Statham, 'John Baret of Bury', *The Ricardian* 13 (2003), pp. 420–31, on p. 426. Bishop Stratford dedicated the chapel in London's West Smithfield plague cemetery to the Virgin Mary in January 1349, before 'a great multitude and with solemn procession': Sloane, *Black Death in London*, p. 47.

[186] *RPBC*, pp. 102–3.

adopted in Dover of delivering a 'trendyll', or great candle wound around a wheel, to the shrine of St Thomas Becket at Canterbury every three years. Being equivalent in length to 'the circumference of the town' (presumably as defined by the walls), this votive offering performed a similar function to Elys's statues; and although it probably predated the Black Death it must have seemed to bestow particular immunity in light of a miracle reported in the plague year of 1467, whereby the martyr vanquished 'a dragon with fyry flamys of helle' and dispelled 'horryble ayere'.[187] These prophylactic measures promised to safeguard communal health as effectively as the more mundane provisions of men like Ralph Hunt (d. 1432) and Thomas Blount (d. 1441), who were both MPs. Hunt left a substantial sum for the repair of Bath's conduits, and Blount bequeathed 500 lb of lead for the construction of pipes to improve Bristol's water supply.[188] Yet they, too, believed that they were sponsoring pious works to the greater glory of God. Indeed, as we shall see in Chapter 4, conduits were frequently embellished with crosses and statues of saints as a further guarantee that their contents would be pure and good to drink.

The fact that particular features of urban topography resonated with Christian symbolism, and, indeed, with latent spiritual power, was recognised with varying degrees of sophistication throughout society, not least because of the many processions and other religious ceremonies which interspersed the liturgical year. On the one hand, the routes taken by participants served to reinforce the intimate connection between the human body, the civic body and the body of the Church, both on earth and in heaven; on the other, the act of procession offered an opportunity for collective supplication and repentance for the many times the inhabitants had faltered on their journey to the celestial Jerusalem.[189] Given the assumption that epidemic disease was ultimately sent by God to chastise, admonish and test sinful humanity, one obvious response was to stage public displays of contrition through the medium of penitential processions. In July 1348 Archbishop Zouche of York decreed that such events should take place twice-weekly throughout his diocese, along with special prayers and masses beseeching divine mercy. He thus apparently became the first English prelate to institute measures against the 'pestilence and infection of the air' then spreading rapidly across continental Europe.[190] Other northern bishops followed his example, and in August Edward III called for similar displays of communal 'entreaty, humility and fasting' in the province of Canterbury. Although, once plague arrived, the emphasis gradually shifted from expiation to straightforward appeals for clemency,

---

[187] S. Sweetinburgh, 'Wax, Stone and Iron: Dover's Town Defences in the Late Middle Ages', *Archaeologia Cantiana* 124 (2004), pp. 183–207, on p. 187; M. Connor, ed., *John Stone's Chronicle, Christ Church Priory, Canterbury, 1417–1472* (Kalamazoo, MI, 2010), p. 118. I am most grateful to Dr Sweetinburgh for drawing my attention to these references. For the 1467 epidemic, see Appendix.

[188] E. Jacob, ed., *The Register of Henry Chichele, Archbishop of Canterbury, 1414–1443*, vol. 2 (Oxford, 1937), p. 464; Roskell, Clark and Rawcliffe, *Commons, 1386–1421*, II.258.

[189] Lilley, 'Cities of God?', pp. 304–7; Lilley, *City and Cosmos*, pp. 159–63.

[190] Horrox, *Black Death*, pp. 111–12.

the practice continued.[191] As late as 1528, by which time rudimentary quarantine measures were in operation for the isolation of victims, Henry VIII gave orders for 'general processions to be made throughout the realm for good weather and for the plague'.[192] Twelve years later the attacks made by Protestant reformers on these 'uplandyshe processions and gangynges about' encountered a considerable setback when the king repeated his instructions during another pestilence.[193] Rituals of this kind have been described as 'corporate strategies for collective health', being little different in their ultimate objective from the more ostensibly pragmatic attempts to create a salubrious urban environment that are discussed later in this book.[194]

Civic processions and the elaborate theatrical productions that often accompanied them also constituted a 'show of unity' or model of how the elite believed the urban body *should* function, very much as the *regimen sanitatis* presented its readers with a tantalising prospect of robust physical health. Corpus Christi day celebrations, in particular, gave magistrates an ideal opportunity to legitimise and reinforce earthly hierarchies through collective devotion to the Eucharist as it was solemnly transported through the streets. In Beverley, for example, 'the worshipful men of a wealthier sort' met in 1411 to discuss the plays that were to be performed not only 'to the praise and honour of God and of the Body of Christ', but also 'for the peaceful union [*unitate*] of the worthier and lesser commons of the town'.[195] How far these rituals actually succeeded in diffusing conflict and cementing 'the wholeness of the social body' is, however, a moot point that has been debated by historians since the appearance in 1983 of a pioneering article by Mervyn James.[196] His contention that Corpus Christi festivities provided the perfect vehicle for resolving the often bitter disputes that erupted between participants, thereby containing far wider social and economic problems, has not gained universal acceptance.[197] And although some of these disagreements do, indeed, appear to have been effectively settled through the medium of arbitration, others proved more intractable and divisive.[198]

[191] Horrox, *Black Death*, pp. 113–19; Dohar, *Black Death and Pastoral Leadership*, pp. 4–5. Asserting that the population of Carlisle had already been 'in great part destroyed' by previous epidemics, in 1369 the bishop once again ordered 'prayers and processions to avert God's wrath': Summerson, *Medieval Carlisle*, I.299.

[192] *LPFD*, IV, part 2, no. 4467.

[193] Duffy, *Stripping of the Altars*, p. 426.

[194] Horden, 'Ritual and Public Health', p. 24.

[195] *BTD*, p. 34. See also James, 'Ritual, Drama and Social Body', p. 10; Lilley, *City and Cosmos*, pp. 135, 170–1.

[196] James, 'Ritual, Drama and Social Body', pp. 3–29. See also Phythian-Adams, 'Ceremony and the Citizen', p. 69.

[197] Most notably by S. Beckwith, *Signifying God: Social Relation and Symbolic Act in the York Corpus Christi Plays* (Chicago, 2001), chap. 3.

[198] In Beverley and Chester, for example, disputes over precedence were settled by the authorities reasonably quickly (*BTD*, p. 35; CCA, M/B/5k, fol. 216), but in late fifteenth-century York the crown had twice to intervene to end a longstanding conflict which threatened 'the perversion and breche of our peas and inquietacon of our subgiets' (*YCR*, II.70–1, 90, 93, 97–100).

According to Miri Rubin, the history of Corpus Christi is as much one of exclusion and instability as it is of cohesion, since the ostensibly 'natural' image of the 'well functioning and harmonious' body invoked by the ruling elite was clearly conceived in its own image, reinforcing a scale of values that marginalised women, the poor and the forces of unskilled labour.[199] But these plays and processions served a wider purpose than simply underwriting the authority of urban oligarchs. As we shall see, the powerful message of the Last Judgement, especially as conveyed in the York pageant, brought home forcibly to spectators the importance of good works in achieving salvation.[200] Mutual support and compassion, the hallmark of a healthy body, extended a promise of paradise. If properly observed, and accompanied by the necessary displays of charity and contrition, the sacramental rituals of Corpus Christi would also safeguard the urban population against disease. Often encircling city walls or perimeters, the route taken by participants appeared, like that of Rogationtide processions, to establish a *cordon sanitaire* around component parts of the built environment. In York the procession and pageant together traced the sign of the cross (the head of which was the Minster), thereby placing the city directly under the protection of Christ, whose body was symbolically superimposed upon it.[201]

More than any other religious ritual, the mass – itself the focal point of Corpus Christi celebrations – promised to heal fractured communities and dispel pestiferous miasmas. Manifest in the Host through the process of transubstantiation, the 'richchest medisyn' of Christ's body constituted a 'cheef restauratyff ... geynst al seeknesse'.[202] John Lydgate described it as the spiritual equivalent of theriac, or 'treacle', a costly prophylactic that was consumed in considerable quantities during plague time:

> Goostely tryacle and our lyves boote,
> Ageynst the sorowes of wordely pestylence,
> Alle infect ayres it puttethe vnder foote
> Of hem that take this bred with reuerence.[203]

During the decades following the Black Death two new masses were introduced for 'turning away plague', one, for the health of the people (*salus populi*), being adopted in southern England by 1382.[204] Many congregations also enlisted the protection of particular saints and of *Christus Medicus* himself by offering masses in their honour. Not surprisingly, appeals to the celestial physician proliferated. In 1468, for example, the Drapers of Coventry secured papal approval for a new

---

[199] M. Rubin, *Corpus Christi: The Eucharist in Late Medieval Culture* (Cambridge, 1992), pp. 247, 260, 263, 269–70. For the exclusive nature of the guild system, see H. Swanson, 'The Illusion of Economic Structure: Craft Guilds in Late Medieval English Towns', *P&P* 121 (1988), pp. 31–48.

[200] Beckwith, *Signifying God*, pp. 112–13; see section 6.6 below.

[201] Lilley, *City and Cosmos*, pp. 172–4.

[202] Lydgate, *Minor Poems*, I.41; J. Bossy, 'The Mass as a Social Institution, 1200–1700', *P&P* 100 (1983), pp. 29–61, on pp. 50–6.

[203] Lydgate, *Minor Poems*, I.39. For the attributes of theriac, see Rawcliffe, *Leprosy in Medieval England*, pp. 220–2.

[204] Horrox, *Black Death*, pp. 120–4; Thomas, *Religion and the Decline of Magic*, p. 37.

altar at the church of St Michael, erected by them specifically for the celebration every Friday of a mass dedicated to Jesus. This weekly ceremony had first been introduced during an outbreak of pestilence some three years earlier by one of their members 'to the end that Almighty God, appeased by the prayers of the faithful, might deliver the said city from the said plague'. Persuaded of its efficacy, the townspeople established a confraternity of Jesus there in 1469; during the epidemic of 1479 a similar mass was instituted at the church of Holy Trinity.[205]

The sanitary, social and religious agendas pursued by the rulers of late medieval and early Tudor English towns formed a coherent and inseparable whole, as closely interconnected as the networks of natural, vital and animal spirits that coursed around the human body. The importance of regarding them in this light will be apparent from the last two sections of this chapter, which examine responses to the specific and interrelated problems of indolence and prostitution. It is, indeed, far easier to understand the growing, but far from novel, tendency to police the more private aspects of human behaviour that many historians have observed from the 1470s onwards if we bear in mind the repeated outbreaks of infectious disease then faced by the urban population. An objective analysis would reveal that, from a national perspective, the demographic impact of these more localised epidemics was considerably less dramatic than that of many earlier pestilences. Yet the combined effect of frequent eruptions of plague in major urban centres and of 'strange and new diseases', such as the Great Pox and sweating sickness, encouraged a belief that mankind had embarked upon an irreversible process of physical and spiritual decline.[206] While attempting to tackle a growing roster of sanitary nuisances, the rulers of English towns and cities were painfully aware of the need to address the problem of moral degeneracy.

2.5 The disease of idleness

Because these communities depended upon their economic health and productivity for survival, it was essential that every able-bodied resident should contribute to the best of his or her ability towards the common profit.[207] Far from marking the advent of a new Protestant work ethic, fear of idleness and a staunch belief in the redemptive powers of honest toil had long exercised a profound influence upon the ruling elites of medieval Europe.[208] It was, after all, to expiate

---

[205] J. A. Twemlow, ed., *Calendar of Papal Letters*, vol. 12: *1458–1471* (London, 1933), pp. 644, 761–2, 772; Phythian-Adams, *Desolation of a City*, p. 118 n. 2.

[206] Slack, *Impact of Plague*, p. 25. See Appendix for a chronological list of epidemics which helps to explain this assumption.

[207] As John Lydgate warned the commons of the realm, 'where slovth hath place there welth es faint and small': R. H. Robbins, ed., *Historical Poems of the XIVth and XVth Centuries* (New York, 1959), p. 233.

[208] J. M. Bowers, 'Piers Plowman and the Unwillingness to Work', *Mediaevalia* 9 (1983), pp. 239–49; M. K. McIntosh, *Controlling Misbehavior in England, 1370–1600* (Cambridge, 1998), pp. 199–200. The interconnected problems, or perceived problems, of idleness and sexual promiscuity are considered at length by Frank Rexroth in the context of official fears about a subversive underworld in late medieval London: *Deviance and Power*, part 1. While there can be little doubt

the Original Sin of its first parents, Adam and Eve, that mankind had to endure an unending sentence of hard labour. According to the regimen allegedly composed by Thomas Aquinas for Hugh III of Cyprus, the ability to eliminate indolence and lead his subjects 'to virtuous works by his laws and precepts, penalties and rewards' ranked as one of the three principal achievements of any successful ruler.[209] And, as we have already seen, the Holy Roman Emperor was advised, in his capacity as 'an expert physician', to purge his realm of the phlegmatic humours that inhibited 'virtuous efforts to gain a livelihood'.[210] Exhortations of this kind drew ample support from the pages of both vernacular and Latin medical literature, where sloth and sickness were frequently linked. Their relevance in an urban context is clearly apparent from royal letters patent of 1352, drawing attention to the army of shiftless vagrants and piles of filth that had accumulated in the streets of Norwich after the Black Death. Although, in this particular instance, any unemployed indigents over sixty were excused from the task of cleaning and repairing public thoroughfares, we should not assume that older men and women were customarily exempt from manual or mental labour.[211] Even elderly and disabled paupers were expected to perform sedentary tasks, such as spinning or sewing, while members of the ruling elite, however advanced in years, could not abandon their responsibilities without good reason.

Notwithstanding the almost universal stipulation that they ought no longer to be capable of gainful employment, the inmates of late medieval urban almshouses were rarely allowed to remain unoccupied. That even the most decrepit could offer daily prayers for the salvation of their benefactors was clearly understood, but some physical exertion might well be required too.[212] For example, statutes marking the refoundation in 1386 of the hospital of St Mary, Yarmouth, assumed that the fitter residents would 'usyn hyr craftys that thei han lernyd, so that thei ben honeste', but forbade them to dissipate their energies in games, idle gossip and drink. In addition, the warden was authorised to compel those brothers and sisters who still remained active 'for to deluyn & wedyn in the gardeyn & to do odyr layth [light] werkys'.[213] At the *maison Dieu* established in Hull almost thirty years later by the wealthy merchant John Gregg, all but the bedridden were required to undertake gardening duties 'by thair best avyle for the welfare of them alle', perhaps as much for therapeutic as moral and economic reasons.[214]

that the authorities exploited contemporary anxieties about disease 'to repress undesirable elements in the population' (p. 3), their campaign against moral miasmas clearly had a wider dimension.

[209] J. M. Blythe, ed. and trans., *On the Government of Rulers: De regimina principium: Ptolemy of Lucca with Portions attributed to Thomas Aquinas* (Philadelphia, 1997), p. 103.

[210] See p. 59 above.

[211] *CPR, 1350–1354*, pp. 283–4.

[212] For the 'labour' of prayer, see section 6.9 below.

[213] Bodleian Library, Oxford, MS Gough Norfolk 20, fol. 30r.

[214] J. Tickell, *History of the Town and County of Kingston-upon-Hull* (Hull, 1798), p. 758. Despite the prohibition placed upon 'servile, manual or labouring work' in the statutes of the almshouse founded in Stamford by the merchant William Browne (d. 1489), residents were employed in quite strenuous activities, such as building

It was, moreover, usual for men and women who seemed relatively 'hole of body' to be enlisted as carers to 'helpe and ministre into their felawes' until they, in turn, needed assistance. The regulations devised in 1442 by the Mercers Company of London for the management of Richard Whittington's almshouse, and early Tudor ordinances for St John's hospital in Lichfield both incorporated such measures, along with predictable strictures about lounging around in taverns and the dangers of any 'ydil wordes' that might fester upon elderly lips.[215]

At the other end of the social spectrum, freedom from the cares of public office was accorded only to those who could present an overwhelming case, and even they might have to provide financial reparation. In York, for example, sick as well as elderly occupants of the aldermanic bench had often to pay heavily for leave to resign, in part because they presented an easy target for the cash-strapped council, but also because of the importance placed upon civic duty.[216] This approach was fairly typical, especially when the pool of available candidates was quite small and it proved difficult to find suitably fit and energetic volunteers. The mayor of Lincoln elected in 1535 had been a widower for many years without much in the way of domestic support and was himself reputedly of 'great age'. The rulers of Norwich at this time were just as inflexible, expecting any sickly or nervous alderman who wished 'to kepe in the country for his helthe' to pay heavily for leave of absence.[217] It was, moreover, a common practice to fine any officials who missed assemblies or arrived late, in order to instil a sense of collective responsibility in leading members of the urban body.[218]

Sloth took many forms, being a deadly sin and thus a threat to the health of the immortal soul as well as the body. Lucianus of Chester's conviction that collective misfortunes were usually attributable to some temporary loss of enthusiasm for almsgiving on the part of the citizens serves as a reminder that spiritual inertia had potentially fatal ramifications for whole communities as well as individuals.[219] Referring specifically to the importance of pious works, but clearly annunciating wider assumptions about the physical dangers of indolence, medieval preachers warmed to this theme. One observed that:

> it is of oure liffe here in this world as it is of the watur of the see, and as of othur watur that stondeth in podels [puddles]. The watur of the see is euermore in contynue mevynge and sterynge, ebbynge and flowynge; but the watur

walls: M. K. McIntosh, *Poor Relief in England, 1300–1600* (Cambridge, 2012), p. 87; Bodleian Library, Oxford, MS Rawl. B.352, fol. 88v. The rulers of Sandwich likewise expected the almsmen and women of St Bartholomew's hospital to weave, plant vegetables and assist at harvest time if their health allowed: BL, MS Cotton Julius B IV, fol. 93r).

[215] J. Imray, *The Charity of Richard Whittington* (London, 1968), pp. 114, 116, 117; Bodleian Library, Oxford, MS Ashmole 855, fols 150v–161r.

[216] Kermode, 'Urban Decline? The Flight from Office', pp. 192–3.

[217] HMC, *Fourteenth Report*, appendix 8, p. 34; NRO, NCR, 16C/2, Assembly Minute Book, 1510–1550, fol. 243v.

[218] Maddern, 'Order and Disorder', p. 195; NRO, Y/C18/1, fols 26r, 28v; Kermode, 'Urban Decline? The Flight from Office', p. 189.

[219] Lucianus of Chester, *Liber Luciani*, p. 42.

against sloth/ languores

that stondeth in podels meves not, but is in reste. Where-fore it vaxes sone corrupte and stynkynge ... ryght so man that is not goyinge ne wirchynge in good verkes vexeth corrupte and stynkynge thorowe dedelye synne.[220]

The conventional assumption that the idle would forfeit 'reste in the liffe that euermore shall laste in the blisse of heven' is here rendered all the more persuasive when clothed in the language of the contemporary plague tract. Not surprisingly, fear of the miasmatic exhalations arising from the stagnant depths of filthy, polluted souls found frequent expression in ecclesiastical propaganda, most notably in the years following the Black Death. And by the same process of cross-fertilisation, the physicians who composed plague *concilia* increasingly warned their readers that divine wrath would surely light upon those who proved negligent in the discharge of their pious obligations. Thomas Forestier's solemn caveat at the start of his treatise against 'the venymous feuer of pestilens' – that there was little point in adopting prophylactic measures unless one had first attended with due diligence to the business of prayer and almsgiving – is representative of many.[221]

Humoral theory provided moralists and physicians alike with yet more powerful ammunition in their ongoing battle against physical and spiritual lassitude. Ranking along with relaxation as one of the six 'non-naturals' itemised in the *regimen sanitatis*, exercise was regarded as essential for physical and mental health, notably by stimulating the production of wholesome humoral matter, assisting the effective absorption of food, enabling the body to eliminate any potential superfluity or source of putrefaction and strengthening the musculature.[222] Inertia would inevitably lead to sickness, if not death, as these vital mechanisms ceased to function and the system was overwhelmed by phlegmatic torpor. At the very least, feckless 'ale drinkers and taverne haunters', who 'heped up in their bodies moche evill matter', would more readily succumb to infection when epidemics struck.[223] Elaborating this point, John Mirfield (d. 1407), a London priest who produced two *regimina*, probably for use in St Bartholomew's hospital, Smithfield, explained that, 'just as stagnant waters putrefy and iron and all other metal rusts from lack of use, so is excessive rest the creator, nurse and multiplier of evil humours and the begetter of corruption in members of the body and in the human blood'.[224] It was,

[220] W. O. Ross, ed., *Middle English Sermons Edited from British Museum MS Royal 18 B XXIII*, EETS o.s. 209 (London, 1940), p. 75.

[221] BL, Add. MS 27582, fol. 71r. See also *Here Begynneth A Litill Boke Necessarye & Behouefull agenst the Pestilence* (London, 1485), fol. 3v; R. Palmer, 'The Church, Leprosy and Plague in Medieval and Early Modern Europe', *SCH* 19 (1982), pp. 79–99, on pp. 86, 89.

[222] Gil-Sotres, 'Regimens of Health', pp. 304–8. By the same token, overindulgence, as manifest in 'rere soperis [suppers] of grete excesse, of nodding hedis & of candel lyght', would inevitably result in 'slouth at morowe & slumbryng ydilnysse, which of al vyces is chef norysse [nurse]': Wellcome Institute Library, Western MS 411, fol. 3r.

[223] John Caius, *A Boke, or Conseill against the Disease Commonly Called the Sweate, or Sweatyng Sicknesse* (London, 1552), fols 20v, 29v. His argument was then centuries old: see sections 5.1 and 5.5 below.

[224] BL, MS Royal 7 F XI, fol. 129v.

therefore, vital to set the young on the right track. In a powerful sermon clearly directed at an urban congregation, Robert Rypon warned self-indulgent parents that they were setting a lethal example to their children:

> These people eat and drink, not to restore their natural heat but rather to slake the unnatural heat that is generated by too great an excess in their gullet ... And further, it is commonly the case that such people are sleepy and consequently lazy and accidious, not by nature, as children are, but from too great an excess, like pigs. Now since this disposition comes to children from their natural complexion, nature has also provided a remedy, because from natural love their parents *want to keep them in bodily health* [my italics]. Hence, good parents do not allow their children to be idle, but keep them busy in some craft, work or labour against *accidia*, and they give them food and drink in moderation against gluttony.[225]

The dangers of idleness figure even more prominently in the vernacular *Regiment de la cosa publica* composed in 1383 by the Franciscan friar Francesc Eiximenis for the guidance of the magistrates of Valencia. In it he urged all citizens, whatever their rank, to play an active part in promoting the health of the urban body, lest it succumb to the dropsy of sloth. The wealthy and literate should spend their time learning about 'the regimen of the community and its life, or something equally profitable', in order to become wise and moral rulers.[226] Nobody should lack employment, since the improvident drone would have the same effect upon society as a useless limb that withers and dies. For this reason, Eiximenis favoured a system subsequently developed by sixteenth-century reformers, whereby support would be denied to all but the most deserving cases.[227] In many respects his recommendations anticipate the ideal community depicted by Sir Thomas More over 130 years later in *Utopia*. Although, in accordance with current literature on health, the magistrates of this model republic recognised the manifold benefits of recreation, they abhorred idleness or indulgence, expecting the inhabitants to devote their leisure to gardening, study and other inherently *useful* activities.[228]

The deployment of medical metaphors sprang readily to other humanist scholars such as Thomas Starkey, whose stay in early sixteenth-century Padua would have exposed him to the work of many 'experte physycyonys'. Hoping to remedy the chronic 'faute & sykenes' that had afflicted the entire country during the 1520s, he warned that the 'polytyke body' had become 'replenyschyd & over fulfyllyd wyth many yl humorys, wych I cal idul & unprofytabul personys'.[229]

---

[225] S. Wenzel, 'Preaching the Seven Deadly Sins', in R. Newhauser, ed., *In the Garden of Evil: The Vices and Culture in the Middle Ages* (Toronto, 2005), p. 167.

[226] Francesc Eiximenis, *Regiment de la Cosa Publica*, ed. P. D. de Molins de Rei (Barcelona, 1927), p. 128.

[227] Eiximenis, *Regiment de la Cosa Publica*, pp. 124–5, 127. See, for example, Salter, *Some Early Tracts on Poor Relief*, p. 65.

[228] More, *Utopia*, pp. 40–1.

[229] Starkey, *Dialogue between Pole and Lupset*, p. 52. For Starkey's use of anatomical and medical imagery, see J. G. Harris, *Foreign Bodies and the Body Politic:*

Although he blamed a parasitic horde of baronial retainers and underemployed clergy rather than improvident paupers for undermining the health of the nation, Starkey identified the same debilitating symptoms:

> For lyke as in a dropcy the body ys unweldy, unlusty & slo, no thyng quyke to move, nother apte nor mete to any maner of exercyse, but solve wyth yl humorys lyth idul & unprofytabul to al utward labur, so ys a commynalty replenyschyd wyth neclygent & idul pepul as unlusty & unweldy, no thyng quyke in the exercyse of artys & craftys, wherby hyr welth schold be mayntenyd & supportyd, but ... boyllyth out wyth al vyce, myschefe & mysery, the wych out of idulnes as out of a fountayn yssuth & spryngyth.[230]

His diagnosis was eloquent but far from original. Well before this date, historians have observed a growing preoccupation on the part of urban magistrates with the corrosive effects of indolence and attendant misrule.[231] When attempting to discriminate between the respectable and feckless poor in the later fourteenth century, prominent Londoners blamed the 'ill governance' (*malam gubernationem*) of the latter, very much as a physician might bewail the intemperate behaviour of an uncooperative patient.[232]

In late medieval Nottingham, too, David Marcombe detects 'an increased effort directed against patterns of perceived antisocial behaviour which it was believed might undermine the moral basis or economic wellbeing of the community'.[233] Beginning in about 1463 with a 'comprehensive set of orders' directed against brothels, suspicious alehouses and other presumed dens of iniquity, this crusade extended to games and sporting activities that lured impressionable apprentices and servants away from more reputable pursuits. Here, as elsewhere, the enthusiasm with which a statute of 1388, forbidding the playing of dice and other '*jeues importunes*' by working men, was enforced owed more to a vendetta against the workshy than the desire to maintain regular archery practice (which was the original intention).[234] Before too long, anyone given to 'myspendyng hys tyme in ydelnesse', or simply lounging about, faced an uncomfortable interview with Nottingham's magistrates. In 1482, for example, two local men were indicted on the charge that, on Monday 24 June 'and divers other days and occasions, commonly and usually', they had wandered around 'unemployed in the streets and

Discourses of Social Pathology in Early Modern England (Cambridge, 1998), pp. 30–40; and Hale, *The Body Politic*, pp. 61–8.

[230] Starkey, *Dialogue between Pole and Lupset*, p. 54.

[231] McIntosh detects a sharp rise from the 1460s onwards: *Controlling Misbehavior*, pp. 88–93.

[232] Barron, *London in the Later Middle Ages*, pp. 276–7.

[233] D. Marcombe, 'The Late Medieval Town, 1149–1560', in J. Beckett, ed., *A Centenary History of Nottingham* (Manchester, 1997), p. 93.

[234] *SR*, vol. 2, 12 Richard II, cap. 6, p. 57; 11 Henry IV, cap. 4, p. 163. Urban guilds played a major role in disciplining their members. In 1490, for example, the Shoemakers of Norwich imposed a substantial fine of 6s. 8d. upon journeymen and servants who were 'gretly disposed to riot and idelnes', sleeping late on Sundays and missing divine service as a result: *RCN*, II.104.

roads of the said town, and will not work although they be able in body to labour, to the pernicious example of other lieges of our Lord the King'.[235]

In parallel with measures for the elimination of sturdy beggars and other undesirables, many towns and cities took active steps to prevent temporarily unemployed artisans from lapsing into lazy ways. In a ruling designed to curb the independence of potentially unruly 'wyfes, doughtours and maidens', as well as to prevent skilled craftsmen from languishing 'vagaraunt and vnoccupied', Bristol's magistrates introduced measures in 1461 to restrict the employment of female weavers when men were available.[236] Those who lacked motivation had to be galvanised into activity. The constables of Lincoln were instructed in 1518 to round up all 'idle persons' and bring them before the mayor so that they could be suitably admonished and either put to work or expelled from the city.[237] Shortly afterwards, every journeyman or labourer who reached the end of his contract in King's Lynn was obliged to present himself at a designated spot in the Tuesday Market for one hour at the start of each working day in the hope of finding a new master. Anyone who failed to appear or otherwise proved reluctant 'to wurke & labour dayly, if God send hym his helthe, for th'entent to get his lyvyng' was to be regarded as a vagabond and punished accordingly.[238]

Reflecting the author's conviction that it was better to stifle temptation at birth, Thomas More's *Utopia* is notable for the lack of opportunities for the young to 'loaf or kill time', especially in alehouses, taverns, gambling dens and brothels, all of which were strictly prohibited.[239] For idleness was not only a threat to the spiritual and physical health of individuals and communities alike, but also a first step on the road to far greater dangers, of which inebriation was by no means the worst. Orders enacted in London in 1417 (a plague year) for the closure of public stews, or bath-houses, stressed not only the potential for crime and disorder wherever 'lewd men and women' congregated, but the likelihood that vulnerable young people with time on their hands would be enticed there to explore 'the illicit works of their lewd flesh'. The imposition of hefty fines of £20 upon anyone who contravened measures intended for 'the pleasing of God, the salvation of their own souls, the removal of the evils aforesaid and the *purifying* and decency of the said City' underscores the seriousness with which the ruling elite embarked upon its mission.[240] As was so often the case, however, the inflated scale of penalties also suggests a keen awareness, born of experience, that attempts to eliminate

---

[235] Stevenson, *Records of the Borough of Nottingham*, II.325; and also III.372. A list of suspect persons to be reported by the Yarmouth leet courts at this time included 'all vacabondes that be idyll & use none ocupacion, but excersise tavernes and alehouses & use unleffull pleyes, as dise, cardes, coytes, etc', anyone who slept in daytime (and thus shunned honest work), and the people who received them: NRO, Y/C18/1, fol. 16v.

[236] *LRBB*, II.127–8. For the wider background to this ordinance, see Goldberg, 'Coventry's "Lollard" Programme', p. 98.

[237] HMC, *Fourteenth Report*, appendix 8, p. 27.

[238] KLBA, KL/C7/5, Hall Book, 1497–1544, fol. 229r.

[239] More, *Utopia*, p. 49.

[240] *CLB*, I, p. 178; Riley, *Memorials of London*, p. 647.

the moral and physical dangers of prostitution would prove as daunting as other efforts to sanitise the urban environment.[241]

2.6 Prostitution

Much has been written about the social and economic history of the sex trade in medieval English towns, not least with regard to the information that it yields about attitudes to gender. While recognising that beliefs about male and female physiology helped to frame responses to prostitution, scholars have paid less attention to the ways in which considerations of health and hygiene may have influenced the efforts made by magistrates to control the behaviour of 'commune strumpetes, bawdes, or ony other otherwyse mysrewlyd'.[242] As Ruth Karras observes in her comprehensive study of 'common women', these 'ill-governed' creatures not only subverted the norms of acceptable female conduct, but also appeared to spread crime and discord throughout the civic body.[243] Since, however, they were widely recognised as a necessary evil, providing an outlet for male sexuality while preserving the honesty of decent women, most authorities took the practical step of regulation rather than vainly attempting to eradicate the problem altogether. The relative freedom enjoyed by the north European female labour force, at least in comparison with the south, meant that prostitution was a more transient, casual activity, to which women turned when times were hard, rather than regarding it as a permanent source of employment. As a result, institutionalised brothels were rare, and the main challenge faced by magistrates was to ensure that any potential hazards posed by street-walkers and suspect houses were contained, very much in the way of other insalubrious civic nuisances, including drains, vagrant pigs, dung hills and noxious industries.[244] Steps were taken to confine prostitution to the urban periphery, where such environmental pollutants as tanneries, slaughterhouses, smithies and lime kilns were also to be found, well away from the sensitive nostrils of the elite.[245]

---

[241] Sure enough, this complete ban was replaced by a more realistic licensing system in 1428: Barron, *London in the Later Middle Ages*, p. 259.

[242] HMC, *Ninth Report*, part 1, Royal Commission on Historical Manuscripts 8 (London, 1883), appendix, p. 288.

[243] R. M. Karras, *Common Women: Prostitution and Sexuality in Medieval England* (Oxford, 1996), pp. 5, 16–19, 31, 40. See also McIntosh, *Controlling Misbehavior*, pp. 69–74.

[244] P. J. P. Goldberg, 'Pigs and Prostitutes: Streetwalking in Comparative Perspective', in K. J. Lewis, N. J. Menuge and K. M. Phillips, eds, *Young Medieval Women* (Stroud, 1999), pp. 172–93; Karras, *Common Women*, p. 66. For an account of the Bankside Stews, where the sex trade was regulated, see Carlin, *Medieval Southwark*, chap. 9.

[245] Françoise Choay observes tellingly that the use of anatomical metaphors in an urban context never extended to the sexual organs, which remained '*en marge du texte*': 'La Ville et le domaine', p. 246. The zoning of prostitutes and baths was not a medieval development, having been adopted by the Romans: Horden, 'Ritual and Public Health', pp. 36–7. Indeed, the intimate relationship between physical and moral hygiene was clearly apparent in Roman towns: A. Wallace-Hadrill, 'Public

With characteristic pragmatism, the rulers of Hull banned prostitutes (*meretrices*) from the town centre, while renting accommodation to them on the foreland and in the towers round the walls. As in so many other English towns, these women were expected to wear coloured hoods, which in 1444–5 were supplied out of public funds, perhaps in recognition of the fact that they occupied a recognised – albeit marginal – position in society, but principally, as we will see, because it was important that they should be easily identifiable.[246] The jurats of Winchelsea, too, appear to have accepted that, since commercial sex could never be entirely eliminated, some of the profits might at least be diverted into the common coffers through a substantial quarterly rate levied upon any 'common woman' who worked within the walls. Additional fines of 3s. 4d. imposed in 1472 for soliciting after curfew would effectively have confined most activity to daylight hours and thus have reduced the likelihood of disorder even further.[247] In Southampton, one of the very few English towns to sanction the provision of an official brothel (ostensibly for the sole use of 'galleymen' and other sailors visiting the port), the authorities actually derived their largest single source of income from fines for immoral behaviour imposed upon married residents found there and on prostitutes who entered the town without wearing the prescribed dress.[248]

More sweeping offensives against prostitution grew apace during the later fifteenth century, but were certainly not a new phenomenon, being recorded at such times of crisis as the famine years of the early fourteenth century and in 1439, when acute food shortages increased the number of 'strumpetys' attempting to earn a crust on the streets of English cities.[249] Jeremy Goldberg has drawn attention to the close proximity in urban regulations from at least the fourteenth century of measures against wandering pigs and 'women of evil name', stressing the shared imagery of gluttony, lust and vagrancy that linked one with the other, the swine as agents of physical pollution and the females as a moral menace.[250] Deriving from a rather free rendition of a passage in St Augustine's *De ordine*, the analogy between 'common women' and public sewers was equally widespread. However noisome and unpleasant they might be, the removal of either would create a

Honour and Private Shame: The Urban Texture of Pompeii', in T. J. Cornell and K. Lomas, eds, *Urban Society in Roman Italy* (London, 1995), pp. 50–1.

[246] K. J. Allison, ed., *VCH York, East Riding*, vol. 1 (London, 1969), p. 75.

[247] BL, MS Cotton Julius B IV, fol. 25v. The Chester authorities also favoured a type of licensing during the fifteenth century: Laughton, *Life in a Late Medieval City*, pp. 125, 160–1.

[248] Butler, *Book of Fines*, pp. xx–xxi. Having established a brothel for the confinement of the town's prostitutes, the rulers of Sandwich embarked in 1523 upon a policy designed to contain all licensed beggars in St John's hospital, while rounding up any other undesirables and expelling them altogether: Clarke *et al.*, *Sandwich: A Study of the Town and Port*, p. 135; S. Sweetinburgh, *The Role of the Hospital in Medieval England* (Dublin, 2004), pp. 208 n. 14, 238–9.

[249] Hudson, *Leet Jurisdiction*, pp. 58–9; R. F. Isaacson and H. Ingleby, eds, *The Red Register of King's Lynn*, 2 vols (King's Lynn, n.d.), I.64; Kingsford, *Chronicles of London*, p. 146.

[250] Goldberg, 'Pigs and Prostitutes', pp. 172–4; Goldberg, 'Coventry's 'Lollard' Programme', pp. 104–5, 107. For the regulation of swine, see section 3.6 below.

flood of noxious waste that threatened to engulf the entire community.[251] Such a pungent choice of simile is hardly surprising, given the connection made at all social levels between the moral miasma of lechery and the disease-bearing stench of excrement, sometimes in the most literal of contexts.[252] In 1422, for example, just five years after the above-mentioned attempt to close down London's stews, the jurors of Cripplegate Ward Without indicted once such place as

> a common house of harlotry and bawdry, and a great resort of thieves and also of priests and their concubines, to the great disgrace of the city and the danger and mischief of the neighbours and passers-by, and likewise ... the privy of the stew-house as a nuisance because of the great corruption coming therefrom.[253]

We should also note the frequency with which ordinances about street-walking appear in tandem with provisions for purging the urban body of infectious matter. In fourteenth-century Bristol, bye-laws to do with 'common women' were recorded alongside edicts concerning the removal of lepers and disposal of dung.[254] Shortly afterwards, the compiler of London's *Liber albus* indexed rules about prostitutes and brothels together with measures for the avoidance of health hazards such as polluted wells.[255] In contemporary eyes these kinds of nuisance seemed remarkably similar.

Following complaints made to the crown during the plague year of 1459 by the Cambridge university authorities, the chancellor was authorised to punish anyone who blocked roads or polluted waterways in the town 'by casting of dung, corrupt earth, foetid water, garbage, and intestines of slain beasts, carcasses and other filth'. He was also empowered to expel 'all prostitutes and immodest and incontinent women' living within a radius of four miles.[256] Orders promulgated in

---

[251] Augustine, *De ordine*, in *Contra academicos; De beata vita; De ordine; De magistro; De libero arbitrio*, ed. W. M. Green and K. D. Daur, Corpus Christianorum Series Latina 29 (Turnhout, 1970), II.iv.12, p. 114. For the most celebrated reiteration of this argument, frequently misquoted by historians of prostitution, see Blythe, *On the Government of Rulers*, p. 254.

[252] William of Conches describes the uterus of a prostitute 'after frequent acts of coitus' as being 'clogged with dirt' (D. Jacquart and C. Thomasset, *Sexuality and Medicine in the Middle Ages* (Oxford, 1985), p. 25), while Chaucer's Parson in *The Canterbury Tales* compares 'fool woomen' in brothels to ' a commune gong [privy], where as men purgen hire ordure' (Geoffrey Chaucer, *The Riverside Chaucer*, ed. L. D. Benson (Oxford, 1987), p. 319, l. 884). The 'turpis vicus' or 'dyrt vicus' noted in a late medieval tourist's guide to Norwich was so named because of the prostitutes who congregated there: E. Rutledge, 'Economic Life', in Rawcliffe and Wilson, *Medieval Norwich*, p. 182.

[253] *CPMRL, 1413–1417*, p. 154.

[254] *LRBB*, II.229; E. W. W. Veale, ed., *The Great Red Book of Bristol*, vol. 1, Bristol Record Society 4 (Bristol, 1933), p. 143. Legislation introduced in Florence to curb the spread of plague in April 1348 restricted both the emptying of privies and soliciting by prostitutes to specific times and places: Park, *Doctors and Medicine*, p. 4.

[255] *MGL*, III.234.

[256] Cooper, *Annals of Cambridge*, pp. 209–10. In Sandwich, the first sustained efforts to remove 'badly goverened' women can also be dated to the 1460s, when the town

Leicester in 1467 (when there was another epidemic) for the elimination of similar threats extended not just to 'corrupcion in the strettes', 'fylthe and swepynges' and 'muke', but also to brothels, bawds and general immorality. Offenders reported to the court by watchful residents were to be ejected 'at the fyrst warnyng in payne of imprisonment and fyne'.[257] Having introduced measures for the compulsory removal of waste to extramural 'muckhylles', the rulers of Stamford turned predictably at this time to 'the greatt occasyon of synn and mysruell' presented by tapsters, or barmaids, and other loose women. They decreed that:

> every tapester in this towne nowe beyng, every woman sogerrant [sojourning] whos guydyng and rule hath nott ben knowen goodd, every woman vacabound, every woman inhabyte gyven to idylnes, unto whom the said tapesters and the other woman hath ben coadherent, that they and iche of them departe and avoyd owt of the towne by Sundaye in senytt [next] uppon payn … to be ledde abought the towne with hoodds of sey [silk] upon ther heds unto the cukestole [ducking stool] and ther to be sowsid, and so shamefullye to be dryven owt of this towne withowt any specyall grace or pardon.[258]

It was, significantly, in preparation for the penitential season of Lent (and in the aftermath of the first outbreak of sweating sickness) that the rulers of York issued directives a couple of decades later for cleaning the streets, along with a proclamation requiring all 'misruled people to avode evere parish out of the citie to the utter partes of the suburbs'.[259] In the Durham borough of Crossgate, too, court orders regarding stray pigs, noisome latrines and the dumping of garbage merged seamlessly with others forbidding the reception or accommodation of any woman 'badly and dishonestly governed of her body' ('male et inhoneste gubernacionis sui corporis') and of idle vagabonds. Fears of this nature were compounded in 1498 by anxiety lest travellers might bring with them the pestilence then raging in Bishop Auckland, but there were other, more alarming ways in which resort to 'common women' might spread epidemics.[260]

Stringent measures for the removal of 'comyn qwenys', 'baudys' and female yarn pickers from the streets of Gloucester were introduced in about 1500 by the ruling elite as a necessary means of restoring public order. Prompt action seemed especially desirable because the city had become a byword for scandal,

was struggling to recover from heavy losses inflicted by the plague of 1457: Clarke et al., *Sandwich: A Study of the Town and Port*, pp. 135, 137.

[257] *RBL*, II.290–1.

[258] A. Rogers, ed., *William Browne's Town: The Stamford Hall Book*, vol. 1: *1465–1492* (Stamford, 2005), p. 36, and p. 99 for further injunctions against the accommodation of 'suspect women'.

[259] L. C. Attreed, ed., *York House Books, 1461–1490*, 2 vols (Stroud, 1991), II.465–6.

[260] *RBC*, nos 140, 699, 706, 712. See also nos 155, 270, 325, 458, 483, 534, 556, 573, 625, 630, 642, 654, 668, 672, 676, 688. Concern that vagrants would spread infection were subsequently voiced in Edinburgh in 1505 (Marwick, *Records of the Burgh of Edinburgh*, p. 107) and at Basingstoke in 1521, when they were ordered to return to the places of their birth, lest 'lest the disease should come by them or any other misfortune, till it please God to send it' (Baigent and Millard, *History of the Town and Manor of Basingstoke*, p. 325).

being 'abomynable spokyn of in alle England and Walys' because of 'the vicyous lyvyng of dyvers personez, as well spyrtuell as temperall, with to[o] excidyng nowmbre of commyn strompettes and bawdes dwellyng in every ward'.[261] In light of its unenviable reputation as the Sodom or Gomorrah of the early Tudor commonwealth, Gloucester's magistrates also 'feryd leste Alle Myghty God wole caste his greate vengeaunce uppon the said towne in shorte tyme'. As a result, they decided to adopt the practice of imprisoning flagrant offenders and of parading shaven-headed prostitutes as a public spectacle through the streets 'as hit is usid in the worshipfull citie of London and in the towne of Bristow'.[262] We shall encounter many similar examples of concern for collective 'fame' and of the conscious borrowing of regulations that had been successfully adopted elsewhere in subsequent chapters of this book. Of more immediate interest is the assumption that lechery would rapidly incur divine retribution.[263]

The Cities of the Plain had been destroyed by fire, which remained a constant hazard in all pre-modern towns.[264] Yet epidemic disease must have seemed a more likely prospect, especially as 'fleschely lust with wymmen' ranked as one of the principal sources of 'putrifacion & stinking' likely to generate pestilence in communities as well as individuals.[265] The causes of infection were both moral and physical. On the one hand, as preachers and the authors of many plague *concilia* warned, epidemic diseases were the arrows discharged by God as a specific punishment for idleness and debauchery, which were even deadlier than the mephitic air from rotting garbage and noxious drains. In a sermon delivered during the pestilence of 1375, Bishop Thomas Brinton exhorted his congregation to repentance on the ground that, just as God had wrecked vengeance upon sinners in the Old Testament, so too the people of England were being punished for a vicious combination of sloth and 'the corruption of lechery'.[266]

[261] HMC, *Twelfth Report*, appendix 9: *The manuscripts of the Duke of Beaufort, K. G., the Earl of Donoughmore, and others*, Royal Commission on Historical Manuscripts 27 (London, 1891), p. 435. Ordinances were then also introduced for the expulsion of beggars and the cleaning of the streets.

[262] The ritual of public humiliation, which was similar to that employed for the punishment of men and women who sold contaminated food and drink, is described in *MGL*, III.180–8.

[263] Minutes recording the interrogation of two procuresses before the mayor of Lynn in 1312 describe them as plying their trade '*ad damnum et periculum totius communitatis*', which clearly suggests fear of divine wrath: Isaacson and Ingleby, *Red Register of King's Lynn*, I.64. Voicing his own Protestant suspicions of clerical negligence and avarice, John Stow claimed that the people of London themselves took action against 'such filthinesse' in 1383 because they feared 'least through God's vengeance, either the pestilence or sworde should happen to them': John Stow, *Survey of London*, ed. C. L. Kingsford, 2 vols (Oxford, 1908), II.189–90. Certainly, a bawd convicted in 1385 was said to have placed the City 'in great peril': Riley, *Memorials of London*, pp. 484–6.

[264] See section 3.8 below.

[265] *Here Begynneth A Litill Boke*, fol. 3v.

[266] Horrox, *Black Death*, pp. 143–9. Significantly, one of the government's first responses to the cholera epidemic of 1832 was to institute a 'National Day of Fasting and Humiliation'. The outbreak was widely blamed upon the 'bad, dirty,

On the other, Erasmus' warning that the vigilant Christian should 'eschewe as a certayne pestylence the communycacion of corrupte and wanton persons' assumed a real as well as a metaphorical significance, since his readers would have understood the physical risks posed by association with prostitutes in times of plague.[267]

As we have seen, bath houses were often a byword for sexual licence, but even their more legitimate services prompted concern during epidemics, when it was important to keep as cool as possible and abstain from any form of activity likely to generate heat. Not surprisingly, given his monastic background, John Lydgate highlighted both the spiritual and somatic dangers of 'stiwes' in his *Dietary and Doctrine for Pestilence*. Whoever wished to remain 'holle & kepe hym from sekenesse' was urged to shun both the 'incontynence' and exposure to warm, infected air that would occur when frequenting them.[268] A vernacular version of John of Burgundy's popular plague tract, transcribed in the commonplace book of a fifteenth-century Yorkshire gentleman, also advises the reader to 'vse none excesse nor surfete in mete & drynke, nor bathes, nor [to] swete noghte gretly', since open pores would allow 'venomous ayere' to seep throughout the entire body. Couched in the original Latin, almost certainly for greater emphasis, there follows a solemn warning against sexual intercourse because of its tendency to weaken the vital spirits just as they were most needed to combat infection.[269] It is surely no coincidence that a campaign against disorderly houses in Ipswich began during the pestilence of 1465, leading to at least fifteen prosecutions in 1468 and the introduction five years later (after another major epidemic) of orders for the expulsion of all 'harlots and bawds'.[270] Measures for the removal of procurers and prostitutes from the wards of London had long been regarded as essential for 'the *cleanliness* and honesty of the said City', but references to the pervasive miasmas of sexual depravity likewise became more explicit at this time.[271] One order for the arrest and expulsion of all 'common women' from the

---

drunken and idle people': P. K. Gilbert, *Cholera and Nation: Doctoring the Social Body in Victorian England* (Albany, NY, 2008), pp. 20–1.

[267] Desiderius Erasmus, *Enchiridion militis Christiani*, ed. A. M. O'Donnell, EETS o.s. 282 (London, 1981), p. 191.

[268] Lydgate, *The Minor Poems*, II.702.

[269] 'Et super omnia alia nocet coitus & accelerat ad hunc morbum quod maxime aperit poros et destruit spiritus vitales': M. S. Ogden, ed., *The liber de diversis medicinis*, EETS o.s. 207 (London, 1938), p. 51. Some plague tracts were more overtly moral, observing that 'men that abusen them self with wymmen or vsen ofte times bathes … be more disposed to this sekenes' (*Here Begynneth A Litill Boke*, fol. 3r), or singling out 'those who were too full and plethoric, idle and base, performing the venereal act without discretion and measure' (C. Nockels Fabbri, 'Continuity and Change in Late Medieval Plague Medicine' (PhD thesis, Yale University, 2006), pp. 55–6).

[270] Only three presentments against the promotion of fornication and adultery are recorded before 1465 (in 1416 and 1419): SROI, C/2/8/1/3–4. After 1465 they became quite regular: C/2/8/1/13, 15–16, 19, 21; C/2/10/1/2–5, 7. For the ordinance, see Nicholas Bacon, *Annalls of Ipswiche*, ed. W. H. Richardson (Ipswich, 1884), p. 135. For the pestilence, see Appendix.

[271] *MGL*, III.179; McSheffrey, *Marriage, Sex and Civic Culture*, p. 179.

capital refers specifically to the 'the stynkyng and horrible synne of lechery, the whiche daily groweth and is used more than it hath been in the daies past, by the meanes of strumpettes, mysguyded and idil women, daily vagraunt and walkyng aboute'.[272]

Whereas pestilence might be regarded as collective punishment periodically inflicted by God upon whole communities, sexually transmitted disease was a more immediate and individual consequence of recourse to infected prostitutes. By the later Middle Ages the dangers of consorting with 'common women' were well known and comprehensively documented. Vernacular remedy books and surgical texts prescribed numerous ointments and potions for occasions when 'a man is sumtyme seke in his yerde [penis] be cause of a foule woman ... so that the corupcioun is', noting such different symptoms as 'pymplys or aposteem [swelling] ... gret heet & brennyng & pricking & ache & reednesse', as well as the generally corrosive effects of 'venimous mater'.[273] In order to provide some rudimentary safeguards for patrons, fifteenth-century regulations for the Southwark stews prohibited the employment of women with 'any sikeness of brennynge', which is generally believed to have been gonorrhoea, or the 'perilous infirmite'.[274] This unspecified complaint may well have been endemic or venereal syphilis, but there were other possibilities. While stressing that all manner of unpleasant venereal diseases could arise from coitus with a woman whose vagina was 'full of impure and virulent matter', moralists tended to focus upon the danger of contracting leprosy, largely because it provided such powerful propaganda against the snares of lust.[275]

The comparative immunity apparently enjoyed by women in this regard was explained in terms of their denser and colder complexions, which rendered the uterus 'hard and extremely resistant to male corruption'. The semen produced from the contaminated blood of a leper would thus remain secure within its protective walls, transforming into a toxic vapour that would be readily absorbed by another sexual partner. Since men were temperamentally far hotter than women, the poisonous miasma would be drawn through the open pores of the penis into the bloodstream and thence throughout the entire body.[276] Women who frequently engaged in sexual relations with lepers were deemed to become more vulnerable, as the jurors who in 1500 indicted the notorious Yarmouth prostitute and brothel-keeper Alice Dymok for being *leprosa* must smugly have

---

[272] *CLB*, L, p. 206.

[273] Glasgow University Library Special Collections, MS Hunter 95, fols 132r–133r; MS Hunter 307, fols 145v–146r; MS Hunter 509, fols 161v–162v.

[274] J. Post, 'A Fifteenth-Century Customary for the Southwark Stews', *Journal of the Society of Archivists* 5 (1977), pp. 418–28, on p. 426. One chronicler reported grimly that, on his 1475 expedition to France, Edward IV 'lost many a man that fylle to the lust of women, & wer brent be them; & there membrys rottyd away, & they dyed': F. W. D. Brie, ed., *The Brut*, vol. 1, EETS o.s. 131 (London, 1906), p. 604. For the army's resort to infected prostitutes, see also *PL*, II.414.

[275] Robert of Brunne, *Robert of Brunne's 'Handlyng Synne'*, ed. F. J. Furnivall, 2 vols, EETS o.s. 119, 123 (London, 1901, 1903; repr. in 1 vol., 1973), pp. 237–8; Jacquart and Thomasset, *Sexuality and Medicine*, chap. 5.

[276] Rawcliffe, *Leprosy in Medieval England*, pp. 82–3.

observed.[277] And since leprosy was regarded as a progressive condition that might be successfully treated, or at least kept in remission, if it were caught early enough, it is easy to see why so many of the transient symptoms today associated with sexually transmitted diseases were then regarded as incipient signs of the disease. Predictably, in view of these assumptions, some medical authorities described the Great Pox, or 'French disease', as an unusually contagious type of *lepra*.[278]

Late medieval physicians and surgeons warned of the risks posed by sexual congress with women like Alice, who were known to consort with suspect or known lepers. They itemised the various symptoms likely to follow such a reckless encounter, noting fluctuations in colour from redness to pallor and back again, dramatic chills and hot flushes, stiffness, crawling sensations and abscesses. Initially confined to scholastic texts, information of this kind soon became widespread, not least through the didactic medium of sermons and the confessional.[279] Having been born into the ruling elite of Lynn, the mystic Margery Kempe (*fl.* 1373–1440) would have been well aware of the efforts made by members of the merchant class to prevent young men from frequenting prostitutes when they travelled abroad unsupervised on business.[280] She records in her spiritual autobiography the anxiety occasioned by her son's dissolute lifestyle and her desire that God would punish his failure to remain 'clene'. To her evident satisfaction, his lapse into 'the synne of letchery' when overseas incurred its just reward as his face erupted 'ful of whelys and bloberys as it had ben a lepyr'.[281] But Margery's dose of abject penitence was not for all. Adopting a non-judgemental approach characteristic of his profession, the English physician John of Gaddesden (d. 1348–9) itemised the prophylactic measures that a man might take immediately after having sex with a suspect woman, while also offering practical advice designed to guard against the further spread of infection.[282]

Evidence of this kind confirms the existence of a direct and widespread connection between prostitution and disease, especially as the suburban stews, alehouses and taverns associated with commercial sex were widely believed to attract lepers.[283] In a move designed to remove 'malefactors and disturbers of the peace' from the London area before he left for France in 1346, Edward III warned the mayor and aldermen that leprous individuals were maliciously attempting to

---

[277] Rawcliffe, *Leprosy in Medieval England*, pp. 252–3. She was said to have caused a public nuisance by mixing freely among the population, and was bound over in securities of £10 to leave, this being the highest indemnity hitherto recorded in the Yarmouth leet rolls: NRO, Y/C4/202, rot. 4v. See also McSheffrey, *Marriage, Sex and Civic Culture*, pp. 144–5.

[278] Rawcliffe, *Leprosy in Medieval England*, pp. 87–8.

[279] Rawcliffe, *Leprosy in Medieval England*, p. 84.

[280] See, for example, rules for 'yong men' living in Danzig: D. M. Owen, ed., *The Making of King's Lynn: A Documentary Survey*, Records of Social and Economic History n.s. 9 (Oxford, 1984), p. 279.

[281] Margery Kempe, *The Book of Margery Kempe*, ed. S. B. Meech, EETS o.s. 212 (London, 1940), pp. 221–3.

[282] John of Gaddesden, *Rosa Anglica practica medicine a capite ad pedes* (Pavia, 1492), fol. 61r–v. See also Bodleian Library, MS Ashmole 1505, fol. 30v.

[283] Rawcliffe, *Leprosy in Medieval England*, pp. 285–6.

infect others 'as well in the way of mutual communications and by the contagion of their polluted breath, as by carnal intercourse with women in the stews and other secret places'.[284] Anxiety on this score may help to explain the ubiquity of measures designed to ensure that 'common queans' would be easily recognisable, most often by means of a striped hood or other readily identifiable items of clothing.[285] While hoping to protect 'honest' men from infection and respectable women from unwelcome sexual advances, magistrates were also increasingly alarmed by the ostentatious way in which the more successful prostitutes chose to dress, not only subverting the social and moral order but also luring impressionable young girls into a life that evidently promised far richer rewards than domestic service. From the 1280s onwards, the rulers of London fought an intermittent battle against brazen 'harlots' who aped the garb of 'good and noble dames and damsels', thereby concealing the rottenness within. Wider concerns about the collapse of the social hierarchy after the Black Death intensified their efforts. In 1351, for example, any 'lewd woman going about in the said City' was required to advertise herself 'openly with a hood or cloth of ray, single' on pain of forty days' imprisonment. The wearing of fur and other costly trimmings was similarly puished.[286] If, as was demonstrably the case, it proved impossible to confine such women to the suburbs, they had at least to submit to official surveillance and control.

Nervousness on all scores is clearly apparent in plague-ridden Yarmouth, a sea port which attracted a significant number of prostitutes, many of whom hailed originally from the Low Countries, and were thus already viewed with suspicion. In 1384–5, for example, the aptly named Magna Haughoe (Great Whore) was presented on the three counts of continuing to live within the walls despite an exclusion order, of failing to wear the compulsory striped hood of a harlot and, significantly, of offering 'hospitality' to known lepers. The latter were by this date expected to remove themselves to the dunes just north of the town, which was also the designated abode of 'common women', such as Licebet Janpetressen, who was dispatched there a decade later on account of her 'wicked and shameful behaviour'.[287] As the next century reached its close and urban epidemics became more frequent, anxiety about the sexual transmission of leprosy was not only directed at prostitutes. In 1486, a year marked by a comprehensive offensive against gambling, brothel-keeping and other misbehaviour, as well as a variety of sanitary offences, John Cook the younger was indicted for 'illicitly keeping and frequenting the wife of a leper, through which infection may occur'.[288]

---

[284] *CCR, 1346–1349*, pp. 54, 61–2; Riley, *Memorials of London*, pp. 365–6; Rexroth, *Deviance and Power*, pp. 6–7, 93–5.

[285] Karras, *Common Women*, pp. 21, 37; *LRBB*, II.229; Veale, *Great Red Book of Bristol*, I.143; DRO, ECA, Chamber Act Book 1, 1508–1538, fol. 110r. In Winchelsea, however, they had to go bareheaded: HMC, *Ninth Report*, part 1, appendix, p. 288.

[286] Riley, *Memorials of London*, p. 267, and also pp. 20, 458; *MLG*, III.102.

[287] NRO, Y/C4/96, rot. 10r; Y/C4/105, rot. 6v. Grimsby magistrates shared these concerns, ordering the proctor of the port's leper house to ensure that it was not used as a brothel: Rigby, *Medieval Grimsby*, p. 99.

[288] NRO, Y/C4/191, rot. 15r–v.

It was against this background of fear and suspicion that an even greater source of physical and moral contagion, the above-mentioned Alice Dymock, was finally expelled from the borough a decade later, no doubt after infecting many others.

Alice may in fact have been one of Yarmouth's first – but by no means last – victims of the Great Pox, which swept across Europe during the later 1490s. Spreading north quite rapidly from Italy, it soon reached Shrewsbury, where a local chronicle records the onset of 'the fowle scabbe and horryble syckness called the freanche pocks'.[289] Its initial impact is more fully documented in Scotland. In April 1497, the rulers of Aberdeen issued a decree for the avoidance 'of the infirmitey cumm out of Franche and strang [foreign] partis'. All 'licht weman', or prostitutes, were instructed 'to decist fra thar vicis and syne of venerie', leave the booths and houses where they plied their trade and henceforward to support themselves by honest labour, upon pain of expulsion and branding on the cheek.[290] However, the new epidemic could not be contained, and five months later James IV promulgated draconian measures to protect the people of Edinburgh from 'the greit appearand dainger' of infection from 'this contagius seiknes callit the *grandgor*'. All suspects were to be shipped at once to an island in the Firth of Forth, along with anyone purporting to offer successful treatment, or face disfigurement with a hot iron followed by permanent exile.[291] In the event, this brutal ordinance proved unenforceable, although, as Claude Quétel observes, it provides a striking example of the terror that the new epidemic inspired.[292]

In their initial struggle to provide a convincing explanation for the outbreak (which posed as great an etiological problem as the Black Death had done generations earlier), some Continental physicians immediately blamed contact with infected prostitutes and other women who had engaged in sexual relations with suspects.[293] It is therefore tempting to regard the Aberdeen edict, along with an unsuccessful move by Henry VII to close the Southwark stews in 1506,

---

[289] W. A. Leighton, ed., 'Early Chronicles of Shrewsbury, 1372–1603', *Transactions of the Shropshire Archaeological and Natural History Society*, 1st series 3 (1880), pp. 239–352, on p. 250.

[290] J. Stuart, ed., *Extracts from the Council Register of the Burgh of Aberdeen, 1398–1570* (Aberdeen, 1844), p. 425. In 1507, the authorities proposed to make a 'diligent inquisitioun of ale infect personis, with this strange seiknes of Nappillis', as the Great Pox was also known (p. 437). Suspects were ordered to remain at home and to avoid any premises that sold food, as well as contact with laundry workers. The latter prohibition probably related less to the association between laundresses and prostitution than to the assumption that infectious miasmas would cling to clothing.

[291] Marwick, *Records of the Burgh of Edinburgh*, pp. 71–2.

[292] C. Quétel, *History of Syphilis*, trans. J. Braddock and B. Pike (Oxford, 1990), p. 15.

[293] Quetel, *History of Syphilis*, pp. 20–4; J. Arrizabalaga, J. Henderson and R. French, *The Great Pox: The French Disease in Renaissance Europe* (New Haven, CT, 1997), pp. 36–7; W. Schleiner, 'Infection and Cure through Women: Renaissance Constructions of Syphilis', *Journal of Medieval and Renaissance Studies* 24 (1994), pp. 499–517.

as early attempts to remove the principal agents of transmission.[294] However, as this chapter has shown, epidemic disease was rarely, if ever, viewed in such simple, mono-causal terms, and it is just as likely that the authorities sought to eliminate a source of *moral* contamination as well as physical contagion, while also combating the dual menace of vagrancy and sloth. Indeed, during its first two decades, when it was at its most virulent, the Great Pox prompted a wide range of theories and responses in keeping with conventional medical wisdom.[295] Following a pattern already established in the case of leprosy, sexual transmission was regarded as one among many potential causes, along with divine wrath, poor food and hygiene, bad air and celestial forces, only gradually emerging as the principal culprit.[296] As late as 1547, the English physician Andrew Boorde counselled his readers that the pox could be contracted in many ways, from infected sheets and lavatory seats, shared drinking vessels, breastfeeding and protracted exposure to the breath of 'a pocky person'. He nevertheless warned explicitly against 'synne in lechery'.[297]

In fact, vagrant paupers and other indigents caused far greater concern than prostitutes, largely because they were the most obvious victims of the disease. Anxiety focussed primarily upon the sanitary threat posed by a growing army of beggars 'vexed with the frensshe pockes, poore and nedy, lyenge by the hye wayes, stynkynge and almoost roten aboue the grounde'.[298] The challenge of containing such a dangerous source of noisome miasmas was not the only problem, as the authorities had also to provide an effective type of relief that would not only care for the terminally sick, but also offer effective treatment to those who might eventually resume work. One answer lay in the utilisation of suburban leper houses, although in London, where the need was correspondingly greater, other hospitals, such as St Bartholomew's, were requisitioned as well. In 1517–18 the mayor and aldermen ruled that 'all such poore people as been visited with the great pokkes outwardly apperyng, or with other great sores or maladyes tedious, lothsome or abhorrible to be loked vppon & seen to the great anoyaunce of the people', should no longer be allowed to beg in public places, but dispatched immediately 'to th'ospytalles'.[299] How far these institutions were able to cope with a sudden influx of desperate cases we shall see in Chapter 6.

Along with fear of unrest, idleness and sexual depravity went a growing conviction that 'the poor, dirty and morally degenerate' were most likely to fall sick because of their vicious habits and squalid living conditions, and then to infect

---

[294] J. Fabricus, *Syphilis in Shakespeare's England* (London, 1994), p. 61. Carlin suggests that this offensive was part of a campaign to eliminate crime and vagrancy: *Medieval Southwark*, pp. 223–4.

[295] Arrizabalaga, Henderson and French, *Great Pox*, pp. 11–123.

[296] Rawcliffe, *Leprosy in Medieval England*, pp. 87–8.

[297] Andrew Boorde, *The Breviary of Helthe* (London, 1547), fol. 96v.

[298] John Fisher, *The English Works of John Fisher*, ed. J. E. B. Mayor, EETS e.s. 27 (London, 1876), p. 240. Fisher was writing in about 1509.

[299] Fabricius, *Syphilis in Shakespeare's England*, p. 60. In 1549, the city's six former lazar houses were officially assigned as 'outhouses' to St Bartholomew's, two aldermen being delegated to oversee their management: M. B. Honeybourne, 'The Leper Hospitals of the London Area', *TLMAS* 21 (1967), pp. 4–54, on p. 9.

other, more innocent victims.[300] Taking these ideas to their ultimate conclusion, the humanist courtier Sir John Cheeke (d. 1557) described the 'multitudes of vagabonds' who allegedly roamed England in the aftermath of Kett's Rebellion as a pestiferous rabble, like to a toxin spreading inexorably through the veins and arteries of the body politic:

> When we see a great number of flies in a yeare, we naturallie iudge it like to be a great plague, and hauing so great a swarming of loitering vagabonds, readie to beg and brall at euerie mans doore, which declare a greater infection, can we not looke for a greeuouser and perillouser danger than the plague is? Who can therefore otherwise deeme, but this one deadlie hurt, wherewith the commonwelth of our nation is wounded, beside all other is so pestilent, that there can be no more hurtfull thing in a well gouerned estate, nor more throwne into all kind of vice and vnrulinesse …[301]

Here, as in so many other examples presented in this chapter, the symbiotic connection between body and soul, individual and society, provides a key not only to understanding the basic principles of late medieval and early Tudor medicine but also the *rationale* behind many of the environmental improvements adopted in English towns and cities.

The ubiquitous influence of religious belief does not mean that we should underplay the impact of Classical and Islamic ideas about disease, which gained widespread currency in the aftermath of the Black Death. The assumption that urban magistrates considered it pointless to implement sanitary measures because they believed that 'epidemics were God's punishments for human sin, and that the only effective action possible was to intercede with Him by fasts and processions', runs contrary to much of the evidence presented in the rest of this book.[302] It also ignores the sophisticated relationship between morality and hygiene characteristic of medieval attitudes to disease. With their stress upon the quality of the air and the importance of a wholesome diet, the vernacular guides to health that circulated widely in later medieval Europe clearly played an important part in arming the ruling elite in their battle against pollution and pestilence. But we should not forget that these texts achieved general acceptance precisely because their underlying principles of restraint and moderation accorded so well with the basic tenets of Christianity. And it was for this reason that urban health was never a simple matter of drains, privies and conduits, however important they might be, but also of rich and poor alike behaving in a manner that seemed both appropriate and pleasing to God.[303]

---

[300] M. Healy, '"Seeing" Contagious Bodies in Early Modern London', in D. Grantley and N. Taunton, eds, *The Body in Late Medieval and Early Modern Culture* (Aldershot, 2000), p. 165.

[301] Cheeke, 'Hurt of Sedition', pp. 1002–3.

[302] Palliser, 'Epidemics in Tudor York', pp. 57–8. For a conclusive rebuttal of such arguments, see S. K. Cohn, 'Triumph over Plague: Culture and Memory after the Black Death', in T. van Bueren, ed., *Care for the Here and the Hereafter: Memoria, Art and Ritual in the Middle Ages* (Turnhout, 2005), pp. 35–54.

[303] Or, in Peregrine Horden's words, 'sewers and skeletons are not quite enough': 'Ritual and Public Health', p. 18.

✎ Chapter 3
Environmental Health

The Cities of England in the Middle Ages were too small to keep their inhabitants week after week, month after month, in one deadly vapour-bath of foul gas; and though the mortality among infants was probably excessive, yet we should have seen among the adult survivors few or none of those stunted and etiolated figures so common now in England ... But there was another side to this genial and healthy picture ... Every now and then epidemic disease entered the jolly city – and then down went strong and weak, rich and poor, before the invisible and seemingly supernatural arrows of that angel of death whom they had been pampering unwittingly in every bedroom. They fasted and prayed; but in vain. They called the pestilence a judgement of God; and they called it by a true name. But they knew not (and who are we to blame them for not knowing?) what it was that God was judging thereby – foul air, foul water, unclean backyards, stifling attics, houses hanging over the narrow street till light and air were alike shut out – that there lay the sin; and that to amend that was the repentance which God demanded.

Charles Kingsley, 'Great Cities and Their Influence for Good and Evil' (1857)[1]

In December 1421 jurors from the London ward of Farringdon Without indicted a local trader named William atte Wode for causing 'a great nuisance and discomfort to his neighbours by throwing out horrible filth on to the highway, the stench of which is so odious and infectious that none [of them] can remain in their shops'. Their other carefully itemised grievances included dangerous buildings and traffic hazards, whereby pedestrians were 'likely to be dismembered and lose their lives as well by day as by night', at least four blocked gutters and two thoroughfares that were 'flooded and heaped with filth'.[2] Similar problems were reported elsewhere in the City at this time: residents of Cordwainer Street Ward protested about 'the stinking filth thrown out by the wife of Sutton, grocer', while the state of the pavements, as well as nine 'defective, noisome and putrid' sewers, concerned the householders of Bishopsgate. Presentments from Bassishaw Ward began with a complaint about draymen who persistently dumped 'horrible noisome things outside the gate', and went on to report with unconcealed distaste that certain 'rents' lacked privies, thereby obliging the tenants to 'cast their ordure and other horrible filth and liquids before their doors, to the great nuisance of Holy Church and all people passing there'.[3]

On the face of things, evidence of this kind lends eloquent support to the longstanding assumption that 'the thoroughfares and byways of towns and cities

---

[1] This public address, delivered in Bristol, appeared three decades later in Kingsley, *Sanitary and Social Lectures*, pp. 194–6.

[2] *CPMRL, 1413–1437*, pp. 129–30.

[3] *CPMRL, 1413–1437*, pp. 126, 117–18, 121–4.

were loathsome and deep with offensive matter'.[4] Miscreants such as William atte Wode certainly highlight the apparent refusal of individual citizens to shoulder responsibility for the state of their surroundings that so many Victorian and Edwardian authors regarded as the principal cause of urban squalor. From their perspective, such stubborn indifference to basic matters of hygiene rendered medieval streets 'a constant danger to health and life', and explained why so little progress could be made towards the great goal of sanitary reform. Writing in 1906, Sir Walter Besant assumed that fourteenth-century London was only prevented from becoming completely 'defiled and impassable' by the rain, which flushed away much of the garbage, excrement and slops, and by airborne scavengers:

> ... they swoop down out of the sky, they alight in the street, they tear the offal with their beaks and claws, they carry it to the house-tops; these are the kites and crows who build their nests on the church towers and roofs, and find their food in the refuse thrown out into the streets. Were it not for these birds, London streets would be intolerable.[5]

Although Besant conceded that 'public opinion' demanded rather more than the unpredictable services of avian refuse collectors, his gothic imagery, borrowed without acknowledgment from a short story by Charles Dickens, caught the popular imagination.[6] Almost a century later, in 2003, Anthony Quiney painted an equally lurid picture of life in the medieval Capital, observing that:

> As in most towns, the mess of refuse and excrement was aggravated by horse dung, fertilizing a rich breeding ground for insects and beetles and a feeding ground for mice and rats. Crows pecked at putrid garbage, while, overhead, hawks hovered on the lookout for lunchtime snacks, and kites wheeled in the heavy air to prey on carrion.[7]

---

[4] T. P. Cooper, 'The Mediaeval Highways, Streets, Open Ditches, and Sanitary Conditions of the City of York', *Yorkshire Archaeological Journal* 22 (1912), pp. 270–86, on p. 271.

[5] Sir Walter Besant, *Mediaeval London*, vol. 1: *Historical and Social* (London, 1906), p. 171. But see also pp. 177, 346.

[6] Dickens believed that Jacobean London was 'a perfect quagmire, which the splashing water-spouts from the gables, and the filth and offal cast from the different houses, swelled in no small degree'. He described the 'insupportable stench' of 'odious matters being left to putrefy in the close and heavy air' and the 'kites and ravens feeding in the streets (the only scavengers the City kept)': *Master Humphrey's Clock* (Oxford, 1958), p. 71.

[7] A. Quiney, *Town Houses of Medieval Britain* (New Haven, CT, 2003), p. 93. In his defence we might, however, cite an Italian visitor to England, who noted in 1497 that the English protected ravens because they kept 'the streets of the towns free from all filth': C. A. Sneyd, ed., *A Relation of the Island of England*, CS 37 (London, 1847), p. 11. Moreover, some raven remains have been found in a late medieval refuse dump near Smithfield market in London: A. Telfer, 'Medieval Drainage near Smithfield Market: Excavations at Hosier Lane, EC1', *London Archaeologist* 10.5 (2003), pp. 115–20, on p. 119; Schofield, *London, 1100–1600*, p. 219.

As we saw in Chapter 1, not all historians have adopted such a negative stance, or succumbed so readily to the temptations of purple prose. In a reflective article of 1937, E. L. Sabine argued that the worst nuisances reported by early fifteenth-century London ward moots were generally confined to the suburbs, and that 'people were for the most part disgusted with such conditions when they came in contact with them'.[8] By dwelling upon the most flagrant cases of insanitary behaviour, he maintained, scholars had hitherto not only ignored wider questions of time and place, but had also disregarded – or at best dismissed – the many initiatives taken at both national and local levels to grapple with these problems.[9] An analysis of archival material has more recently prompted Caroline Barron to conclude that 'one cannot read the records of medieval London without being made aware of a restless pursuit of high communal standards of public health and safety'.[10] We shall examine the ways in which magistrates throughout England sought to improve the urban environment later in this chapter, but it is first worth noting two important factors that fostered growing anxiety on this score.

The list of criticisms directed at William atte Wode by his neighbours ended with the telling charge that his behaviour constituted 'a great reproof to all this honourable city, because of the lords and other gentlemen and men of the court who pass there'.[11] It is hardly surprising that Londoners should be sensitive on this score, since any failure to uphold acceptable standards of cleanliness invariably prompted a sharply worded reprimand from the crown.[12] Recognising that 'they were bound to preserve the *good name* of the City', the mayor and aldermen responded quickly to protests voiced in 1422 by the Franciscans of Newgate and others who lived in close proximity to the butchers' shambles by St Nicholas's church. In order to prevent the eponymous 'stinking lane' from being blocked with 'dung and foul intestines', they arranged for the construction of a gate to exclude the cattle that were herded there before slaughter, while also providing higher pavements and deeper gutters to facilitate the elimination of waste.[13] We should note, too, that by the fifteenth century the officials responsible for removing refuse from each ward had to swear on oath that 'the weyys, stretes and lanys [would] be clensid of dunge and all maner of filthe *for honeste* of the Cite'.[14]

Even though they were less often exposed to a censorious royal gaze, the residents of other towns and cities also regarded dirty streets and polluted watercourses as a source of collective shame. In 1439, for instance, a Yarmouth jury presented various people for depositing rubbish, blubber, and the blood of slaughtered animals in a major thoroughfare by the gates. The ensuing stench was described as both a threat to health and a 'public *rebuke*' to the entire community.[15] In the same spirit, plans for a comprehensive inspection of the streets, privies,

---

[8] Sabine, 'City Cleaning in Mediaeval London', p. 26.

[9] See pp. 17–18 above.

[10] Barron, *London in the Later Middle Ages*, p. 266.

[11] *CPMRL, 1413–1437*, p. 129.

[12] See sections 1.3 and 1.4 above.

[13] *CPMRL, 1413–1437*, pp. 147–8.

[14] *CLB*, D, pp. 192, 201.

[15] NRO, Y/C4/147, rot. 16r.

ditches, sewers and gutters of Salisbury were announced a couple of decades later in the hope that, once properly cleansed and repaired, they would again serve 'to the *adornment* of the city'.[16] These sentiments emerge so often in the records of late medieval English towns as to appear almost platitudinous. Protests voiced in early sixteenth-century Canterbury that, although the streets were well paved, lack of proper refuse collection rendered them 'foule and full of myre to the *grete dishonour* of the Cite and the grete damage of the inhabitaunts by the corrupte and infectuose heires', were certainly far from unusual.[17] Shortly afterwards a Nottingham jury castigated 'maister mayre' and his brethren in similar terms, begging them 'to remember the clensyng of the lanys at the coming in off the towne, for the townys *wirship* and profyte'.[18] Significantly, because of the deference and respect due to them by virtue of their high office, future mayors of Lynn were empowered at this time to demand the removal of any laystall, or dung-hill, should they happen to live near one at the time of their election.[19]

It might be argued that concerns of this kind were largely cosmetic, in so far that they tended to focus upon superficial appearances.[20] But such an assumption fails to account for the second and far more pressing reason for mounting vigilance. Notwithstanding an obvious anxiety about the impression that heaps of rotting garbage and other signs of urban decay might convey to high status visitors, the chief priority in each of the above-mentioned cases was to eliminate 'corrupt exhalations and other abominable and infectious smells'.[21] Our Yarmouth jurors, for instance, must have been desperate to avoid the 'infirmite most infectif' then spreading throughout England, which they would have associated with rank and contaminated air.[22] Sabine's 'hypothesis' that the dramatic and unprecedented rise in the number of sanitary measures recorded in the London Letter Books between 1350 and 1400 constituted a response to repeated onslaughts of plague was surely correct.[23] However, he did not venture beyond the suggestion that 'a genuine and serious-minded' effort was being made to combat disease. Nor did he consider the impact that current beliefs about the spread of epidemics might have had upon the regulation of urban nuisances. While doing much to refashion our image of late medieval cities, Sabine's successors have also fought shy of a more systematic

---

[16] Carr, *First General Entry Book*, no. 453.

[17] HMC, *Ninth Report*, part 1, appendix, p. 174. A carter was duly appointed to remove waste from the streets.

[18] Stevenson, *Records of the Borough of Nottingham*, III.338.

[19] KLBA, KL/C7/5, Hall Book, 1497–1544, fol. 35v.

[20] In his discussion of sanitary measures in seventeenth-century Prescot, for example, Walter King asserts that the residents adopted this approach because they 'had no concept of germs and were less concerned about odors and being odor free than we [are]': 'How High is too High? The Disposal of Dung in Seventeenth-Century Prescot', *Sixteenth-Century Journal* 23 (1992), pp. 443–57, on p. 454.

[21] *CPMRL, 1413–1437*, p. 147.

[22] See Appendix.

[23] Sixteen such entries are recorded between 1300 and 1350 and four times as many (sixty-five) during the next half-century: Sabine, 'City Cleaning in Mediaeval London', p. 28.

exploration of the medical rationale behind the impetus for a healthier urban environment. To conclude that such activity simply reflects 'a universal impulse shared by all communities' is to ignore the specific circumstances which gave rise to a spate of initiatives for cleaner streets and purer air.[24]

3.1 Medical beliefs

In order to understand the late medieval preoccupation with 'infectif' matter and the avoidance of miasmas, we should briefly return to the physiological theories of the Ancient Greeks, as mediated through the work of Muslim physicians such as Al-Majusi (Haly Abbas) and Ibn-Sina (Avicenna). Whereas, in the first instance, the preservation of humoral balance, and thus of good health, depended largely upon diet, which determined the composition and quality of the natural or nutritive spirits, air had a more immediate impact upon the animal and vital spirits. These flighty, nervous creatures were responsive to odours, both bad and good, and if perturbed could retreat rapidly into the heart or brain, causing such alarming symptoms as palpitations, breathlessness, paralysis, or fainting. They could also play havoc with the body's internal thermostat, in extreme cases draining it of warmth, and thus of life itself, or suffusing it with dangerous levels of heat.[25] While agreeing that scent could have either a malign or beneficial effect, Greek physicians and natural scientists offered two rather different explanations for the phenomenon. For some, smells were composed of extremely fine particles which coalesced into a type of 'fumosity', or smoky vapour, somewhere between air and moisture. This misty substance was invisible to the naked eye, but able easily to enter the body through the nostrils, mouth and open pores of the skin. Odours absorbed through the spongy and permeable receptors of the nose would pass rapidly up the olfactory tract to the brain, transmitting to the animal spirit the 'prynte and liknes' – along with all the properties or attributes – of the things from whence they came.[26] Another school of thought regarded smells as *species* or immaterial forms which conveyed the very essence, rather than a mere copy, of whatever had produced them. According to both Aristotle and Galen, they were identical to 'the odoriferous body' in 'substance and qualities', and therefore just as potent.[27]

The practical implications of these theories were frighteningly obvious. In the words of the thirteenth-century encyclopaedist Bartholomaeus Anglicus: 'yif the vapour is malicious, stinkinge, and corrupt, it corrumpith the spirit that hatte [is called] *animalis* and often bringith and gendrith pestilence'.[28] There were other ways in which polluted air could precipitate a rapid descent into sickness, if not

---

[24] Carr, 'From Pollution to Prostitution', p. 41.

[25] *OPT*, I.105–7; II.1298–9; Harvey, *Inward Wits*, pp. 16–17; see p. 56 above.

[26] R. Palmer, 'In Bad Odour: Smell and its Significance in Medicine from Antiquity to the Seventeenth Century', in W. F. Bynum and R. Porter, eds, *Medicine and the Five Senses* (Cambridge, 1993), pp. 61–8; Harvey, *Inward Wits*, p. 19; *OPT*, II.1297, 1301.

[27] R. E. Siegel, *Galen on Sense Perception* (Basel, 1970), pp. 155–6; Woolgar, *The Senses*, pp. 14–15; S. Kemp, 'A Medieval Controversy about Odor', *Journal of the History of the Behavioral Sciences* 33 (1997), pp. 211–19.

[28] *OPT*, I.116.

miasmas

death, since whatever was inhaled into the lungs would contaminate the *pneuma*, or vital spirit that carried heat from the heart along the arteries to the other vital organs. At the same time, noisome air drawn through the open pores would pass from the capillaries into the venous system, obstructing the transmission of humoral matter throughout the body and poisoning its source of nourishment. As a general rule, however, the essential purity and sweetness of a fragrant aroma seemed to render it more powerful than anything unpleasant or toxic.[29] The scent of a rose or lily, for example, would be 'good to [the] brayne, for he comfortith the spiritis of the brest and of the herte and restorith the heed ... and cometh inward to comforte senewis'.[30] For this reason, well-stocked gardens offered a welcome resort for men and women who felt sick or lethargic, and were highly prized as a prophylactic by those town-dwellers who could afford to maintain them.[31]

Ever since the appearance of Al-Majusi's *Liber pantegni* in Europe during the late eleventh century, miasmatic air had been recognised as a major cause of illness.[32] It was, however, during the century before the Black Death that the authors of *regimina* and medical text books began to focus more specifically upon the correlation between environment and disease. Their interest was fuelled by a growing appreciation of the ideas discussed above, most notably regarding the crucial role of *pneuma* as a source of heat and life. The frothy mixture of air and venous blood that had been warmed and refined in the heart was essential for survival, but dangerously vulnerable to 'the stynch and fylthye sauours that corrupte that ayre whyche we lyue in'.[33] As the physician Arnald of Villanova (d. 1311) advised one of his royal patients:

> The first item or consideration with regard to the preservation of health concerns the choice of air. For among the things which, by necessity, affect the human body nothing changes it more than that which, inhaled by the mouth and nostrils ... and mixed with the spirit of the heart, travels along all the arteries, by which means all the activities of daily life are accomplished.[34]

Already by this date medical authorities had not only begun to consider the physiological impact of environmental factors, but also to recommend the most salubrious towns in which to live. Drawing upon the concepts first advanced in Hippocratic texts such as *Airs, Waters, Places*, which dealt at length with these issues, the authors of medieval *regimina* generally agreed that an easterly location would be 'more temperate than others' and the inhabitants 'more healthy', especially if they enjoyed the advantage of pure sea breezes.[35] Sometimes quoting verbatim, if selectively, from these works, the authors of England's earliest urban

[29] Harvey, *Inward Wits*, p. 27.

[30] *OPT*, I.562; and also II.1299–1300.

[31] C. Rawcliffe, '"Delectable Sightes and Fragrant Smelles": Gardens and Health in Late Medieval and Early Modern England', *Garden History* 36 (2008), pp. 1–21.

[32] Al-Majusi, *Liber pantegni*, 'Theorica', book 5, cap. 11, fol. 20r.

[33] Thomas Phaer, *A Treatyse of the Pestylence* (London, 1544), fol. 10r.

[34] Arnald de Villanova, *Regimen sanitatis ad regem Aragonum*, p. 423.

[35] Hippocrates, *The Medical Works of Hippocrates*, ed. J. Chadwick and W. N. Mann (Oxford, 1950), pp. 90–4; Pierpont Morgan Library, New York, MS M.165, fols 34r–36v.

histories made much of the beneficial qualities of the towns and cities about which they wrote, temporarily forgetting the devastating effects of pestilence.[36] Henry Manship's early seventeenth-century *History of Great Yarmouth* provides a classic example of the continuity of ideas first developed almost two millennia earlier. Because of its position on the east coast, he observed, the port basked in the 'the first rising of the sun ... which doth disperse the mists and vapours from off the earth, whereby it purgeth and cleanseth the air'. Indeed, being 'as wholesome for situation as any town in the kingdom', it had come to enjoy a unique reputation among physicians for its healthy and invigorating climate.[37] Generations of sick and aged Norwich monks, schooled in the principles of the *regimen sanitatis*, had certainly enjoyed the therapeutic effects of 'recreations' in its bracing air, being regularly dispatched to the mother house's cells there and at King's Lynn for periods of rest and convalescence.[38]

However, few men and women were free to follow this advice, and not even they could escape the hazards of daily life. All too often 'perceptible corruptions' from 'animal dung, corpses and other stinking putrefactions' were carried on the wind, multiplying and spreading as they travelled.[39] In 1252, for example, Henry III arranged for one of his servants, 'afflicted with insanity by the evil nature of the air', to enjoy the healthier environment of Wiltshire until he recovered. He may, perhaps, have fallen victim to the stench arising from the kitchens at Westminster, since eight years later considerable sums were assigned for the construction of a conduit to carry malodorous refuse directly to the Thames and thus avoid the likelihood of infection sweeping through the royal palace.[40] An influential passage in book four of Ibn-Sīna's *Canon of Medicine* provided the rationale for such measures:

> Vapours and fumes rise [into the air] and spread in it, and putrefy it with their debilitating warmth. And when air of this kind reaches the heart, it corrupts the complexion of the [vital] spirit that dwells within it; and, surrounding the heart, it then putrefies it with humidity. And there arises an unnatural heat; and it spreads throughout the body, as a result of which pestilential fever will occur, and will spread to a multitude of men who likewise have vulnerable dispositions.[41]

[36] 'Bad air' was just as interesting to early modern topographers and physicians: Dobson, *Contours of Death and Disease*, p. 10, and chap. 1, *passim*; A. Wear, 'Making Sense of Health and the Environment in Early Modern England', in A. Wear, ed., *Medicine and Society: Historical Essays* (Cambridge, 1992), pp. 119–47.

[37] Henry Manship, *The History of Great Yarmouth*, ed. C. J. Palmer (Yarmouth, 1854), pp. 103–4.

[38] C. Rawcliffe, '"On the Threshold of Eternity": Care for the Sick in East Anglian Monasteries', in C. Harper-Bill, C. Rawcliffe and R. G. Wilson, eds, *East Anglia's History* (Woodbridge, 2002), pp. 71–2.

[39] Arrizabalaga, 'Facing the Black Death', pp. 255, 275.

[40] *Calendar of Liberate Rolls, 1251–1260* (London, 1960), pp. 59, 507.

[41] Ibn-Sīna (Avicenna), *Liber canonis medicine* (Lyon, 1522), book 4, fol. 329r. See also Arrizabalaga, 'Facing the Black Death', pp. 252, 255. According to the tenets of Galenic medicine, powerful odours were characterised by their innate heat, which was especially dangerous in epidemics.

Though shorn of their theoretical underpinnings, these ideas began to percolate downwards through society at a comparatively early date, their transmission hastened by renewed outbreaks of plague from the 1360s onwards. In many cases, urban magistrates simply repeated the unambiguous wording of royal directives such as that dispatched in 1332 to the rulers of York with regard to 'the abominable smell abounding in the said city', thereby embedding in their own ordinances the association between air pollution and pestilential disease.[42] Echoing Edward III's complaint about the 'noisome smells arising from the streets and river', a proclamation of 1357 issued by the mayor and aldermen of London for improving cleanliness in the City refers explicitly to the 'corruptions', 'abomination and damage' occasioned by the dung, filth and other noxious detritus that littered the streets and clogged the Thames. These new prohibitions on the dumping of miasmatic waste were reinforced by stiff fines of 2s. for each offence, along with imprisonment in some cases, obliging even the most sceptical or obtuse Londoners to reflect upon their behaviour.[43] Letters close of 1372 for the removal of dung-heaps and other malodorous rubbish deposited on Tower Hill similarly refer to the 'manifest peril' likely to arise from such 'corruption and stench', especially as the air was 'so tainted thereby as to strike the men dwelling all about and the passers by with disgust and loathing'. These phrases were duly noted in the civic record and reappear in the wording of an inquiry designed to name and punish offenders. Not surprisingly, they, and similar warnings about other threats to survival, began to appear regularly in the presentments made by local juries.[44]

From the late thirteenth century onwards Norwich leet courts sometimes went beyond the usual terse description of insanitary nuisances such as the dumping of dung and rubbish in the streets, and noted the environmental hazards that they presented. In 1288–9, for example, one Roger Benjamin was indicted for burying offal in a public muck-heap which badly polluted the surrounding air ('per quod aer pessime corrumpitur'), while a skinner faced similar charges arising from his thoughtless disposal of dead cats.[45] Mounting concern about the risks posed by miasmatic air is especially apparent in the case of presumed lepers, whose presence in towns and cities had to be reported so that appropriate measures could be taken for their removal to a hospital or lodging beyond the walls. Originally justified by the canonical ruling that suspects should live 'outside the camp', and thus based upon religious and cultural, rather than medical, criteria, this requirement gradually became a matter of public health.[46] A growing awareness that 'from infected bodies comme ... infectious and venomous fumes and vapours, the whiche do infecte and corrupte the aire' made people nervous, especially of the 'stinking breath' associated with the leprous. Alarm spread during times of pestilence, when physicians urged the need to 'avoyde and eschewe all suche' as a precautionary measure.[47] The effect of their warnings is strikingly apparent

---

[42] *CCR, 1330–1333*, p. 610.

[43] *CCR, 1354–1360*, p. 422; Riley, *Memorials of London*, p. 299.

[44] *CCR, 1369–1374*, p. 365; *CLB*, G, pp. 291–2; *CPMRL, 1364–1381*, pp. 140–1.

[45] Hudson, *Leet Jurisdiction*, pp. 23, 29.

[46] See section 6.7 below.

[47] Rawcliffe, *Leprosy in Medieval England*, p. 276.

from an analysis of the 113 presentments for leprosy made by Yarmouth juries between 1369 (the date of England's 'third pestilence') and 1501. Although other motives besides fear of infection are clearly apparent, intense bouts of surveillance invariably coincided with local or national epidemics, when the risks seemed particularly great. Moreover, from the 1390s onwards we can detect a shift in vocabulary, as Yarmouth jurors – or the scribes who recorded their complaints – began to indict specific individuals 'propter fetorem' (on account of the stench), and because of the likelihood of infection ('ad periculum et infeccionem populi').[48] Increasingly, too, in the records of cities as far apart as London and Berwick-on-Tweed, ordinances for the removal of lepers were inscribed alongside others for the elimination of noxious waste.[49]

We should note in this context that it was the 'odious and infectious' smell of the refuse deposited by William atte Wode in 1421 that so incensed the residents of Farringdon Ward Without. Already by then a significant, if not overwhelming, proportion of the urban population recognised that 'wholesome aire' was 'faire and cleare without vapours and mistes ... lightsome and open, not darke, troublous and close ... not infected with carrian lying long above ground ... [nor] stinking or corrupted with ill vapours, as being neere to draughts, sinckes, dunghills, gutters, chanels, kitchings, church-yardes, or standing waters'.[50] The following pages furnish many examples of the ways in which these ideas affected the working practices of urban craftsmen. In 1455, for instance, the Horners of London undertook 'in eschuyng of the grete and corrupt stenche and grievous noyance of neyghbours' that they would no longer dismember carcasses within the City.[51] On occasion, fear of miasmatic vapours even overcame the customary desire for elaborate funerary rituals, especially in plague time. Such was the level of anxiety in King's Lynn during the pestilence of 1528 that local magistrates were able to insist upon a dramatic curtailment of obsequies for the Christian departed. Because 'the corses & dede bodyes of ... inhabitauntes' brought to church on these occasions had 'enfected & putrefied the same churche & chapelles & the people resortyng theder to the grete perill, infection & hurtt of the same', a rapid transit from deathbed to grave, with no intervening ceremonial, seemed the most obvious precaution.[52]

Although Classical ideas about the sense and nature of smell were effectively challenged during the seventeenth century, the conviction that epidemics spread

---

[48] Rawcliffe, *Leprosy in Medieval England*, pp. 282–3; NRO, Y/C4/103, rot. 10v; 186, rot. 15r.

[49] Smith, Smith and Brentano, *English Gilds*, p. 341; *CLB*, G, p. 301; Corporation of London Records, Journal 8, fols 21v–22r.

[50] Thomas Cogan, *The Haven of Health* (London, 1584), pp. 7, 262.

[51] F. J. Fisher, *A Short History of the Worshipful Company of Horners* (London, 1936), pp. 22–3.

[52] KBLA, KL/C7/5, Hall Book 1497–1544, fol. 276r. A century earlier, the master and clergy of St Michael *in Riola*, London, closed the cemetery on the east side of the church because 'the smells and infections of the bodies of the dead buried there' obliged them to vacate the premises in plague time: Twemlow, *Calendar of Papal Letters*, vol. 8: *1427–1447* (London, 1909), p. 341.

through the medium of polluted air remained unshaken until the reign of Queen Victoria.[53] The tenacity of this belief owed much to the fact that it offered a rational and intelligible explanation for the frequently observed connection between dirt and disease, while according perfectly with current interpretations of human physiology. However, the nose and lungs were not the only organs vulnerable to external attack. That complaints about dung-heaps, offensive latrines and the like so often refer to their unpleasant *appearance* as well as their disgusting smell may surprise a modern reader. During the plague of 1369 the 'abominable' and 'loathsome' spectacle of the offal dumped by London butchers caused just as much offence as the ensuing 'corruption and grievous stench'.[54] The catalogue of grievances presented by London ward moots in the early 1420s likewise includes several apparently aesthetic objections to sanitary hazards, such as a dilapidated privy in Ludgate. The 'horrible stench and *foul sight*' of overflowing ordure together contributed 'to the great discomfort and nuisance of all folk dwelling thereabout and passing thereby', besides constituting 'a disgrace to all the City'. No less abhorrent were the waste dumps from common latrines and 'other *horrible sights*' in Watergate Street.[55]

Lepers, too, were feared not only because of their miasmatic odour but also the disfiguring effect of symptoms which so often rendered them physically repugnant. Indeed, it was only when a leper had become intolerable to the beholder ('tam deformis quod aspectus eum sustinere non posit') that he or she lost the right to plead in a court of law.[56] Significantly, this ruling was made during the thirteenth century, when Aristotelian theories about optics were gaining ground in the West through the work of Ibn-Sīna and Ibn al-Haytham (Al-Hacen). According to these authors, the eye was a passive organ which absorbed the impressions, 'forms', 'virtues' or 'similitudes' that radiated outwards in a continuous sequence of multiple images from all visible objects and had a similar impact upon the body to smells.[57] Thus a beautiful or spiritually uplifting sight would conserve or even promote health, while that of a decaying corpse, stagnant gutter or mutilated beggar would have the opposite effect.[58] The physician Gilbertus Anglicus (d. *c.* 1250) regarded the *aspectus*, or appearance, of lepers as a potential source of infection, warning that the *species* of the disease might enter the eye of anyone who stared at them,

---

[53] Jenner, 'Civilization and Deodorization?', pp. 134–6.

[54] *CPMRL, 1364–1381*, p. 93; *CCR, 1369–1374*, pp. 31–2. In April 1370 offenders were threatened with imprisonment and a massive fine of £100: *CCR, 1369–1374*, pp. 177–9; *RP*, II.460.

[55] *CPMRL, 1413–1437*, pp. 141, 157.

[56] S. E. Thorne, ed., *Bracton on the Laws and Customs of England*, 4 vols (Cambridge, MA, 1968–77), IV.309.

[57] K. H. Tachau, *Vision and Certitude in the Age of Ockham: Optics, Epistemology and the Foundations of Semantics, 1250–1345* (Leiden, 1988), pp. 8–10, 94–5; D. G. Denery, *Seeing and Being in the Later Medieval World* (Cambridge, 2005), pp. 82–9.

[58] The clerk who described the refurbishment of the Colchester moot hall (see p. 84 above) observed that 'it rejoices the eyesight of the whole of the common people', thus implicitly doing them good: *RPBC*, p. 10.

polluting the animal spirit and eventually suffusing the entire venous system with corruption.[59] Following Galen, some physicians assigned a more dynamic role to the eye, maintaining that it could transmit as well as receive matter, notably in the case of plague victims, whose gaze was contaminated by toxic emissions in search of a new 'dwelling place'.[60] Basic information along these lines had already reached the general populace by 1344, when one Scottish chronicler observed that, during an epidemic affecting poultry, 'men utterly shrank from eating, or *even looking upon* a cock or hen, as though unclean and smitten with leprosy'.[61]

Anxieties about sight and smell alike were reinforced by the powerful religious imagery used to evoke the joys and torments of the next life. The aroma of sanctity, which enveloped so many saints in a delicious perfume, contrasted sharply with the feculent stench of evil. Populated by an army of physically repugnant devils, hell reeked with the sulphurous fumes of eternal damnation, while heaven exceeded all mortal concepts of sensory perfection.[62] Purgatory, too, was envisaged in terms of disfigurement and filth. One fifteenth-century English translation of the *Vision of the Monk of Eynsham* describes the 'ful horrable clowde' of poison hovering above its frozen lakes and furnaces. Here, 'myxte and medylde to-gedir', arose 'a fume of brymstone wyth a myste, a gret stenche and a flame blak as pycche', while the deformed inhabitants breathed fire through their noses and exhaled foul breath from gaping mouths.[63] There was, as many preachers warned, a striking difference between superficial cleanliness and inner purity, but the association between dirt, disfigurement and sin still remained overwhelming. When the play of *The Last Judgement*, which brought the York Corpus Christi cycle to an end, reached its final station in the great marketplace known as The Pavement, hell (on stage left) looked onto the butchers' shambles, while paradise (on the right) lay reassuringly close to the church of All Saints where former mayors were buried.[64]

As we shall see in the rest of this chapter, the practical application of these concepts in crowded towns and cities was rarely so straightforward (3.2). One of the first steps towards the creation of a more salubrious environment was to provide adequately paved streets, which were both safer and easier to keep clean. They also represented the public face of a community, and, as such, could provoke

[59] Gilbertus Anglicus, *Compendium medicine* (Lyon, 1510), fols 337v, 339r.

[60] Siegel, *Galen on Sense Perception*, pp. 71–8; Arrizabalaga, 'Facing the Black Death', pp. 263–4; Horrox, *Black Death*, pp. 183–4; Berger, 'Mice, Arrows and Tumours', p. 51. One option was to blindfold the patient: Aberth, *From the Brink of the Apocalypse*, p. 111.

[61] John of Fordun, *John of Fordun's Chronicle of the Scottish Nation*, ed. W. F. Skene (Edinburgh, 1872), p. 358.

[62] C. Classen, D. Howes and A. Synnott, *Aroma: The Cultural History of Smell* (London, 1994), pp. 52–4.

[63] R. Easting, ed., *The Revelation of the Monk of Eynsham*, EETS o.s. 318 (London, 2002), pp. 45, 49. Other visions dwell upon the 'fyr so horrible and stynkynge that all the creatures in the world myght not telle the wikked smyllynge ther-of': M. Powell Harley, ed., *A Revelation of Purgatory by an Unknown, Fifteenth-Century Woman Visionary*, Studies in Women and Religion 18 (New York, 1985), p. 59.

[64] A. Higgins, 'Streets and Markets', in J. D. Cox and D. S. Kastan, eds, *A New History of Early English Drama* (New York, 1997), p. 91.

shame as well as pride. Acknowledging the 'disworshipp' occasioned by their failure 'to maynteyne that thing which heretofore by ther predecessors have ben well maynteyned and lokyed unto', the rulers of Norwich observed ruefully in 1559 that from

> tyme oute of mynde there hathe bene a comely and decent order used within this cittye for the pavyng of the stretes ... whiche thing hath not only bene a great ease and helthefull commodyte to the inhabitauntes of the same, but also a goodly bewtefyng and an occasyon that dyuerse [visitors] havyng accesse to the same cittye from ffare and strange places haue moche comended and praysed.[65]

In addition to its obvious benefits, street paving facilitated schemes for refuse collection and the creation of communal dumps well away from residential areas (3.3). London, predictably, had the most complex and labour-intensive system, but many other towns opted to pay salaried cleaners, while at the same time imposing stringent penalties on householders who failed to discharge their personal responsibilities.

Even when the population was falling, the production of daunting quantities of human and animal waste, as well as dirt and rubbish, constantly threatened to contaminate thoroughfares and watercourses. Nevertheless, it would be mistaken to assume that people were oblivious to the need for better sanitation, if only because of their desire to avoid miasmatic air. Communal latrines, often of considerable size, were to be found in almost all late medieval towns; and private dwellings were increasingly equipped with privies whose location might well be determined by stringent building regulations (3.4). The growing appetite for meat gave rise to a similar problem with regard to the slaughtering of animals and disposal of carcasses, which attracted mounting concern in the aftermath of epidemics (3.5). Tighter controls on butchery were accompanied by efforts to tackle the thorny issue of urban livestock, most notably vagrant dogs and pigs, which not only endangered health, but all too often seemed to replicate the behaviour of the idle, feckless poor (3.6). We then turn to the growing preoccupation with man-made pollution, especially through the use of sea coal and the proliferation of noisy, unpleasant industrial processes (3.7), before finally considering the many practical steps taken to avoid the spread of fires, one of the greatest perils of urban life (3.8).

3.2 The problem of urban waste

As the sheer volume of records dealing with the problem confirms, the removal of mountainous quantities of waste was one of the greatest challenges to face the rulers and residents of medieval English towns. Alongside the ever growing heaps of human excrement, domestic refuse, cinders and garbage from shops, taverns, markets and workplaces, lay piles of filthy straw and dung produced by a surprising variety of animals and poultry, noisome mounds of offal, blood and entrails from urban slaughterhouses, yards full of rubble, timber, clay and thatch left by builders,

---

[65] *RCN*, II.133–4.

garden rubbish, and wheelbarrows crammed with the dirty rushes that had once been strewn on the floors of town houses. Muddy, unpaved thoroughfares made matters worse, since they were hard to clean, dangerous for pedestrians and irresistible to the casual fly-tipper.[66] Yet all this spoil could, on occasion, prove a valuable asset rather than a liability. Archaeological evidence of waterfront reclamation in towns and cities throughout Europe reveals that substantial areas of land were recovered from the sea or rivers by constructing timber revetments and filling the area behind them with compacted rubbish. Activity has been discovered in at least sixteen English towns, as well as London, whose size increased by at least ten per cent between the eleventh and sixteenth centuries as a result of riverside developments, sometimes involving deposits of garbage over ten metres deep.[67] Work on this scale would clearly have accounted for a great deal of the refuse generated by ordinary householders, and may in some instances have been undertaken specifically as a means of disposal.[68] Domestic refuse was also utilised in other structural projects, such as the raising and levelling of large public spaces, including Shrewsbury market and the site of the Augustinian friary in Hull, as well as for creating stable road surfaces in preparation for metalling with flints and cobbles.[69]

There was, in addition, a constant demand for manure, both human and animal, on the part of local farmers, at least during periods of population growth when agricultural produce remained at a premium. The cost of transportation by cart or boat could easily be offset when food prices soared, but once the market began to contract so too did the need for intensive fertilisation. At St Giles's hospital, Norwich, dung from the precinct and adjacent properties was initially carried away to outlying manors in the empty carts that had brought in produce, while residents of Winchester were, for a time, able to sell manure for use on the nearby episcopal estates. The shift from demesne farming to a scaled-down *rentier* economy after the Black Death significantly curtailed such operations, although since urban populations were also in decline less waste was generally being produced.[70] Contraction was nonetheless a mixed blessing: on the one hand, marginal land became available for the creation of communal rubbish tips and dung-hills not too far away from residential areas, but, on the other, householders were inclined to take the easy option by dumping their waste on

[66] Keene, 'Rubbish in Medieval Towns', pp. 26–30.

[67] G. Milne, 'Medieval Riverfront Reclamation in London', in G. Milne and B. Hobley, eds, *Waterfront Archaeology in Britain and Northern Europe*, CBA research report 41 (London, 1981), pp. 32–6. See also B. Hobley, 'The London Waterfront – The Exception or the Rule?', in *ibid.*, pp. 1–9.

[68] Keene, 'Rubbish in Medieval Towns', p. 28; D. H. Evans, 'The Infrastructure of Hull between 1270 and 1700', in Gläser, *Lübecker Kolloquium*, p. 63.

[69] M. O. H. Carver, 'Early Shrewsbury: An Archaeological Definition in 1975', *Transactions of the Shropshire Archaeological Society* 59 (1973–4), pp. 225–63, on p. 247; Jørgensen, 'Cooperative Sanitation', p. 560.

[70] Rawcliffe, 'Sickness and Health', p. 312; B. Ayers, *Norwich: Archaeology of a Fine City* (Stroud, 2009), p. 100; Keene, *Survey of Medieval Winchester*, I.53. In London, boats took manure out of the City for agricultural use: Sabine, 'City Cleaning in Mediaeval London', pp. 24–5.

the nearest unoccupied plot. In 1521, the residents of King's Lynn were ordered to cease the antisocial practice of leaving garbage 'wher as houses or groundes stand speryd & buletten [bolted]'.[71] As we shall see in the concluding section of this chapter, fire damage also tended to encourage this kind of insanitary behaviour.

The contemporary ring of many late medieval ordinances for waste disposal inevitably prompts a comparison with the practices deployed in modern British cities. We should, nevertheless, resist the temptation to evaluate these measures by our own standards, or to frame them within what Mark Jenner describes as 'a narrative of progress and deodorization'.[72] Cultural attitudes to dirt and, indeed, the degree of offence caused by specific nuisances are subject to a wide and shifting range of priorities, which during the later Middle Ages hinged primarily – but not exclusively – upon a desire to eliminate 'those unsavory and noysome smells and stenches ... which hath a pestiferous influence on mans body'.[73] They were also tempered by a strong dose of pragmatism. Simply depositing rubbish in the road, for instance, was rarely regarded as an offence unless it seemed especially noxious or obtrusive. After all, since most refuse collections were made in this way, some measure of compromise was essential, even in cities such as York, where the heaping of dung in public places had been prohibited as early as 1301.[74] An ordinance of 1467 'for clensyng the strettes' in the borough of Leicester allowed residents three days in which to leave 'muke or fylthe' outside their front doors before facing a fine, although from 1508 builders were permitted greater leeway.[75] Norwich householders enjoyed four days' grace, but faced a draconian penalty of 40*d.* a day thereafter, in order to keep the market and major thoroughfares free of rotting garbage.[76] Contention generally arose only if a midden stood for too long, posed an obstacle to traffic, spilled in a 'disorderly' fashion onto the pavement, blocked drains or gutters, created a dangerous miasma or threatened to contaminate wells or watercourses.[77] Local juries frequently voiced specific

---

[71] KLBA, KL/C7/5, Hall Book, 1497–1544, fol. 232v. For the use of depopulated areas for waste disposal, see Keene, *Survey of Medieval Winchester*, I.53.

[72] Jenner, 'Civilization and Deodorization?', pp. 127–44.

[73] Jenner, 'Civilization and Deodorization?', p. 131.

[74] YCO, p. 17. This ruling was reiterated in 1364 and 1371: *YMB*, I.lxvi. From 1372 onwards, Londoners faced a fine of 2*s.* for leaving dung in front of their houses, and of 4*s.* for dumping it outside neighbouring property at any time (Riley, *Liber albus*, p. 289). A ruling of 1385 established that rubbish could only be placed in the streets when a cart was available to collect it (*CLB*, H, p. 255).

[75] *RBL*, II.291, 380. The early fourteenth-century customs of Southampton made a similar provision: Studer, *Oak Book of Southampton*, I.52–3, 131. Residents of the Durham borough of Crossgate had about a week in which to remove dung-heaps (*RBC*, nos 389, 393, 429, 483), as did those of Beverley (*BTD*, pp. 4–5), Cambridge (Cooper, *Annals of Cambridge*, p. 148), and Henley (P. M. Briers, ed., *Henley Borough Records: Assembly Books i–iv, 1395–1543*, Oxfordshire Record Society 41 (Banbury, 1960), p. 41).

[76] *RCN*, II.84.

[77] King, 'How High is too High?'.

objections to dung-hills that hindered pedestrians or, even worse, filled them with nausea because of the unbearable stench.[78]

Some towns, such as Ipswich, routinely imposed modest fines of 2*d*. or 3*d*. on about a score of residents for 'casting muck' and household waste in the highway and on common land. This practice may have constituted a form of licensing, akin to that imposed on brewers and bakers, rather than an attempt to penalise recidivists for polluting the environment. Quite possibly both factors came into play. An unusually full, but not continuous, set of leet court records for the borough reveals that between 1415 and 1470 the number of individuals presented in any one year never exceeded thirty-six and only reached thirty on four occasions. Some of these people were clearly deemed more reprehensible than others, being charged with dumping 'large quantities' of 'noxious' dung and, in quite a few cases, facing steep fines were it not quickly removed.[79] In the aftermath of the 1471 epidemic the authorities appear to have adopted a tougher line, since fifty-three offenders were then indicted. The number remained high during the plague year of 1479, rose again during the sweating sickness of 1485 and reached an unprecedented total of ninety-three in 1487. This striking burst of activity was also marked by growing vigilance in the matters of vagrant pigs, blocked drains, noisome gutters and offences such as brothel keeping, which undermined the moral health of the borough.[80] Since Ipswich was then experiencing a nascent economic revival after years of recession, some evidence of demographic growth might be expected, but it also seems likely that magistrates and juries recognised the sanitary implications of allowing even small quantities of refuse to contaminate the streets.[81]

Entrenched resistance to court orders could certainly incur serious punishment, especially if it involved the abuse of a senior official whose rank commanded respect. The woman who called alderman Simon de Worstede 'a false thief and broken-down old yokel' when he arrested her in 1364 for depositing filth into a London street was promptly dispatched to the sheriff's counter to contemplate the enormity of her offence. The astronomical – and clearly unfeasible – damages of £100 demanded from one of the city's dyers in similar circumstances some twenty years earlier reflect the same culture of deference to social superiors, but it is worth noting that an assault in 1390 on a lowly ward constable who had been collecting the street cleaners' quarterly wages earned both a fine *and* imprisonment.[82] Each of these cases underscores the fact that the quest for a healthier environment not only cost money, but was also a collaborative undertaking whose success demanded the active participation of all, or at least most, citizens.

---

[78] Hudson, *Leet Jurisdiction*, pp. 3, 6, 7, 11, 23–4, 26–7, 29.

[79] SROI, C/2/8/1/2–13, 15, 16; C/2/10/1/2–5.

[80] See section 2.6 above, and sections 3.6 and 4.2 below.

[81] SROI, C/2/8/1/14, 17–21; C/2/10/1/7. Amor documents the port's revival in the later fifteenth century: *Late Medieval Ipswich*, chaps. 6 and 7.

[82] *CPMRL, 1323–1364*, p. 162; *CPMRL, 1364–1381*, p. 15; *CLB*, H, p. 360.

3.3 Paving and cleaning the streets

Contrary to popular belief, English towns and cities began paving their streets from an early date. The laying of cobblestones in alleyways, as well as major thoroughfares, seems already to have been adopted in twelfth-century York, while Norwich was by then using large quantities of locally excavated gravel.[83] Both materials were employed together in London, where a shift from predominantly gravel to predominantly stone composites occurred during the fifteenth century.[84] As noted in Chapter 1, the cost of this exercise might at first be supported by a royal grant, but the burden of repairing and replacing road surfaces more often fell upon those residents whose properties abutted onto the streets in question. Instead of undertaking the task themselves, they were increasingly expected to pay skilled craftsmen to 'make goode & sufficient pavyng' that would be uniform and even (plate 6).[85] During the early fourteenth century the corporation of London retained first four and then six master paviors on a permanent basis; indeed, there was such demand for paviors' services that by 1479 they had formed their own guild to regulate working practices.[86] In provincial towns such as Newcastle on Tyne one expert, along with his journeymen or 'fellows', could generally keep on top of routine maintenance.[87] Nevertheless, striking variations occurred, not only from town to town but also, crucially, from one neighbourhood to another.

In Winchester it appears that, despite the reluctance of some householders to discharge their obligations, major roads were initially maintained 'at least to a minimum standard'. Archaeological evidence suggests that regular metalling took place from before the Norman Conquest and that surfaces were renewed at frequent intervals thereafter. Flint and chalk would usually be deposited over a bed of impacted brushwood and rubbish, which may either have accumulated because of illicit dumping or have been placed there deliberately to consolidate the subsoil.[88] However, as so often happened, depopulation and recession took their toll on the condition of the streets, and thus upon trade, with the result that, in 1485–6, the mayor and bailiffs followed the example of other magistrates by securing a parliamentary act which empowered them to rectify the potholed and dangerous

---

[83] Jørgensen, 'Cooperative Sanitation', p. 560; Ayers, *Norwich: Archaeology of a Fine City*, p. 74; B. Ayers, 'The Infrastructure of Norwich from the Twelfth to the Seventeenth Centuries', in Gläser, *Lübecker Kolloquium*, p. 37.

[84] Martin, 'Transport for London', pp. 94–101.

[85] *Coventry Leet Book*, I.199; II.389. As Londoners often complained, 'freelance' repairs could be worse than none at all: *LAN*, nos 140, 142; *CPMRL, 1458–1482*, p. 117. See also Salusbury-Jones, *Street Life in Medieval England*, pp. 35–7.

[86] *CLB*, C, pp. 11, 115; Martin, 'Transport for London', chap. 2.

[87] C. M. Fraser, ed., *The Accounts of the Chamberlains of Newcastle upon Tyne, 1508–1511*, The Society of Antiquaries of Newcastle upon Tyne Records Series 3 (Newcastle, 1987), p. xxiv. A contract of 1502 awarded the town pavior of Nottingham 33s. 4d. a year, with a gown, for repairing and maintaining all the pavements with stone and sand provided by the chamberlain: Stevenson, *Records of the Borough of Nottingham*, III.309.

[88] Jørgensen, 'Cooperative Sanitation', p. 560; see section 1.1 above.

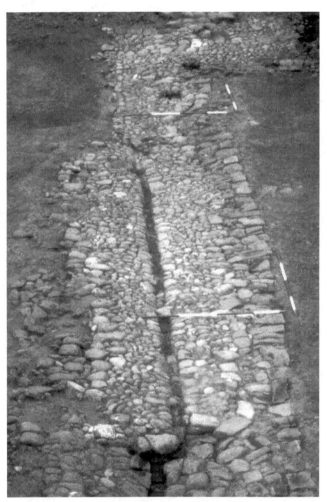

6 A fine example of a late medieval cobbled street excavated at the Royal Infirmary site, Chester. A central channel carried away water and liquid waste, while blocks of local sandstone made up the right hand curb.

state of Winchester's major roads. Henceforward, the owners or occupiers of any adjacent tenements could be compelled to lay a 'sufficiant pavement' whenever necessary, upon pain of distraint to cover the cost.[89] Rather than risk the delays and disagreements likely to arise over personal contributions, some urban authorities were prepared to divert corporate funds for this purpose.[90] Despite his protests to the parliament of 1477 that no revenues could be spared, the mayor of Southampton managed to finance various 'cawsey' repairs and similar public works from his own budget. In 1488–9, for example, he spent over £4 on mending the East Street pavements, and slightly less in 1496 on those near God's House.[91] But otherwise the burgesses remained responsible for the upkeep of roads, as we can see from the appointment in 1482 of a salaried pavior, who was employed 'to survey the state of the paving and to undertake repairs at the cost of the householders'.[92]

[89] *RP*, VI.333–4. See also Vowell, *Description of the Citie of Excester*, p. 922; section 1.4 above.

[90] Jørgensen, 'Cooperative Sanitation', p. 556; Barron, *London in the Later Middle Ages*, p. 261.

[91] His accounts reveal that in most years money was spent on road repairs, the removal of dung-hills and cleaning: Butler, *Book of Fines*, pp. 5, 44, 71, 78, 82, 109, 120.

[92] *RP*, VI.180–1; C. Platt, *Medieval Southampton: The Port and Trading Community, AD 1000–1600* (London, 1973), p. 171.

The ubiquity of bye-laws and presentments on the subject of pavements suggests that evasion was common, regardless of whether an act had been obtained. Public-spirited citizens such as the Londoner William Wollechirchehawe (d. 1301), whose executors assigned the handsome sum of £80 for civic projects including repairs to the highway in Bishopsgate, appear to have been outnumbered by less generous souls.[93] As noted above, the much-vaunted 'use and custome' that from at least 1428 required residents of Norwich to lay and maintain stone pavements was eventually undermined by 'the great gredynes and obstynacy growne into dyuerse mens hartes, whiche neyther regarde the comodyte of helth, ther owne eses and ther naybors, nor yet the bewtefyng of the cittie'.[94] Coercive measures were adopted in towns such as Coventry, where, in 1423, burgesses who failed to repair their street frontages from the door to the gutter within six months faced a blanket fine of 40*d.*[95] In King's Lynn, on the other hand, the aldermen and ward constables who routinely inspected the streets and pavements charged negligent home owners at a rate of 1*d.* a yard, or 2*d.* if they proved recalcitrant.[96] Far harsher sanctions seemed necessary in Southwark, not least because the volume of traffic passing through the borough on its way to and from London took such a heavy toll on road surfaces. During the early sixteenth century some residents faced 'savage' penalties of as much as £10 for non-compliance (among them prominent figures such as the abbot of Hyde, who kept a town house there and was sufficiently affluent to disregard conventional fines).[97] Across the river, where, in theory, the pavements of each ward were regularly surveyed from the 1270s onwards, the mayor could order repairs to be undertaken within forty days or send in one of the City's paviors, who would charge the owner of the adjacent property for his services.[98]

Yet even here complaints about pavements that were 'defective, dangerous and a nuisance to passers-by' seem to have been frequent, especially in the outlying wards and areas near the Thames, where narrow, insalubrious lanes ran down to

---

[93] *CEMCRL*, p. 151; Martin, 'Transport for London', p. 136; *CLB*, C, p. 130. In the event, only £19 was actually handed over, being either pocketed by the mayor or spent elsewhere: *CLB*, E, pp. 25–6. Perhaps for this reason some testators left building materials rather than cash, as we can see from the will of Robert Hardyng of Eye (d. 1470), who provided 120 loads of clay for road repairs in the town: P. Northeast and H. Falvey, eds, *Wills of the Archdeaconry of Sudbury, 1439–1474: Wills from the Register 'Baldwyne'*, vol. 2, Suffolk Records Society 53 (Woodbridge, 2010), no. 457.

[94] *RCN*, II.cxxix, 96–8, 133–4.

[95] *Coventry Leet Book*, I.58. In some boroughs, such as Lyme in Dorset, a blanket fine would be imposed on the entire community should roads not be repaired by a specific date: Dorset Record Office, DC/LR B1/2 nos 8, 19.

[96] KLBA, KL/C7/4, Hall Book, 1453–1497, p. 464.

[97] Carlin, *Medieval Southwark*, p. 234.

[98] Barron, *London in the Later Middle Ages*, pp. 261–2; *CLB*, L, pp. 84–5; *LAN*, no. 249. In 1495 a similar policy was adopted in Coventry, the common sergeant being authorised to charge anyone who failed to maintain his pavement for the cost of repairs, and also to issue a fine: *Coventry Leet Book*, II.568–9.

the quays.[99] To Continental observers, accustomed to higher standards or simply disposed to carp, there was undoubtedly room for improvement. Although he found much to praise about its 'pleasant and delightful' situation, an Italian who visited London at the turn of the fifteenth century was shocked by the impassability of major thoroughfares, noting that 'all the streets are so badly paved that they get wet at the slightest quantity of water'. Because of the constant press of draught animals and the incessant rain, he complained, 'a vast amount of evil-smelling mud is formed, which does not disappear quickly, but lasts a long time, in fact nearly the whole year round'.[100] We might note in this context that the popular English translation of the French romance *Partonopeu de Blois* begins in a magical walled city, celebrated for the cleanliness of its paved streets and the health of its inhabitants.[101] Sometimes both must have seemed the stuff of fairy tales.

However imperfectly it may have been enforced, individual responsibility for the state of urban thoroughfares went far beyond the need to ensure that pavements were well maintained and roads free from potholes. Ordinances for the regular removal of noxious and unsightly heaps of muck and rubble from street frontages proliferated from the thirteenth century onwards, those of Bristol instituting an unusually steep fine of 40*d.* for every dereliction.[102] From 1421 onwards each Coventry householder was expected to 'make clene the streyte before hur place' on Saturdays, while resisting the temptation to sweep domestic waste onto a neighbour's patch whenever it rained.[103] Similar arrangements were adopted in Leicester in 1467 and in early sixteenth-century Winchester, where it proved necessary to establish a communal rubbish dump on unoccupied land within the walls.[104] By then the rulers of Worcester had promulgated a rather optimistic ordinance for the daily cleansing of the streets, their principal concern being that refuse should be promptly 'caried awey' before it clogged up the gutters.[105] In the Durham borough of Crossgate residents were customarily required to clear the front of their houses of any garbage, cinders, dung and builders' rubble between

[99] *LAN*, nos 141, 175–6, 186, 369; *CPMRL, 1413–1437*, pp. 118, 121–4, 132–3, 135–7, 139, 151, 156. Some of these nuisances had already been 'several times indicted'.

[100] C. H. Williams, ed., *EHD*, vol. 5: *1485–1558* (London, 1967), p. 189. A compatriot, who arrived sixty years later, reported that 'the streets are spacious and well paved with limestone and flint': C. Barron, C. Coleman and C. Gobbi, 'The London Journal of Alessandro Magno 1562', *London Journal* 9 (1983), pp. 136–52, on p. 142.

[101] A. F. Trampe Bödtker, ed., *The Middle English Versions of 'Partonope of Blois'*, EETS e.s. 109 (London, 1911), p. 25.

[102] *LRBB*, II.31. Exasperated by the number of 'dunghylles in the stretes', the jurats of Winchelsea doubled this penalty, 'to be paide withoute any pardon' by recidivists: BL, MS Cotton Julius B IV, fol. 26v.

[103] *Coventry Leet Book*, I.23. Disposing of dung in wet weather, when it would turn into malodorous sludge, was specifically forbidden under a penalty of 40*d.* in York from 1371 onwards: *YMB*, I.lxvi.

[104] *RBL*, II.290; W. H. B. Bird, ed., *The Black Book of Winchester* (Winchester, 1925), pp. 124, 128. Weekly waste removal was also adopted in Dover by 1384–5 (BL, MS Egerton 2091, fol. 91r), and Faversham by 1446 (Harrington and Hyde, *Early Town Books of Faversham*, p. 85).

[105] HMC, *Twelfth Report*, appendix 9, p. 435.

each session of the bishop's court, which might also insist upon the removal of dirt from common lanes within a specific time on pain of fines ranging from a few pence to several shillings.[106] As many historians have observed, rules of this kind depended for their success upon a strong sense of community, although policing by neighbours, through presentments to local courts, and, increasingly, by officials with a specific brief to enforce sanitary regulations, must have curbed the activities of all but the most brazen individuals. In 1497, for example, the common sergeant and town crier of Coventry began patrolling the town on Sundays and Mondays to ensure that the residents had, indeed, disposed of all unsightly waste.[107]

London's comprehensive network of officials and salaried employees with responsibility for the state of the streets provided a model which other towns could adapt to fit their own more limited budgets and requirements. Oversight of the City and its twenty-five wards lay with the mayor, aldermen and councillors, who possessed the authority to raise the necessary capital, introduce and enforce the relevant ordinances and manage the growing roster of cleaners. Supervision at a more local level was undertaken from 1293 by teams of scavengers, whose oath required them to ensure that pavements were properly repaired 'and that the weyys, stretes and lanys be clensid of dunge and all maner of filthe for honeste of the Cite'. They were also expected to report any potential fire hazards.[108] By this date, each ward employed at least one raker to remove rubbish and manure from public places. When necessary, the ward beadles, assisted by the constables, had to lend a hand, while also helping to collect the rates levied from all householders for this service. The appointment in 1385 of a sergeant of the channel, with a specific brief to ensure that the banks of the Thames, markets and streets were 'wel and honestly clensid of filthis and dungehill' and to fine any delinquents, reflects the seriousness with which the authorities viewed matters of public health.[109]

Not surprisingly, given their proximity to the capital, the rulers of Westminster opted for a scaled-down version of this system, employing six scavengers to keep the streets free of garbage by 1508.[110] Elsewhere arrangements were more fluid. In Coventry, the common sergeant and deputy bailiff shouldered much of the burden, while the chamberlains might take charge of specific tasks such as cleaning the market.[111] From 1436 the rulers of Lynn assigned 26s. 8d. a year for a

[106] *RBC*, nos 160, 187, 236, 256, 259, 276, 371, 425, 441, 461, 473, 493, 521, 523, 551, 568, 573, 585, 591, 600, 642, 713.

[107] *Coventry Leet Book*, III.587.

[108] Barron, *London in the Later Middle Ages*, p. 262; Sabine, 'City Cleaning in Mediaeval London', pp. 21–3; *MGL*, III.125–6; *CLB*, D, p. 192. There were initially four scavengers per ward, but numbers later rose to as many as thirteen in some cases: Martin, 'Transport for London', pp. 188–90.

[109] *MGL*, III.135; *CLB*, A, p. 183; *CLB*, D, p. 201; *CLB*, H, p. 275; Barron, *London in the Later Middle Ages*, pp. 193–4.

[110] Rosser, *Medieval Westminster*, p. 237. A scavenger's contract of 1561 may be found in A. L. Merson, ed., *The Third Book of Remembrance of Southampton*, vol. 2, Southampton Records Series 3 (Southampton, 1955), no. 247.

[111] *Coventry Leet Book*, I.113, 217; II.425.

raker to deal with the watergates and the town's two principal markets, the ward constables being otherwise accountable for any 'defautes of the ffylthines in the stretes'.[112] In Beverley, too, the burgesses paid a salaried cleaner specifically to tidy up the markets and the pavements along 'the Beck', where waste was often dumped, as well as two keepers for overseeing and dredging watercourses.[113] The hiring of labourers for *ad hoc* cleaning tasks fell in Southampton to the stewards, who appear to have recruited workmen whenever it was necessary to clear heavily frequented areas, such as the gates, quays and conduits.[114] Magistrates and residents alike made considerable demands of these officers, who could be removed if they proved negligent. In February 1485, for example, the rulers of York decreed that the streets were to 'be clenely kepid and wekely sweped at the sight of the officers of the maire in there wards upon payne of fforfaitting of ther office'.[115] Shortly afterwards the common sergeant of Coventry received a terse reminder that he would be discharged unless he cleared heaps of dung from one of the gates, as previously requested.[116] Following the introduction of heavy fines for 'lyeng muck in the markyttes', in 1500, the chamberlains of Leicester were made personally liable for every uncollected sum.[117] The London ward moots were similarly quick to blame anyone whom they deemed to be lax or incompetent. In 1421 the chamberlain was roundly criticised for failing to pay a raker to cleanse the grates at London Wall, which had become 'evilly and horribly stopped up with mud and ordure to the great nuisance of all'.[118]

Activity on this scale required the creation of common laystalls, or dung-hills, where householders and street cleaners could dispose of their garbage well away from densely populated areas. Having already appointed a phalanx of scavengers and rakers, in 1378 the Common Council of London addressed various matters relating to civic health, including the need for designated places for the 'deposit of rubbish and filth'. This measure assumed particular urgency because of ongoing plans to cleanse the Thames and other waterways of malodorous waste.[119] Even in a relatively small borough, such as Stafford, the introduction of bye-laws to curb 'the indiscriminate dumping of filth' led rapidly to the provision of a communal tip in 1397, followed by others outside the gates.[120] By the late 1420s Coventry had established five 'official' extramural waste pits and dumps, while the residents of

---

[112] KLBA, KL/C7/3, Hall Book, 1431–1450, fol. 60v; C7/4, Hall Book, 1453–1497, p. 300; C7/5, Hall Book, 1497–1544, fol. 335r.

[113] Allison, *VCH York, East Riding*, VI.225; *BTD*, pp. 22–3.

[114] H. W. Gidden, ed., *The Stewards' Books of Southampton from 1428*, vol. 1: *1428–1434*, Southampton Record Society 35 (Southampton, 1935), pp. 13–15.

[115] Attreed, *York House Books*, i, p. 352. From the early fourteenth century the streets were to be inspected 'twice a term' in order to ensure that they were free from dung: *YCO*, p. 17.

[116] *Coventry Leet Book*, III.622.

[117] *RBL, II*, p. 359.

[118] *CPMRL, 1413–1437*, p. 117.

[119] *CLB*, H, p. 108; see section 4.3 below.

[120] M. W. Greenslade and D. A. Johnson, eds, *VCH Stafford*, vol. 6 (Oxford, 1979), p. 231.

both Hull and King's Lynn could choose between at least three.[121] In 1466 each parish in the Lincolnshire town of Stamford was assigned a designated spot for its own 'dunghylle', separate provision being made for local butchers, who were warned not to stray elsewhere.[122] The acquisition of dung carts accelerated the move towards the development of authorised sites and the imposition of heavy fines upon those who persistently littered the streets or neighbouring properties when more acceptable alternatives were readily available.[123] For example, orders of 1500–1 for the purchase of a refuse cart in every ward of York were accompanied by restrictions confining the deposit of dung to pre-arranged collection points where agricultural workers could easily remove it.[124] Rather than leave residents to make their own *ad hoc* arrangements, magistrates increasingly favoured regular services funded from communal resources or by special rates levied upon all but the poorest householders.

As might be expected, London appears to have been the first English city to institute a ward-based system for refuse collection. By 1357 an unspecified number of horses and wagons had been supplied for this task, any official who appropriated them for other purposes being threatened with automatic dismissal. More were clearly needed: as part of a wider campaign for environmental health, an additional twelve tumbrels and twenty-four draught horses were purchased in 1372 for use in the central wards of the City alone; and a few years later civic officers were empowered to commandeer any cart that had brought building materials (but nothing else) into London for the transport of dung and rubbish on its return journey.[125] Other towns adopted similar practices according to their needs. In 1420, for example, the rulers of Coventry imposed a quarterly charge of 1*d.* upon every household and a half-penny upon each shop to pay a carter for weekly collections. Extra help was recruited on a daily basis to assist with the cleansing of ditches and gutters.[126] When considering the acquisition of two communal refuse carts at about this time, Salisbury's magistrates appear initially to have favoured a type of means test for contributors, but by 1443 had approved an identical rate based on fixed quarterly

---

[121] Jørgensen, 'Cooperative Sanitation', p. 562; Evans, 'Infrastructure of Hull', pp. 60, 62; KLBA, KL/C7/4, Hall Book, 1453–1497, p. 388.

[122] Rogers, *William Browne's Town*, pp. 18–19.

[123] In London, casting 'urine and filth' onto other people's property fell within the remit of the assize of nuisance (*LAN*, nos 525, 566, 644), as did depositing 'dung and other refuse' on the streets 'in abomination to the common people passing along the road at night' (*LAN*, nos 493, 494). See also Keene, 'Rubbish in Medieval Towns', p. 29.

[124] *YCR*, II.165. By 1491 the mayor of Southampton had designated specific places 'for castyng of dunge': Butler, *Book of Fines*, p. 18.

[125] Riley, *Memorials of London*, pp. 435–6; Sabine, 'City Cleaning in Mediaeval London', pp. 23–4; Barron, *London in the Later Middle Ages*, p. 262. When the city's carters formed a fraternity in 1517, they agreed to provide a supplementary refuse collection service: Martin, 'Transport for London', pp. 239–42.

[126] *Coventry Leet Book*, I.21; II.361, 552–3.

payments.[127] The Norwich Assembly, by contrast, preferred to allocate revenues directly from the civic treasury, voting £10 in 1517 for a tumbrel and a further 40*s.* a year for the 'canel raker' who made the weekly refuse collection and kept the gutters free from rubbish. Thanks to an additional yearly levy, it proved possible to acquire two more 'comon cartes for the avoyding of fylthye and vile mater', which had to be put out by residents on the appointed day 'ayenst ther own groundes … upon rounde hepys redye to the carte'.[128] The householders of Leicester were less persuaded by the merits of communal action. The threat of imprisonment at the mayor's pleasure for those who failed to 'ordeyne a carte' for the removal of 'muk and swepynges and othere fylthes and corripcions' certainly suggests that consensus had yet to be reached during the 1460s.[129]

Implementing these schemes required both patience and flexibility, as we can see from the records of King's Lynn, where investment in a costly new water supply was accompanied by a vigorous campaign to cleanse the streets and ditches of accumulated dirt.[130] Following their inspection of the existing facilities in November 1444, the mayor and aldermen instituted a twice-weekly round by the town's muck-cart, and recruited another carter specifically to ferry rubbish to a common pit (*puteus*) north of the town at 'Doucehill' (Map 1). In order to fund this greatly improved service, a rate of between one half-penny and 2*d.* a quarter was introduced, depending upon the amount of garbage generated by each household. Aware that people might seek to avoid payment by fly-tipping in unauthorised places, the mayor imposed a series of escalating penalties, as much as 4*d.* being forfeit for 'euery grete lepe' (large container) used. A further ordinance, in March 1445, restricted the disposal of waste to three designated spots, upon pain of a 12*d.* fine or imprisonment for each offence. At first all went well, and by November there were sufficient funds to appoint another cleaner. But within five years filth had again begun to accumulate in the streets because the carters were not being paid. The ward constables were duly instructed to confer with residents about alternative types of levy, the overall preference being for assessment on the basis of wealth. Perhaps because it seemed more equitable, this system worked better. No further problems occurred until 1478, when the mayor was obliged to issue a new scale of

---

[127] Carr, *First General Entry Book*, nos 271, 388. In 1445 the mayor entered a five-year contract with one carter for the removal of refuse (no. 396), but eventually, in 1485, the citizens decided to acquire a cart of their own and hire a man to drive it (Wiltshire Record Office, G23/1/2, Salisbury Ledger Book 2, fol. 159r).

[128] NRO, NCR, 16C/1, Assembly Minute Book, 1492–1510, fol. 62r; 16C/2, Assembly Minute Book, 1510–1550, fol. 52r; *RCN*, II.109–10. Further help came from Alderman Robert Jannys, whose 'memoriall' acts (see p. 71 above) included the provision of a rental income specifically for this purpose, and to assist in cleansing the River Wensum: NCR, 16D/2, Assembly Proceedings, 1491–1553, fol. 102r. Individual donations, such as the sum of £10 left in 1518 by Elizabeth Thorsby 'to the continuans of a comyn carte for the fowyng (cleaning) of the stretes', were also readily forthcoming: NRO, NCC Gyles, fol. 98v.

[129] *RBL*, II.290.

[130] See section 4.1 below. From at least the 1380s onwards the chamberlains of Lynn spent sums of up to 35*s.* a year on cleaning the streets and ditches, but this may no longer have sufficed: KLBA, KL/C39/39–45.

fines for the illicit disposal of 'synders' and other domestic waste, and to provide a fourth communal rubbish dump outside the east gate. Having finally secured a degree of compliance, magistrates had now simply to monitor the use of the existing laystalls, when necessary creating new ones or, as happened in 1519, moving some of the older, more unsightly and malodorous dumps to unoccupied ground further away.[131]

The incessant transport of tons of waste in heavy carts with iron-bound wheels created its own problems, as the authorities of York complained in 1524, when exculpating themselves from blame over the lamentable state of the streets. These cumbersome vehicles had caused so much damage to thoroughfares 'newe pavyd to the great costs and chargs of the inhabitaunts' that cleaning operations had ground to a halt and conditions seemed far worse than before (plate 7). Henceforward, refuse was to be carried 'oonely [in] waines that hathe woulne [wooden] whellys or els uppon sledds'.[132] York was, in fact, rather behind the times, since iron-shod carts had already been banned or obliged to pay substantial tolls in London (1277), Beverley (1367), Cambridge (1402), Lincoln (1423), King's Lynn (1449), Chester (by 1493) and Gloucester (1500) for this very reason, as well as from a desire to reduce noise levels at night.[133] In Salisbury in 1452 the authorities placed restrictions upon the use of trailers attached to the backs of wagons, and upon large packs transported on wooden poles, because of the harm that was being done to highways, gutters and ditches, not least by the mud churned up in their wake.[134] Even worse were the refuse collectors who worked for private hire. They were liable not only to leave behind an offensive trail of manure and garbage, but even to ditch their loads at the first opportunity, rather than go to the trouble of taking them away. In Ipswich during the 1440s, one John Plunket was fined for removing 'dung and soil from various households' only to dump it in the highway and other inappropriate places.[135] However tolerant they may have been of minor peccadilloes, communities were not prepared to countenance offences of this kind. Indeed, from 1405 onwards the tumbrels used in London had to be fitted

---

[131] KLBA, KL/C7/2, Hall Book, 1422–1429 (addendum), p. 319; C7/3, Hall Book, 1431–1450, fols 194v, 195v, 197r–v, 200r, 212v, 271v, 274v, 278v; C7/4, Hall Book, 1453–1497, p. 395; C7/5, Hall Book, 1497–1544, fols 201v, 202r, 232v; Owen, *Making of King's Lynn*, pp. 218–19. In 1530 two additional dumps were established on staithes along the River Ouse, presumably so that refuse could more easily be removed by boat: C7/5, fol. 284r.

[132] *YCR*, III.90–1. From 1489 onwards the driver of every 'bound wain' entering the city was supposed to pay 4*d*. towards the repair of the pavements and bridges, although the money may have been diverted for other purposes: *YCR*, II.165.

[133] *CLB*, A, p. 217; *CLB*, H, p. 352; *CPMRL, 1364–1381*, p. 196; Martin, 'Transport for London', pp. 86, 126–7, 226–30; *BTD*, p. 21; Cooper, *Annals of Cambridge*, p. 148; HMC, *Fourteenth Report*, appendix 8, p. 21; KLBA, KL/C7/3, Hall Book, 1431–1450, fol. 272v; CCA, ZS/B/4c, Sheriffs' Book, 1493, fols 30r–33r; HMC, *Twelfth Report*, appendix 9, p. 434. From 1445 carters in Lynn had to make good any damage that they might cause to the gates: KLBA, KL/C7/3, Hall Book, 1431–1450, fol. 197v.

[134] Carr, *First General Entry Book*, no. 453.

[135] SROI, C/2/8/1/7, 10, 12. It was not unknown for London rakers to deposit dung and garbage in another ward, rather than removing it from the City as they were supposed to do: *CPMRL, 1381–1412*, p. 71.

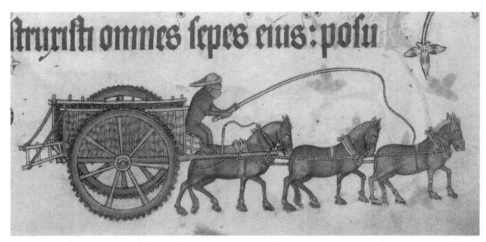

7 An engaging illumination from the Luttrell Psalter of *c*. 1320–45 depicts a heavy cart with iron-bound wheels, of the kind so often banned from late medieval cities. The studded nails used to attach the metal rims to the wood improved traction, but caused great damage to paved streets.

with a tall backboard to prevent the malodorous contents from spilling onto clean pavements.[136]

3.4 Latrines, cesspits and privies

The common assumption that the streets of medieval towns were submerged under a morass of human excrement is confounded by an incident of 1307 in which one of the king's grooms became embroiled in a fight with two indignant Londoners who found him relieving himself in a side road. They upbraided him, remarking 'that it would be more decent to go to the common privies of the City', and were assaulted for their pains.[137] Although it was hardly uncommon – if increasingly unacceptable – for people to urinate in public thoroughfares, considerations of hygiene and common decency alike demanded that men, women and children should defecate in more private places, preferably those designed for the purpose.[138] A beggar child killed in 1339 by a cart when squatting in a London street ('secreta nature faciendo sedentem') is censoriously described in the record as little more than a savage.[139] With such considerations in mind, and in sharp

---

[136] *CLB*, I, p. 45; *CPMRL, 1413–1437*, p. 133.

[137] *CEMCRL*, p. 255.

[138] Urination in the environs of important civic buildings, such as the London Guildhall, could prove especially contentious, as Paul Strohm has demonstrated: *Hochon's Arrow: The Social Imagination of Fourteenth-Century Texts* (Princeton, NJ, 1992), pp. 11–31, 173–7. Significantly, the guild merchant at Berwick-on-Tweed fined anyone who relieved himself at the gates or against the walls of the guildhall (Smith, Smith and Brentano, *English Gilds*, p. 340), while both the council chamber and the guildhall at Shrewsbury were equipped with 'urine tubs', which, when full, were presumably utilised by local tanners (Champion, *Everyday Life in Tudor Shrewsbury*, p. 17).

[139] Barron, *London in the Later Middle Ages*, pp. 260–1; *CCRCL*, p. 220.

contrast to the gloomy view of medieval sanitation espoused by most of his contemporaries, Ernest Sabine concluded his 1934 assessment of London's cesspits and latrines by suggesting that the citizenry deserved 'wholehearted praise and respect' for their efforts to maintain 'comfortable, clean and sanitary' facilities for both common and domestic use.[140] On his very conservative estimate, fifteenth-century residents and visitors enjoyed the benefit of just over a dozen public conveniences situated in the busiest parts of the capital. Some, such as the privies flushed with running water in the Stocks Market and in the aptly named 'long house' built on the bank of the Thames by the executors of Richard Whittington (d. 1423), catered for significant numbers at a time.[141]

Whittington's posthumous concern for the physical needs of his fellow citizens was far from unusual. Whereas some of the philanthropists who left money for the construction or upkeep of 'houses of easement' belonged, like Sir John Philipot (d. 1384), to the mercantile elite, or even royalty, others were less affluent.[142] Indeed, the construction of public conveniences was often a communal venture. Although the type of prestigious building erected in 1382–3 by the wardens of London Bridge at a cost of £11 was clearly beyond the means of most people, a smaller latrine required fewer resources, especially if it could be placed over or near a watercourse, thereby obviating the need for an expensive stone-lined cesspit. And even those with just a few pence to spare could contribute towards cleaning and maintenance. It is interesting to note that a public privy near St Margaret's church, Lynn, built by John de Walton in 1309, was still attracting legacies eighty years later, when one elderly widow left a small bequest for repairs.[143] Family pride, as well as zeal for good works, no doubt prompted the wealthy London mercer John Woodcock to provide in his will for the upkeep of the 'common latrine' and market cross that his father had erected in his native Doncaster.[144] But rather than wait for donations to materialise, the residents of Buck Street in Winchester, which already boasted a number of shared privies, clubbed together to build a new one of their own over a culverted stream.[145]

Evidence of this kind confirms that, although we know most about arrangements in the capital, a desire for better sanitation was certainly not confined to the elite of medieval London.[146] Often situated on heavily frequented

---

[140] Sabine, 'Latrines and Cesspools of Mediaeval London', p. 321.

[141] Sabine, 'Latrines and Cesspools of Mediaeval London', pp. 307–9; P. E. Jones, 'Whittington's Long House', *London Topographical Record* 23 (1974 for 1972), pp. 27–34. For the remains of a substantial stone-built public latrine near the Guildhall, see B. Sloane, 'Archaeological Evidence for the Infrastructure of the Medieval City of London', in Gläser, *Lübecker Kolloquium*, p. 92.

[142] *CWCHL*, II.276. A 'necessary house' was erected at Queenhithe by Matilda, the widow of Henry I, and extended in 1237 so that it continued to empty into the Thames: L. F. Salzman, *Building in England* (Oxford, 1967), p. 282.

[143] Owen, *Making of King's Lynn*, p. 214; KLBA, KL/C/50/63.

[144] *CWCHL*, II.398.

[145] Keene, *Survey of Medieval Winchester*, I.179–80.

[146] For a survey of the archaeological evidence for latrines and privies, see D. H. Evans, 'A Good Riddance to Bad Rubbish? Scatological Musings on Rubbish Disposal

bridges, where high demand combined with an easy means of flushing waste away, public conveniences are documented in almost all late medieval English towns and cities.[147] The colloquially named 'pissyngholes' and privies over the Ouse Bridge in York were maintained, like their equivalents in London, by bridge wardens, who were also responsible for cleaning and repairing the domestic privies in their various tenements throughout the city.[148] The contract made in 1544 with a local widow 'for keping cleyn' the conveniences on the bridge and allowing 'none to lye any wodd or other noysaunce in the same, nor caste no fylthe nor other ramell [rubbish] furthe ... into watter of Owse' continued the medieval practice of providing lavatory attendants and adequate lighting.[149] At Coventry the authorities rented out at least one of the common 'sege houses', along with a neighbouring bridge, on the understanding that the tenant would 'kepe & repair theym sufficiently' in return for any attendant profits.[150]

Once magistrates began to invest in cleaner, well-paved marketplaces, the need for accessible facilities that could be used by traders as well as shoppers and sightseers became apparent. In 1411–12 the treasurers of Norwich recorded a substantial outlay on 'scouring and making new' the privies at the fish market and nearby Guildhall, where the mayor's court met; and over £10 was spent in the 1450s on the gutters leading from another latrine on the north-west approaches to this crowded area.[151] Busy ports such as Southampton erected privies on the quays, while also ensuring that the constant flow of travellers entering the gates

and the Handling of "Filth" in Medieval and Early Post-Medieval Towns', in K. de Groote, D. Tys and M. Pieters, eds, *Exchanging Medieval Material Culture*, Relicta Monografiëen 4 (2010), pp. 267–78.

[147] Reading had at least one 'common latrine' by 1420: HMC, *Eleventh Report*, appendix 7: *Supplementary report on the manuscripts of the Duke of Leeds, the Bridgewater trust, Reading corporation, the Inner Temple, etc.*, Royal Commission on Historical Manuscripts 22 (London, 1888), p. 173. In Exeter there was a long vaulted latrine, known as 'the fairy house', on the Exe bridge and another over the mill fleet during the 1460s: D. Portman, *Exeter Houses, 1400–1700* (Exeter, 1966), p. 15. In Salisbury a public convenience stood from 1406 on Fisherton Bridge: Carr, *First General Entry Book*, nos 71, 89, 127, 136. William of Worcester approvingly noted a 'privey' for women and men near Aylward's gate and another on the Avon bridge, Bristol, in c. 1480: J. Dallaway, ed., *Antiquities of Bristow* (Bristol, 1834), pp. 68, 72–3. Sixteen years later the town of Shrewsbury erected 'come[n] pryveys bothe for men and women for theyre eassments' on Welsh Bridge: Leighton, 'Early Chronicles of Shrewsbury', p. 251.

[148] P. M. Stell, trans., *The York Bridgemasters' Accounts* (York, 2003), pp. 122, 128, 209, 256, 257. In 1301 it was decreed that public latrines should be available in each of the four wards of York: *YCO*, p. 17.

[149] *YCR*, IV.122; Stell, *York Bridgemasters' Accounts*, pp. 204, 226, 243, 253, 296, 348, 375, 400, 435, 448. As at Whittington's 'long house' in London, a civic almshouse was situated above the latrines: Stell, *York Bridgemasters' Accounts*, pp. 204, 226, 243.

[150] *Coventry Leet Book*, I.194.

[151] NRO, NCR, 7C, Treasurers' Account, 1411–1412; 7D, Chamberlains' Account, 1457–1458. By 1411 the city employed a designated 'fower latrinarum', or lavatory cleaner.

would not have far to search for a 'comyn wedraft housse'. In 1495–6, a small one was constructed in the walls at a cost of 30s., and regular sums were voted for the upkeep of various other conveniences throughout the town.[152] Quite probably they were timber-framed and tiled like those used by visitors to Dover and Sandwich.[153] By the fifteenth century five rather more impressive 'places of easement for the common people' stood at regular intervals along the Hull waterfront, each being built and maintained from the public purse.[154] Well aware of the effect that unfavourable first impressions might have upon their collective reputation, in 1431 the rulers of Lynn appointed a committee of no fewer than ten leading burgesses to oversee repairs to a troublesome *cloaca* at the main eastern gate.[155]

From a comparatively early date the more affluent residents of English towns opted to construct their own privies, while poorer people who rented lodgings in tenement blocks were increasingly able to share with other families.[156] Both decency and hygiene required that all latrines should be situated as far as possible 'out of the wey from syght and smellynge', but crowded urban life often made this impossible.[157] Many householders had little choice but to dig cesspits for the deposit of waste in backyards and cellars, often by means of intramural chutes or pipes, but those whose properties enjoyed access to streams or rivers understandably preferred to use running water. By the late fourteenth century, however, anxiety on the part of urban magistrates about the pollution and blockage of waterways heralded a shift away from privately owned riparian privies, which invited removal orders and stringent financial penalties. First set at 6s. 8d. in 1433, the fine imposed in Coventry rose to a substantial 20s. in just three years as the scale of the problem became glaringly apparent.[158] Given their often fraught relations with the university authorities, who complained repeatedly about their shortcomings, the burgesses of Cambridge must have derived considerable satisfaction from naming several scholars among the offenders with 'seges or privies overhanging the common river'.[159]

Having initially sanctioned the construction of latrines over the Fleet and Walbrook rivers, the rulers of London performed a similar *volte face* in the fifteenth century, not least because of concern lest the inmates of the Fleet prison

[152] C. Platt and R. Coleman-Smith, *Excavations in Medieval Southampton, 1953–1969*, vol. 1 (Leicester, 1975), p. 34; H. W. Gidden, ed., *The Stewards' Books of Southampton, from 1428*: vol. 2: *1434–1439*, Southampton Record Society 39 (Southampton, 1939), p. 90; Butler, *Book of Fines*, pp. 42, 46, 109, 115.

[153] BL, MS Egerton 2107, fols 9v, 14v; Clarke *et al.*, *Sandwich: A Study of the Town and Port*, p. 134.

[154] One alone cost £5 to build in 1442 and was, apparently, 'quite an elaborate structure': Evans, 'Infrastructure of Hull', pp. 57 (fig. 5b), 60.

[155] KLBA, KL/C7/3, Hall Book, 1431–1450, fols 9v–10v.

[156] By the fifteenth century, at least, the lack of an accessible privy was regarded as a 'defect' to be amended: *CPMRL, 1413–1437*, p. 118.

[157] Salzman, *Building in England*, p. 283.

[158] *Coventry Leet Book*, I.202, 227.

[159] Cooper, *Annals of Cambridge*, p. 258; Williams, 'Plague in Cambridge', pp. 53–5; see section 1.4 above.

might succumb to 'abominable stenches'.[160] By contrast, some of the City's other restrictions dated back to the reign of King John, if not before. The late twelfth-century *assisa de edificis*, which regulated the design and use of buildings, laid down precise rules for the situation of private cesspits, especially with regard to their proximity to neighbouring properties. Those that were simply lined with earth, and thus liable to seep into the surrounding soil, had to be sunk at a greater distance (3.5 feet) from party walls than pits with solid stone or timber linings (2.5 feet).[161] Infringements generally resulted in an order for the removal of the offending nuisance within forty days, although the solution was, inevitably, less straightforward when neighbours shared the same pit. In such cases both parties might be ordered to empty it at their joint cost, or pay a hefty fee to the sheriff's officers for undertaking this thankless task.[162] Whereas complaints regarding mephitic vapours from noisome latrines and cesspits were generally dealt with in London by the ward moots, rather than the assize, exceptions would be made if a breach of the building regulations had also been committed.[163]

As we discovered in Chapter 1, archaeological excavations in Southampton have established a striking connection between changes in sanitary practice and increased sensitivity to the risks posed by noxious odours, most notably after the Black Death. Before the thirteenth century 'cesspits and rubbish pits of all kinds [were] scattered in a disorderly and unsystematic way', but from then onwards the construction of new and improved stone houses meant that 'the whole pattern of waste disposal changed'.[164] As in London, building regulations determined exactly where pits might be dug, while encouraging a trend towards the use of solid stone or timber, both to prevent seepage and to facilitate cleaning (plate 8). Some even possessed vaulted stone roofs in order to provide better ventilation and eliminate miasmatic air.[165] Even so, by the 1400s Southampton's wealthier householders seem to have favoured the immediate removal of waste by the night carts that regularly patrolled their streets. A similar picture emerges in Hull, where the introduction of weekly – and from 1481 thrice-weekly – refuse collections has been linked by archaeologists to the disappearance of back-yard middens. These developments, together with the growing popularity of purpose-built latrines, made the borough a far cleaner place to live.[166] The same is true of Norwich, where at least one ingenious fourteenth-century resident solved the problem of lining

---

[160] Sabine, 'Street Cleaning in Mediaeval London', pp. 33–6. Concern on this score began in the aftermath of the Black Death: E. Williams, ed., *Early Holborn and the Legal Quarter of London*, 2 vols (London, 1927), no. 209; see section 4.3 below.

[161] *MGL*, I.323–4; J. Schofield, *Medieval London Houses* (New Haven, CT, 1995), pp. 33, 86–7; Schofield, *London, 1100–1600*, pp. 76 (fig. 4.9), 90.

[162] *LAN*, p. xxv, nos 2, 3, 44, 60, 96, 98, 165, 191, 297, 384.

[163] *LAN*, nos 214, 364, 585, 644.

[164] Platt and Coleman Smith, *Excavations in Medieval Southampton*, p. 34. It is, however, likely that householders had more space for the hygienic disposal of rubbish before tenement boundaries were defined in the 1200s.

[165] Salzman provides some interesting examples of the construction of vents 'to voyd the heyr a wey' from privies: *Building in England*, p. 284.

[166] Evans, 'Infrastructure of Hull', pp. 60, 62, 65 (fig. 8).

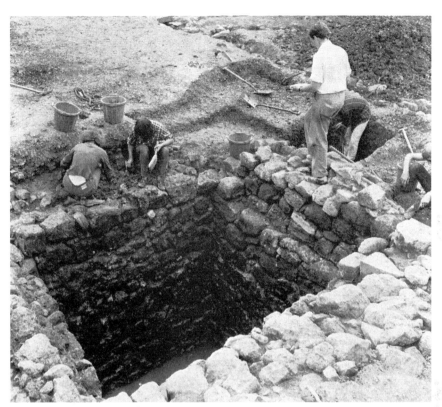

8 This fine example of a late thirteenth-century stone-lined cesspit, excavated in Cuckoo Lane, Southampton, reveals that well before the Black Death more affluent home owners were taking steps to improve domestic sanitation.

his cesspit by sinking a large and solid wooden barrel into the ground (plate 9).[167] More prosperous citizens in the residential areas of Pottergate and King Street enjoyed the benefit of stone-lined pits filled by means of chutes or chimneys that speedily conveyed waste from upper-storey privies.[168] As in London and Lincoln, the town houses of leading merchants boasted separate, stoutly built flint and brick-rubble garderobes constructed as external features adjacent to, but safely apart from, the main range.[169]

That effective sanitation was becoming a priority for many less affluent

[167] B. Ayers, ed., *Excavations at Fishergate, Norwich, 1985*, EAA 68 (Norwich, 1994), pp. 11–12, 49–50. For the use of casks or barrels as linings for cess pits, see also Greig, 'Investigation of a Medieval Barrel-Latrine', pp. 265–82. In 1278 two Londoners were killed while sinking a cesspit made of five wine casks stacked together: *CLB*, B, pp. 277–8.

[168] Ayers, *Norwich: Archaeology of a Fine City*, pp. 100, 121, 123–4.

[169] A. Shelley, *Dragon Hall, King Street, Norwich*, EAA 112 (Norwich, 2005), pp. 58–9. See also R. H. Jones, *Medieval Houses at Flaxengate, Lincoln:* The Archaeology of Lincoln 11.1 (London, 1980), p. 12 and fig. 9. Proximity to kitchens meant that domestic privies were also used for the disposal of food waste: Schofield, *Medieval London Houses*, p. 70.

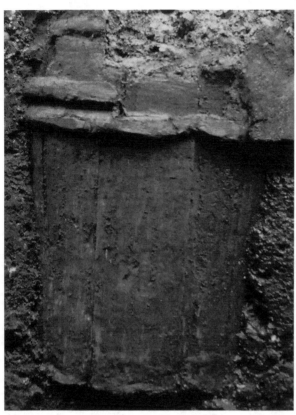

9 Large barrels served as a cheaper alternative to stone-lined cesspits. This effective, if rudimentary, fourteenth-century latrine was excavated, complete with human fecal remains, from domestic premises in Fishergate, Norwich.

people is apparent from the wills of men like the Londoner Alexander Heyrun, who left a house to his step-children in 1308 on the condition that they would regularly clean and maintain the privy that was shared with another property. Leases frequently imposed the same obligation upon tenants.[170] This was no mean requirement, as the emptying of cesspits could prove both expensive and unpleasant, being generally delegated to 'gongfermours', whose high rate of pay reflects the disagreeable nature of the work.[171] Their scale of charges was customarily based upon the number of tuns, or large barrels, of waste removed, although institutional land-owners such as the wardens of London Bridge were sometimes able to negotiate lower rates. Costs (which often included the wages of a master mason to breach and replace part of the stonework) were sufficiently high to explain why private householders tended to postpone the day of reckoning and accidentally let their cesspits overflow. The extraction of nineteen barrels of waste from a single latrine pit in 1461–2 cost the wardens 47s. 6d.; and even at a cut price of just 20d. a barrel they still had to pay over £8 in 1501–2 for the removal of almost a hundred tuns of ordure from various dwellings.[172] But despite the size of the bill, property owners who tried to economise by shirking their responsibilities might end up in court. In Durham, for example, the owners of latrines that annoyed their neighbours or polluted the water supply were expected to rectify the problem immediately

[170] *CWCH*, I.197 (see also the will of John Walpol, p. 564); *CPMRL, 1413–1437*, p. 297; Schofield, *Medieval London Houses*, pp. 205–6.

[171] For the problem of cleaning domestic latrines, see Portman, *Exeter Houses*, p. 15.

[172] V. Harding and L. Wright, eds, *London Bridge: Selected Accounts and Rentals, 1381–1538*, LRS 31 (London, 1995), pp. 135, 156. See also, Salzman, *Building in England*, pp. 284–5. In 1466, the appropriately named John Lovegold contracted with the mayor of London to empty all the city's public latrines for the next ten years at a rate of 2s. 2d. a tun: *CLB*, L, pp. 67–8.

under threat of a cumulative fine.[173] Although, in comparison with their volubility about the dumping of waste in public places, Ipswich jurors made far fewer presentments on this score, offenders could still face stringent penalties. In 1436, for instance, one householder who had built his privy too close to the town ditch stood to forfeit 40s. for resisting a demolition order. Not surprisingly, he duly complied.[174]

As a general rule, the landlords of multi-storey 'slum' dwellings in crowded side-roads proved most resistant to change. The catalogue of nuisances listed by London jurors in the 1420s included several offensive privies, as well as others that appeared 'defective and perilous' and likely to cause serious accidents. The note of exasperation apparent in some indictments, especially regarding the filthy narrow lanes leading down to the Thames, was clearly warranted, given that similar complaints had been voiced on and off since at least the 1270s.[175] An inquiry of 1343 into the blockage of these dank and malodorous alleyways had already painted an unsavoury picture of leaking and obstructive latrines, as well as garderobe chutes emptying directly from upper storeys into the street, sometimes upon the heads of unfortunate passers by ('super capita hominum transeuntium').[176] However vigorously they may have been expressed, official sanctions and peer pressure could only achieve so much. The challenge proved even greater in the case of butchers, whose capacity for polluting the urban environment was matched only by their notorious truculence in the face of authority.

3.5   Butchers and butchery

By the early fourteenth century butchers had established a significant presence in most English towns: both York and Norwich then supported about fifty, while Durham, which was far smaller and less affluent, could muster at least seventeen.[177] Their successors were among the first to benefit from the rise in standards of living discernible after the Black Death, when they secured a dominant position among the victualling trades as the demand for their products escalated.[178] This trend was accompanied by growing anxiety, clearly apparent before the first outbreak of plague, about the keeping and slaughtering of animals in residential areas, the contamination of surrounding streets and watercourses with blood, offal and carcasses, and the hazards posed by such offensive matter. Most plague tracts and *regimina* made a direct connection between the spread of pestilence and the noxious effluvia arising from 'the corruption of deed carreyne, the whiche dothe fortune often tymes in corrupte places'.[179] As a result, although

---

[173] *RBC*, nos 211, 413, 547, 580, 699.

[174] SROI, C/2/8/1/7, 9, 13; C/2/10/1/2.

[175] *CPMRL, 1413–1437*, pp. 124, 129, 132–3, 135, 141, 152, 154–7; *CLB*, A, p. 218.

[176] *MGL*, II.ii.444–53; Sabine, 'City Cleaning in Mediaeval London', pp. 32–3, 39.

[177] Bonney, *Lordship and Urban Community*, p. 151; *YCO*, p. 24; Rutledge, 'Economic Life', p. 171.

[178] See section 5.2 below.

[179] Horrox, *Black Death*, p. 176; Thomas Paynell, *A Moche Profitable Treatise against the Pestilence* (London, 1534), sig. Aiij.

slaughterhouses such as St Nicholas Shambles in London were often situated in peripheral areas (Map 2), they still occasioned such concern that, by the 1360s, if not well before, systematic attempts were being made to impose stricter controls or to remove their 'grievous corruption and foulness' to the outer suburbs.[180] The uncharacteristic silence of Norwich's ruling elite on this topic is due to the fact that the resident butchers congregated on high ground to the extreme south-west of the city, where there was plenty of grazing land, easy access to the river for waste disposal downstream of more densely populated areas and a strong breeze to disperse any miasmas (plate 10).[181] Elsewhere, however, the struggle to regulate an essential but potentially dangerous component of urban life gave rise to a battery of ordinances and complaints that provide a fascinating insight into the spread of medical knowledge, as well, perhaps, as growing sensibilities regarding the use of public space. Envisaged in 1515–16, Thomas More's Utopia is notable for its extramural slaughterhouses, where waste could safely be flushed away in streams and rivers. 'They don't allow anything dirty or filthy to be brought into the city', the narrator reports approvingly, 'lest the air become tainted by putrefaction and thus infectious.'[182]

Since they had such a major impact upon the City's water supply, we shall explore the activities of London's butchers more fully in the next chapter. But it is worth quoting here from a parliamentary petition presented in the plague year of 1379 by a group of influential courtiers and other 'residents of the streets of Holborn and Smithfield', who protested that:

> because of the great and horrible stenches and deadly abominations which arise there from day to day from the corrupt blood [*sank corrupt*] and entrails of cattle, sheep and pigs killed in the butchery next to the church of St Nicholas in Newgate and thrown in various ditches in two gardens near to Holborn Bridge, the said courtiers, frequenting and dwelling there, contract various ailments, and are grievously exposed to disease [*trop grevousement mys a disease*] as a result of the infection of the air, the abominations and stenches above-said, and also by many evils that notoriously ensue.[183]

The royal response simply emphasised the need to enforce earlier directives against the pollution of the highways and river, but was followed, nine years and at least one regional epidemic later, by a statute comprehensively forbidding the deposit of butchers' waste and similar refuse in or near *any* English towns or cities because of the threat posed by miasmatic air.[184] Since the residents of Cambridge, where this parliament met, had recently been subject to an order from King Richard for the removal of all swine, dirt, dung and rubbish from the streets, it has been suggested that 'the filthy state' of the town gave rise to this particular item of legislation.[185]

---

[180] *CCR, 1369–1374*, pp. 31–2.

[181] Rawcliffe, 'Sickness and Health', p. 204; Kirkpatrick, *Streets and Lanes*, p. 16.

[182] More, *Utopia*, p. 46.

[183] *PROME*, VI.181.

[184] *SR*, vol. 2, 12 Richard II, cap. 13, p. 59. For the East Anglian plague of 1383, see Appendix.

[185] Cooper, *Annals of Cambridge*, pp. 133, 134.

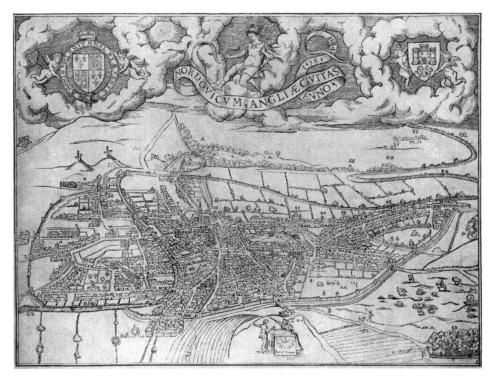

10 A somewhat idealised depiction of Norwich produced in 1558 by the physician William Cuningham emphasises its healthy situation, in accordance with Hippocratic ideas about the environment. The butchers had been consigned for centuries to the southern periphery (on the right of this west-facing map), with easy access to grazing land and the River Wensum.

But fear of pestilence transcended the merely local, placing the general problem of urban nuisances high on the political agenda. Edward III had initially prohibited the slaughtering of animals in London during the second great national epidemic of 1361, although his attempts to remove its butchers to Knightsbridge (in the west) and Stratford (in the east) clearly had unwelcome consequences. Whereas some of them took the easy option of dumping their offal immediately outside the walls in the fields and ditches of Holborn, others raised their prices to allow for the cost of transport, thereby occasioning an outcry in the City.[186] As we shall see, the obvious solution lay in the construction of proper facilities for the disposal of processed waste into the tidal waters of the Thames, thereby making it possible to supply London markets with cheap, fresh meat on demand.[187]

The proximity of the royal court inevitably exposed London's butchers to particular scrutiny, although alarm about the insalubrious activities associated with urban slaughterhouses was certainly not confined to the capital. As early as 1301, the customs of Sandwich imposed a ban upon butchering in shops and streets, an insanitary practice against which other towns and cities (including

---

[186] Sabine, 'Butchering in Mediaeval London'; P. E. Jones, *The Butchers of London* (London, 1976), pp. 78–80.

[187] See section 4.3 below.

Chester, Lynn, Northampton, Winchelsea and York) also took action, not least because of the filth and congestion caused by animals awaiting slaughter.[188] By the 1380s Yarmouth butchers faced heavy fines for herding and killing their beasts in public highways 'to the great prejudice and defilement [*turpitudinem*]' of the town. They were also in trouble for pasturing animals on the dunes immediately outside the walls and thereby depriving others of a valuable resource.[189] Although it posed only an indirect risk to public health, the overgrazing of common land by butchers fattening their stock for slaughter often went hand in hand with a propensity to deposit offal, dung and other noxious waste there as well. For this reason, the subletting of land to butchers who might use it to dispose of 'entrails and other filth causing foul smells' was prohibited in both York and Westminster. Furthermore, since animals sometimes escaped, causing accidents and even fatalities, in 1422 and again in the 1480s Westminster's butchers were ordered to pen their sheep, pigs and cattle safely at all times.[190]

Some towns opted for the obligatory use of common scalding houses, where butchers could kill animals and prepare their carcasses out of sight, without polluting neighbouring highways and gutters (plate 11). In 1421 the rulers of Coventry proposed to construct one, but had to concede that butchers might continue using their own premises in the interim, on the condition that each of them kept 'his durre [doorway] clene fro bloode and other fylthis', promised not to raise pigs at home and refrained from tethering or slaughtering any beasts in the street. By 1447 all these disagreeable activities had been confined to two designated places and forbidden elsewhere in the borough.[191] Alarmed by the 'abomination, filth and *viliditatem putredorum*' in front of 'Butcher Row', Salisbury's magistrates decreed in 1423 that the slaughtering of animals should henceforth be relegated to the back, and that no offal should be carried away or fat rendered into tallow by day 'on account of the stench'. Some twenty years later, the mayor himself built a new 'skaldynghous' at his own cost, so that, as in Coventry, the butchers could be restricted to one spot.[192] Similar rules obtained in Gloucester, largely

---

[188] W. Boys, *Collections for a History of Sandwich*, 2 vols (Canterbury, 1792), II.501; CCA, ZS/B/5b, Sheriffs' Book, 1504–1505, fol. 35r; KLBA, KL/C7/2, Hall Book, 1422–1429, p. 64; *RBN*, I.335; Markham, *Liber custumarum*, p. 35; BL, MS Cotton Julius B IV, fol. 26r; *YMB*, I.83; R. B. Dobson, ed., *York City Chamberlains' Account Rolls, 1396–1500*, Surtees Society 192 (Gateshead, 1980), pp. 145–6.

[189] NRO, Y/C4/ 93, rot. 4r; 171, rot. 18r.

[190] Rosser, *Medieval Westminster*, p. 242; *YMB*, III.58.

[191] *Coventry Leet Book*, I.32, 42–3, 58, 232.

[192] Carr, *First General Entry Book*, nos 236, 398. The shambles in Hull was equipped with a well to facilitate cleaning after solid waste had been removed to the main rubbish dump outside the town (Evans, 'Infrastructure of Hull', p. 62), while the new slaughterhouse built in Reading in the 1420s had both a well and gutters (C. Slade, ed., *Reading Gild Accounts, 1357–1516*, part 1, Berkshire Record Society 6 (Reading, 2002), pp. lxxi–lxxii). This municipal 'scleynge house' was effectively rebuilt by 1459, leading to a rent strike on the part of the butchers. Five years later the mayor ordered all burgesses to cease buying meat until a satisfactory agreement could be reached: J. M. Guilding, ed., *Reading Records: Diary of the Corporation*, vol. 1 (London, 1892), p. 58.

to preserve the cleanliness of public thoroughfares. Although it was not until 1516 that the rearing of pigs near the official scalding house in Grass Lane became illegal, the authorities had by then instituted special measures for the compulsory disposal of butchers' waste by night in order to avoid the 'inordinate savour and stynche that the comen gorreour [raker] makith by daye when he carieth awey innewardes of bestes, filthi vessels and other filthy thynges out of the Bocher Rewe'.[193] Arrangements of this kind were designed to reduce the transmission of contaminated air, and offered residents some level of protection against infection.

The safe removal of carcasses, especially in hot weather, taxed the ingenuity of urban authorities to the limit. It was easy to fine or even imprison offenders who endangered others by littering streets, gardens and yards with the 'annoyable' remains of slaughtered animals, but harder to offer a viable alternative.[194] Private arrangements were fraught with difficulties, as one Nottingham butcher discovered

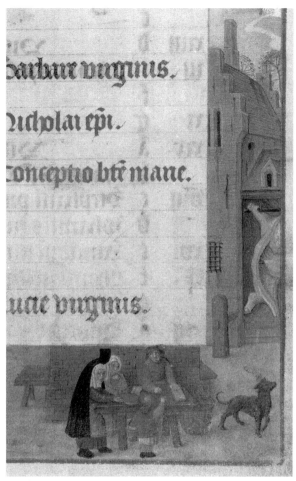

11 This street scene from an early sixteenth-century Flemish liturgical manuscript depicts a stall, a butcher's dog and, in the background, a freshly butchered carcass, hanging in full public view.

in 1378–9 when the carter with whom he had contracted for the disposal of entrails and other detritus took umbrage at the disrespect shown to his wife and

[193] HMC, *Twelfth Report*, appendix 9, pp. 433–4, 440–1. Nocturnal disposal of offal was compulsory in Sandwich by 1301 at the latest (BL, MS Cotton Julius B IV, fol. 75v), but was not apparently adopted in Westminster until 1505 (Rosser, *Medieval Westminster*, pp. 242–3).

[194] For complaints about negligent butchers, see, for example: D. Hutton, 'Women in Fourteenth-Century Shrewsbury', in L. Charles and L. Duffin, eds, *Women and Work in Pre-Industrial England* (London, 1985), p. 95; DRO, ECA, Chamber Act Book 1, 1508–1538, fol. 25r; NRO, Y/C4/191, rot. 16v; A. Raine, *Mediaeval York* (London, 1955), p. 83; Studer, *Oak Book of Southampton*, I.52–3, 131; Laughton, *Life in a Late Medieval City*, p. 85.

left a pile of stinking waste behind him.[195] In general, it seemed better to insist upon collective responsibility. Probably influenced by the system for street cleaning already adopted in London, York's magistrates ruled at this time that offal should always be transported in covered wagons, in order to prevent airborne pollution.[196] The rulers of Lynn openly acknowledged their debt when, in 1439, they instructed the resident butchers to equip themselves with 'covered barrows or carts according to the practice of London'. Notwithstanding the threatened fine of 20s. for non-compliance, they were obliged to repeat the demand seven years later (when plague was raging not far away in Lincoln), and to insist that intestines and other unpleasant matter should only be conveyed through the town after dark. At the turn of the fifteenth century they lit upon the more effective stratagem of forcing any butcher who left filth in the streets or withheld his contribution towards the cost of transport to slaughter his animals outside the walls, and thus to forfeit a valuable commercial advantage.[197]

In order to render their waste marginally less offensive, butchers would also sink pits in which the remains and blood of animals could either be stored, pending removal, or safely buried. As in the case of urban cesspits, the cleansing process was profoundly disagreeable, with the result that some authorities deemed it necessary to regulate this activity, too. In Worcester a decree of 1466 established 'that no intraillez of eny manner bestes, nor no puttes [pits] of bloode, be clansed or caryed awey on the day, but ouer nights in due tyme ... and that no blode putte be vnclensyd ouer [for more than] a day and a night, be it wynter or somer'.[198] Meanwhile in Coventry, the mounting problem of noxious refuse demanded the creation of a large communal pit, or series of pits, specifically for the deposit of carrion from butchery. Understandably reluctant to linger over his work, the carter responsible for this unpleasant task received stern orders in 1474 to cease tipping offal around the edges, and to cast it into the middle, out of the reach of scavenging pigs.[199] Many of these intimidating creatures belonged to the town's butchers, whose misdemeanours all too often extended to the ownership of potentially dangerous animals.

[195] Stevenson, *Records of the Borough of Nottingham*, III.181–2.

[196] *YMB*, I.lxix, 17–18. For Colchester, see below pp. 268–9.

[197] KLBA, KL/C7/3, Hall Book, 1431–1450, fols 103r, 271v; C7/5, Hall Book, 1497–1544, fol. 35v; Owen, *Making of King's Lynn*, p. 21. For the 1446–7 plague, see Appendix.

[198] Smith, Smith and Brentano, *English Gilds*, p. 385. In Stamford, ditches 'withowt the towne' served for the dumping of all 'intrales of flesshe or fysche or bowells', which were to be removed promptly from the borough: Rogers, *William Browne's Town*, pp. 11–12.

[199] *Coventry Leet Book*, II.271–2, 389. The construction and daily use of large pits for the deposit of entrails was one of the many grievances voiced by the residents of Holborn in the late fourteenth century: Sabine, 'City Cleaning in Mediaeval London', pp. 41–2.

3.6 Vicious dogs and marauding pigs

The assumption that baiting a bull with dogs would improve the taste and digestibility of its flesh encouraged many authorities to fine any butchers who failed to do so.[200] Hugely popular with spectators (who shared few, if any, of the modern reader's sensibilities about cruelty to animals), these spectacles were often staged in open thoroughfares, where security might well be minimal. One of the most dramatic of Thomas Becket's reputed miracles provides a vivid account of the pandemonium that ensued when an enraged beast ran amok among the London crowds. About to gore a child to death, the escaped bull – and the pack of yelping dogs that pursued it – froze immobile when the boy's mother invoked St Thomas's name and disaster was narrowly averted.[201] It was, no doubt, in the interests of public safety, as well as to guarantee the quality of the meat supply, that in 1423 the rulers of Coventry decided to construct a proper bull-ring.[202] However, such measures did not protect pedestrians from the general menace of butchers' dogs, which were needed to drive cattle as well as bait them, and also to satisfy the incessant public craving for dog fights, boar and bear baiting and other blood sports (plate 12). Sharing many of their owners' less amiable characteristics, these large and aggressive animals were frequently allowed to roam the streets, where they caused a serious nuisance. But any householder, shopkeeper or artisan might well acquire a fierce guard dog to scare away thieves, and they, too, were liable to run wild given the opportunity. Many others were strays that hunted in packs.

Since flocks of sheep were frequently herded through English towns on their way to market or the slaughterhouse, while others grazed on suburban smallholdings or even on grassy plots within the walls, we should not be surprised by the number of cases of sheep-worrying heard in urban courts.[203] In both London and Durham

---

[200] As, for example, in Basingstoke (Baigent and Millard, *History of the Town and Manor of Basingstoke*, pp. 307, 318, 321), Beverley (*BTD*, p. 129), Bristol (Veale, *Great Red Book of Bristol*, I.144), Chester (Laughton, *Life in a Late Medieval City*, p. 185), Colchester (*RPBC*, pp. 18–19), Faversham (Harrington and Hyde, *Early Town Books of Faversham*, p. 85), Ipswich (Bacon, *Annalls of Ipswiche*, p. 128), King's Lynn (KLBA, KL/C7/4, Hall Book, 1453–1457, p. 547), Leicester (*RBL*, II.289, 322), Southampton (Butler, *Book of Fines*, pp. 88, 99–100), Winchester (Keene, *Survey of Medieval Winchester*, I.257) and Yarmouth (NRO, Y/C18/1, fol. 21v). For the medical rationale behind these rulings, see section 5.2 below.

[201] R. C. Finucane, *The Rescue of the Innocents: Endangered Children in Medieval Miracles* (New York, 1997), p. 110.

[202] *Coventry Leet Book*, I.58, 83. Grimsby's bull-ring was in the market (Rigby, *Medieval Grimsby*, pp. 70, 171 n. 115), while Shrewsbury's lay safely outside the Stone Gate (Owen and Blakeway, *History of Shrewsbury*, I.271). By the sixteenth century both Southampton and Winchester had permanent rings in their respective High Streets: Butler, *Book of Fines*, pp. xliii, 120; Keene, *Survey of Medieval Winchester*, I.257.

[203] Even after the Black Death, sheep were free to roam the streets of Beverley (*BTD*, p. 19), whereas residents of Winchelsea could be fined for allowing them to 'renne at large' (BL, MS Cotton Julius B IV, fol. 26r).

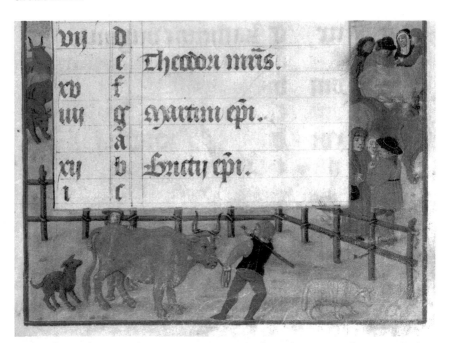

12 Another early sixteenth-century street scene reflects the congested nature of urban markets as cattle, a dog and a sheep jostled for space alongside people.

heavy damages were awarded against the owners of dogs that mauled sheep.[204] In Durham, where nearby rabbit warrens offered further temptation, local courts insisted that all dogs should be tied up or kept indoors at night and adequately muzzled during the day. Negligence in this respect could incur a fine of up to 6s. 8d. and an order for the destruction of the animal in question, partly because of the threat of rabies.[205] Regulations of this kind were common. Whereas the rulers of Northampton were prepared, in 1381, to exempt well-behaved dogs ('malum non facientem') from a rule demanding the compulsory use of leashes in public places, Coventry's magistrates simply banned 'grett houndes' and bitches from the city's streets altogether. Half a century later, in 1470, they repeated the order, along with another for the restraint of 'bochour dogges' at night.[206] Measures were already in place in Bristol for the chaining of all large hounds after dark, while Beverley magistrates responded to complaints directed specifically at butchers by imposing a blanket fine of 40d. on the owners of any stray or vicious dogs.[207] But, as the residents of Winchester discovered in the 1360s, it was one thing to issue proclamations and quite another to enforce them.[208] In 1377 the mayor of London

[204] *CPMRL, 1364–1381*, pp. 68–9; *RBC*, nos 242, 258.

[205] *RBC*, nos 23, 292, 300, 453, 458, 483, 518, 521, 528, 538, 547, 580, 668, 683, 699, 706, 709, 712, 714.

[206] *RBN*, I.248; *Coventry Leet Book*, I.27, 361.

[207] *LRBB*, II.227; Veale, *Great Red Book of Bristol*, I.142; *BTD*, p. 29.

[208] J. S. Furley, ed., *Town Life in the XIV Century as Seen in the Court Rolls of Winchester* (Winchester, 1946), pp. 136–7. In 1380 and 1405 respectively local

actually imprisoned a barber for repeatedly defying court orders, his previous record of intransigence towards the civic authorities confirming that belligerent humans are usually to blame for canine delinquency.[209]

The ubiquity of remedies for 'howndis bytinge' in late medieval leech books and surgical treatises confirms that the risk of personal injury was serious.[210] In an age without antibiotics, septicaemia could easily prove fatal, even following an apparently innocuous bite. And, although it was probably less common than some sources suggest, rabies remained endemic in England until the early twentieth century. Significantly in this context, medical authorities attributed the onset of madness to the dog's production of black choler, which (as in the case of leprosy) would rapidly become 'corrupt and i-rotid' through the consumption of rancid or contaminated meat. Hounds, like humans, were thus vulnerable to a poor diet, most notably during the oppressive 'dogs days' (*canicularis dies*) of summer, when their humours were most likely to overheat and their food to go bad.[211]

There is, however, surprisingly little evidence of the explicit association between dogs and the transmission of plague that led to the 'massacres' of the early modern period, so graphically described by Mark Jenner.[212] One of the earliest signs that English magistrates had begun to blame strays for the spread of miasmatic infection apparently occurred in Exeter. According to the antiquary John Hooker (d. 1601), in 1433–4 the mayor ruled that:

> forasmiche as great damages do growe within this citie, aswell in the night tymes as specially in the infectiouse tymes of sycknes, by keepinge of dogges within this citie, which doe not only in the night tymes barke & fight in the streetes to the noysaunce of the people in there beddes, as also do in the daye tyme rvnne from house to howse where the sycknes ys, that therefore no man shall hensforthe keepe any suche dogg or dogges ... vpon payne to pay xij*d*.[213]

As originally transcribed by Hooker in his commonplace book, the directive stipulated that any vagrant animals were to be killed, but made no explicit

    magistrates demanded that dogs should be restrained until a specific time of day, when they might be released: Keene, *Survey of Medieval Winchester*, I.257–8.

[209] *CPMRL, 1364–1381*, pp. 252–3. See also Carlin, *Medieval Southwark*, p. 240.

[210] See, for example, BL, MS Harley 2390, fol. 148v; MS Sloane 5, fol. 25v (pencil foliation); MS Sloane 983 fols 24v, 72v; Wellcome Institute Library, Western MS 411, fols 57r–58r; Western MS 564, fols 82v–84r; Hunt, *Popular Medicine*, pp. 212, 283, 284, 304; Henri de Mondeville, *Chirurgie de Maitre Henri de Mondeville*, ed. E. Nicaise (Paris, 1893), pp. 439, 447–50; Lanfrank, *Science of Cirurgie*, pp. 59–62.

[211] *OPT*, I.430–4; J. D. Blaisdell, 'Rabies in Shakespeare's England', *Historia medicinae veterinariae* 16 (1991), pp. 1–48, on p. 18. The author of one late fourteenth-century 'book of operacioun' observed that 'ofte times men ben bitten with wodde houndes ... replete of euyl humours': Glasgow University Library Special Collections, MS Hunter 95, fol. 148r, which also furnishes a remarkably accurate description of a rabid dog.

[212] M. S. R. Jenner, 'The Great Dog Massacre', in W. G. Naphy and P. Roberts, eds, *Fear in Early Modern Society* (Manchester, 1997), pp. 44–61.

[213] Vowell, *Description of the Citie of Excester*, p. 898.

reference to 'sycknes', even though plague was then raging in London. Quite possibly Hooker embroidered the text in light of his experience of the culls ordered by Tudor magistrates during later epidemics.[214] Less uncertainty attaches to an offensive of October 1512, when the bailiffs and council of Edinburgh introduced a number of sanitary regulations 'for to eschew by Goddis grace this contagious seiknes of pestilence laitlie rissin', including a complete prohibition on the ownership of dogs, 'vnder payne of slawchter of thame'. As the disease spread, orders went out in the following January for the immediate extermination of 'all vile and suspect bestis, as doggis, swyn and cattis', without compensation, although securely chained hounds were to be spared.[215]

As Jenner points out, such brutal exercises served more than a sanitary purpose, being of a piece with the strict controls aimed by Tudor magistrates at sturdy beggars and other undesirables whose behaviour threatened to undermine the stability of a well-ordered commonwealth.[216] In this respect at least, medieval civic authorities shared the same overriding commitment to a code of conduct that dictated exactly how animals as well as humans of all classes should behave. An ordinance of 1354, which reflects the unsettled state of Norwich during the years after the Black Death, describes the 'great injury and contentions' occasioned by untethered, masterless dogs running wild in the city, just like the feckless poor whose idle ways had recently been condemned by the king. However, while death awaited the stray cur or mongrel, elite greyhounds, spaniels and small hunting dogs could still roam freely.[217] In a similar concession to status, the rulers of London opted in 1387 to fine negligent owners, except for those of sufficient rank or wealth to possess *chiens gentilz*. The ordinance was repeated in 1475, although in this instance butchers' dogs who worked for a living, and thus ranked as honest, if truculent, labourers, joined 'gentil houndes' on the list of exemptions.[218] Attempts in early sixteenth-century Coventry to restrict the keeping of greyhounds to more prosperous householders were clearly aimed at rowdy apprentices and journeymen with a penchant for illicit sports, and had far less to do with issues of public health or safety.[219] In each of these cases we can clearly detect the anxiety

[214] DRO, ECA, Book 51, fol. 304v. The killing of dogs during epidemics was not adopted in Florence as a routine precautionary measure until the 1460s: Carmichael, *Plague and the Poor*, pp. 105, 159 n. 44.

[215] Marwick, *Records of the Burgh of Edinburgh*, pp. 137, 140; J. F. D. Shrewsbury, *A History of Bubonic Plague in the British Isles* (Cambridge, 1970), pp. 165–6.

[216] Jenner, 'Great Dog Massacre', pp. 53–6.

[217] *RCN*, II.205–7; *CPR, 1350–1354*, pp. 283–4. In Northampton 'gentle', or high status, dogs were also exempted from the rule about leashes, which was passed in the year of the Peasants' Revolt: see n. 206 above.

[218] *MGL*, III.178; *CLB*, H, p. 311; *CLB*, L, pp. 130–1; Barron, *London in the Later Middle Ages*, p. 255.

[219] *Coventry Leet Book*, III.630. An act of 1389 had originally imposed this ban: *RP*, III.273; *SR*, vol. 2, 13 Richard II, statute 1, cap. 13, p. 65. Basingstoke jurors complained in 1518 about the 'great trouble' caused by hunting dogs, especially those owned by people who were 'scant of power to keep themselves' – in other words, the disorderly poor: Baigent and Millard, *History of the Town and Manor of Basingstoke*, pp. 321–2.

about social breakdown that prompted increasingly draconian legislation against troublesome members of the civic body.

The same combination of social, sanitary and cultural factors prompted an even greater corpus of urban bye-laws and regulations concerned with the ubiquitous problem of wandering swine. As we have seen, some of these measures were specifically directed against butchers, yet they were not the only culprits. A significant proportion of ordinary householders kept at least one pig, often in such cramped conditions that it was tempting to let them root about freely in the gutters and rubbish heaps of neighbouring streets. Others escaped as they were being herded on their way to or from common land.[220] A Colchester tax assessment of 1301 reveals that about 40 per cent of taxpaying households owned pigs (155 out of 389); in many cases a plump porker or two must have represented the family's principal investment.[221] But not all these swine were raised for domestic consumption. Some residents of early fifteenth-century Westminster regarded pig husbandry as a lucrative sideline; and, given their numbers, it is hardly surprising that marauding animals threatened the lives of local children, as well as posing an environmental hazard. In 1404, for example, one infant was rescued in the nick of time from the mouth of a hungry sow, being lucky to escape the fate of others who were less fortunate.[222] Perhaps, as happened in the case of the young John atte Brok, whose ear was bitten off in similar circumstances, it was necessary to secure a testimonial for use in adulthood, 'lest sinister suspicion' arise because his injury resembled the mutilation inflicted upon criminals in the pillory.[223]

Although we should not exaggerate the number of fatalities, enough evidence survives to confirm that pigs were a recognised peril of urban life.[224] In 1322 a London coroner investigated the tragic case of Margaret de Irlaunde's one-month-old baby daughter who was attacked in her cradle by a stray sow and expired the following day.[225] Seventy years later another small child died in Oxford, her head consumed 'even to the nose' as she lay unattended.[226] Such gruesome accidents were, however, sufficiently rare to attract comment, and often occurred

[220] For this reason the rulers of Coventry appointed a swine herd in 1434: *Coventry Leet Book*, I.170.

[221] M. Carlin, 'Fast Food and Urban Living Standards in Medieval England', in M. Carlin and J. T. Rosenthal, eds, *Food and Eating in Medieval Europe* (London, 1998), p. 44. An inventory of goods owned by a London shopkeeper in 1321 recorded possessions worth 6s. 11d., of which 'two small pigs' accounted for half: *CCRCL*, p. 47.

[222] Rosser, *Medieval Westminster*, pp. 140–1.

[223] *CPR, 1266–1272*, p. 193. See also *CPR, 1301–1307*, p. 141.

[224] For another alleged attack, see J. Gairdner, ed., *The Historical Collections of a Citizen of London*, CS n.s. 17 (London, 1876), p. 75. According to Chaucer's Knight in *The Canterbury Tales*, one of the gruesome images decorating the shrine of Mars depicted a sow devouring a child 'right in the cradel': *Riverside Chaucer*, p. 52.

[225] *CCRCL*, pp. 56–7. In 1254 a one year old girl had met a similar fate: M. Weinbaum, ed., *The London Eyre of 1276*, LRS 12 (London, 1976), p. 14.

[226] H. E. Salter, ed., *Records of Medieval Oxford: Coroners' Inquests* (Oxford, 1912), p. 46.

during epidemics and other times of crisis, when owners died or grew negligent. The potential risk to youngsters was but one of many issues addressed in 1354 by the magistrates of Norwich, to whom foraging pigs represented a far greater menace than stray dogs. The ensuing ordinance paints an alarming picture of savage herds roaming the streets:

> whereby divers persons and children have thus been hurt by boars, children killed and eaten, and others [when] buried exhumed and others maimed, and many persons of the said city have received great injuries, as wrecking of houses, destruction of gardens … upon which great complaint is often brought before the bailiffs.[227]

Henceforward, swine were to be securely penned at all times, save for a brief period on Saturdays while their sties were being cleaned. Not only did owners now risk losing any strays, which could be slaughtered on sight, but they also became legally liable for injuries or damage caused by unsupervised animals.[228] These regulations were partly a pragmatic response to the deteriorating standards of hygiene occasioned by the upheavals of 1349–50. But they also reveal the same underlying fear of rootless beggars that prompted action against dogs, compounded, in this instance, by the uncomfortable connection between 'misgoverned' women and swine already explored in Chapter 2.[229]

Stray pigs could also transgress by scavenging on human remains. Even before the plague, urban graveyards were so crowded that decomposing bodies sometimes became exposed, causing alarm and abhorrence among the living. Along with predictable anxiety about the release of miasmatic vapours went very real revulsion at the sacrilege involved. In 1304 the priest and parishioners of St Benet Fink in London complained of the 'enormities in contempt of God' committed in their cemetery by wandering swine; similar concerns were still being voiced in Durham during the early sixteenth century.[230]

It did not, however, require either a major epidemic or an outbreak of moral rectitude for magistrates to instigate measures against such a serious nuisance and threat to communal health. As early as 1272, the owner of any 'hogge' taken at large in the streets of Portsmouth stood to pay 4*d.* for each offence up to the fourth, when the butcher's axe would fall.[231] Similar rules were adopted in London by the end of the decade, followed in 1292 by the election of four officials charged with collecting fines and culling strays. The post was certainly no sinecure, especially as some owners contravened a further ordinance of 1297 by allowing their pigsties to encroach on neighbouring tenements or overhang watercourses. A civic custom

---

[227] *RCN*, II.205.

[228] *RCN*, II.205–7. This regulation was repeated in 1437, although any pigs or ducks then found 'wandering in the streets … to the nuisance of the neighbours' were to be driven from the city rather than killed (p. 88). Already in 1331 the rulers of Lynn had insisted that swine might only be released on Saturdays, to permit mucking-out: Isaacson and Ingleby, *Red Register of King's Lynn*, I.203.

[229] In Southampton, fines for allowing pigs to wander and for accommodating vagabonds were recorded together: Butler, *Book of Fines*, pp. 116, 118, 120.

[230] *LAN*, no. 63; *RBC*, nos 256, 309.

[231] Bateson, *Borough Customs*, p. 87.

permitting St Anthony's hospital to claim any vagrant pigs, which wore bells to denote their special status, undermined so much of this legislation that, in 1311, the master was ordered to take only those animals donated specifically to the house.[232] In contrast, St John's hospital, Sandwich, benefited directly from the appointment at this time of a common sergeant with orders to kill any hogs, poultry or cattle found roaming through the town or fouling the water supply, since some of the meat went to feed the patients.[233] In London the offensive against vagrant pigs may have owed something to royal intervention, as was certainly the case in York. A complaint addressed by Edward I to the bailiffs of St Mary's abbey in 1298 focussed upon the 'corrupted and infected' air emanating from 'the pigsties situate in the king's highways and ... the swine feeding and frequently wandering about in the streets and lanes'.[234] Not surprisingly, one of a catalogue of hygienic measures introduced before the royal court arrived in the city prohibited residents from letting their animals run loose within the walls.[235]

By the later fifteenth century, and often far earlier, most English towns had placed severe restrictions, if not outright embargoes, on 'bores, sowes or any other maner hoggs wandryng or wrotyng in the comen strets'.[236] Whereas the magistrates of Beverley were prepared, in 1356, to allow sows with litters the freedom to roam,[237] a blanket ban on the keeping of swine, even in sties or stalls, was introduced in Coventry in 1423, modified in 1444 under the threat of harsh penalties for any alleged nuisances, and then reintroduced in the 1490s.[238] Did such restrictions actually succeed in containing the problems

---

[232] *MGL*, III.88; Riley, *Memorials of London*, pp. 20, 28, 35, 83; *CLB*, A, pp. 216–17, 220; *CLB*, C, p. 5; *CLB*, D, p. 251. The assize of nuisance dealt with complaints about pigsties that were built too near to party walls or water supplies: *LAN*, nos 263, 332, 382–3.

[233] Boys, *History of Sandwich*, I.129; II.501, 503.

[234] *CCR, 1296–1302*, p. 218.

[235] *YCO*, p. 16. The ordinance *de porcis euntibus* was repeated in 1377 and 1398 (*YMB*, I.lxix, 18, 164), and again in 1482 (Goldberg, 'Pigs and Prostitutes', p. 172). The city's butchers were among the worst offenders: York City Archives, Chamberlains' Account Book 2, 1520–1525, fols 13r–14r, 18r, 51r, 52r, 137v.

[236] *RPBC*, pp. 98, 181–2. See, for example, prohibitions in Bristol (Veale, *Great Red Book of Bristol*, I.144; *LRBB*, II.31–2), Cambridge (Cooper, *Annals of Cambridge*, p. 258), Carlisle (Summerson, *Medieval Carlisle*, II.670), Dover (BL, MS Egerton 2091, fol. 91r), Gloucester (HMC, *Twelfth Report*, appendix 9, p. 434), Henley (Briers, *Henley Borough Records*, pp. 34, 57, 75, 124), Leicester (*RBL*, II.21–2, 103–4, 292), Northampton (*RBN*, I.247–8), Nottingham (Stevenson, *Records of the Borough of Nottingham*, I.356–8), Reading (Guilding, *Reading Records*, pp. 67, 68; Slade, *Reading Gild Accounts*, pp. l–li), Salisbury (Carr, *First General Entry Book*, nos 203, 419A), Scarborough (I. H. Jeayes, ed., *Description of Documents Contained in the White Vellum Book of Scarborough* (Scarborough, 1914), p. 53), Southampton (Studer, *Oak Book of Southampton*, I.52–3), Winchelsea (BL, MS Cotton Julius B IV, fol. 26r), and Winchester (Keene, *Survey of Medieval Winchester*, I.153; Bird, *Black Book of Winchester*, p. 149).

[237] *BTD*, p. 19.

[238] During the plague year of 1421 residents had been forbidden both from keeping pigsties near streets and from letting their animals roam, but this ordinance

caused by urban livestock? It is interesting to note that in 1425 the rulers of Lynn threatened anyone who hindered the bellman in removing vagrant animals with imprisonment.[239] This was quite possibly a response to resistance of the sort documented in Leicester during the 1350s, when a goldsmith and his son had been bound over in heavy securities for assaulting the official who had confiscated their errant pigs.[240] There can, however, be little doubt of the vigour with which some borough courts pursued offenders, especially from the 1470s onwards. In Ipswich, for example, the number of annual presentments for permitting swine to roam at large increased dramatically from an average of fewer than three or four before the 1440s to twelve in 1468, twenty-three in the plague year of 1471 and twenty-five in 1482. By 1488 the total had reached no fewer than forty, heavier fines being imposed upon those residents who allowed their swine to forage along the quays and contaminate the river.[241] Had the borough authorities simply accepted the situation and decided to impose a tax upon anyone who wished to rear pigs, similar perhaps to that paid by the owners of some urban dung-heaps? Since many offenders were bound over in heavy securities to restrain their animals in future it seems unlikely that such a steep rise in numbers can simply be explained in fiscal terms. Indeed, the general offensive then being waged across England against other forms of pollution, both moral and physical, would suggest otherwise.

Even the most docile and sedentary pigs added appreciably to the quantities of dung and filthy straw deposited in urban thoroughfares, while also generating a pungent aroma that, in extreme cases, ranked as a serious health hazard. Thus, for example, during the sweating sickness of 1485 one Yarmouth man was charged with keeping his pigs in such squalid conditions that people passing by risked infection from the mephitic air.[242] London ward moots were also expected to report anyone whose swine or cattle offended their neighbours, which no doubt explains why, in 1365, William Baldwyn was bound over in the remarkable sum of £100 to remove his pigs from the City within seven days and fined 20s. for the nuisance they had already caused.[243]

Other animals could prove just as annoying and potentially dangerous. Setting aside such exotica as the lion for which the burgesses of Southampton had to buy a secure cage, collar and chain at considerable expense in 1438–9, a surprising number of creatures were placed under restraint in late medieval English towns.[244]

evidently proved insufficient: *Coventry Leet Book*, I.27, 58, 217; II.544; III.652.

[239] KLBA, KL/C7/2, Hall Book, 1422–1429, p. 104. In 1427 and 1428 residents were ordered to keep pigs securely in their sties, on pain of a fine of 12*d.*, or imprisonment (pp. 165, 178).

[240] *RBL*, II.104. Pigs were banned from the streets in 1335–6, 1355 and 1467 (pp. 21–2, 103–4, 292).

[241] SROI, C/2/8/1/11, 13, 15, 17–22; C/2/10/1/5. Ordinances against vagrant swine were enacted in 1473, 1476 and 1482: Bacon, *Annalls of Ipswiche*, pp. 134, 140, 147.

[242] NRO, Y/C4/190, rot. 17r. It was at about this time that the leet courts were instructed to present 'alle thos persones that keppe anny sweyne or lett them goo a brood in the towne': Y/C18/1, fol. 17r.

[243] *MGL*, III.134, 137; *CPMRL, 1364–1381*, p. 39.

[244] Gidden, *Stewards' Books of Southampton*, I.90. In Coventry, for example, goats were banned from the streets in 1470: *Coventry Leet Book*, II.360–1.

Many householders kept a few geese, ducks or hens, while poultry sellers, who operated on a commercial basis, might well rear birds in significant quantities at home. Magistrates took understandable exception to the noise, mess and aggravation (as well as the 'gret rebuke, shame & slaunder') caused by flocks of poultry in busy thoroughfares, although penalties of the sort imposed in Bristol, Leicester and Norwich must have been hard to enforce.[245] Ducks and geese, as well as pigs, were banned in 1380 from the streets of Winchester, while hens, which had been pecking open corn merchants' sacks and devouring the contents, were henceforth excluded from the marketplace.[246] Having for too long endured the 'the evel rule and demenyng' of poultry sellers in the area near the Stocks market and other 'principal' thoroughfares, a group of concerned Londoners petitioned the mayor in 1444 about the risks posed by so many

> swannes, gees, heronsewes [young herons] and other pultre, wherof the ordure and standyng of hem is of grete stenche and so evel savour that it causeth grete and parlous infectyng of the people and long hath done ... which pulters myght purvey and have houses and places in oute weyes nygh London Wall and elleswere in this Citee, kepyng ther her said pultrye ... [so] that the ordure of hem myght be voided oute of her houses and forthwyth oute of the stretes twies in the week, and that in due tymes whan fewe people passe by.[247]

Nor was it easy to control the large number of horses that were ridden or driven into towns, where they not only fouled the streets and watercourses but were also likely to cause serious accidents. Adults as well as youngsters could easily be bitten, kicked or trampled underfoot by temperamental animals, especially at crowded watering places.[248] Following what looks to have been a spate of nasty incidents, the rulers of York decreed in 1377 that horses should always be led by the reins when on their way to drink in the river because of 'the great danger to children going about in the city'.[249] The practice of tethering

[245] Veale, *Great Red Book of Bristol*, I.144; *RBL*, II.292–3; NRO, NCR, 16D/1, Assembly Proceedings, 1434–1491, fol. 5r; 16D/2, Assembly Proceedings, 1491–1553, fol. 202r; 16C/2, Assembly Minute Book, 1510–1550, fol. 237r–v.

[246] Keene, *Survey of Medieval Winchester*, I.153.

[247] *CLB*, K, p. 289. Already in 1366 the authorities had forbidden the plucking of birds in the streets, which were littered with feathers (*CLB*, G, p. 207). In 1422 a poulterer was presented for dumping goose, heron and horse dung (*CPMRL, 1413–1437*, p. 153).

[248] See, for example, H. M. Chew and M. Weinbaum, eds, *London Eyre of 1244*, LRS 6 (London, 1970), no. 166; Riley, *Memorials of London*, pp. 4–5; R. R. Sharpe, ed., *Calendar of Letters from the Mayor and Corporation of the City of London, 1350–1370* (London, 1885), no. 265; Keene, *Survey of Medieval Winchester*, I.154; Hanawalt, *Growing Up in Medieval London*, pp. 62–3, 65. In 1503 a commission of aldermen and commoners was set up in Norwich to examine the state of the principal watering place on the Wensum, which had become 'filled with mud & myre': Kirkpatrick, *Streets and Lanes*, pp. 73–4.

[249] *YMB*, I.18. A similar ruling of 1426 insisted upon the leading of horses in the streets of Nottingham: Salusbury-Jones, *Street Life in Medieval England*, p. 64.

horses in public places obstructed busy city centres, leading some authorities, such as those of Bristol and Stamford, to insist that all mounts should be stabled on arrival, 'for parell of children and noying the kynges strets'.[250] Such was the congestion of traffic in Salisbury, that in 1416 traders coming to market with pack horses or carts were ordered to remove their animals beyond the walls immediately after unloading because of the nuisance they caused to passers-by and the damage likely to result. A decade later the livestock market was transferred to the urban periphery, thereby reducing levels of dirt and disturbance even further.[251]

Long after death, livestock continued to pollute the urban environment. We need not take too seriously John Stow's claim that London's Houndsditch derived its name from the number of 'dead dogges' left to rot there, but the disposal of animal remains certainly posed a serious threat to water supplies.[252] In 1464–5 alone the chamberlains of Kingston-upon-Hull had to remove three dead horses from the canal bringing fresh water into the town, and it was far from unusual for owners to dump the bodies of domestic animals in nearby dikes or sewers.[253] Shortly afterwards the mayor of Leicester deemed it necessary to reinforce his warning that all such carcasses should be safely conveyed beyond the gates on pain of indefinite imprisonment for each offence.[254] So bad had the problem become in Winchester by the 1480s, that anyone who blocked the drains and gutters with 'donge, strawe, dede hogge, dogge or cate' stood to pay a 12*d.* fine for each offence.[255] The disposal of dead animals, as well as the watering of live ones, was likewise forbidden in the Milburn, the main water source of the Durham borough of Crossgate.[256] As a rule, however, neighbours were quick to report the most flagrant transgressors. At the beginning of the fourteenth century, following a series of complaints by irritated Londoners, Richard de Houndeslowe was ordered to cease killing and skinning horses and burying their carcasses near his premises in the City; and in 1390 a Norwich jury protested volubly about the abandonment

---

[250] Veale, *Great Red Book of Bristol*, I.143; Rogers, *William Browne's Town*, pp. 27, 70. As an additional control on the number of animals at large, Bristol's butchers were forbidden from buying livestock within the walls: *LRBB*, II.230. 'Country' butchers who brought their horses into the shambles at Leicester faced imprisonment from 1467 onwards (*RBL*, II.292). In Lynn from at least 1533 a fine of 4*d.* per animal was imposed on anyone who let a horse or calf loose in the street (KLBA, KL/C7/5, Hall Book, 1497–1544, fol. 293r).

[251] Carr, *First General Entry Book*, nos 167, 236, 260. The arrival of large numbers of animals on market days posed a major sanitary problem. Having been awarded two new fairs, or 'free marts', by the crown in 1482, the rulers of Norwich issued proclamations specifying exactly where livestock could 'lie and walk' in the city at such times: *RCN*, II.102–3.

[252] Stow, *Survey of London*, I.128. For similar nuisances, see Carlin, *Medieval Southwark*, p. 240.

[253] R. Horrox, ed., *Selected Rentals and Accounts of Medieval Hull, 1293–1528*, YASRS 141 (Leeds, 1983), p. 103.

[254] *RBL*, II.290.

[255] Bird, *Black Book of Winchester*, p. 121.

[256] *RBC*, no. 413.

of a dead horse in a public thoroughfare 'to the abominable offence and poisoning of the air'.[257]

3.7 Smoke and noise

In the popular English version of the *The Liber celestis* by St Bridget of Sweden, the world with all its travails and temptations is compared to a 'pore house' contaminated by 'foule wallis, mekill sote, and smoke'.[258] The force of this metaphor is apparent from the widespread skeletal evidence of maxillary sinusitis caused by air pollution in low status medieval urban populations, especially among children.[259] Members of the elite, both lay and religious, lived in cleaner, better ventilated homes, but still found it difficult to escape the unpleasant consequences of industrial activity and inconsiderate neighbours. Affluent merchants in Mercers' Row, Chester, complained about the harmful effects of the smoke rising from the cellars beneath them, where poorer people (including single elderly women) lived.[260] Not even monastic communities could avoid this problem, at least if they occupied marginal land on the edge of towns. We can more readily understand why a fourteenth-century Norwich Benedictine should copy verses about the incessant din of 'swart smoky smiths, smirched with smoke' into one of the priory's books if we bear in mind that the area around the cathedral precinct was colonised by blacksmiths, lime-burners and foundries. The constant hammering and acrid smoke of neighbouring workshops must have lent verisimilitude to his contemplation of the Last Judgement.[261] The burgesses of Beverley made a 'healthful' (*salubriter*) decision to prohibit the construction of brick kilns near the town, partly to protect the fruit in their earthly paradise, although they clearly recognised that atmospheric pollution would affect human beings as well as trees.[262] Similarly, the 'grave nuisance' occasioned by lime-burning prompted a complete ban upon such activities in Bridgwater by 1388, and the imposition of draconian fines on those who disobeyed.[263]

Whereas Classical authorities such as Galen had concentrated upon the

---

[257] *CPMRL, 1298–1307*, pp. 161–2; p. 206 below; Hudson, *Leet Jurisdiction*, p. 75.

[258] St Bridget of Sweden, *The Liber Celestis*, ed. R. Ellis, vol. 1: *Text*, EETS o.s. 291 (Oxford, 1987), pp. 387–8.

[259] Lewis, *Urbanisation and Child Health*, p. 2.

[260] CCA, ZS/B/5a, Sheriffs' Book, 1502–1503, fol. 7v; ZS/B/5d, Sheriffs' Book, 1508–1509, fol. 59v; ZS/B/5f, Sheriffs' Book, 1510–1511, fol. 109v.

[261] Rawcliffe, *Medicine for the Soul*, p. 39.

[262] *BTD*, p. 58.

[263] T. B. Dilks, ed., *Bridgwater Borough Archives, 1377–1399*, Somerset Record Society 53 (Bridgwater, 1938), no. 439. During the early sixteenth century, the borough court at Lyme ordered the removal of dangerous 'lyme pyttes' under threat of a 20s. fine: Dorset Record Office, DC/LR B1/2 no. 16. This was not, however, a universal trend. In Norwich, lime-burning was still undertaken in relatively close proximity to the homes of wealthy residents: C. Rawcliffe, 'Health and Safety at Work in Late Medieval East Anglia', in C. Harper-Bill, ed., *Medieval East Anglia* (Woodbridge, 2005), p. 145.

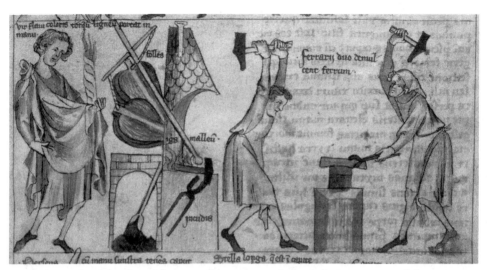

13 Smiths working metal at a forge, as depicted in a fourteenth-century text of the *Tractatus astronomicus* attributed to Abu-Ma'shar

transformative effect of rotting matter upon the quality of the air, late medieval practitioners and educated laymen became increasingly conscious of the additional risks posed by man-made environmental hazards.[264] Indeed, activities like smelting and metal working seemed doubly dangerous, since they not only created an unpleasant stench but often gave rise to a level of noise that was itself deemed injurious to health (plate 13). In his *De decem ingeniis curandorum morborum* of 1299, the celebrated Montpellier physician Bernard Gordon adapted traditional Galenic recommendations about the *regimen* to accord more closely with the contemporary urban *milieu* in which his students would have to practise. They were advised to ask if their patients had been 'disturbed by an adjoining shop occupied by a carpenter, hammerer, tanner of hides, melter of tallow, or by persons who work with sulphur and the like'. Loud drunks, barking dogs and anxiety about crime, the blight of life in towns throughout the ages, seemed just as likely to cause illness because of their capacity to destabilise the body's sensitive animal spirits.[265] Not long afterwards, in 1311, the royal surgeon Henri de Mondeville undertook as part of his official duties to deliver a series of public lectures on anatomy and surgery in Paris. Whether the audience actually included craftsmen, as has been suggested, remains a moot point, but his graphic warning about the potentially fatal consequences for the sick of 'the noise of neighbouring workmen, such as smiths, carpenters and others, the bad air, the foul stench [and] the smoke of coal from the earth' clearly spread far beyond the university.[266]

[264] L. García-Ballester, 'The Construction of a New Form of Learning and Practising Medicine in Medieval Latin Europe', *Science in Context* 8.1 (1995), pp. 75–102.

[265] L. Demaitre, *Doctor Bernard Gordon: Professor and Practitioner* (Toronto, 1980), pp. 47, 157.

[266] Henri de Mondeville, *Chirurgie*, pp. xxv, 179; García-Ballester, 'Construction of a New Form of Learning', pp. 90–1. De Mondeville, whose work was widely admired in England, urged that convalescents should be moved to the country.

Smoke posed such a threat because once it reached the inner recesses of the brain the attendant 'derknesse and stenche' could disrupt the vulnerable processes of thought and movement, while also damaging the eyes. Bartholomaeus Anglicus described how 'the scharpnesse therof ... greuyth yghen [eyes] and maketh hem droppe out teeres and greueth the sight notabelyche, and ... cometh in by his scharpnesse to the brayne and greueth the spirit of felynge'.[267] He probably had in mind the unpleasant effects of sea coal (so called because it came by ship from Newcastle), which was burnt in London and other English cities during the later Middle Ages. Industrial consumers, such as lime-burners, braziers, smiths and bell-founders, welcomed it as a cheaper, if dirtier, alternative to wood or charcoal, especially during fuel shortages, although others were less enthusiastic.[268] As early as 1257, Queen Eleanor allegedly left Nottingham for the purer air of Tutbury because the fumes from burning sea coal made life there insupportable.[269] Since her mother had recently commissioned a vernacular regimen for her benefit from the physician Aldobrandino of Siena (d. 1287), we may assume that she was well versed in such matters.[270]

Awareness of the dangers of inhaling thick smoke was not confined to the elite.[271] At the end of the thirteenth century, just as Bernard Gordon began writing on this very subject, a group of London smiths set out to regulate their craft, unanimously agreeing 'that none should work at night on account of the unhealthiness of the sea coal [*propter putridinem carbonis marine*] and damage to their neighbours'.[272]

[267] *OPT*, I.52. For a remedy specifically for 'yen that be hurte in the smoke', see BL, MS Sloane 122, fol. 59v.

[268] W. H. TeBrake, 'Air Pollution and Fuel Crises in Pre-Industrial London, 1250–1650', *Technology and Culture* 16 (1975), pp. 337–59, on pp. 340–2; J. A. Galloway, D. Keene and M. Murphy, 'Fuelling the City: Production and Distribution of Firewood and Fuel in London's Region, 1290–1400', *EconHR*, 2nd series 49 (1996), pp. 447–72; J. Hatcher, *The History of the British Coal Industry*, vol. 1 (Oxford, 1993), pp. 22–6. The extent of domestic use is unknown, although coal was sold by the sack from at least 1360 in London, and was allocated to prisoners in Ludgate and Newgate gaols: Schofield, *London, 1100–1600*, p. 76.

[269] H. R. Luard, ed., *Annales monastici*, 5 vols, RS 36 (London, 1866), III.203–4.

[270] BL, MS Sloane 2435. This fine presentation copy, which was given to Eleanor by Beatrice of Savoy in 1256, is discussed by P. Murray Jones, *Medieval Medical Miniatures in Illuminated Manuscripts*, rev. edn (London, 1998), pp. 103–7. The text, which became extremely popular, contains advice on avoiding 'pestilence and the corruption of the air', and draws attention to the dangers of fumes and smoke: Aldobrandino of Siena, *Le Régime du corps de Maître Aldebrandin de Sienne*, ed. L. Landouzy and R. Pépin (Paris, 1911), pp. 59–61.

[271] See, for example, a short fifteenth-century vernacular regimen, allegedly based upon one 'that was sent to Dame Isabelle, qwene of Engelond, be prayer of the kyng of Fraunse hir brother', which warns against the effects of smoke: Wellcome Institute Library, Western MS 408, fol. 14r.

[272] *CEMCRL*, pp. 33–4; Barron, *London in the Later Middle Ages*, p. 264. According to Peter Brimblecombe, they understood that 'stable atmospheric conditions at night could lead to severe pollution': 'Early Urban Climate and Atmosphere', in Hall and Kenward, *Environmental Archaeology*, p. 19.

They may well have recalled a couple of royal commissions set up in 1285 and 1288 to investigate complaints about lime-burning with sea coal (as opposed to wood) in Southwark and the suburbs, whereby the air had become 'infected and corrupted to the peril of those frequenting and dwelling in those parts'.[273] Demonstrating considerably less regard for the sensibilities – and respiratory organs – of others, the civic authorities had managed from a comparatively early date to banish unduly noisome or intrusive processes to the south bank of the Thames, though smoke could less easily be confined or excluded.[274]

The problem of atmospheric pollution had not yet reached the proportions so apparent during the mid-seventeenth century, when John Evelyn compared London to 'the face rather of *Mount Ætna*, the *Court of Vulcan, Stromboli*, or the Suburbs of Hell', but it did prove a major irritant in places where lime-burning (which released carbon dioxide) and other heavy industries were carried out.[275] In 1307 Edward I forbade the use of sea coal by workmen anywhere in the City or adjacent suburbs, apparently as a result of further protests by 'prelates and magnates of the realm' about the 'intolerable stench' wafting into their residences from kilns in Southwark, Wapping and East Smithfield. The crown had its own vested interest in promulgating such measures: because of the perceived risk to Queen Margaret's health posed by 'the infection and corruption of the air' a temporary prohibition was imposed on lime-burning and similar activities, even with wood, while she stayed in the Tower at this time. Three years later a more effective *cordon sanitaire* was established through the compulsory removal of all neighbouring kilns.[276]

Ordinary Londoners were just as vocal, if sometimes less successful, in their campaign for cleaner air. In 1371, for example, residents of St Clement's Lane objected to local plumbers soldering lead on a nearby plot of land 'to the great damage and peril of death of all who shall smell the smoke from such melting – as may be proved by some of the trade and other good folks'. Their demand that the lease should be revoked 'for the saving of human life' was rejected by the mayor's court, although the plumbers, who mounted a strenuous defence, were obliged to raise the height of the chimney on their furnace in order to disperse the fumes more effectively. As in so many areas of urban life, it was clearly necessary to strike a compromise between communal health and commercial profit.[277] The burning of sea coal also figured in a litany of complaints made a few years later

[273] *CPR, 1281–1292*, pp. 207, 296.

[274] Carlin, *Medieval Southwark*, pp. 44, 223; H. E. Malden, ed., *VCH Surrey*, vol. 2 (London, 1905), p. 249. On a visitation of St Thomas's hospital, Southwark, in 1387, Bishop Wykeham complained about workmen 'exercising mechanical arts in the precincts ... both night and day, making a clamour and noise to the great nuisance of the poor and infirm': New College, Oxford, MS 3691, fols 91v–92r.

[275] Evelyn, *Fumifugium*, p. 6; P. Brimblecombe, *The Big Smoke: A History of Air Pollution in London since Medieval Times* (London, 1987), pp. 6–11.

[276] *CPR, 1301–1307*, p. 549; *CCR, 1302–1307*, pp. 537, 539; *CCR, 1307–1313*, p. 330.

[277] Riley, *Memorials of London*, pp. 355–6. See also the appeal made to the mayor's court two years later against a plasterer who generated 'obnoxious' fumes: *CPMRL, 1364–1381*, p. 166. The outcome is unrecorded

about an armourers' workshop in Watling Street, where a combination of noxious smoke and the constant pounding of sledge hammers proved intolerable for the couple next door, disturbing their sleep, reducing the value of their property and even spoiling the wine and ale in their cellar. Against the claim that they had contravened a number of building regulations designed to avoid the risks of fire and air-borne pollution, the armourers cited an 'ancient custom', which allowed them 'to carry on their trade anywhere in the City, adapting their premises as [was] most convenient for their work'.[278]

As we shall see in the next chapter, industrial activity was, where possible, confined to the outlying areas of most English towns, but noise was a ubiquitous problem that affected the rich as well as the poor, to the detriment of both physical and mental health. Bracketed together among the six 'non-naturals' whose proper management was essential for survival, relaxation and repose assumed particular importance in the medieval *regimen* because of their role in facilitating the absorption of nutritive matter. By drawing heat away from the brain towards the stomach and liver, sleep acted as 'noryce of digestioun', promoting the conversion of food into natural spirit, especially after a heavy meal.[279] It also facilitated the release of moist vapours, which hydrated the principal organs and allowed the over-active animal spirit a period of tranquillity. Loud and persistent noise of the sort described by Bernard Gordon and Henri de Mondeville (and, most eloquently, by the satirist Juvenal in his account of the cacophonous hell of Ancient Rome) was therefore harmful as well as irritating, and prompted an appropriate response.[280]

In order to protect the citizenry from constant vexation, the rulers of London imposed restrictions on certain craftsmen, such as horners, wiredrawers and blacksmiths, who were prohibited from 'knokkyng, filyinng or any other noyfulle werk whereby [their] neighbours might be noyed or diseased' at night.[281] But no sooner had one racket ceased than another began. In 1422, jurors from Bassishaw ward, who had clearly endured many sleepless nights, indicted some recent arrivals, 'new come from Coventry' and thus apparently unused to the more civilised ways of the capital. Their habit of holding open house for strangers until the small hours and of 'making violent and grievous noises to the nuisance of all dwelling around' earned them few friends. Nor were raucous provincials the only problem. Despite the prohibition on their use, heavy iron-shod carts trundling through the streets 'beyond the due and proper hour' left the same insomniacs 'grieved of their repose and quiet at night', while the quacking and crowing of urban poultry proved yet

---

[278] *LAN*, no. 617.

[279] John Lydgate, *Lydgate and Burgh's 'Secrees of Old Philisoffres'*, ed. R. Steele, EETS e.s. 66 (London, 1894), p. 40; R. Steele, ed., *Three Prose Versions of the 'Secreta Secretorum'*, EETS e.s. 74 (London, 1898), p. 71.

[280] Juvenal, 'Satire Three', in *The Sixteen Satires*, trans. P. Green, rev. edn (Harmondsworth, 1974), notably lines 222–38.

[281] Riley, *Memorials of London*, p. 238; *CLB*, H, pp. 363–4; Fisher, *History of the Worshipful Company of Horners*, p. 19–20; Barron, *London in the Later Middle Ages*, p. 265.

another source of 'discomfort and nuisance'.[282] The nocturnal 'affrayes and debates' reputedly made by drunken clergy carousing in one of the better residential areas of Exeter during the late 1440s likewise occasioned an anguished protest from householders who were so 'foule accombred therof and y-lette of theire nyghte reste' that resort to violence seemed inevitable.[283]

Whether or not they had taken holy orders, those who spent too long in the tavern or alehouse posed a serious risk both to themselves and others. Few twelfth-century readers would have disagreed with William Fitz Stephen's assertion that 'the only plagues of London are the immoderate drinking of fools and the frequency of fires'.[284] As medieval coroners' rolls so often attest, a fatal combination of alcohol, candles, straw mattresses and inflammable building materials meant that inebriation and conflagration were, quite literally, common bedfellows. Having returned to his lodgings 'very drunk' from a civic feast in 1275, John de Hancrete collapsed before dousing his light and was incinerated when his bed caught fire.[285] Within the space of a few months in 1297–8, an Oxford coroner recorded the death of one woman and the serious injury of her husband in a similar incident, and the destruction of two houses by an intoxicated servant who perished in the blaze.[286] Other factors were also to blame for this most unpredictable and devastating hazard of urban life, which gave rise to constant anxiety on the part of magistrates and residents alike. According to Sir Keith Thomas, the vulnerability of men and women who lived in such crowded conditions, and the lack of effective measures to combat fires once they had started, provided fruitful ground for belief in the supernatural. There can, indeed, be little doubt that the residents of medieval towns frequently invoked divine protection on this score.[287] They were, however, far from supine in the face of adversity and could muster an impressive battery of safeguards besides prayers and charms to protect their property.

3.8 Fire prevention

Fire was an essential precondition of urbanisation. It was needed for cooking, heating and lighting, as well as in a plethora of crafts from brewing and baking to pottery-making and metalworking. All but the meanest of hovels maintained some kind of naked flame, if only a rush candle or brazier, the sparks from which could rapidly catch alight.[288] The close proximity of dwellings, the juxtaposition

---

[282] *CPMRL, 1413–1437*, pp. 117–19, 154; Barron, *London in the Later Middle Ages*, pp. 264–5.

[283] S. A. Moore, ed., *Letters and Papers of John Shillingford*, CS n.s. 2 (London, 1871), pp. 90–1. Under normal circumstances, anyone who created disturbances at night would be presented to the local courts. See, for example, Stevenson, *Records of the Borough of Nottingham*, III.94–7.

[284] D. C. Douglas and G. W. Greenaway, eds, *EHD*, vol. 2: *1042–1189* (Oxford, 1981), p. 1027.

[285] Riley, *Memorials of London*, p. 8.

[286] Salter, *Records of Medieval Oxford*, pp. 5, 7.

[287] Thomas, *Religion and the Decline of Magic*, pp. 17–20.

[288] Friedrichs, *Early Modern City*, p. 276.

of industrial workshops and domestic housing and the widespread use of straw combined to increase the risk. Although smiths, lime-burners, potters and the practitioners of other potentially dangerous occupations gradually withdrew to the suburbs, inner cities still remained unsafe.[289] The number of complaints made in London about stacks of firewood heaped against party walls and in other inappropriate places reveals how easy it must have been for flames to spread from one house to another.[290] Fitz Stephen can hardly be charged with exaggeration, as there may have been as many as five 'major conflagrations' in London between *c.* 1050 and the end of the twelfth century, followed by another that devastated large areas of Southwark as well as the City in July 1212. The response to this particular disaster reveals that official action could, in fact, prove remarkably effective.[291] The stringent building regulations then introduced to eliminate such obvious dangers as thatched roofs, combustible chimney stacks and wooden houses, along with the restrictions placed upon the activities of bakers and brewers (who were forbidden from working at night and from using reeds, straw and stubble as fuel), ensured that the next four centuries passed without major incident.[292]

Provisions for the avoidance of fire hazards were subsequently incorporated into the London assize of buildings, with the result that infringements ranked alongside other nuisances, such as the noxious cesspits described above.[293] It was, for instance, possible for householders to demand the removal of chimneys that stood too close to their property or seemed defective, while local juries were instructed every year just before summer to report any possible trouble spots 'perilous for mischief that might befall of fire'.[294] Enforcement was, inevitably, far from perfect, but, once they had been identified, offenders would be bound over to implement the necessary repairs within a specific time, after which the authorities could levy a standard fine of 40s. in order to complete whatever work remained. Thus, for example, certain householders in Colman Street ward, who had been presented to the mayor in 1376 for ignoring the prohibition on thatch, were ordered to tile their roofs within forty days, or pay the sheriff to do so.[295]

---

[289] D. J. Keene, 'Suburban Growth', in R. Holt and G. Rosser, eds, *The Medieval Town: A Reader in English Urban History, 1200–1540* (London, 1990), p. 116; D. Cromarty, *Everyday Life in Medieval Shrewsbury* (Shrewsbury, 1991), pp. 11, 57–8.

[290] *LAN*, nos 16, 55, 60, 183, 199, 312. The fourteenth-century court rolls of Bridgwater furnish many presentments of this nature: Dilks, *Bridgwater Borough Archives*, *passim.*

[291] *LAN*, pp. ix–xi; Barron, *London in the Later Middle Ages*, pp. 247–8; D. M. Palliser, T. R. Slater and E. P. Dennison, 'The Topography of Towns, 600–1300', *CUHB1*, p. 184.

[292] *MGL*, II.i.xxxii–xxxiii, 86–8; III.132–7. Earlier regulations had apparently been promulgated in 1189: Schofield, *Medieval London Houses*, pp. 32–3.

[293] *LAN*, pp. ix–xi.

[294] *LAN*, nos 77, 658; *MGL*, III.132–7; *CPMRL, 1413–1437*, pp. xxv, 118, 139.

[295] *CPMRL, 1364–1381*, p. 237. See also Riley, *Memorials of London*, pp. 46–7; *CLB*, C, p. 105; *CPMRL, 1413–1437*, p. 125. The City's scavengers were also responsible for inspecting buildings and reporting fire hazards: *CLB*, D, p. 192.

Other towns and cities adopted similar measures. As Robert Ricart explained when copying the 'laudable customes' of London into his calendar of *c.* 1479, since Bristol had long followed the 'grete president of the noble Citee' its officials needed 'to know and vnderstonde' these 'auncient vsages'. His interest extended to building regulations designed to prevent the spread of fire, notably with regard to the mandatory use of approved roofing materials and the scale of fines imposed for infractions.[296] In general, however, magistrates tended to act in the aftermath of major conflagrations, if only because it was then easier to rebuild housing stock from scratch on safer lines. Just as an outbreak of plague invariably prompted renewed interest in environmental health, the loss of lives, homes and possessions concentrated the minds of urban populations, making them more receptive to change. It was under such distressing circumstances that Reynold, Lord Grey, promulgated four new ordinances in 1364 for the prevention of future fires in his borough of Ruthin on the Welsh March. As in London, it appears that the highly combustible fuel used by brewers and bakers represented a serious hazard, and had now to be stored well away from built-up areas. Although no specific reference was made to the introduction of slate or tile, a significant shift away from thatch at this time also offered householders greater protection.[297]

In Chester, too, tilers replaced thatchers, who rapidly declined in number from the fourteenth century onwards. Faced, like the people of Ruthin, with the additional threat of arson attacks from the Welsh, Chester's merchants stored their more valuable goods in secure stone undercrofts, while curtailing the risk of domestic accidents through the construction of detached kitchens, kilns and bake houses, and by placing the hearths of public cook-shops outside in the open air.[298] Notwithstanding the rudimentary arrangements for hearths and heating adopted in most Winchester houses until the sixteenth century, it looks as if the striking reduction in the number of serious fires from the 1250s onwards was also due to pre-emptive action. By the 1360s thatched roofs had given way to tile, and flint walls were being built to contain the risk of fire from industrial premises.[299] Salisbury followed suit in 1431 with a ban on the use of straw for roofing; and in 1466 and 1493 respectively the rulers of Worcester and Coventry imposed heavy penalties of up to 100s. upon anyone who retained or constructed a chimney made of timber, rather than the compulsory brick or stone.[300] We should, however,

[296] Ricart, *Maire of Bristowe Is Kalendar*, pp. 93, 113. Even in a small town like Basingstoke, residents could be presented to the court for failing to repair their chimneys: Baigent and Millard, *History of the Town and Manor of Basingstoke*, p. 321.

[297] R. I. Jack, 'The Fire Ordinances of Ruthin, 1364', *Transactions of the Denbighshire Historical Society* 28 (1979), pp. 5–17. Fired clay tiles were used in York from the thirteenth century onwards: Addyman, 'Archaeology of Public Health', p. 258.

[298] A. Brown, ed., *The Rows of Chester*, English Heritage Archaeological Report, 16 (London, 1999), pp. 11, 72, 74. Leases stipulated that any rebuilding should involve slate or tile roofs: Laughton, *Life in a Late Medieval City*, p. 87.

[299] Keene, *Survey of Medieval Winchester*, I.178; Furley, *Town Life*, pp. 136–7.

[300] Carr, *First General Entry Book*, no. 275; *Coventry Leet Book*, II.549; Smith, Smith and Brentano, *English Gilds*, p. 386. Properties owned by the borough of Nottingham had solid stone chimneys from at least the 1480s, although thatch was

bear in mind that breaches of these regulations must have been common, while in smaller towns thatch remained popular well into the Elizabethan period if not later.[301]

Whatever their size, most communities attempted to provide effective and accessible fire-fighting equipment, along with a ready supply of water to dowse the flames. As we shall see in the next chapter, measures for the compulsory repair of wells, either from official revenues or at a parochial level, were in part intended for this purpose.[302] Individual householders were also expected to keep tubs of water by their doors, especially in hot weather. The Custumal of Sandwich, which was transcribed in the early fourteenth century, made such a ruling, as did the mayor of London during the 'intensely hot and dry' summers of the late 1370s and 1381.[303] After the conflagration of 1364, the burgesses of Ruthin deemed it expedient to provide a large vat for the storage of water in each of the town's four main streets, charging the local water-carriers with the task of filling them every week.[304] Throughout England these otherwise obscure figures played a major role in protecting their neighbourhoods. The 'bitters', or water-bearers, of Worcester appear to have constituted an embryonic fire brigade by the 1460s, when they had to 'be ready with hur horses and bittes [buckets] to brynge water vnto euery citezen when … required by eny man or child when eny parelle of fuyre ys withyn the cite'.[305] In Coventry, the obligation to supply leather buckets fell upon senior office holders, who faced a fine of 6s. 8d. in 1493 should they fail to do so at their own expense. Arrangements had already been made (or perhaps reiterated) some twenty years earlier for the necessary 'ffyrehokes, rynges, ropes & ladders' to be kept in each ward, so that buildings could be pulled down quickly and roofs stripped in order to prevent fires from spreading.[306] This, too, was a common practice, having been adopted in London during the thirteenth century, when local juries were first required to check that each ward possessed an adequate supply of chains, cords and hooks, that the beadle had 'a good horn and loudly sounding' to raise the alarm, and that the owners of 'great houses' could provide a ladder or two, as well as the essential buckets of water. Significantly, the quality of street paving also came under review in this context, since badly maintained

---

still then being used: Stevenson, *Records of the Borough of Nottingham*, III.257–8, 292–3.

[301] J. Schofield and G. Stell, 'The Built Environment, 1300–1540', *CUHB1*, p. 391; Quiney, *Town Houses*, p. 106.

[302] See section 4.4 below.

[303] Boys, *History of Sandwich*, II.504; *CLB*, H, pp. 28, 92, 128, 165. Hitherto in London, the keeping of water barrels had been recommended but was not obligatory: *MGL*, II.i.88.

[304] Jack, 'Fire Ordinances of Ruthin', pp. 7–8, 16.

[305] Smith, Smith and Brentano, *English Gilds*, p. 382.

[306] *Coventry Leet Book*, II.414, 549. Similarly, in 1506 the rulers of Canterbury decreed that each ward should possess an iron hook and a ladder with thirty rungs 'for suerte and savegard of the cite': HMC, *Ninth Report*, part 1, appendix, p. 174. For the use of fire-hooks, see Jack, 'Fire Ordinances of Ruthin', pp. 6–7, 16–17.

roads could hamper accessibility.[307] That regular, if not always productive, reports were made by concerned Londoners is apparent from presentments filed in both January and December 1422 about the continuing lack of crooks and iron chains for use in Bridge ward 'in case a fire should happen, which God forbid'.[308] Rather than delegate the acquisition of such vital equipment, the rulers of Lynn made the necessary purchases themselves from the public purse.[309] In Worcester, too, the chamberlains were personally responsible for ensuring that 'ther be v fuyre hokes, to drawe at euery thynge wher paryle of fuyre ys in eny parte of the cite'.[310]

Negligent householders might well face serious reprisals. Residents charged with *affraria ignis* were regularly hauled before the courts in Chester, where the ravages of marcher warfare made juries particularly unsympathetic towards home-grown arsonists and accident-prone workmen.[311] But vigilance was not confined to the borders. From 1419 onwards any Londoner whose fire was large enough to be seen from outside his or her dwelling could incur a substantial penalty of 40s., which had, appropriately, to be surrendered in a *red* purse.[312] The rulers of Lynn not only fined individuals such as Frederick Beerbrewer, who caused two minor conflagrations in 1457, but also took action against those who failed to extinguish their fires at night.[313] Offenders in Norwich faced the prospect of a year's imprisonment or a 100s. fine, imposed by the Assembly in 1423, when eight officers of the watch were appointed in each of the city's four wards to see that the curfew was duly observed. Orders were also then issued for the provision of a ladder and two pairs of 'feerhoks' in every parish, although their reiteration some fourteen years later suggests that people had grown casual about the need for precautions.[314]

Norwich was notoriously prone to fires, a fact apparent from the names of two of its many churches, one being known as St Mary 'the unbrent', or unburned, in memory of its miraculous escape from the fire that had ravaged part of the city just after the Conquest, and the other St Margaret *in Combusto*.[315] Dramatic conflagrations occurred there in the early sixteenth century: following an

---

[307] *MGL*, II.i.xxxiii, 87–8; *MGL*, III.134.

[308] The residents of Walbrook ward also needed a ladder, grappling hooks and ropes: *CPMRL, 1413–1437*, pp. 135, 139, 152, 158.

[309] In 1390–1, for example, the corporation bought seven new ladders, ranging in height from 11 to 43 feet, for fighting fires: Isaacson and Ingleby, *Red Register of King's Lynn*, II.134v.

[310] Smith, Smith and Brentano, *English Gilds*, pp. 385–6.

[311] Brown, *Rows of Chester*, p. 72. See also Jack, 'Fire Ordinances of Ruthin', p. 13.

[312] Bateson, *Borough Customs*, pp. 81–2.

[313] KLBA, KL/C7/2, Hall Book, 1422–1429, p. 128; C7/4, Hall Book, 1453–1497, p. 85. Heavy fines were also imposed in Winchester upon those who caused fires: Keene, *Survey of Medieval Winchester*, I.178.

[314] *RCN*, I.279–80; II.87; NRO, NCR, 16D/1, Assembly Proceedings, 1434–1491, fol. 6r.

[315] Blomefield, *Topographical History of the County of Norfolk*, IV.439; B. Ayers, *Digging Deeper: Recent Archaeology in Norwich* (Norwich, 1987), p. 11.

unspecified but quite serious blaze in 1505, two fires in rapid succession during the spring and early summer of 1507 together destroyed at least 40 per cent of the entire housing stock.[316] The long-term consequences of this disaster were mixed. On the one hand, better dwellings with tiled roofs rather than 'thakke' could be constructed, stricter regulations for building introduced and drains and sewers repaired; on the other, the rental income that funded both private and public schemes for civic improvement fell sharply and derelict areas remained unoccupied for decades. A slump in the worsted trade, upon which the city's wealth depended, exacerbated matters, sparking resentment on the part of the poor towards richer neighbours who exploited the crisis to augment their own holdings.[317] Twenty-eight years after the 1507 fires a parliamentary act 'for the re-edifienge of voyde groundes in the Citie of Norwich' reported that whole tracts of 'desolate and vacant groundes, many of theym nighe and adjoyninge to the high stretes, replenished with moche unclennes and filthe' still blighted the urban landscape, threatening the health of residents and visitors alike.[318] There can be little doubt that members of the ruling elite used this legislation to gain possession of 'grounde decaied by the ffyer' on highly advantageous terms. Yet men such as Augustine Steward, who acquired two plots 'soore accombred ... by divers persons with muk & suche other vile mater', at least possessed the resources to clear away the debris and begin again.[319]

Urban fires could reduce even the rich to penury, creating swathes of depopulation and placing an inordinate strain upon resources that might already be stretched to capacity. As in Norwich, reconstruction often took place slowly, with the result that some towns and cities were defaced by charred ruins, wasteland and building sites for long periods.[320] Although national fund-raising campaigns of the kind documented in the aftermath of late sixteenth- and seventeenth-century fires were not apparently mounted in medieval England, help might be available from the crown in the form of financial concessions or a grant of

---

[316] A. Carter and J. P. Roberts, 'Excavations in Norwich, 1973', *NA* 36 (1973–77), pp. 39–71, on pp. 48, 52.

[317] *RCN*, II.107; NRO, NCR, 16D/2, Assembly Book, 1491–1553, fols 64v, 100r; Rawcliffe, 'Sickness and Health', p. 313; Ayers, *Norwich: Archaeology of a Fine City*, pp. 140–1. In 1530 the Corporation carried out an inspection of the city's housing, fining anyone who had thatched his or her property during the previous decade: NRO, NCR, 16A/2, Mayor's Book, 1510–1532, pp. 236–7.

[318] *SR*, vol. 3, 26 Henry VIII, cap. 8, pp. 504–5. The new occupants of 'grounde decaied by the ffyer' were required to enclose and develop their land: *RCN*, II.122. Similar measures were then adopted in Northampton, where a devastating fire in 1516 had accelerated economic and demographic decline: W. Page, ed., *VCH Northampton*, vol. 3 (London, 1930), pp. 30–1.

[319] *RCN*, II.122; NRO, NCR, 16D/2, Assembly Proceedings, 1491–1553, fol. 163r–v.

[320] As Robert Tittler points out, because there was far less demand for accommodation while urban populations continued to stagnate or even decline, the replacement of lost housing stock only became a priority in the 1530s: 'For the "Re-Edification of Townes": The Rebuilding Statutes of Henry VIII', *Albion* 22 (1990), pp. 591–605, on pp. 595, 597.

building materials.[321] Following yet another arson attack by the Scots, for instance, the people of Carlisle obtained permission from Edward I in 1305 to remove stone from the royal forest of Inglewood in order to construct houses that would be less combustible. Their assurance that the ensuing repairs 'would be better than they had been in the past' confirms that devastation was not only a regular fact of life for the inhabitants of marcher towns, but that hasty rebuilding might well leave much to be desired.[322] Did some communities exaggerate their losses? Petitions to parliament for tax relief in the aftermath of fires inevitably painted a bleak picture, just like modern-day insurance claims. It is now impossible to tell if 'the greater part of the commonalty' of Tamworth was actually rendered homeless after a conflagration in 1345, although the apparent success of the appeal would suggest that serious damage had occurred.[323] Similar requests for allowances and exemptions made by the people of Arundel in 1344 (after two serious fires in six years), of Cambridge (where a hundred burgages were reputedly destroyed in 1385), of Basingstoke in 1392, of Shrewsbury in 1394 and again shortly before 1407, of Hythe in 1401 (when an apocalyptic combination of fire and pestilence struck the town) and of Andover in 1435 underscore the vulnerability of urban populations to sudden and widespread disaster.[324]

Where possible, individual householders were expected to make good any fire damage as quickly as possible, especially as abandoned buildings could be unsafe for passers-by, attracting fly-tippers and generating miasmatic air.[325] Civic pride also demanded that such eyesores should be removed at the first opportunity, like rotten teeth, although, as the Norwich example confirms, this was easier said than done. Londoners, at least, were legally bound to repair their business premises and dwellings within a reasonable period, while the authorities could insist that dangerous structures be demolished and rebuilt.[326] Anyone deemed responsible for destroying adjacent property through negligence might well find himself in

---

[321] P. Roberts, 'Agencies Human and Divine: Fire in French Cities, 1520–1720', in Roberts and Naphy, *Fear in Early Modern Society*, p. 9; Friedrichs, *Early Modern City*, pp. 277–8.

[322] TNA, SC8/1/34; *RP*, I.166. Edward I also made grants of timber to those whose property had been destroyed: TNA, SC8/3/103, 99/4905, 100/4954; *CCR, 1302–1307*, pp. 256, 259, 302. It has been suggested that residents of the borders preferred to rebuild quickly in wood, since their dwellings would soon be destroyed again: Palliser, Slater and Dennison, 'Topography of Towns', pp. 182–3.

[323] TNA, SC8/13/641; *RP*, II.189.

[324] *RP*, II.185–6; *CCR, 1343–1346*, p. 283 (Arundel); F. W. Maitland and M. Bateson, eds, *The Charters of the Borough of Cambridge* (Cambridge, 1901), pp. 32–9; Baigent and Millard, *History of the Town and Manor of Basingstoke*, pp. 75–6; TNA, SC8/299/14935, 14942; *RP*, II.618–19; Owen and Blakeway, *History of Shrewsbury*, I.175, 204; SC8/250/12465; *CPR, 1399–1401*, p. 477 (Hythe); SC8/90/4477 (Andover).

[325] Tittler, 'Re-Edification of Townes', p. 596. In thirteenth-century York, tenants could be required to rebuild after a fire: P. M. Tillott, ed., *VCH York: The City of York* (Oxford, 1961), p. 52. However, it was difficult to enforce this type of obligation and urban landlords, including hospitals, often suffered as a result: Keene, *Survey of Medieval Winchester*, II.806; Rawcliffe, *Medicine for the Soul*, p. 98.

[326] *LAN*, no. 206.

court, as is apparent from a case of 1377, in which a chandler successfully sued his neighbour for compensation because an unsupervised fire had spread out of control into his tenement. It is interesting to note that most of the damage was caused by the removal of tiles and laths 'with chains and hooks' on the command of the constables in order to contain the blaze, which confirms that the fire-fighting measures described above were effectively put into practice.[327]

It seems hard to deny that at least some of the schemes and regulations considered in this chapter had a tangible impact upon the late medieval urban environment. However, not all scholars are persuaded that the residents of English towns and cities were capable of implementing even the most rudimentary health measures. Two arguments in particular have been advanced in support of this thesis. A system that depended so heavily upon voluntary co-operation is deemed to have been unworkable without more robust means of policing and enforcement, while the authorities themselves stand charged with a collective failure to invest the necessary time, money and effort for the creation of better public utilities. Some historians maintain that magistrates and householders alike 'preferred the unpleasantness to the trouble of having to continually carry off their waste', and chose to ignore the mounting heaps of dung and garbage that contaminated their streets.[328] There can, indeed, be little doubt that the problem sometimes seemed intractable, and that, despite strenuous efforts, insanitary nuisances – from noisome latrines to dirty and broken pavements – could never be completely eliminated.

Yet, as the most cursory examination of urban records reveals, the presumption of inertia flies in the face of an overwhelming mass of archival and archaeological evidence. The threat of increasingly draconian fines for antisocial behaviour may reflect desperation, but can hardly be regarded as a sign of indifference. Indeed, in some respects, such as the introduction of refuse collections and communal rubbish tips, the control of vagrant animals, the more systematic removal of butchers' waste and the prevention of fires, many towns and cities could lay claim to modest success against formidable odds. Perhaps the final verdict should rest with G. T. Salusbury-Jones, who observed in 1939 that, whereas 'squalor and filth' might often reach alarming levels, the challenge was generally met by a desire for prompt and effective action rather than passive resignation. 'Judging by the number and vehemence of municipal laws for the cleaning of the streets, particularly in the fifteenth century', he concluded, 'more credit should be given to the townsfolk of the Middle Ages for their sensibility to the dangers and unpleasantness of foul ways than is generally accorded them.'[329] Their concern extended to the provision of clean, unpolluted water, to which we now turn.

---

[327] *CPMRL, 1364–1381*, pp. 235–6. One early sixteenth-century legal formulary records the wording of writs for use in such cases: TNA, C193/1, fol. 22r.

[328] Classen, Howes and Synnott, *Aroma*, p. 57.

[329] Salusbury-Jones, *Street Life in Medieval England*, p. 72.

✒ Chapter 4
Water

'I hold it', said Mr Saunders, 'to be one of the great triumphs of our day, that it has so subordinated all the vaguer and more lawless sentiments to the solid guidance of our sober economical considerations. And not only do I consider a cotton-mill, but I consider a good sewer, to be a far nobler and a far holier thing – for holy in reality does but mean healthy – than the most admired Madonna ever painted.'

'A good sewer', said Mr Herbert, 'is, I admit, an entirely holy thing; and would all our manufacturers and men of science bury themselves underground, and confine their attention to making sewers, I, for one, should have little complaint against them.'

W. H. Mallock, *The New Republic; or Culture, Faith and Philosophy in an English Country House* (1878)[1]

Delivered by Sir George Newman, the Chief Medical Officer for the Ministry of Health, the Heath Clerk lectures for 1931 had little good to say about medieval urban life. Sir George's history of the rise of preventative medicine glossed quickly over the dark period between the Romans and the Renaissance, when European towns and cities had been chiefly distinguished by their 'narrow, unpaved streets, open drains, collections of filth, refuse and offal', and a corresponding 'absence of adequate water supplies'.[2] He probably had in mind the celebrated description of Norwich's Franciscan friary by the Victorian scholar Augustus Jessopp, who believed that the brethren lived 'in a filthy swamp ... through which the drainage of the city sluggishly trickled into the river, never a foot lower than its banks'.[3] This is a powerful image, which Sir George certainly used elsewhere to considerable effect, albeit one that evokes the conditions of Jessopp's youth rather than those of the late medieval city.[4] The friars first settled on land that was, indeed, rather marshy, but a recently published excavation report on the permanent site which soon became their home has revealed an extremely sophisticated scheme of water management. It was planned from the outset as an integral part of the claustral layout, and included no fewer than eleven wells, a network of lead and ceramic piping, and an impressive system of brick and flint-lined underground drains, the chief of which ran into the Dallingflete stream and thence to the river. Moreover,

---

[1] W. H. Mallock, *The New Republic; or Culture, Faith and Philosophy in an English Country House* (London, 1878), p. 46. This satirical exchange, in which Saunders represents the sanitary reformer Kingdon Clifford, and Herbert the distinguished aesthete John Ruskin, has been taken at face value by some medical historians. Compounding the error, Wohl, *Endangered Lives*, p. 101, implausibly attributes Saunders' remark to Ruskin.

[2] Newman's lectures appeared in print as *The Rise of Preventative Medicine* (Oxford, 1932). The quotation is on p. 122.

[3] Jessopp, *Coming of the Friars*, p. 44.

[4] See pp. 11–14 above.

the sewerage system was constructed in such a way as to allow regular flushing with clean water to prevent blockages and the deposit of offensive matter.[5]

The Norwich grey friars were certainly not unusual in this respect. Informed by the growing corpus of literature on medicine and hygiene which occupied a prominent place in their libraries, mendicant communities throughout England did their utmost to improve the surroundings in which they and their neighbours lived. This could be a struggle since, as newcomers to the urban scene, some had been allocated insalubrious, marginal land on which to build. Their efforts thereby permit us a fascinating insight into contemporary notions of environmental health and the best means of promoting it.[6] Having initially sought to enclose and drain the stagnant cesspool which lay next to their church, the Exeter Franciscans won royal approval for a complete change of location in 1285 after their patron, the earl of Hereford, intervened personally on their behalf. A few days spent in the precinct persuaded him that life 'in a horrible drain where the place smelled indoors and out' was not only profoundly unpleasant, but also a cause of high mortality among the brethren. The death of their formidable opponent Bishop Quinel (whose resistance to the move no doubt explains why he was erroneously said to have succumbed to a choking fit on the vigil of the feast of St Francis) enabled them to secure healthier accommodation in the suburbs.[7]

Whether or not they opted for relocation, most English friaries invested heavily in the construction of sewers designed to remove potentially dangerous waste, while also providing a regular supply of fresh, clean water. Sometimes these initiatives were sponsored as works of Christian charity and civic improvement by local burgesses such as John Glovere of Lynn, who left the munificent sum of £40 so that the Austin friars could pipe water through the town to their precinct.

[5] P. A. Emery, 'The Franciscan Friary', *Current Archaeology* 170 (2000), pp. 72–8, on p. 77; P. A. Emery, *Norwich Greyfriars: Pre-Conquest Town and Medieval Friary*, EAA 120 (Dereham, 2007), pp. 58, 75–6, 83, and figs. 3.7, 3.19, 3.21.

[6] The Austin friary at York, for example, occupied a site on the River Ouse that was deemed 'very contagious, as well in winter as in summer, by means of the sundry corrupt and common channels, sinkers and gutters of the said city conveyed under the same': *LPFD*, vol.13, part 2, no. 768.

[7] A. G. Little and R. C. Easterling, *The Franciscans and Dominicans in Exeter* (Exeter, 1927), pp. 14–17; A. Montford, *Health, Sickness, Medicine and the Friars in the Thirteenth and Fourteenth Centuries* (Aldershot, 2004), pp. 47–9. It was accepted that, where feasible, religious houses should move to avoid the threats posed by the miasmatic air arising from foul water. As early as 1110, the monks of the New Minster at Winchester abandoned their original site, on a cramped and unhealthy spot next to the cathedral, where 'water, flowing from the West Gate down the steep streets of the town, came together … in a terrible bog (*paludem horridam*) with mud deposited in a stagnant pond, giving off an intolerable stink, and so infecting the air that the brothers serving God in this place suffered many hardships': M. Biddle, ed., *Winchester in the Early Middle Ages* (Oxford, 1976), p. 317; M. Biddle and R. N. Quirk, 'Excavations near Winchester Cathedral, 1961', *Archaeological Journal* 129 (1962), pp. 150–94, on p. 179. A century later, the brethren of St Thomas's hospital, Southwark, seized the opportunity presented by fire to find a more salubrious site, 'ubi aqua est uberior et aer est sanior', qualities especially needful in a hospital: Luard, *Annales monastici*, III.451, 457.

He clearly intended to benefit the laity as well as the brothers, since before work began, in 1386, it was agreed that a cistern, fed by three pipes, would be set up to the south of the convent by the Grass Market (map 1). Residents would be free to draw water there during daylight hours between Easter and Michaelmas, while the prior recognised an obligation to effect whatever repairs should prove necessary.[8]

Religious houses might themselves take the first steps towards the provision of shared facilities, in part, no doubt, to avoid disputes about the running of pipes through private property, but also for more philanthropic motives.[9] In early fourteenth-century Southampton, for instance, it was the friars minor who funded and built a watercourse and cistern from which the burgesses were permitted to pipe water. Eventually, in 1420, the latter assumed control of the entire system, along with responsibility for its upkeep.[10] The Gloucester Franciscans likewise agreed in 1438 'on account of their affection towards the community' to divert three-quarters of their piped water supply to the town in return for a corresponding level of financial support for installation and repairs, which could prove extremely expensive.[11] Similar examples of collaborative activity may be found in so many English towns – Boston, Bridgnorth, Bristol, Carmarthen, Chichester, Coventry, Lichfield, Lincoln, London, Newcastle-upon-Tyne, Oxford, Richmond, Sandwich and Scarborough – that we might justifiably regard them as an important component of the mendicants' urban mission.[12] While washing clean the souls of the laity through confession, they were, quite literally, assisting their physical ablutions as well.

This chapter begins by questioning the assumption that the ruling elites of medieval English towns and cities were disinclined either to promote schemes

---

[8] Owen, *Making of King's Lynn*, pp. 117–19. The town already possessed an aqueduct in the Tuesday Market, which cost almost £16 to repair in 1365–6, and £9 in 1384–5 (pp. 214–15).

[9] For an examination of the complex negotiations involved in constructing shared pipes and conduits, see R. J. Magnusson, *Water Technology in the Middle Ages* (Baltimore, 2001), chap. 2.

[10] A spring had been granted to the friary for this purpose by a local landowner in 1290: Platt, *Medieval Southampton*, pp. 35, 65, 96, 144; H. W. Gidden, ed., *The Book of Remembrance of Southampton*, vol. 2, Southampton Record Society 28 (Southampton, 1928), pp. 14–16; F. W. Robins, *The Story of Water Supply* (Oxford, 1946), pp. 100–1 and plate 9.

[11] Stevenson, *Records of the Corporation of Gloucester*, pp. 352–3, no. 966 (a dispute of 1357 with St Peter's abbey over the supply), pp. 391–2, no. 1112 (agreement of 1438). In 1391, the Bristol Dominicans had reached a similar understanding with the townspeople, exempting them from the costs of maintenance, while safeguarding their own access: Magnusson, *Water Technology*, pp. 33–4. One year later, the bailiffs of Scarborough agreed with the Franciscan community to shoulder two-thirds of the cost of making an aqueduct and laying pipes for their joint use: Jeayes, *White Vellum Book of Scarborough*, p. 42.

[12] A. R. Martin, *Franciscan Architecture in England* (Manchester, 1937), p. 39; C. J. Bond, 'Water Management in the Urban Monastery', in R. Gilchrist and H. Mytum, eds, *Advances in Monastic Archaeology*, BAR British series 228 (Oxford, 1993), pp. 57–63; Clarke *et al.*, *Sandwich: A Study of the Town and Port*, p. 134.

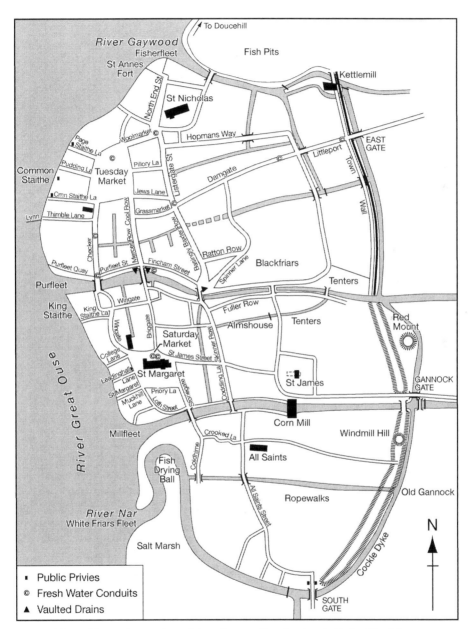

Map 1 The markets and conduits of late medieval and early Tudor King's Lynn

for the amelioration of public water supplies, or even to shoulder the burden of maintaining whatever rudimentary facilities were already in place (4.1). We will then explore the medical rationale that underpinned many of the regulatory measures designed to protect the urban environment from the miasmatic air and risk of disease associated with noxious drains and stagnant water (4.2). The challenge was far from easy, not least because of the quantities of waste and levels of pollution generated by the victualling trades and by the numerous industrial workshops that clustered along the banks of suburban streams and rivers (4.3). Apart from causing contamination, these activities utilised copious amounts of water, often at the expense of domestic consumers, who thus required protection on both fronts (4.4). As Mark Jenner reminds us, 'water was a scarce and valuable resource in all pre-industrial cities', the provision of which engendered 'a well-developed sense of moral economy'.[13]

Although in theory, if not always in practice, common wells and conduits offered the poorer members of society improved access to cleaner water, numerous hazards still lay in wait for those charged with the burdensome and time-consuming task of fetching and carrying it. Magistrates meanwhile had to contend with the daunting problem posed by the obstruction of the streams and rivers that traversed the urban body like veins and arteries (4.5). However draconian they may have seemed, prohibitions on the dumping of dung and rubbish in watercourses were as hard to enforce as other measures for the regulation of waste disposal, being equally dependent upon the creation of more coherent and integrated systems of refuse collection. Yet the quest for material prosperity and health was by no means the only motive behind both public and private investment in better facilities. As the final section of this chapter demonstrates, late medieval benefactors were especially drawn by the prospect of lasting commemoration on earth and an eternal reward in heaven (4.6).

4.1 Investments and improvements

Speculating on the apparent 'failure of most urban authorities to establish more sophisticated supplies of clean water', let alone to embark upon engineering schemes for this purpose, Richard Holt maintained that the profusion of wells, rivers, cisterns and water-carriers in English towns, along with 'the strong cultural prejudice against drinking water', made such an exercise seem unnecessary. It is hard to deny that, with a few notable exceptions, cash-strapped magistrates evinced a general preference for shared ventures of the kind described above, rather than costly public works akin to those undertaken in southern Europe, but less easy to accept 'that the deciding factor was indifference'.[14] Not only did far more towns boast a supply of piped water than Holt's meagre tally of three

---

[13] M. S. R. Jenner, 'From Conduit Community to Commercial Network? Water in London, 1500–1725', in M. S. R. Jenner and P. Griffiths, eds, *Londinopolis: Essays in the Cultural and Social History of Early Modern London* (Manchester, 2000), pp. 250, 254.

[14] R. Holt, 'Medieval England's Water-Related Technologies', in P. Squatriti, ed., *Working with Water in Medieval Europe* (Leiden, 2000), p. 98.

(Gloucester, London and Southampton), but in almost all urban communities the upkeep of gutters, drains, wells and watercourses rapidly became an official priority.[15] Indeed, given the legal difficulties and financial constraints which often frustrated attempts at long-term planning, the achievements of some authorities testify to dogged perseverance rather than apathy.

The struggle to secure an adequate supply of potable water was especially pronounced in coastal towns, whose rivers were too saline either for use in the preparation of food and alcoholic beverages, or in a variety of industrial processes. In low-lying settlements such as Kingston-upon-Hull, even the wells would be contaminated with salt. The ongoing, but only partially successful, efforts of its residents to remedy their difficult situation illustrate some of the many obstacles that hindered large-scale hydraulic projects, among which opposition from local landowners to the running of dikes through productive farmland caused particular problems. Attempts in 1376 to bring water from Anlaby along a series of interconnected watercourses to the town failed on this score, although a renewed campaign at the start of the fifteenth century eventually overcame resistance.[16] Nevertheless, as we shall see in the following pages, open trenches and canals were vulnerable to floods, pollution and blockages, while also requiring frequent dredging. Underground pipes offered a better alternative, and were clearly high on the agenda when, in 1438, Joan Gregg, the widow of a former burgess, left £20 to kick-start the enterprise.[17] Bequests of this kind (which might well impose specific deadlines) provided a much-needed catalyst, besides furnishing the capital to cover such initial expenses as the purchase of springs, wells and rights of way. The obligatory royal letters patent authorising the acquisition of whatever land might be needed did not come cheap. Hull finally secured permission for the transportation of water 'by subterranean leaden pipes and other necessary and suitable engines' in 1447, and an even more generous legacy of £100 from the wealthy merchant Robert Holme made it possible to complete all the work within the next three years.[18] However, the townspeople's pride in what was, by any standard, a significant achievement was not destined to last. Abandoning their efforts to maintain the system, the ruling elite decided to dig up and sell the pipes in 1461, and reverted to the use of water-carriers, or 'bussemen', who plied their trade between the town centre and the freshwater dike beyond the walls.[19] It may have proved impossible to create the gradient necessary to sustain a steady flow of water or to generate the funding needed for maintenance, but, whatever the problem, there had clearly been no lack of commitment before this date.

[15] A point stressed by F. W. Robins, whose survey of 1946 presents a far more positive view of the topic: *Story of Water Supply*, chap. 15.

[16] Allison, *VCH York, East Riding*, I.371. See also Magnusson, *Water Technology*, pp. 26–7, 44; and Robins, *Story of Water Supply*, p. 107.

[17] Borthwick Institute, York, York Registry Wills, iii, fols 555v–556v (Joan's will was made in 1438 and proved a decade later).

[18] J. Raine, ed., *Testamenta Eboracensia*, vol. 3, Surtees Society 44 (London, 1865), p. 182; *CPR, 1446–1452*, pp. 43–4. The town had secured royal letters of incorporation in 1440, which clearly facilitated the acquisition of property.

[19] Allison, *VCH York, East Riding*, I.371.

The experience further down the North Sea coast at King's Lynn proved more encouraging. Despite the fact that it was bordered on the north, south and west by rivers, and traversed from east to west by two broad fleets, or dikes, Lynn faced the same problem as Hull, in so far that none of this water was drinkable. Although they were already served by at least two conduits, the residents still suffered from shortages until, in 1423, the council debated the possibility of following Hull's example by constructing a canal that would feed through sluices into the 'common ditch' at Gannock gate. The need for a more effective source of power to drive the town's corn mill gave the project additional impetus. The MP Bartholomew Petipas busied himself in London by petitioning for an all-important royal licence, while the mayor lavished gifts and hospitality upon the bishop of Norwich, who was not only lord of the borough but also owner of much of the land through which the new dike would carry 'sweet' water from the upper reaches of the River Gay. Several other interested parties had also to be wined, dined and compensated (evidently to better purpose than had been the case in Hull), as had all the farmers whose crops might be destroyed by earthworks. These various charges, along with the cost of a comprehensive programme for cleansing and repairing the town ditch, were met in part by the fortunate remission of £266 in taxes by the royal council.[20] In order to maximise their investment and prevent any part of this network from becoming clogged with filth, the magistrates decreed that all unauthorised dunghills, rubbish tips and the like should immediately be removed, and instituted a quarterly rate for the upkeep of two communal muck-carts. Exemplary fines were also imposed on any householders who failed to maintain adjacent fleets and ditches, or who dumped refuse in them.[21] It is a measure of the importance of this undertaking that one thoughtless individual who, in 1424, allowed sea water to infiltrate the new dike was consigned to the pillory and forced to abjure the town for ever.[22]

Because of the expense and high level of risk involved, it made sense to seek the best professional advice before proceeding further. Having already rejected proposals submitted by an *operarius* from Peterborough, in 1428 the rulers of Lynn invited a specialist who was then working in Boston to pronounce on the feasibility of plans for transporting uncontaminated river water from the

[20] V. Parker, *The Making of King's Lynn: Secular Buildings from the Eleventh to the Seventeenth Century*, King's Lynn Archaeological Survey 1 (London, 1971), pp. 21–3, 132; KLBA, KL/C7/2, Hall Book, 1422–1429, pp. 1, 4, 8, 14–23, 38, 41, 42, 47, 62, 65, 67–9, 73. The royal letters patent of 1424 cite a petition from the burgesses to the effect that 'no fresh water is to be obtained there but by purchase, and with great labour and cost of carriage, for which reason many of the poor inhabitants have left and more intend to do so'. Since identical claims were made by the people of Hull, we can perhaps detect signs of collaboration, as well as a common rhetoric: *CPR, 1422–1429*, pp. 183–4.

[21] KLBA, KL/C7/2, Hall Book, 1422–1429, pp. 24, 56, 103, 126–7, 134, 146, 170. In 1430 it was agreed that the common ditch and fleets would be flushed clean once a week with a combination of fresh and sea water (p. 297). For later measures against fly-tipping, which lost none of their initial force, see C7/3, Hall Book 1431–1450, fols 200r, 212v, 270r, 271v; C7/4, Hall Book, 1453–1497, pp. 388, 395, 468.

[22] KLBA, KL/C7/2, Hall Book, 1422–1429, p. 90.

north-east outskirts of the town to the centre. He was also to demonstrate a novel 'engine' (*ingenium*) that they might use. Clearly intrigued, the mayor retained him to oversee the construction of Lynn's first horse-powered kettle-mill, or vertical wheel with buckets attached, which cost the burgesses at least £26. By this means fresh water could be conveyed in 'a leaden gutter' along or near the walls to designated outlets.[23] Another round of activity followed in 1444, when a 'water-house' and device 'per le castying de le water' were constructed outside the east gate, along with an aqueduct leading thence to the Tuesday Market. The installation of a separate system of pipes from a similar 'water-house' beyond the south gate a few months later pushed up the bill to well over £100.[24] Raising the money to maintain all this equipment and extend the piping was not always easy, especially during periods of economic hardship. In 1475, 1485 and 1496 the authorities followed a royal precedent by appealing for 'benevolences', or voluntary contributions, to repair the heavily used conduit near St Margaret's church and the Saturday Market, while imposing an annual levy of 1*d.* on councillors and one half-penny on other residents to fund the keeper's annual salary of 20*s.* Members of the ruling elite were not only encouraged to make generous provision in their wills for the support of such vital public utilities, but also to set an example to other residents by paying higher rates. For example, each of them was required to contribute towards the £23 needed to replace the stone cistern and aqueduct at St Margaret's in 1520.[25]

Work on this scale had invariably to wait until money became available and stop when it ran out. We do not know how much was spent on the construction of Exeter's impressive network of aqueducts and conduits, or the subterranean tunnels, up to 14 feet high, which allowed easy access to the pipes. But the decision, taken in 1420, to supplement an inadequate water supply shared uneasily with the Benedictine priory and the dean and chapter must have imposed a heavy burden on communal resources.[26] Indeed, although Exeter enjoyed considerably

---

[23] KLBA, KL/C7/2, Hall Book, 1422–1429, pp. 163, 178–9, 190, 206, 225, 229, 256, 260, 281; Owen, *Making of King's Lynn*, p. 196. Supervision of the kettle mill was delegated to a committee in 1458 and a salaried keeper was appointed in 1463: C7/3, Hall Book, 1431–1450, pp. 116, 197. Pipes eventually ran from this source to the Tuesday, Saturday and Grass Markets. Parker, *Making of King's Lynn*, pp. 162–3, underestimates the extent of the fifteenth-century infrastructure.

[24] The burgesses spent at least £10 from the public purse on one water-house 'for lack of a donation'; a legacy of £12 paid for the other; the Trinity Guild offered £15 for pipes; and the bishop of Norwich contributed £66 towards the aqueduct: KLBA, KL/C7/3, Hall Book, 1431–1450, fols 184v, 189r, 190r, 194v. Problems occurred in 1449, when the mayor had to ask the Augustinians to share their supply with the townspeople because of temporary shortages (fol. 273v).

[25] KLBA, KL/C7/4, Hall Book, 1453–1497, pp. 343, 363, 366, 506, 508, 546, 576, 582, 623; C7/5, Hall Book, 1497–1544, fols 213r, 216v, 282v.

[26] Information about this system may be found in C. G. Henderson, 'The City of Exeter from AD 50 to the Early Nineteenth Century', in R. Kain and W. Ravenhill, eds, *Historical Atlas of South-West England* (Exeter, 2000), pp. 489–91; W. Minchinton, *Life to the City: An Illustrated History of Exeter's Water Supply* (Exeter, 1987), pp. 14–17, 92–3. The following account is based upon two

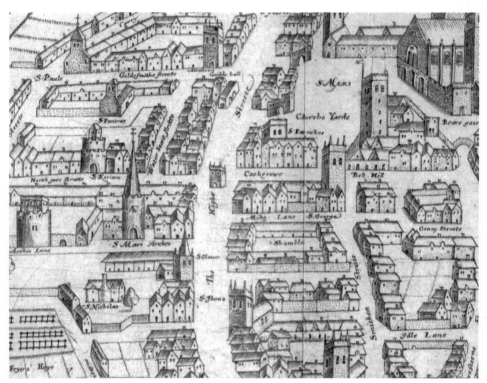

14 A detail of Remigius Hogenberg's 1587 plan of Exeter showing the great conduit at the Carfax or crossroads

better economic health than most fifteenth-century English cities, the various stages of such an ambitious project were necessarily protracted and dependent upon the traditional combination of private donations, legacies and public funding.[27] The first bout of activity saw the creation of a new aqueduct, which by 1429 conveyed fresh water from a well-head some distance to the north-east of the city by lead pipes to what was to become known as the Great Conduit at the Carfax, or central crossroads (plate 14). Within just over a decade, however, the need for improvements became apparent. Since the Dominicans, too, wished to overhaul their own system, a partnership offered the best way forward, and by 1445 the citizens and mendicants had together replaced and extended most of the existing infrastructure. In view of the fact that their joint disbursements reached almost £150 in 1441 alone, it is easy to see why further plans had to be shelved once

unpublished archaeological reports made available to me by John Allan of the Exeter Archaeology Unit, to whom I am extremely grateful: J. Z. Juddery and M. J. Stoyle, 'The Aqueducts of Medieval Exeter', Exeter Archaeology report 95/44; M. J. Stoyle, 'The Underground Aqueduct Passages of Exeter', Exeter Archaeology report 95/45.

[27] Kowaleski, *Local Markets*, p. 91. The initial impetus appears to have come from bequests left by the three wealthy citizens John Talbot (the rents of a shop), William Wilford (£10) and Simon Grendon (£20): Juddery and Stoyle, 'Aqueducts of Medieval Exeter', p. 9; DRO, ECA, Mayor's Court Roll, 1421–1422, rot. 13.

recession started to bite in the third quarter of the century. Work resumed in earnest during the more prosperous 1490s, when labourers began to build some 250 metres of stone-lined vaults to house the pipes more safely, and another joint project with the black friars got underway, this time for the creation of a second aqueduct. It was completed by 1502, and the vaults by the 1530s, when the citizens could reflect with satisfaction upon an undertaking that demonstrably beautified and preserved the urban body (plate 15).

Lynn and Exeter were not the only towns to retain specialist plumbers or metal founders as conduit keepers so that they could attend to repairs and general maintenance on a permanent basis.[28] Remuneration varied considerably. In the 1360s Gloucester allocated its common plumber an unremarkable fee of 13*s*. 4*d*. a year 'pro custodiendo aquaeductu'.[29] A decade later Hugh White of Bristol negotiated more lucrative (but demanding) terms whereby, in return for a substantial lifetime annuity of £10, he contracted with the mayor

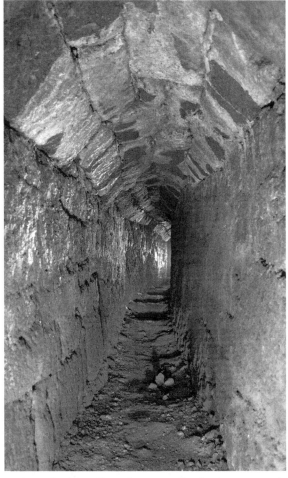

15. An early sixteenth-century stone-lined passage, or vault, constructed in Exeter for the conveyance and protection of water pipes, which could be easily accessed by workmen when repairs were needed without digging up the pavement

to ensure that all three of the town's public conduits remained in good working order, to clean and repair the entire system regularly and to lay 1,000 feet of new or replacement subterranean piping every year, all at his own cost. Since he stood to forfeit the entire annual fee in the event of any protracted stoppages, it would seem that the people of Bristol expected a first-class service.[30] As so many householders learned to their cost, piped water could prove a mixed blessing if

[28] Magnusson, *Water Technology*, pp. 119–20; KLBA, KL/C7/4, Hall Book, 1453–1497, p. 576.

[29] HMC, *Twelfth Report*, appendix 9, p. 424.

[30] Veale, *Great Red Book of Bristol*, I.114–17. For a map of Bristol's water supply, see Bond, 'Water Management', p. 45. For information about the pipes, see Robins, *Story of Water Supply*, pp. 106–7.

cisterns flooded or piping began to leak into workshops and cellars. Although, as we shall see, London boasted the most sophisticated and costly provision of water in late medieval England, accidents were still common. Following a series of 'inundations owing to fractured pipes' the residents of Fleet Street clubbed together in 1388 to build a 'pinnacle' or covering for the conduit house outside the home of John Walworth, who left some of his rental income for its upkeep shortly afterwards.[31] Civic funds were, however, specifically earmarked for the use of the two specialist metalworkers who initially served as keepers of the Great Conduit in Cheapside, since this was one of London's most celebrated landmarks (Map 2).[32] In 1350, when trade must have been severely disrupted in the aftermath of plague, they still managed to raise over £15, mostly from the tolls levied on commercial users who needed to fill large vessels known as 'tankards'. Almost all of this money was spent on running repairs, although it cost 32s. to flush out and cleanse all the pipes following claims that the water had been poisoned.[33] Such allegations proliferated during epidemics, and reflect the close connection then made between water and disease.[34]

The open gutters that channelled water and waste through urban thoroughfares also had to be maintained, usually by recourse to a similar combination of official funding and individual effort. From at least the turn of the fourteenth century, the treasurers and chamberlains of Norwich shouldered a significant part of the cost of scouring and repairing the city's many public conveniences, culverts, sewers and freshwater streams (known locally as 'cockeys'). In 1422–3, for example, almost £5 was spent on rebuilding the gutter in St Cross Lane, which involved the purchase of twenty carts of tile, lime, sand and clay and six of stone. Four years later, three masons and four labourers were between them employed for over seven weeks on extensive repairs to another watercourse in the market.[35] Work of this kind

[31] *CLB*, H, p. 326; Riley, *Memorials of London*, pp. 503–4; *CWCHL*, II.325. For the problem and its symbolic overtones in early modern England, see J. G. Harris, 'This Is Not a Pipe: Water, Supply, Incontinent Sources, and the Leaky Body Politic', in R. Burt and J. M. Archer, eds, *Enclosure Acts: Sexuality, Property and Culture in Early Modern England* (Ithaca, NY, 1994), pp. 203–28. Residents who caused accidental damage could face heavy penalties, as in the case of John More of Exeter, who was fined 20s. in 1525 'for brekyng of the citie pypes & letting owte of the water', and ordered to make good all the damage at his own expense: DRO, ECA, Chamber Act Book, 1508–1538, fol. 110v.

[32] Excavation has disclosed an impressive subterranean stone-vaulted chamber containing a lead tank, from which water could be pumped upwards: Sloane, 'Archaeological Evidence for the Infrastructure of London', pp. 90–1; Schofield, *London, 1100–1600*, pp. 30–1.

[33] Riley, *Memorials of London*, pp. 264–5. In 1368 it was decided to farm out the water supply rather than to appoint keepers. For an account of the City's medieval conduits, which dated from 1245, see Barron, *London in the Later Middle Ages*, pp. 256–8.

[34] Tales of poisoning generally concerned wells rather than pipes: Horrox, *Black Death*, pp. 45, 50, 207, 211–19, 222–5; Aberth, *From the Brink of the Apocalypse*, pp. 156–91.

[35] NRO, NCR, 7D, Treasurers' Accounts, 1422–1423, 1426–1427.

posed few challenges to a master craftsman, but more complex operations like the laying of pipes might require the services of an outside expert. Such was the case in 1451, when the Coventry magistrates allocated an initial sum of £16 15s. to one Lewis Dyker, who may have been Dutch, for cleansing, repairing and shoring up the town's ditches. He was to be paid at a rate of either 5s. or 6s. 8d. per perch (16'6"), depending upon the amount of labour involved in 'rammeng & stoppeng the spayre of ston for the water shuld not issu owt'. The final bill, which included materials as well as labour, must have been nearer £50, since the scale of his operations trebled over the summer.[36]

In line with the practice adopted for street paving, householders were expected to play their part in the routine maintenance of adjacent watercourses, usually under the threat of heavy fines and public censure should they prove remiss.[37] Not surprisingly, given Lynn's dependence upon its network of sluices, fleets and ditches, the authorities kept a constant eye on potential problems. Between 1431 and 1519, the mayor and council issued at least forty-two separate directives for repairs and cleaning either by the burgesses themselves or by workmen funded 'at the common cost'. On paper, at least, the penalties imposed on those who failed to comply ranged from a few pence to as much as 40s., or even imprisonment.[38] Various other sanctions were deployed elsewhere to deal with routine nuisances. In London negligent freeholders such as Alice Wade (who piped sewage into a public gutter in 1314) and Robert atte Haye (accused in 1377 of failing to cleanse the 'gutteram subterraneam' he shared with a neighbour) could face a court order requiring them to take prompt remedial action.[39] Tenants, too, found it increasingly difficult to shirk their liabilities, especially if they were renting from corporations or religious houses. Leases of property made by the rulers of Hull, Ipswich and York, for instance, often included a clause insisting that any neighbouring watercourses should be kept clean; and in Lynn the ownership of certain dwellings carried with it an obligation to maintain public latrines and other common utilities.[40] Inscribed in the 1301 custumal of Sandwich was a memorandum to the effect that responsibility for the upkeep of all gutters carrying public waste lay with those who lived next to them.[41]

[36] *Coventry Leet Book*, II.259–61.

[37] In the port of Lyme, for example, 'all men of the vill' were required to scour the gutters in front of their houses or incur a standard fine of 12d. When trenches had to be dug to drain off flood water, the penalty for non-compliance rose to 100s.: Dorset Record Office, DC/LR B1/2, nos 3, 9, 13.

[38] KLBA, KL/C7/2, Hall Book, 1422–1429, p. 328 (insertion for 1451); C7/3, Hall Book, 1431–1450, fols 3v, 10r–v, 34v, 35v, 36r, 37r, 39v, 43v, 61r, 113r, 170r, 171v, 172v, 174v, 175r–v, 189r, 195r, 196r, 200r, 212r, 254v; C7/4, Hall Book, 1453–1497, pp. 149, 151, 194, 217, 236, 253, 298, 300, 369, 389, 411, 483, 507; C7/5, Hall Book, 1497–1544, fols 38v, 180r, 193v, 195v. See also Owen, *Making of King's Lynn*, pp. 193–200, 216, 218–19.

[39] *LAN*, nos 214, 614.

[40] Evans, 'Infrastructure of Hull', p. 60; Bacon, *Annalls of Ipswiche*, p. 138; *YMB*, III.63; Owen, *Making of King's Lynn*, p. 193.

[41] Boys, *History of Sandwich*, II.539. Residents of Bridgwater were frequently presented by local juries for failing to cover their gutters in order to prevent

However, coercion was not always necessary. Exeter's subterranean vaults far surpassed their basic utilitarian function by effectively advertising the 'wealth and civic confidence' of the ruling elite, as well as communal pride in the provision of a clean and sanitary environment.[42] The multi-storey great conduit in Northampton, erected in 1481, dominated the town's marketplace, no doubt earning plaudits similar to those bestowed at this time by William of Worcester upon the water supply of his native Bristol. He described the castellated conduit on St Stephen's quay as 'a most beautiful house … sumptuously wrought in masonry', while the impressive free-stone well with its elegantly tiled penthouse at the Alyward gate also caught his eye.[43] On a more humdrum domestic level, excavations at Southampton have revealed that wealthier householders lavished substantial sums on the construction of drains that were both efficient and easy to flush clean (plate 16).[44] Evidence of this kind is not simply a reflection of rising standards of living and heightened sensibilities. The dumping of waste, along with any other activities likely to contaminate or obstruct urban watercourses, seemed particularly reprehensible and incurred appropriate punishment whatever one's social status. This was because flooding, itself a recurrent hazard of late medieval life, was directly associated in the medical literature of the period with stagnant water and pools of rotting debris that bred the miasmas of plague and other epidemic diseases.

4.2 Medical beliefs

A representative example of the vernacular texts on preventative medicine that circulated widely among the English reading public – and which were, indeed, produced especially for its benefit – may be found in Thomas Forestier's manual of 1485 on the causes and avoidance of pestilence. It begins with a solemn warning against the evils of water pollution, most notably

> stynken caryn cast in the water nye to the cytees or townes … and the corrupcion of privys, of this the water is corrupt; and when as mete is boyled, and drynke made of this water, many sikenes is gendered in mannes body; and also of the castyng of stynkyng waters and many other foule thinges in the streates the ayre is corrupte; and of kepyng of stynkyng waters in houses or in kechyns long tyme; and then, in nyght, of those thinges vapours ar lyft up in to the ayre, the whiche doth infecte the substance of the ayer, by the whiche sustans of the ayre, corrupte & infecte, men to dy [die] sodenly goyng by the stretes or by the way; of the whiche thinges let every man that *loveth god and his neighbour* amende.[45]

blockages and floods: Dilks, *Bridgwater Borough Archives*, nos 317–26, 328–30, 332.

[42] Stoyle, 'Underground Aqueduct Passages of Exeter', p. 5.

[43] Page, *VCH Northampton*, III.25; Dallaway, *Antiquities of Bristow*, pp. 68–9.

[44] Platt, *Medieval Southampton*, pp. 181–2; Platt and Coleman-Smith, *Excavations in Medieval Southampton*, pp. 273–5, 287 (fig. 94), 289.

[45] BL, Add. MS 27582, fol. 71v. Forestier drew heavily upon over a century of didactic literature on this theme, and there is no evidence to support M. T. Walton's

Three specific points of interest emerge from this quotation. First, we may note the influence and longevity of concepts that were first developed in Classical texts, such as the Hippocratic *Aphorisms* and *Airs, Waters, Places*. These ideas formed the basis of book one of Ibn-Sīna's *Canon of Medicine*, which contains a lengthy section on the risks to health posed by the consumption of 'non commendable waters'. He warned in particular against any that had remained 'a long time putrefying in the channels of the decomposing earth', since they caused a wide range of medical problems, including dropsy, fevers, diseases of the spleen, inflammation of the lungs and other organs, insanity, constipation, stomach upsets, infertility and congenital defects.[46] Of even greater

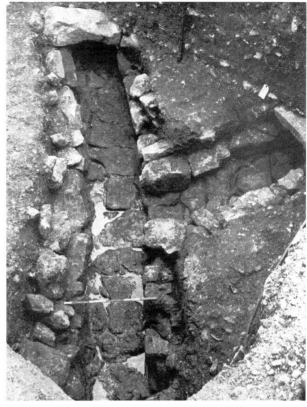

16 The junction of two stone-lined and carefully maintained drains of *c.* 1300 excavated in Cuckoo Lane, Southampton

significance in the present context are the author's observations on the pestilential air generated by the attendant process of putrefaction, this 'degradation of substance' being most likely to occur in the humid climate of late summer and autumn. Such a dramatic transformation in 'the character of the atmosphere' would, in turn, 'induce septic changes in the body fluids' beginning with the vital spirit which lodged in the heart.[47]

From the outset, the authors of treatises on the plague, such as the Leridan physician Jacme d'Agramont, emphasised the danger inherent in fumes arising from 'putrid', 'rotten' or otherwise polluted water.[48] The 'Canutus' plague tract,

suggestion that he was describing conditions then to be found in London: 'Stinking Air, Corrupt Water and the English Sweat', *JHM* 36 (1981), pp. 67–8.

[46] M. H. Shah, ed. and trans., *The General Principles of Avicenna's Canon of Medicine* (Karachi, 1966), pp. 190–1; Cameron Gruner, *Treatise on the Canon of Medicine of Avicenna*, pp. 221–8.

[47] Shah, *Avicenna's Canon of Medicine*, p. 173; Cameron Gruner, *Treatise on the Canon of Medicine of Avicenna*, p. 202; see pp. 120–2 above.

[48] d'Agramont, *Regiment de preservació de pestilència*, p. 57; Aberth, *Black Death*, p. 52.

translations of which circulated widely in late fifteenth-century England, refers to both the 'Amphorismys' of Hippocrates and the work of Ibn-Sīna, emphasising the dangers of 'corrupcyon of stynkyng dyches & watters, [as yt] fortune often tymes in corrupte places'. Filthy streets, dirty houses, miasmas generated by the remains of dead animals and, even worse, the 'grett stynche' arising from stagnant pools were to be shunned by the cautious citizen.[49] That the message so clearly enunciated in these pages reached its intended target is apparent from the wording of numerous administrative and legal documents, such as orders promulgated by the mayor of London in 1415 for the removal of a noisome latrine and other insanitary nuisances near Moorgate. His directive refers to the floods of sewage which had inundated neighbouring properties and the 'many sicknesses and other intolerable maladies arising from the horrible, corrupt and infected atmosphere'. We should also note that orders for the rebuilding of the latrine on a more salubrious site over running water, for the construction of sluices to ensure that waste would be quickly flushed away and for the planting of gardens to improve the surrounding air were expressly designed to safeguard 'the human body as people go, return and pass'.[50]

Although he was, in theory, describing King Priam's 'New Troy' rather than fifteenth-century London, John Lydgate wrote of similar plans, envisaged on a far grander scale, whereby 'fresche stremys clere' were cunningly diverted

> Thorugh condut pipis, large & wyde with-al,
> By certeyn meatis [channels] artificial,
> That it made a ful purgacioun
> Of al ordure & flythes in the toun,
> Waschyng the stretys as thei stod a rowe,
> And the goteris in the erthe lowe,
> That in the cite was no filthe sene;
> For the canel [gutter] skoured was so clene,
> And deuoyded in so secre wyse,
> That no man myght espien nor deuyse
> By what engyn the filthes, fer nor ner,
> Wern born a-wey by cours of the ryuer –
> So couertly euery thing was cured [hidden].
> Wher-by the toun was outterly assured
> From engenderyng of al corrupcioun,
> From wikked eyr & from infeccioun,
> That causyn ofte by her violence
> Mortalite and gret pestilence.[51]

[49] Pickett, 'Translation of the "Canutus" Plague Treatise', pp. 271–2, 274. See also C. Bonfield, 'Medical Advice and Public Health: Contextualising the Supply and Regulation of Water in Medieval London and King's Lynn', *Poetica* 72 (2009), pp. 1–20.

[50] The mayor ordered the removal of another latrine 'by reason of the foulness and infectious nature of the odious and horrible atmosphere ... and manifest perils to human life': Riley, *Memorials of London*, pp. 614–16.

[51] John Lydgate, *Lydgate's Troy Book*, ed. H. Bergen, vol. 1, EETS e.s. 97 (London, 1906), p. 166. See also, Strohm, 'Sovereignty and Sewage', pp. 60–1.

However far removed it may have been from the reality of late medieval urban life, Lydgate's vision of a city cleansed of miasmatic waste and stagnant water represented a goal towards which most magistrates aspired. An agreement made during the 1450s between the rulers of Exeter and the residents of a thoroughfare leading from St John's hospital into the city reflects the ubiquity of these concerns. The authorities' readiness to bear the entire cost of a new stone drainage system followed allegations that, because of flooding, 'the head of the lane was sometimes so obstructed by the waters as to form a great marsh and became a receptacle for filth and putrid carcasses, *exposing the inhabitants to the immediate danger of infection*' (my italics). Given the obvious risk of epidemic disease, prompt and effective action was clearly essential.[52]

Being almost certainly familiar with the vernacular (if not the original Latin) text of Bartholomaeus Anglicus' *De proprietatibus rerum*, the most popular reference work of the later Middle Ages, members of the urban elite would also have understood the secondary threat posed by polluted rain:

> Also whanne corrupt wapours beth ydrawe vp out of mareys [marshes] and dichis and carreynes [carrion] and othir corrupt thinges, of her incorporacioun in substaunce of cloudes there cometh of the cloudes ful gret corrumpcioun and pestilence and infeccioun.[53]

In this respect, as in so many others, Bartholomaeus was influenced by Ancient Greek sources and the Muslim physicians who elaborated upon them. While in principle rating rain water (especially when collected in summer) as 'one of the best' for human consumption, certainly in preference to any drawn from wells, cisterns or pipes, Ibn-Sīna recognised that it was 'easily vitiated by impurities from the earth and atmosphere', and thus likely to induce further 'putrefactive changes in the humours'.[54] These beliefs persisted until the development of germ theory in the late nineteenth century. Although he was writing two millennia after the birth of Hippocrates, the Norwich physician Tobias Whitaker began his *Peri ydrospsias: or, a discourse of waters their qualities, and effects diaeleticall, pathologicall, and pharmacaiticall* of 1634 with a fulsome invocation of Classical authorities. Maintaining that death would follow fast upon 'the ill disposition of water and ayre', he warned his readers 'how dangerous it may be to forsake the beaten roade or path, in which the ancient Worthies have safely walked so many ages'.[55] It is thus hardly surprising that the eighteenth-century Norfolk antiquary

---

[52] HMC, *Report on Records of the City of Exeter*, Royal Commission on Historical Manuscripts 73 (London, 1916), pp. 284–5. The health of the residents rather than that of the hospital patients was clearly at issue here, since the former included members of the cathedral chapter.

[53] *OPT*, I.579.

[54] Shah, *Avicenna's Canon of Medicine*, p. 190. For this reason, rain from 'high' clouds, which were less subject to pollution, seemed safer. See, for example, the popular advice manual based upon Aldobrandino of Siena's regimen: Pierpont Morgan Library, New York, MS M.165, fol. 11v.

[55] Tobias Whitaker, *Peri ydroposias: or, a discourse of waters their qualities, and effects diaeteticall, pathologicall, and pharmacaiticall* (London, 1634), introduction, sig. A.

Francis Blomefield should attribute the 'very pestilential fever' which had swept the county in 1382 to *mal aria* caused by 'extraordinary inundations in the fens'. He was, after all, drawing upon the same intellectual tradition as the men and women who had actually lived through the epidemic.[56]

Even if they did not cause wholesale mortality, the noxious vapours arising from garbage-strewn watercourses and blocked drains could still apparently kill vulnerable individuals, as the Exeter Franciscans had explained in their petition of 1285.[57] Not long afterwards, the Carmelites of London likewise claimed that the disgusting stench of the River Fleet, about a hundred yards to the east of their precinct, 'had occasioned the death of many brethren'. Far worse, in their eyes, it both impeded and polluted the celebration of mass, and thus presented a spiritual as well as a physical hazard. Their immediate neighbours, the bishop of Salisbury and the Dominican friars, who lived right next to the Fleet and thus experienced the full force of the problem, supported their petition, which was approved by parliament.[58] York's Franciscan community was even more eloquent in its appeal to the forces of God, medicine and Mammon. Complaining in 1372 about butchers who dumped their waste in the River Ouse, the brethren lamented that:

> ... the air in their church is poisoned by the stench there generated as well around the altars where the Lord's body is daily ministered as in other houses, and flies and other vermin are thereby bred and enter their church and houses, so that as well the lords and noble persons of the county flocking to the city as the good men of the city who used to come to the church to hear mass and to pray are withdrawing themselves because of the stench and the horrible sights, shrinking from them and avoiding to repair thither, and it is feared that sickness and manifold harm will thereby arise to the friars and other of the people unless speedy remedy be applied.[59]

The Use of York provided a special mass, dedicated to St Anthony, that offered protection from corrupt air and similar hazards, but these pungent exhalations had clearly proved resistant to spiritual prophylaxis.[60]

The friars' predicament brings us, secondly, to the assumption that the preservation of the water supply was a *Christian duty* incumbent upon all

---

[56] Blomefield, *Topographical History of the County of Norfolk*, III.111. For continuing concerns about the threat of corrupt air, see Cockayne, *Hubbub*, pp. 141, 147–8, 155–6, 206–16; for their persistence in the face of late nineteenth-century advances in microbiology, see Stevenson, 'Science Down the Drain', pp. 1–26.

[57] See n. 7 above.

[58] *RP*, I.61; M. Honeybourne, 'The Fleet and its Neighbourhood in Early Medieval Times', *London Topographical Record* 19 (1947), pp. 13–87, on pp. 51–2; Sabine, 'City Cleaning in Mediaeval London', pp. 34–6; Montford, *Health, Sickness, Medicine and the Friars*, p. 48.

[59] *CCR, 1369–1374*, p. 438. The prior of Coventry voiced analogous complaints in 1380, against 'certain evildoers living by the river [who] throw the bones, hides and offal of oxen, swine and sheep, and other things into it, corrupting the water running to a mill in the priory and infecting the air': *CPR, 1377–1381*, p. 579.

[60] W. G. Henderson, ed., *Missale ad usum insignis ecclesiae Eboracensis*, vol. 2, Surtees Society 60 (Durham, 1872), pp. 233–4.

God-fearing citizens, for whom cleanliness and virtue marched hand in hand. Rebuilt at a cost of almost £50 in 1534–5, Exeter's Great Conduit not only stood at a crossroads but was surmounted by eight elaborately designed iron crosses, their 'vayns' brightly gilded to catch the sunshine (see plate 14).[61] One of the three pipes leading from Gloucester's Franciscan friary fed a fountain below the High Cross, which also presided symbolically over a crossing of the four main streets in the town centre. Reserved strictly for domestic use, it was out of bounds to butchers and other potential sources of pollution.[62] From the opposite perspective, the equation of sin with the miasmatic contents of drains, pits and sewers gave rise to the type of arresting metaphor beloved of medieval preachers. Bernard of Clairvaux (d. 1153) had, for example, memorably compared the sinner's vain attempts at penance to the futility of arresting 'a flood of filthy water that contaminates an entire house with its intolerable stench'.[63] And centuries later, in his Constitutions of 1409, Archbishop Thomas Arundel abandoned the traditional analogy between heresy and spiritual leprosy in favour of a more compelling – and immediately relevant – reference to the spread of plague.[64] His campaign to purify the 'infected waters' of Oxford from which the lethal miasmas of lollardy arose would certainly have struck a receptive chord among his contemporaries, especially as part of the town was often blighted by floods which Anthony à Wood, for one, believed to be a prime cause of epidemics.[65]

Finally, the conscientious implementation of sanitary measures was widely regarded as a manifestation of good neighbourliness and concern for the wellbeing of the entire urban body. As health manuals like Forestier's warned, city life demanded a particular degree of vigilance and cooperation on the part of those who dwelled in crowded places, especially during epidemics.[66] We can, for example, readily appreciate why complaints about the failure of certain Ipswich householders to cleanse their drains and gutters should reach an unprecedented

[61] When the previous conduit was completed in 1502, the cathedral choir sang over it in blessing: Juddery and Stoyle, 'Aqueducts of Medieval Exeter', p. xix.

[62] Holt, 'Water-Related Technologies', p. 99. For the *cursus aque* that ran from the high cross in the market at Bridgwater, see Dilks, *Bridgwater Borough Archives*, nos 439–40. For a similar arrangement at Wells, see pp. 227–8 below.

[63] Bernard of Clairvaux, *Œuvres complètes*, vol. 21: *La conversion*, ed. J. Leclercq *et al.* (Paris, 2000), p. 344.

[64] R. I. Moore, 'Heresy as a Disease', in W. Lourdaux and V. Verhelst, eds, *The Concept of Heresy in the Middle Ages*, Mediaevalia Louaniensia 1st series 4 (Leuven, 1976), pp. 1–11.

[65] He claimed to be acting 'ne purgato rivulo maneat fons infectus, et aquam ab eo currentem non sinat esse claram': D. Wilkins, ed., *Concilia Magnae Britanniae*, 3 vols (London, 1737), III.318; J. I. Catto, 'Wyclif and Wycliffism at Oxford, 1356–1430', in Catto and Evans, *History of the University of Oxford*, II.244. Anthony à Wood believed that the early sixteenth-century pestilences resulted from 'the stopping of water courses about Oxford, which causing frequent inundations in the meads and low places, would, for want of due conveyance, putrefy and infect the air': *History and Antiquities of the University of Oxford*, II.13–14 (see also I.596).

[66] S. Sheard and H. Power, 'Body and City: Medical and Urban Histories of Public Health', in Sheard and Power, *Body and City*, p. 1.

peak in the years following the 1485 outbreak of sweating sickness. Whereas in 1483–4 the already rising number of presentments on this score stood at forty-nine (in addition to a further forty-six concerning the pollution of watercourses and similar nuisances), by 1486–7 it had more than doubled to 106, and remained just as high in the following year. At this point, between one third and half of *all* presentments (188 out of 470) related directly to the town's gutters, ditches, pits and river.[67] The four leet courts had dealt harshly with the worst offenders since the 1420s, imposing heavy fines of up to 6s. 8d. for non-compliance,[68] but it appears that, as in the case of fly-tipping and vagrant pigs, less serious cases were now attracting attention too. Insistence on collective responsibility was, however, neither new nor invariably dependent upon the onset of pestilence.

Norwich's earliest surviving leet rolls, which date from 1287–8, confirm that local tithings were by then anxious to name, shame and fine individuals whose behaviour threatened to pollute or otherwise endanger the communal water supply. In that year alone at least eight people were accused of obstructing waterways or contaminating them with 'muck', and in the following year eight more came to notice for the illicit dumping of waste.[69] Nuisances of this kind were, of course, profoundly antisocial, and likely to cause offence whatever the circumstances. As we have seen, they also cast 'manifest shame and reproach' upon an entire community, and, if left unchecked, might well invite royal intervention.[70] Since a significant proportion of the urban housing stock was built of timber, lath and daub, rather than brick and stone, even a modest amount of flood-water could cause extensive damage, which further explains why neighbours reacted with such intemperate language to dripping eaves and defective or broken guttering.[71] At least a fifth, and probably far more, of the complaints investigated by the London assize of nuisance between 1301 and 1407 concerned this type of problem, which proved a constant bone of contention between neighbours.[72] It is also apparent that some plaintiffs were at pains to emphasise the health hazards to which they had been exposed. Not all referred to 'the great corruption of the air' and other such dangers likely to arise from the pools of stagnant water that collected on their property or seeped into wells and cisterns, but some were remarkably specific.

In one of several late fourteenth-century cases of trespass to hinge upon the endangerment of water supplies, Katherine Bishop of Norwich sued her neighbour,

---

[67] SROI, C/2/8/1/19, 21, 22. Although it was less dramatic, an increase in the number of presentments relating to water pollution occurred in Yarmouth at this time: Rawcliffe, 'Health and Safety at Work', p. 152.

[68] See, for example, SROI, C/2/8/1/5 (1421), 8 (1434).

[69] Hudson, *Leet Jurisdiction*, pp. 3, 6–9, 11–2, 23–4, 26–7, 29.

[70] *CCR, 1296–1302*, p. 218. See section 1.4 above.

[71] Schofield, *Medieval London Houses*, p. 118; *LAN*, p. xxii.

[72] *LAN*, pp. xxiii–xxiv and *passim*. Of 659 cases (several of which do not specify the alleged nuisance), a bare minimum of twenty related to gutters at ground level, and 115 to those running along the tops of walls or below eaves. For a discussion of urban housing types, see Biddle, *Winchester in the Early Middle Ages*, pp. 345–8. In Exeter, too, 'an old and an auncient custome' made householders personally liable for any nuisance caused by flooding: DRO, ECA, Book 51, fol. 300r.

Richard Crete, in the court of common pleas. She accused him of 'maliciously' damaging trenches on her land:

> by which the water from a spring of hers, wherein the same Katherine used to prepare her food, was so polluted by the stench and rottenness of the dung [*per fetorem et corruptionem fumorum*] flowing into the spring ... that the same Katherine contracted a grave and virtually incurable sickness so that her life was despaired of, and her men and servants likewise suffered a grave illness from tasting the water [*per gustum aque illius*].[73]

By the date of this lawsuit (1374) widespread awareness that contaminated water, or food prepared in it, might cause illness or even death once it entered the digestive tract, and would at the very least increase an individual's susceptibility to plague, prompted understandable concerns about the *purity*, as well as the *odour*, of the domestic supply. Although most late medieval householders used water primarily for cooking, brewing and washing, rather than immediate consumption, Holt's belief that the English actively avoided drinking it whenever possible requires qualification.[74] The poor had little choice, while the more affluent may have heeded medical advice, which accorded water the two vital functions of facilitating the flow of nourishment around the body and, when necessary, combating the effects of excessive heat.[75] For this reason, authorities such as John of Burgundy maintained that during epidemics 'the best drynke were calde water mengede [mixed] with vynagre or tysayn [barley water]' because of its cooling effect.[76] Even so, popular *regimina* such as the pseudo-Aristotelian *Secreta secretorum* warned against the practice of drinking water either immediately before or after a heavy meal, since it 'coldith thi stomak and quenchith the hete of thi digestioun, and confoundith and grevith the body'. On balance, even if one were very thirsty, it seemed advisable to 'take it attemperatly, and not ouirmoche attones [at once]', in order to avoid destabilising the complex physiological processes whereby food was converted into humoral matter.[77]

Conversely, though, a glass of pure warm water, drunk every morning on rising, promised 'to make a man hoole' and was enthusiastically recommended, along with a moderate daily intake of warm water in winter and cold in summer.[78] Some versions of the *Secreta* even urged the reader to 'drynk no wine but watir be ther among', while others provided a short guide, derived from the Hippocratic

---

[73] M. S. Arnold, ed., *Select Cases of Trespass from the King's Courts, 1307–1399*, vol. 2, Selden Society 103 (London, 1987), pp. 350–1.

[74] See section 4.1 above.

[75] Pierpont Morgan Library, New York, MS M.165, fols 11r–12r, 65v.

[76] Ogden, *Liber de diversis medicinis*, p. 51.

[77] Steele, *Three Prose Versions of the 'Secreta Secretorum'*, p. 25. The humoral balance of the individual was also crucial, in so far that those of a choleric or sanguine temperament appeared less likely to suffer harm from drinking too much water than a person who was phlegmatic or melancholic.

[78] Steele, *Three Prose Versions of the 'Secreta Secretorum'*, p. 32; BL, MS Harley 3, fol. 290r.

corpus, explaining precisely what was safe to ingest.[79] Fresh, running streams near cities, notable for their 'lightnes, clernes, good colour and good sauour', were, predictably, deemed the best, and generally provided the piped water for urban conduits, such as those of London, Exeter and Southampton. By the same token, salty, bitter, cloudy or stagnant water appeared 'euyl' because of its propensity to dry and corrupt the stomach. But whatever its initial source, water that had stood too long in the sun posed the greatest danger, since it threatened to 'engendre the blake colere [burnt yellow bile]', thereby harming the spleen and lungs.[80] Despite these caveats, many well-informed individuals elected to drink water in preference to anything else. In his best-selling version of the *regimen*, which appeared in 1534 as *The Castel of Helthe*, Sir Thomas Elyot attributed the intellectual prowess and longevity of Pythagoras and his followers to the fact that they 'dranke onely water', observing that he himself had 'sene men and women of great age, and stronge of body, wyche neuer, or very seldome, dranke other drynke'.[81]

Such abstemious folk almost certainly enjoyed the benefit of private springs, wells or pipes, since public supplies, especially in large towns, were subject to constant contamination. As in other areas of urban life, ordinary householders were not usually the worst offenders. Or, to be more specific, it was in their occupational capacity as tanners, butchers, dyers, fishmongers and the practitioners of other insalubrious trades that they were likely to inflict the greatest damage. Given the limited technological resources at their disposal, magistrates were unable to eliminate many of the nuisances arising from the commercial and industrial activities upon which they and the rest of the community depended for survival. It might, indeed, be argued that the similarity of complaints voiced so loudly in towns and cities across England, as well as the escalating scale of penalties imposed on offenders, reflects general desperation in the face of an intractable problem. Some lesser fines may even have constituted a form of licensing whereby the authorities, reconciled to the inevitability of low-level pollution, determined at least to derive a modest profit from those responsible. In Coventry from 1421, for instance, dyers and other craftsmen who wished to divert river water by means of a 'waturlade', or wooden channel, could do so in return for 'yeldyng a certen [sum] vnto the chambur'. Although such arrangements might be regarded as an admission of failure, they at least had the merit of obliging workers to operate under strict rules in order to avoid both 'perell of ffloodes' and water shortages.[82] Nonetheless, there

[79] Lydgate, *Secrees of Old Philisoffres*, p. 51. BL, MS Egerton 1995, fol. 72v, recommends that wine should be mixed with 'clene welle water'.

[80] See, for example, 'The Knowynge of Waters', in Steele, *Three Prose Versions of the 'Secreta Secretorum'*, p. 79; M.-T. Lorcin, 'Humeurs, bains et tisanes: l'eau dans la médecine médiévale', in *L'Eau au moyen âge*, Senefiance 15 (Aix-en-Provence, 1985), pp. 259–73. Some versions of the *tacuinum sanitatis*, which presented information about food and drink in a more accessible, often illustrated, format, contained a section on different types of water. Most notable among them is the profusely illustrated New York Public Library, MS Spencer 65, fols 95r–102r.

[81] Sir Thomas Elyot, *The Castel of Helthe* (London, 1539), fol. 33r. Sir Thomas More was reputedly one such: Sir Thomas Elyot, *The Boke Named the Gouernour*, ed. H. H. S. Croft, 2 vols (New York, 1967), II.343–4.

[82] *Coventry Leet Book*, I.31–2.

appears to have been a broad consensus regarding unacceptable practices that demonstrably undermined communal health. And in those cases the response was far less accommodating.

4.3 Trade and industry

Men such as the Norwich barber-surgeon who, in 1390–1, committed the 'abominable offence' of depositing putrid blood into the public gutter could expect little sympathy.[83] The enthusiasm for phlebotomy as a means of removing potentially dangerous matter from the body led to the imposition of stringent penalties upon any practitioner who failed to dispose of surplus blood in a discreet, prompt and hygienic manner.[84] During the reign of Edward I London barbers were ordered to abandon the 'bold and daring' practice of leaving containers of blood on open display in their shops, and henceforward to convey them 'privily' to the Thames, so that their contents could be carried away on the tide.[85] These particular ordinances have been cited in support of the contention that medieval streets must have been flooded with 'sticky and malodorous muck'.[86] Yet anxieties on this score were so great that many magistrates enacted specific measures against the pollution of open drains, thoroughfares and streams with *any* type of liquid waste, whether human, animal or vegetable. Residents of Lyme were reminded in 1501 that all water issuing from their homes should be 'good and pure', lest it contaminate the common supply.[87] Mindful of the risks encountered by innocent pedestrians, the rulers of fourteenth- and fifteenth-century Bristol decreed that 'no manner man caste no vryne ne stynkyng water ne noon other felthe oute at ther wyndowes or dores in the stretes'. Anyone who did so faced a penalty of 40*d.*, while similar fines were imposed in Coventry upon miscreants who 'cast pysse in-to the highway' from the town gaol.[88]

Food markets were especially prone to problems of this kind.[89] Whereas ordinary Londoners were permitted to empty slops into the public gutters, fishmongers had to take all their dirty water directly to the Thames.[90] Notable

[handwritten margin note: fears of contaminating common supply]

---

[83] Hudson, *Leet Jursidiction*, p. 70. Phlebotomy was not only deemed beneficial for humans; in 1424, an Ipswich farrier was fined 4*d.* for letting blood from horses in a public thoroughfare: SROI, C/2/8/1/7.

[84] Pouchelle, *Body and Surgery*, p. 74; P. Gil-Sotres, 'Derivation and Revulsion: The Theory and Practice of Medieval Phlebotomy', in Arrizabalaga *et al.*, *Practical Medicine*, p. 120.

[85] Riley, *Liber albus*, p. 236.

[86] Classen, Howes and Synnott, *Aroma*, p. 57.

[87] Dorset Record Office, DC/LR B1/2 no. 13. Throwing dirty water into London streets had by then been forbidden for almost a century: *CLB*, I, p. 131.

[88] Veale, *Great Red Book of Bristol*, I.142; *LRBB*, II.228; *Coventry Leet Book*, I.254.

[89] See section 5.7 below. Having arranged for the fountain in the marketplace to be 'cleansed of dirt' in 1429, the rulers of Cambridge imposed a fine of 6*s.* 8*d.* on anyone who contaminated it in future: Cooper, *Annals of Cambridge*, p. 180.

[90] Martin, 'Transport for London', p. 184.

among the fines levied in Ipswich upon those charged with the upkeep of common utilities was one of 40*d.* imposed in 1416 on the prior of St Peter's for neglecting to scour the drains which carried noisome waste from the fish market into the Orwell and thence out to sea.[91] Perhaps because of its sizeable Dutch community, the port had by then developed a precocious taste for beer, which was still in many quarters deemed 'unholsom for mannes body'.[92] The malodorous lees left over from the brewing process were certainly regarded as a major hazard when tipped into gutters and other public places. In 1421, for instance, Geoffrey Page incurred an exemplary fine for flooding the area around the water gates with 'the filth, excrement and malt dregs of beer, from whence a very bad smell arose to the nuisance of the people'.[93] The residents of Lynn likewise took exception to the washing of brewers' vats and 'ffoule soys' in streets that were all too often already running with the filthy slops discarded by careless fish-sellers.[94]

Equally unwelcome at the conduit houses and common wells of medieval towns were laundresses, whose presence often seemed disruptive and morally questionable, as well as constituting a source of congestion, spillages and dirt.[95] In Coventry they were forbidden from using any of the public facilities in the town centre in 1461, which effectively confined them to a designated washing place outside the walls that was littered with refuse and garden waste.[96] At about the same time, the rulers of Leicester decreed 'that no woman vse to wasshe no clothes ne none other corripcion at common wellys ... ne in the hye strete in payne of imprisonment', while the laundresses of Sandwich stood to forfeit whatever they were washing, along with any tubs or vessels, should they venture near 'the common stream called le Waterdelf'.[97] Having spent almost £30 in 1491–2 on 'the houndewell, the new well, the watering place for hors and the washing place for woman', the rulers of Southampton imposed heavy fines on those who continued to launder their 'clowtes' anywhere near a common conduit.[98] But not all boroughs recognised the need to provide designated facilities. Among the various measures

---

[91] SROI, C/2/8/1/3.

[92] Amor, 'Trade and Industry of Late Medieval Ipswich', pp. 123–6, 265–8, 350–2. For the perceived hazards of drinking beer, see section 5.5 below.

[93] SROI, C/2/8/1/5. For the analogous case of Simon Bierbrewer, see SROI C/2/8/1/3.

[94] KLBA, KL/C7/5, Hall Book, 1497–1544, fol. 180r (1517). Similar complaints were voiced in London: Riley, *Liber albus*, p. 238.

[95] For attitudes to this generally neglected component of the female labour force, see Rawcliffe, 'A Marginal Occupation? The Medieval Laundress', pp. 147–69.

[96] *Coventry Leet Book*, II.312, 338.

[97] *RBL*, II.291; Boys, *History of Sandwich*, II.503–4; BL, MS Cotton Julius B IV, fol. 77r. The 'Waterdelf' was a canal built and maintained at communal expense for the supply of fresh water to the town: Boys, *History of Sandwich*, II.538; E. Hastead, *The History and Topographical Survey of the County of Kent*, 12 vols (Canterbury, 1797–1801), X.167. See also p. 22 above.

[98] Butler, *Book of Fines*, pp. 22, 29. A prohibition on the cleansing of wool and linen in specific watercourses, imposed in Lyme one year later, may well have been aimed as much at fullers as laundresses. This would explain why fines had risen tenfold from 12*d.* to 10*s.* by 1508: Dorset Record Office, DC/LR B1/2, nos 9, 19.

adopted in early sixteenth-century Durham for cleansing the Milneburn, the removal of 'le wesshyngstonez' seemed as desirable as the destruction of privies and other potential hazards.[99]

Laundresses, whose gender and   low economic status made them an easy target, were by no means the worst culprits, being themselves frequently obliged to contend with sources of pollution that rendered their back-breaking work even more distasteful. The washerwomen of Gloucester must have been heartened by a civic ruling at the turn of the fifteenth century which decreed that 'non person or persons wasshe non podynge, guttes, nor innewardes of bestes att the wesshynge place without the inner norgate [north gate]'.[100] We have already examined the attempts by urban magistrates to regulate the more noisome activities of butchers, but the miasmatic air generated by their unsavoury trade was just one of the environmental hazards that they presented.[101] If the disposal of comparatively modest quantities of phlebotomised human blood exercised the authorities, concern about the impact of shambles, butchers' stalls and piles of stinking offal upon the urban water supply was proportionally greater, especially after the Black Death. The condition of slaughterhouses, which needed a regular supply of water for scalding the hair from carcasses and flushing away waste, thus became a matter of serious concern, since it was essential both to prevent the accumulation of stagnant waste and to avoid the contamination of public watercourses.

As E. L. Sabine has demonstrated, the levels of hygiene in such places varied considerably, depending in part upon the extent of official supervision, but more often upon location. Those at the Stocks Market in London were well drained by water from the Walbrook and regularly cleansed, especially after 1400, when they fell under the aegis of the Bridge Wardens.[102] Standards were far laxer on the eastern margins of the City at St Nicholas Shambles, near Newgate, although the presence of some influential neighbours meant that offensive practices would eventually be brought to book (map 2). Indeed, it was because of vigorous protests by members of the Franciscan community and other persons of note that, in the two plague years of 1361 and 1369, Edward III prohibited the slaughtering of animals anywhere in the City, along with the removal of carcasses through public thoroughfares for disposal in the Thames. Significantly, his directives drew particular attention to the fact that, 'by the shedding of ... blood which runs down from the said shambles to the river through the midst of the said streets and lanes, grievous corruption and foulness is gendered as well in the river as in the said streets'.[103] Judging from a case heard by the assize of nuisance in the following year, the friars had ample cause for grievance. In it, they presented the owners of a 'skaldynghous', whence 'the water mixed with the blood and hair of the slaughtered animals, and with other filth from the washing of the carcasses, flows into the

---

[99] Bonney, *Lordship and the Urban Community*, pp. 51, 222.

[100] HMC, *Twelfth Report*, appendix 9, p. 434. Each offence incurred a penalty of 40*d*.

[101] See section 3.5 above.

[102] Sabine, 'Butchering in Mediaeval London', pp. 341–2.

[103] *CCR, 1360–1364*, p. 248; *CCR, 1369–1374*, pp. 31–2.

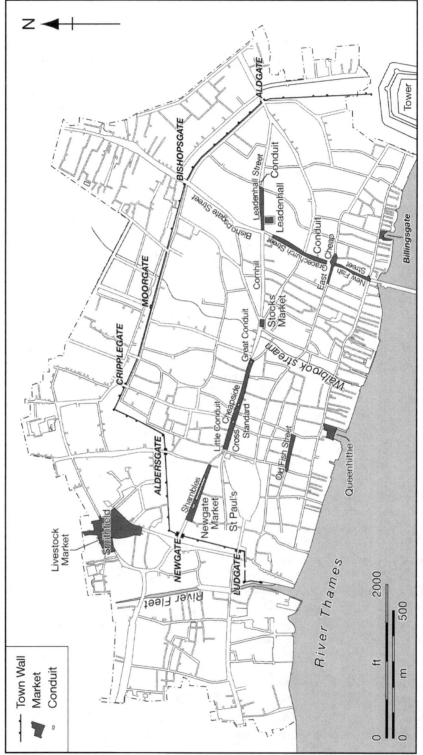

Map 2 The principal markets and conduits of late medieval London

ditch or kennel in the street, through which it is carried into the [precinct] garden, causing a stench in many places there.'[104]

Whereas, with adequate drainage, blood could be flushed away relatively quickly and easily, the water-borne disposal of carcasses, intestines and other solid waste required far more specific and draconian regulation. Here the butchers of St Nicholas's incurred a further battery of complaints, in part because the places initially assigned to them in the 1340s and 1350s 'for the decency and cleanliness of the City' were clearly unsuitable, at least at a time of heightened sensitivity to such matters. Although 'Bochersbrigge' at Blackfriars was supposed to give direct access to the tidal flow of the Thames, those who lived nearby maintained that the water remained clogged with entrails, which, in turn, poisoned both the river and the air, 'making a foul corruption and abominable sight and nuisance to all dwelling near'.[105] The impracticality and unpopularity of subsequent attempts to remove the slaughterhouses of St Nicholas's to the genteel suburb of Holborn led the civic authorities to request parliamentary approval in 1393 for a more viable and hygienic alternative, involving a 'place or pier' at Queenhithe, where butchers' waste could be stored and processed, ready for disposal well away from the shoreline by boat at ebb tide.[106] Clearly successful, the experiment prompted the erection of a second pier, in 1402, for use by the butchers of East Cheap. Stringent penalties (of as much as £40) for the dumping of offal at any other spot apparently served to keep the butchers in check and their neighbours relatively happy for several decades.[107]

By the 1480s, however, a mounting chorus of indignation about the 'unclene and putrified waters' polluted 'by occasion of blod and other fouler thynges' issuing from St Nicholas's culminated in a petition to parliament by the residents of two riverside parishes. Shrewdly voicing particular concern about the health threat posed to royal and aristocratic worshippers attending St Paul's cathedral, they demanded that the fourteenth-century ban upon slaughtering within the walls should be revived.[108] This time, the butchers opted for a more radical solution by investing 'at theyr great and ymportunate costes and charges' in the construction of stone-lined subterranean vaults for the safe removal of 'corrupte waters' and other noxious matter from the shambles directly into the Thames. At last, after a long struggle, the problem of miasmatic air and contaminated water seemed to have been effectively eliminated, and in 1532 the restrictions on civic butchering, which had long since lapsed, were formally repealed.[109]

Since, in principle, fast-flowing streams and rivers presented the most effective means of disposal, most English towns and cities sought to control exactly when,

---

[104] *LAN*, no. 569.

[105] *CPMRL, 1364–1381*, pp. 93, 94. Significantly, these complaints were voiced in midsummer when the 1368 pestilence was at its height.

[106] *RP*, III.306; *CCR, 1392–1396*, p. 133.

[107] Sabine, 'Butchering in Mediaeval London', pp. 346–50.

[108] Jones, *Butchers of London*, p. 81; *CLB*, L, pp. 180, 260; *SR*, vol. 2, 4 Henry VII, cap.3, pp. 527–8.

[109] *SR*, vol. 3, 24 Henry VIII, cap.16, p. 435. The butchers undertook to maintain and clean these vaults at regular intervals under the direction of the mayor.

how and where butchers could jettison their waste, in order to ensure the least possible aggravation to others. We have already seen how measures such as removal by night and the use of covered wagons could protect the atmosphere from noxious exhalations. In order to safeguard water supplies, it became customary to insist that butchers should confine themselves to approved sites, which usually lay down-stream of major residential areas, or at least on opposite banks. Precept did not, however, always translate smoothly into practice. In 1371, evidently in response to an opening salvo from the Franciscan community, the rulers of York set aside a staithe on the River Ouse well below the friary for the construction of a pier, like that subsequently built at Queenhithe by London's butchers. A blanket ban was also imposed on the dumping of 'refuse of pigs or offal or any other noisome stuff' in parts of the river where water might be drawn by brewers or bakers, while leather-workers were specifically forbidden to wash their hides anywhere near the Greyfriars.[110] Demonstrating the intransigence characteristic of their craft, York's butchers proved resistant to change, and, as we have seen, were still causing a major nuisance in the following year. It was then that the crown stepped in, threatening recidivists with a draconian fine of 100s. for each offence.[111] Although some offenders remained obdurate, the mayor's decision to reduce this exemplary sum in line with civic custom clearly exasperated the mendicants, who sought royal assistance for a second time 1380 and once again in 1428, having perhaps found members of the ruling elite more concerned to protect the environment of their inner-city residences than they were to deal with problems on the urban periphery. Plans to make this malodorous waste available to local farmers for use on their land do, however, appear to have proved more successful.[112]

The proliferation of similar ordinances throughout fourteenth- and fifteenth-century England reflects both the extent of the problem caused by the growing demand for meat and hides, and a keen awareness of the need for regulation. Worcester's butchers and leather-workers were warned in 1467 to 'caste non intrelle [entrails] ne fylth of bestes donge ne doust over Severne brygge, ne beyond the seid brugge in the streme', and to 'wasshe none heare [hair] but benethe the brugge, and that on the ferther syde of Severne'.[113] At Lynn, which benefited from the strong tidal flow of the Great Ouse, offal had to be transported under cover to either 'le Balle' on the south-western outskirts of town or 'Doucehill' to the north, ready for disposal at 'half ebbe and half floode' tide.[114] Comparable measures had

---

[110] *YMB*, I.lxvii, 15. A fine of 6s. 8d. was then imposed upon all offenders. Measures were also introduced on behalf of the makers of sausages and blood puddings, who washed entrails nearby: see section 5.2 below.

[111] *CCR, 1369–1374*, p. 438; see section 3.5 above.

[112] *YMB*, I.17–18 (the fine was cut to a mere 6d.); *CPR, 1377–1381*, p. 524; *YMB*, II.70. For York's somewhat fraught dealings with its butchers, see H. Swanson, *Medieval Artisans: An Urban Class in Late Medieval England* (Oxford, 1989), pp. 14–17; and section 5.8 below.

[113] Smith, Smith and Brentano, *English Gilds*, p. 396. See also *RBN*, I.336, for similar regulations against the contamination of rivers.

[114] KLBA, KL/C7/3, Hall Book, 1431–1450, fols 103r, 271v; C7/4, Hall Book, 1453–1497, pp. 362, 530; Owen, *Making of King's Lynn*, pp. 217–19. In 1500 a labourer was

been in place in Winchester since at least the 1370s, although (as in York) the butchers were inclined to save their legs by taking a short cut to the river through the cathedral cemetery, leaving a pungent trail of ordure in their wake, or simply to offload their waste into the city's many brooks and streams. One notorious offender was found not only to have deposited pools of blood in the High Street, but even to have washed his tubs and bowls at a common well![115] Measures of 1409 appear to have curbed the worst abuses, by insisting that all carcasses should be chopped into small pieces before disposal (following the practice in London), while making the wardens of the butchers' guild personally liable to the tune of 3*s*. 4*d*. for each dereliction.[116] As was generally the case in matters of public health and safety, the watchful eyes and twitching noses of neighbours served to police the more heinous breaches of these sanitary regulations.

The noxious detritus abandoned by fullers and dyers was another source of irritation, not least because it had such an obvious impact upon the urban environment. Andrée Guillerme has calculated that it took approximately 2 cubic metres of water to produce a standard measure of coloured cloth in thirteenth-century France. In England, too, the complex processes of fulling and dyeing required a prolific supply. Having been soaked in muddy pits of fuller's earth mixed with water to give it body and texture, the carefully rinsed cloth was 'mordanted' in vats of boiling water containing a fixative, such as alum (plate 17). It was then ready for immersion in a bath of the appropriate dye, and, after a second wash in clean running water, would be stretched on river-side frames known as tenters (which were themselves often regarded as a serious nuisance).[117] The excavation of a late medieval dyer's workshop in north-western Norwich has revealed an industrial complex of four groups of brick-lined furnaces for heating vats, two wells, and a substantial drain for discharging effluent straight into the Wensum, which then meandered slowly eastwards through the city.[118] Guillerme's contention that none of these procedures would have caused significant pollution may have held true for suburban developments with access to fast-flowing streams and rivers, but is less

retained at the butchers' expense to remove 'theyr bones, blode, intrayles & other offall' to the haven 'soo that it anoyeth no man': C7/5, Hall Book, 1497–1544, fol. 35v. At Sandwich butchers' waste had to be deposited in the haven at low water by night, 'in such a cautious manner as may give no public offence': Boys, *History of Sandwich*, II.499, 501.

[115] Keene, *Survey of Medieval Winchester*, I.64, 258. An attempt to safeguard the common water supply in 1299 forbade its use for flushing away dyestuffs, carcasses and dung, as well as for washing tanned hides and infants' soiled clothes: Furley, *Town Life*, pp. 134–5.

[116] Bird, *Black Book of Winchester*, p. 18. However, it was necessary to renew the ordinance in 1513 (p. 124). The butchers of Beverley had been prohibited from depositing 'offal, blood or any tainted thing' in the waterway known as the Welbeck since 1365, but in 1510 regulations allowed them to dispose of waste that had been suitably processed: *BTD*, pp. 29, 129.

[117] Guillerme, *Age of Water*, pp. 96–8. See also, P. Walton, 'Textiles', in J. Blair and N. Ramsay, eds, *English Medieval Industries* (London, 1991), pp. 319–54.

[118] A. Carter and J. P. Roberts, 'Excavations in Norwich, 1972', *NA* 35 (1970–2), pp. 443–68, on pp. 461–2.

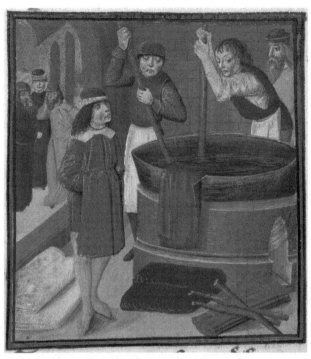

17 The dyeing of cloth in a heated vat illustrates the section on 'colour' in a French translation of Barthomolaeus Anglicus, *Liber de proprietatibus rerum*, produced in Bruges in 1482, possibly for Edward IV.

convincing in the context of many late medieval English towns and the particular sensibilities of their residents. Indeed, notwithstanding the 'extreme cleanliness' of these particular premises, which were neatly tiled and kept free of rubbish, it is clear that operations on this scale frequently caused friction.

In 1390–1, for example, three Norwich dyers were fined for dumping cinders, paste and other filth in the river and streets, while at about the same time residents of Nottingham protested about dyers whose attempts to flush away 'the waters of their art' generated unacceptable levels of airborne corruption likely to infect the public.[119] In order to keep one of the city's main watercourses clean during the day, the rulers of Winchester decreed in 1370 that dyers might only dispose of 'wodgor' (woad-based waste, which would have been dark blue) and similar material at night.[120] Offenders who persisted in emptying tubs of madder and woad into the River Orwell at Ipswich incurred a particularly heavy penalty of 6s. 8d. because of the threat to the town's fish supply. Local juries were also moved to complain intermittently about the diversion of common streams, pollution of wells and creation of 'perilous pits' by dyers, as well as their overflowing, noxious drains which flooded the streets with dyestuffs.[121] Such practices strained neighbourly relations to the limit, as one exasperated Londoner revealed in 1417,

[119] Stevenson, *Records of the Borough of Nottingham*, I.272–3; Hudson, *Leet Jurisdiction*, pp. 70, 73, 75. Not all dyers were irresponsible, though. In 1276, a London 'teynturer' died when attempting to flush out his drains with scalding water: *CLB*, B, pp. 268–9.

[120] Keene, *Survey of Medieval Winchester*, I.64. The ruling was repeated in 1416–17: Bird, *Black Book of Winchester*, p. 8. Basingstoke courts followed suit, imposing a 40d. fine upon any dyer who emptied his 'woad vat' between 3 a.m. and 9 p.m.: Baigent and Millard, *History of the Town and Manor of Basingstoke*, p. 310.

[121] See, for instance, SROI, C/2/8/1/3 (flooding the highway), C/2/8/1/6 (diverting the water supply, polluting wells and dangerous pits), C/2/8/1/7 (flooding the streets and polluting common wells), C/2/8/1/8 (endangering the fish supply); C/2/10/1/7 (noxious drains and woad waste).

when petitioning the mayor about the noisome pit outside his front door in which hot cloths were routinely left to soak.[122] Four years later, the residents of Dowgate ward claimed that the dyers who congregated nearby were throwing bark into the Thames 'to the destruction of the stream and the nuisance of the community'. Moreover, it was often impossible for ordinary people to draw water or even exercise their rights of access because of the congestion caused when fullers came to wash their cloth.[123] Such evidence lends verisimilitude to one of John Bromyard's famous *exempla*, in which he contrasted thirsty pilgrims refreshed by the pure wellspring of divine wisdom with heedless travellers who risked sickness or even death by making do with feculent, polluted river water.[124]

It is sobering to reflect that many of London's water-carriers drew their supplies from this very stretch of river, where the Walbrook debouched into the Thames, and where levels of human, animal and industrial waste must often have been dangerously high.[125] Previously, in 1345, when the filth in Dowgate dock reached such an unacceptable level that the carriers were unable to ply their trade, the rulers of London had imposed a tax on the carts that transported goods to and from ships in order to finance a cleansing operation. Being held partly responsible for causing so much mess, the carters were themselves ordered to effect the necessary improvements, under pain of imprisonment.[126] Just as serious was the constant contamination of the Walbrook itself with 'dung, rotten matter and other wastes and nuisances', which the City's magistrates had sought to prevent from at least the late thirteenth century (when records begin) and probably far earlier. One pragmatic solution, adopted in 1288, involved the compulsory insertion of gratings (*rastalli*) by all residents whose houses and workshops abutted the stream, although this did little to solve the long-term problem posed by irresponsible disposal of rubbish.[127] The appointment of a keeper, in

---

[122] *CPMRL, 1413–1437*, p. 62; Barron, *London in the Later Middle Ages*, p. 265. Evidently reluctant to curb production altogether, the mayor ruled that cloth might be soaked there after it had cooled. See also *LAN*, no. 488.

[123] *CPMRL, 1413–1437*, pp. 134, 156.

[124] John Bromyard, *Summa praedicantium*, 2 vols (Venice, 1586), I.184 (*Delectationum*, cap. v. 2). Significantly, the rulers of Bristol insisted that 'waterleders' should draw only 'pure and clear' water from the Rivers Frome and Avon: *LRBB*, II.230.

[125] Riley, *Memorials of London*, p. 254; *CLB*, G, p. 206; Drummond-Murray and Liddle, 'Medieval Industry', pp. 87–94. That the rights to dispose of dung (for removal by boat) and to draw water often went together is reflected in complaints made in 1356 about obstructed access to a wharf on the Thames at Baynard's Castle: *LAN*, no. 459.

[126] Riley, *Memorials of London*, p. 223. Sabine describes subsequent attempts to cleanse the dock: 'City Cleaning in Mediaeval London', p. 38. Carts posed a particular problem on the approaches to quays and landing stages. Because of the mud and filth they generated, in 1456–7 the Norwich assembly closed a lane leading to the staithe on the River Wensum that served as a designated 'washyng place': Kirkpatrick, *Streets and Lanes*, p. 8.

[127] *CLB*, A, pp. 212–13; Riley, *Liber albus*, p. 237; Sabine, 'City Cleaning in Mediaeval London', pp. 33–4. Failure to comply with this ruling incurred a steep fine of 40s. Nevertheless, during the fourteenth century residents still protested regularly about blockages to the Walbrook: *LAN*, nos 15–16, 109, 188, 198–200, 382–3.

1374, charged with removing blockages and levying an annual rate of 12*d*. on anyone who wished to site a private latrine over the water, enjoyed only limited success.[128] By 1415 the authorities began walling the banks in the more crowded residential areas near the Thames, thereby setting in train a building programme that led to the vaulting-over of almost the entire stretch of the Walbrook by the late sixteenth century.[129] In 1478, following repeated complaints about the quantities of 'dung, rubbish and filth' being deposited in the water by local tawyers, the civic authorities ordered their removal to Bermondsey or Southwark, in yet another eloquent demonstration of what Caroline Barron describes as 'the cavalier attitude that the city adopted to its outlying neighbours'.[130]

Tawyers, who processed the skins of smaller animals such as calves and lambs with alum or oil, and thus operated at the 'lighter' end of the leather trade, often worked in partnership with furriers and skinners.[131] Like butchers, skinners could be remarkably casual when disposing of the remains of slaughtered animals, as we can see from the case of William le Skinnere of Norwich, who in 1288 incurred public opprobrium for throwing dead cats into the pool which fed one of the city's major watercourses, 'ita quod aer corrumpitur' (whereby the air is contaminated).[132] About a third of the seventy-nine feline skeletons discovered in one of Cambridge's medieval wells show signs of skinning; and although the well in question may already have been abandoned and used for dumping refuse, the attendant stench must still have been a serious nuisance.[133] The 'drenchyngfats' in which skins were soaked in a solution of water and lime proved equally uncongenial to neighbours, again because of the smell and risks of water-borne

---

[128] *CLB*, G, p. 324; Riley, *Memorials of London*, pp. 379–80; Barron, *London in the Later Middle Ages*, p. 260. For the growing opposition to riparian privies, see section 3.4 above.

[129] *CLB*, I, pp. 137–8; Stow, *Survey of London*, I.27. In addition to a legacy of £26 13*s*. 4*d*. for improvements to the City's water supply, the former mayor, Robert Large (d. 1441), bequeathed £133 6*s*. 8*d*. for repairs to the Walbrook: TNA, PROB 11/1, fols 121v–122v. Private latrines over the river were finally banned altogether in 1463, when householders were ordered by the mayor to cleanse their part of the stream and vault it: *CLB*, L, pp. 21–2; Sabine, 'Latrines and Cesspits of Mediaeval London', pp. 309–10.

[130] *CLB*, L, pp. 149, 155; Barron, *London in the Later Middle Ages*, p. 264.

[131] J. Cherry, 'Leather', in Blair and Ramsay, *English Medieval Industries*, p. 299.

[132] Hudson, *Leet Jurisdiction*, p. 29. Nor was he the first to offend in this way. Recent excavations in the city have unearthed the remains of twelfth-century felines in a well shaft in the parish of St Stephen, where leather-workers are known to have congregated. I am grateful to Giles Emery of the Norfolk Archaeology Unit for providing me with this information.

[133] R. M. Luff and M. Garcia, 'Killing Cats in the Medieval Period: An Unusual Episode in the History of Cambridge', *Archaeofauna* 4 (1995), pp. 93–114. Feline remains have also been unearthed in significant quantities in Exeter, Lynn and the Walbrook valley, confirming the validity of complaints about pollution: Drummond-Murray and Liddle, 'Medieval Industry', p. 92. In 1304, the skinning of animals and burial of carcasses within the walls of London were forbidden, along with the disposal of remains in ditches 'either within or outside the City': *CEMCRL*, pp. 162–3.

pollution. Indeed, in Winchester these large vessels were banned altogether from the commercial and residential areas around the High Street. Although skinners only needed ready access to water in the early stages of production, their close association with parchment-makers, who were more demanding, meant that they tended to congregate together on the banks of urban watercourses; if anything, Winchester jurors were even more indignant about the washing of 'foul sheep skins and calf skins' in the city's many open streams.[134] An unsuccessful attempt by the University of Oxford (which must, ironically, have consumed enormous quantities of parchment) to remove all such activities outside the walls 'propter corruptionem' (because of pollution) in 1305 underscores both the disagreeable nature of much medieval industry and the level of anxiety that it caused.[135]

Because they deployed a malodorous combination of oak bark, alum, ashes, lime, saltpetre, faeces and urine to treat the hides of cattle and pigs, tanners ranked among the worst culprits in this respect.[136] The tanning process required the immersion of hides for long periods in timber-lined pits of increasingly noisome liquids, which could easily seep into neighbouring wells and streams.[137] Moreover, since the hides had to be washed clean at each stage of the procedure, a regular supply of fresh running water was essential, if not always legally available. In Ipswich – where from at least 1466 pits for industrial use were licensed and inspected by the authorities – tanners were frequently in trouble for defying a prohibition against the pollution of the town ditch and other waterways, and for siting their operations too close to them.[138] In 1471 alone five leather-workers were fined for soaking hides in a common well, while another two stood accused of keeping noxious *barkepits* and mixing 'filth called barkerstan' in a public watercourse.[139] Some Norwich tanners were equally flagrant offenders, not only immersing their hides in the River Wensum, but even diverting it into trenches and blocking it with stakes.[140]

The irritation caused by these nuisances is more easily understood when we consider the close proximity of domestic and industrial space characteristic of the medieval town.[141] The Newland Survey of Lynn shows that by about 1250 fullers

---

[134] Keene, *Survey of Medieval Winchester*, I.286–8.

[135] F. W. Maitland, ed., *Memoranda de Parliamento*, RS 98 (London, 1893), p. 47.

[136] As Guillerme points out, both alum and tannin have anti-pollutant properties, but this fact was unknown to medieval men and women, who were more concerned about miasmatic air and filthy water: *Age of Water*, p. 98.

[137] Cherry, 'Leather', pp. 295–9. London tanners were prohibited from placing their pits too near to other dwellings for this reason, and might be obliged to move them: *LAN* no. 251.

[138] See, for instance, SROI, C/2/8/1/4 (washing hides in the town ditch and polluting other water supplies), C/2/8/1/5 (washing hides in 'common water'), C/2/8/1/10 and C/2/8/1/11 (polluting ditches), C/2/8/1/12 (pits flooding the highway); C/2/10/1/3 (illicit pits).

[139] SROI, C/2/8/1/13.

[140] NRO, NCR, 16C/2, Assembly Minute Book, 1510–1550, fol. 2r–v.

[141] The Southwark waterfront provides a striking example of this cheek by jowl relationship, where Sir John Fastolf's grand town house lay next to a water mill, a brewery and dyers' workshops: Schofield, *London, 1100–1600*, pp. 142–3.

and tanners congregated along the major watercourses leading into the River Ouse on land that had once been marginal, but was rapidly becoming developed as the population rose. One of these streams was even known as Barkers' Fleet, although the tidal flow probably kept levels of pollution at a minimum until the onset of silting in the sixteenth century.[142] Patterns of zoning constantly shifted because of urban growth, so that by the fifteenth century workshops that had once been almost rural were scattered across the poorer residential areas 'apparently at random'.[143] As noted in Chapter 1, it was easier for those towns and cities with a centralised and relatively autonomous system of government to determine where, as well as how, particular crafts might be practised. Whereas in 1344 the rulers of Bristol simply prohibited any tanners or girdlers from working 'within the walls, to wit in the highways where the majority of the people pass',[144] Durham's leather-workers were subject to a more 'informal development control' by the city's various overlords and their courts. Even so, they, too, had decamped to better-watered and more distant places well away from the centre before the Black Death struck.[145]

As a result of this gradual process of regulation, consensus and 'piecemeal aggregation', tanners in most late medieval English towns were generally to be found in extramural or at least peripheral locations, where they were less likely to cause annoyance.[146] At Exeter, for instance, they settled outside the west gate, conveniently near the river Exe and beyond the control of the civic authorities.[147] Similarly, in Norwich some tanneries were consigned to suburban Heigham from a fairly early date, while others sprang up, along with smithies and other heavy industries, to the north and east of the city (map 3).[148] According to the 1381 poll tax returns, all but three of York's forty-four tanners lived in the parish of All Saints, North Street, on the north bank of the Ouse, thereby respecting the sensitivities of wealthier residents. Although they were more widely dispersed, other leather-workers such as skinners and cordwainers also colonised this part of the

---

[142] In 1424 the barkers successfully petitioned for access to the common water supply, which was to be diverted under close supervision through sluices into a ditch of their own making: KLBA, KL/C7/2, Hall Book, 1422–1429, p. 56.

[143] Parker, *Making of King's Lynn*, pp. 36–7, 161, and fig. 7.

[144] *LRBB*, I.34.

[145] Bonney, *Lordship and the Urban Community*, pp. 164–6.

[146] Keene, *Survey of Medieval Winchester*, I.287. This also happened at Carlisle: Summerson, *Medieval Carlisle*, I.116. As the population fell, some workers may have been tempted to move back. In 1457, the leather-finishers of Coventry were ordered 'to curre their ledder withoute the walles as was of olde tyme vsed', or face a fine of 20s.: *Coventry Leet Book*, II.302, 312 (the ruling had to be repeated in 1461).

[147] M. Kowaleski, 'Town and Country in Late Medieval England: The Hide and Leather Trade', in P. Corfield and D. Keene, eds, *Work in Towns, 850–1850* (Leicester, 1990), p. 61. Similarly, in Chester tanneries moved progressively further east: Laughton, *Life in a Late Medieval City*, pp. 145–6.

[148] M. Atkin and D. H. Evans, *Excavations in Norwich, 1971–1978*, part 3, EAA 100 (Norwich, 2002), p. 234; Rutledge, 'Economic Life', pp. 160, 162, 170. At Lincoln, too, the tanners opted to settle in a suburb where there was plenty of water: J. Schofield and A. Vince, *Medieval Towns* (London, 1994), p. 99.

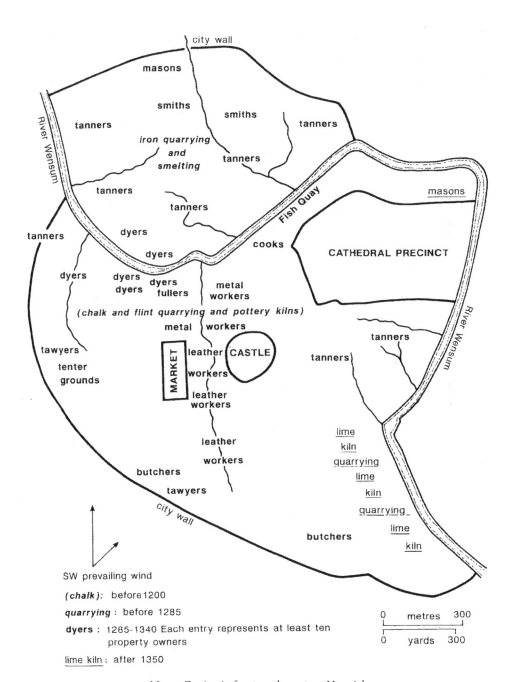

city wall

masons

smiths

smiths

tanners

*iron quarrying
and
smelting*

tanners

tanners

River Wensum

tanners

tanners

Fish Quay

masons

CATHEDRAL PRECINCT

dyers

cooks

tanners

dyers

dyers

dyers

dyers
dyers

dyers
fullers

metal
workers

(chalk and flint quarrying and pottery kilns)

metal workers

tanners

River Wensum

tawyers

tenter
grounds

MARKET

leather
workers

CASTLE

tanners

leather
workers

lime
kiln
quarrying
lime
kiln
quarrying
lime
kiln

leather
workers

butchers

tawyers

city wall

butchers

SW prevailing wind

(chalk): before 1200

quarrying : before 1285

dyers : 1285-1340 Each entry represents at least ten
property owners

lime kiln : after 1350

| 0 | metres | 300 |
| 0 | yards | 300 |

Map 3 Zoning in fourteenth-century Norwich

river.[149] Winchester's tanners actually gave their name to a street which lay to the east of the city and enjoyed a copious provision of water. Excavation has revealed that supplies for their workshops flowed through specially constructed timber-lined channels, diverted from the 'brook' or gutter which ran down the middle of 'Tannerestret', and thence into the river. Significantly, though, a combination of population growth and demands on the part of cloth workers for cleaner water led the tanners and parchment-makers to move even further eastwards during the twelfth century, in response to public pressure.[150]

Since they needed a constant supply of hides, as well as water, many London tanners established themselves immediately to the west of the City in the parish of St Sepulchre, which lay conveniently near to the river Fleet and the butchers' shambles in Newgate. It also gave easy access to Cheapside, where finished leather could be sold.[151] But their close proximity both to the residences of affluent newcomers and to the Fleet prison proved more controversial. The contamination of the river, about which the London Carmelites had protested so vociferously in the late thirteenth century, was in part due to their insalubrious activities, which inevitably attracted even more attention during plague time.[152] Understandable fears about the 'infection of the air' prompted Edward III to instigate a general inquiry in 1355 into the 'abominable stench' arising from the tanners' waste, excrement and rubbish that had been dumped in the prison moat, in some cases by neighbouring householders.[153] A comprehensive programme of repairs and cleansing (which cost the crown £20 in 1356 alone) and an agreement by local residents to provide financial support for seven river wardens may have prevented the worst pollution, but nuisances still occurred from time to time.[154] In 1422, for example, the parishioners of St Sepulchre's and St Andrew's complained to the mayor's court about offences committed by four named tanners, who were not only washing ox hides in Turnmill Brook, a tributary of the Fleet, but had actually driven stakes into the riverbed and constructed 'deep weirs' to facilitate the process.[155]

---

[149] N. Bartlett, 'Lay Poll Tax Returns for the City of York in 1381', *Transactions of the East Riding Antiquarian Society* 30 (1953), pp. 1–91, on pp. 8–9.

[150] Biddle, *Winchester in the Early Middle Ages*, pp. 284, 345, 434, 436, 438; Keene, *Survey of Medieval Winchester*, I.287–9; Magnusson, *Water Technology*, p. 154.

[151] Honeybourne, 'The Fleet and its Neighbourhood', pp. 54–5. Other communities settled outside Cripplegate and Bishopsgate, and south of the Thames in Bermondsey, where water was also abundant: D. Keene, 'Tanners' Widows', in C. M. Barron and A. F. Sutton, eds, *Medieval London Widows, 1300–1500* (London, 1994), pp. 1–27, esp. pp. 9–13.

[152] See p. 192 above. A complaint about blockages in the Fleet, addressed to Parliament a few years later, in 1306, specifically blamed tanners' waste: *RP*, I.200.

[153] Honeybourne, 'The Fleet and its Neighbourhood', pp. 39–40; *CLB*, G, pp. 49–50; Riley, *Memorials of London*, pp. 279–80; C. T. Flower, ed., *Public Works in Medieval Law*, vol. 2, Selden Society 40 (London, 1923), pp. 32–6. It was, significantly, in 1354 that the rulers of Beverley prohibited the washing of hides and 'other tainted things' in or near the town ditch and wells: *BTD*, pp. 43–4.

[154] *CCR, 1354–1360*, p. 379; Honeybourne, 'The Fleet and its Neighbourhood', p. 57.

[155] *CPMRL, 1413–1437*, pp. 125–6.

4.4 Providing access

Tanners, like dyers, fishmongers, butchers and brewers, were as notorious for their heavy use of urban water supplies as they were for the health hazards that they caused. It was therefore essential to regulate large-scale commercial and industrial consumers to ensure that ordinary householders did not suffer.[156] The construction of conduits, whereby fresh water could be piped from extramural streams to a 'house' or 'standard', was designed to overcome both these problems, although abuses were common. Built, as we have seen, at considerable effort and expense, the conduits at Lynn were envisaged as a charitable work for the benefit of the poorer residents. Yet such was the demand upon them that as early as 1390 the stonework of one had been badly damaged and the plugs removed. Having been impressed by 'the good rule' (*bonum regimen*) successfully adopted in London, the mayor and his associates instigated an orderly queuing system along the same lines. Further to prevent the disputes that had erupted between householders and those needing large quantities of water for commercial purposes, a fine of 12*d*. was imposed on anyone attempting to fill large containers, or 'sogs', ahead of those carrying jugs and ewers for domestic use. Compensation was also promised to vulnerable people whose vessels were broken in the general free for all.[157]

Similar measures were adopted in Coventry, where the appointment of conduit-keepers, who policed the system, and the introduction of 'grates & lokkes' to prevent illicit raids under cover of darkness, deterred all but the most resolute offenders.[158] Even so, some traders resorted to ingenious stratagems to divert supplies. In 1478, for example, William Campion of London was found to have 'tapped' the conduit at Fleet Street with small pipes or 'suspirals' leading to his home. His punishment was both ingenious and appropriate, being designed as a public spectacle to impress upon his fellow citizens the antisocial nature of the crime. Mounted upon a horse, he was to be paraded through the streets 'with a vessel like unto a conduyt full of water uppon his hede, the same water rennyng by smale pipes oute of the same vessell'.[159] As a further indignity, the container was

---

[156] For problems in London, see Magnusson, *Water Technology*, pp. 139–41, 144, and Jenner, 'From Conduit Community to Commercial Network', pp. 253–4. For the regulation of Coventry's brewers between 1444 and 1451, see *Coventry Leet Book*, I.208, 232, 255; and for those of Bristol, see *LRBB*, II.229–30. The importance of 'an equable and measured' distribution of water in framing Italian concepts of the 'buon governo', or good ruler, is considered by P. Boucheron, 'Water and Power in Milan, c. 1200–1500', *Urban History* 28 (2001), pp. 180–93.

[157] Isaacson and Ingleby, *Red Register of King's Lynn*, II.50. The order was repeated in 1426: KLBA, KL/C7/2, Hall Book, 1422–1429, p. 124. In 1470 the town's maltsters were forbidden from removing water by means of carts or 'sleddes': C7/4, Hall Book, 1453–1497, p. 286.

[158] *Coventry Leet Book*, I.208; II.517; III.584. Ipswich appointed keepers 'for the upholding and repairing of the conduit' from at least 1482: Bacon, *Annalls of Ipswiche*, p. 145. The early history of this conduit remains obscure, but it had become a local landmark by the 1390s: D. Allen, 'The Public Water Supply of Ipswich before the Municipal Corporation Act', *Proceedings of the Suffolk Institute of Archaeology* 40 (2001), pp. 31–54, on p. 36.

[159] *CLB*, I, p. 160.

to be constantly refilled during the procession, after which Campion was to reflect upon his misdeeds in prison at the mayor's pleasure. Less inventive methods were employed, either to punish or to profit from those who sought to exploit the system. Soon afterwards the Coventry authorities inaugurated a house to house search throughout the town for illegal water pipes, accompanied by an appeal for informers (who stood to earn 8*d*. for each successful prosecution).[160]

Bowing to the inevitable, some magistrates – beginning with those of London in the fourteenth century – resorted to a water rate, whereby brewers, cooks and the like actually paid for controlled access to conduits or wells, or else agreed to share the cost of repairs.[161] From 1465 onwards, for instance, the mayor and council of King's Lynn began leasing out the right to run pipes from the town's various aqueducts and conduits. Higher rates, sometimes as much as 40s. a year, were charged to commercial users, while ordinary householders paid considerably less. By 1542 at least fifty separate contracts had been sealed, earning the authorities a significant sum for investment in public works. Fittingly, under the circumstances, the alderman who negotiated the purchase of the piped water systems owned by the Augustinian, Dominican and Franciscan friaries for communal use at the Dissolution was allowed his own private supply at a token rent.[162]

Squabbles and breakages were by no means the worst of the problems encountered by those who were obliged to fetch and carry water for their families or employers. Drawing water was a potentially dangerous business, especially for the poor, whose lodgings rarely enjoyed direct access to private wells or conduits.[163] The records of most English cities reveal that the risk of drowning was considerable, not least because children and young female servants were often entrusted with the task of hauling heavy pots and buckets out of pits, streams and rivers.[164] One such was Horengia, the servant of Benedict Key, who was sent in 1274–5 to bring water from the pool in the Old Swine Market, Norwich. The cord on her vessel broke, and, as she lent forward to retrieve it, the weight dragged her to the bottom.[165] Her fate was far from unusual: between 1264 and 1282 local coroners investigated at least twenty-three cases of accidental drowning, many in similar circumstances.[166] London's professional water-carriers, who used metal-bound vessels with a capacity of about three gallons, were also vulnerable,

---

[160] *Coventry Leet Book*, III.584. Resort to informers seems to have been common. In 1414, for example, a substantial reward was offered to Londoners who provided information about fly-tipping: *CLB*, I, p. 131.

[161] Magnusson, *Water Technology*, pp. 127–8; *Coventry Leet Book*, III.548–9.

[162] KLBA, KL/C7/4, Hall Book, 1453–1497, pp. 221, 227, 385, 424, 490, 535, 561a, 566, 575, 606; C7/5, Hall Book, 1497–1544, fols 37r, 39r, 47r, 78r, 82v, 84v, 90v, 107r, 208r, 212r, 217r, 268v, 278r, 283r, 293v, 296v, 306r, 321v, 331v, 336v, 343v.

[163] Keene, 'Issues of Water', p. 173.

[164] See, for example, B. A. Hanawalt, 'Childrearing among the Lower Classes in Late Medieval England', *Journal of Interdisciplinary History* 8 (1977–78), pp. 1–22; Hanawalt, *Growing up in Medieval London*, pp. 62–7, 75, 81–2; *CCRCL*, pp. 252–3; Salter, *Records of Medieval Oxford*, p. 26.

[165] NRO, NCR, 8A/2, m. 3r. William Aubyn of London met an identical fate in 1235–6: Chew and Weinbaum, *London Eyre of 1244*, no. 101.

[166] NRO, NCR, 8A/1–2, *passim*.

especially as some of these 'poore tankard slaves' appear to have operated from boats and thus to have run the risk of falling into the Thames.[167] We know less about the long-term physical damage caused by such back-breaking activities, but occasional references survive to the plight of servants like Thomas Bunny, who had the misfortune to work for the owner of a Southwark bath house. In 1366 he addressed an appeal to the mayor of London, on the ground that he had sustained permanent injury while being forced to carry water in a 'tyne' or large tub.[168]

Spiritual considerations apart, it is easy to see why the mercantile elite of English towns and cities regarded the provision of piped water as such a meritorious exercise. When they were properly equipped with buckets, windlasses and ropes, wells also made the lot of the urban workforce much easier. They could, nonetheless, still prove lethal, particularly for small children.[169] Covers or gates were essential, as the residents of Portsoken ward in London recognised when protesting in 1422 about 'a certain well' in the public highway, which lay 'uncovered and not sufficiently enclosed to the peril of men and beasts passing'.[170] Alarm at the likelihood of serious accidents in the City's bustling streets prompted complaints about at least five other wells at this time, either because their owners had failed to implement the necessary repairs or because they were not safely secured at night.[171] Ibn-Sīna had expressed some reservations about the quality of water that collected through seepage and 'remained in prolonged contact with earthly matter', although he considered it safer for human consumption than that which was stored in tanks or cisterns, or had passed for any distance through lead pipes.[172] Underlying anxiety on this score was intensified by the ease with which unprotected wells could be polluted, either accidentally or on purpose. It is interesting that presentments were also filed in 1422 against two London bakers who made their bread with filthy well-water, 'to the great danger and nuisance of all men who eat of it'.[173]

---

[167] Riley, *Memorials of London*, p. 7. The water-carriers formed a guild in 1496, with about forty named members. They were, significantly, based at the Austin friary: H. C. Coote, 'The Ordinances of Some Secular Guilds of London', *TLMAS* 4 (1871), pp. 1–59, on pp. 55–9; T. Flaxman and T. Jackson, *Sweet and Wholesome Water: Five Centuries of History of Water-Bearers in the City of London* (Cottisford, 2004), pp. 1–12, and appendix A.

[168] *CPMRL, 1364–1381*, p. 54. Wagons and horses were widely used (Stevenson, *Records of the Borough of Nottingham*, I.114–16), but many carriers still worked on foot.

[169] Finucane, *Rescue of the Innocents*, pp. 103–4; Owen, *Making of King's Lynn*, p. 425. Faulty equipment put adults as well as children at risk. In 1267–8, for example, two Londoners were killed when the rope on which they were hauling water from a deep well broke, and they both fell to the bottom: Weinbaum, *London Eyre of 1276*, no. 191. See also, *CCRCL*, pp. 94, 100–1, 265–6; *CLB*, B, p. 270; Salter, *Records of Medieval Oxford*, pp. 31, 42.

[170] *CPMRL, 1413–1437*, p. 120.

[171] *CPMRL, 1413–1437*, pp. 123–4, 126–7. Even in a small town the size of Basingstoke negligent householders might be fined on this score: Baigent and Millard, *History of the Town and Manor of Basingstoke*, p. 292.

[172] Shah, *Avicenna's Canon of Medicine*, p. 190.

[173] *CPMRL, 1413–1437*, pp. 135, 152.

The apparently malicious contamination of a hospital well used by the burgesses of Bamburgh, in Northumberland, whenever those in the town ran dry even merited the attention of a royal commission of inquiry, set up in 1393. Claims that a woman who had unknowingly drunk the water 'was poisoned and prematurely delivered of a still-born child' are alone unlikely to have warranted action at this level, but more sensational allegations that 'certain friars preachers' had deliberately killed a pet dog and thrown it down the shaft suggest an ongoing vendetta that could hardly be ignored.[174] As a general rule, magistrates dealt with such matters by punishing offenders and either investing public funds in cleansing projects or delegating the task to local communities. We can see the latter approach at work in Norwich, in 1474, when complaints about the blockage of two common wells led the Assembly to appoint a sub-committee with powers to suggest remedial action. Predictable concerns about health were here compounded by the need to provide safeguards against the fires which broke out with depressing regularity in the more crowded areas.[175] No doubt for this reason, nine months later, in January 1475, city-wide orders were promulgated for the removal of filth and detritus from any wells that had become inoperative. Responsibility for this task was assigned to the appropriate parishes, whose residents faced a collective fine of 100s. should they fail to comply within the time allowed.[176] By contrast, liability in Coventry fell upon individual aldermen, who stood to forfeit as much as 40s. if the wells in their wards remained unrepaired.[177]

Intensive use by those needing large quantities of water for industrial purposes inflicted serious damage upon the stonework and lifting mechanisms of wells, which likewise had to be made good. Local leet courts would generally name, and if necessary penalise, the persons responsible. Rising from 20d. to a daunting 10s., the fines threatened in mid-fifteenth-century Ipswich reveal the scale of the perceived nuisance and the tight deadline imposed for repairs.[178] Sanctions were necessary because of the heavy costs involved, sometimes in human as well as financial terms. Given the lack of protective equipment and difficult working conditions, it is hardly surprising that accidents were common. In 1278, for example, the labourer who was cementing the shaft of a private well owned by Henry de Senges of Norwich died when the rope suspending him in a bucket snapped and he crashed to the bottom. Significantly, the jurors who gave evidence maintained that he had expired through the inhalation of corrupt vapours ('per corrupcionem aeris'), which in this instance may well have been the case.[179] A similar accident

---

[174] *CPR, 1391–1396*, p. 353.

[175] See section 3.8 above.

[176] NRO, NCR, 16D/1, Assembly Proceedings, 1434–1491, fols 97r, 98r (the initial deadline of August 1475 was extended to Michaelmas). The obligation to clean communal wells and ponds was often, as in Durham and Yarmouth, subject to enforcement by local leet courts through the imposition of escalating fines: *RBC*, nos 259, 305, 309, 358, 360, 473, 493, 528; NRO, Y/C4/191, rot. 15r. In London problems concerning shared private wells fell within the remit of the assize of nuisance: *LAN*, no. 633.

[177] *Coventry Leet Book*, II.548.

[178] SROI, C/2/8/1/13; C/2/10/1/5.

[179] NRO, NCR, 8A/2, m. 3r. At least two other Norwich workmen were killed at about this time when attempting to sink wells or pits (mm. 2v, 3v).

occurred in London at about this time because the hoops of the barrels that had been used to line a well shaft were too 'old and rotten' to support the weight of the man who climbed down to retrieve a bucket. He, too, was reputedly 'asphyxiated by bad air' after his fall.[180]

During the later Middle Ages, the practice of lining urban wells with timber (often by stacking large casks on top of each other) gave way to the construction of more permanent stone-lined shafts.[181] A graphic sense of the effort involved is conveyed by the fifteenth-century author of *Jacob's Well*, a protracted meditation on the purification of the soul through confession, which is compared to the difficult process of excavation. Describing the 'long labour' required to turn a noisome pit of stagnant mud into a 'depe welle' of limpid water, he explains:

> Whanne youre pytt is scowryd clene fro the watyr of curs [Original Sin], & fro the wose [ooze] of dedly synnes ... it muste be dolvyn deppere wyth the spade of clennesse, and there-wyth castyn out the sande & the grauel ... and thanne ley in the welle by-nethe the courbyls [corbels] of the artycles of the feyth. Thanne take sande, that is mynde of youre synne, take watyr of weepyng here-to & lyim brent [lime burnt] in fyir, that is crist, whygt as chalk ... wyth brennyng loue for thi lyme .... & medle [mix] hem to-gedere wyth watyr of wepyng, and late this be thy mortere.[182]

Once they had been built, wells needed regular maintenance to keep the equipment in working order and to prevent contamination through seepage.[183] Here, too, a wealthy philanthropist could assist his or her neighbours. In his will of 1463, John Baret of Bury St Edmunds, whose desire for personal commemoration appears remarkable, even by the standards of the age, instructed that

> the well before my house is to be newly repaired, along with the tackle, and the stone work is to be made safe. Item, I wish that my executors, by the advice of Thomas Ide, should surmount it with such a construction of timber, with four posts and a cross, as there is at Eye, or else better, so that it will be in a sufficiently well covered and substantial state to remain in use.[184]

Given his obsessive quest for personal redemption, Baret would have been familiar with that strain of contemporary devotional literature which required the penitent

---

[180] *CLB*, B, p. 276. See also *CCRCL*, pp. 198–9. Following the deaths of two men in identical circumstances in Oxford in 1389, the well in question was deemed a health hazard, and filled up: Salter, *Records of Medieval Oxford*, p. 48.

[181] Keene, 'Issues of Water', p. 172; Schofield, *Medieval London Houses*, pp. 117–18; Carter and Roberts, 'Excavations in Norwich, 1972', p. 461. An example of a fifteenth-century barrel-well from the High Street in Hull may be found in Evans, 'Infrastructure of Hull', p. 59 (fig. 6a). For the transition from timber to stone in York, see Addyman, 'Archaeology of Public Health', pp. 253 (plates 7 and 8), 259. For an impressive stone-lined well with an elaborate timber pump, see Brennand and Stringer, *Making of Carlisle*, pp. 126–7 (fig. 8.4).

[182] A. Brandeis, ed., *Jacob's Well*, EETS o.s. 115 (London, 1890), pp. 2–3.

[183] For repairs to the common well at Nottingham, which resulted in litigation in 1396, see Stevenson, *Records of the Borough of Nottingham*, I.332–5.

[184] Tymms, *Wills and Inventories*, p. 20.

reader to 'make a well of teeris in the middis of [his] hert' in order to wash away the stains of sin.[185] We will return to the spiritual merit of such bequests at the end of this chapter. Of more immediate interest is Baret's desire to emulate (and if possible outdo) the nearby town of Eye, and, by implication, to provide an even more striking advertisement of both his own and his community's commitment to the upkeep of public works.

4.5 The arteries of the civic body

As the state of London's Walbrook reveals, it was extremely difficult to keep the watercourses which flowed through English towns and cities free from obstruction. That resistance to campaigns against fly-tipping and similar nuisances may, in some quarters, have been entrenched is apparent from cases such as the imprisonment in 1364 of a London apprentice for assaulting the constable who tried to stop him from throwing quantities of 'rubbish and filth' into the Thames. Since the master who sent him on this errand was himself bound over to await trial before the mayor, there can be little doubt of the determination, if not necessarily the success, with which the authorities set about their task.[186] Londoners could, at least, rely upon the powerful ebb flow of the Thames, which carried quantities of detritus out to sea, but other cities were less fortunate.[187] Galvanised into action by royal complaints about the clogged and sluggish state of the Wensum, in 1380 the common council of Norwich threatened anyone who attempted to remove refuse privately by boat along the river 'by night or day' with a punitive fine of 20s., rising to 40s. for a second offence and 60s. for a third, along with the loss of citizenship or expulsion in the case of 'foreigners'.[188] As a more positive step, it was decided to tackle the root of the problem. The city treasurer's account for 1398–9 records the travelling expenses of an expert coming to Norwich from Lynn 'to examine the defects of the common river', while 'a man called Blaumester' was recruited from Colchester at fee of 20s. three years later to provide yet more technical advice.[189] Such evidence provides yet another interesting insight into the ways in which specialist knowledge might be shared by different urban communities.

[185] C. W. Marx, 'British Library Harley MS 1740 and Popular Devotion', in N. Rogers, ed., *England in the Fifteenth Century* (Stamford, 1994), p. 221.

[186] *CPMRL, 1364–1381*, p. 2.

[187] Keene, 'Issues of Water', p. 168.

[188] *RCN*, II.84. In February 1378 the bailiffs had been ordered by the crown 'to view the river on one side of the city, which is choked with grass growing therein, and the dry ditches on the other side, obstructed with mud and filth thrown into them' and force all residents to contribute to the necessary repairs and improvements: *CPR, 1377–1381*, p. 121.

[189] *RCN*, II.52–4; Lilley, *Urban Life in the Middle Ages*, p. 174. The construction of new water mills on the Wensum demanded a comprehensive cleansing programme, which, along with other work on the river, lasted thirty-five weeks. Urban mills were vulnerable to damage as a result of careless waste disposal. In 1419, for instance, six Ipswich butchers were fined for dumping dung and offal near the mill dam, thereby raising the water level: SROI, C/2/8/1/4.

The effective application of this knowledge was, of course, more difficult. Yet here, too, we can detect a degree of common purpose, and, perhaps, of consultation and collaboration among the governors of England's towns and cities. We might, for example, compare the steps taken in 1422 by Norwich magistrates to force all those who lived by the river to cleanse it themselves, or pay labourers to do so, with similar orders promulgated in Coventry a year earlier.[190] Among the comprehensive range of sanitary measures then introduced was a ruling that:

> The ryuer and the brokes that comyth and rennyth in to this Cyte & allso the Red-dyche be enlargid of the breed [to the breadth] he owithe to haue of ryght cours, the wiche, be encrochment of dwellers of both sydes, be strayted and narrowid, & with filthe, dong and stonys the watur stoppyd of his cours; [and] that euery man voide afor his ground thorugh the watur, and dyche and clense hym vnto his old ground, to th'end the waters in flod tyme may the lyghtlyer passe, eschewyng dyuers perels had afortyme by floodys thurgh stopping and strayting of the same ryuers & dyches …[191]

More specific regulations followed in 1426, when the rulers of Coventry demanded the immediate removal of all riparian pigsties and stables, under a penalty of 20s. They also appointed a team of overseers to patrol the river Sherbourne, apparently in response to complaints from 'the worthy men of the leet'.[192] No doubt on their insistence, a standard amercement of 40d. was introduced shortly afterwards for the illicit disposal of rubbish into any stretch of common water.[193] As was all too often the case, however, an initial burst of concerted activity, usually undertaken in the aftermath of an epidemic or before a royal visit, eventually gave way to inertia and a gradual return to bad habits. Certainly, by 1469 a new initiative seemed necessary to deal with recent 'encroachments' and the reckless dumping of 'dust, donge, swepyng or eny other fylthe', which now incurred double the fine.[194] By the end of the century, any resident of Coventry whose riverside property was not kept clean, or who contravened the previous ordinances, stood to forfeit 6s. 8d., the money being assigned, significantly, for repairs to the public conduit.[195]

However steep the penalties may have been, the knotty problem of waste disposal remained. If streams and rivers were out of bounds, where was all this urban refuse to go? As the century progressed provincial magistrates became increasingly persuaded that escalating fines alone were at worst counterproductive, and at best only part of a solution which could not be achieved without a sustained investment in communal facilities of the kind described in the previous chapter. Such a policy seemed particularly desirable in a city like Norwich, which not

---

[190] *RCN*, I.277–8. See also Jørgensen, 'All Good Rule of the Citee', pp. 300–15.

[191] *Coventry Leet Book*, I.31. See also pp. 29–30.

[192] *Coventry Leet Book*, I.107–8. At Totnes in Devon wardens of the town's 'wells' or springs were appointed for similar purposes throughout the fifteenth century: H. R. Warkin, *Totnes Priory and Town*, 3 vols (Torquay, 1911–17), II.946–7.

[193] *Coventry Leet Book*, I.119.

[194] *Coventry Leet Book*, II.347–8. Not coincidentally, plague epidemics are recorded in both 1467 and 1468: see Appendix.

[195] *Coventry Leet Book*, III.586.

only had particular reason to fear plague but also depended for its water supply upon its cockeys and river rather than public conduits (map 4).[196] Accordingly, in 1453, almost certainly in response to the recommendations of another royal commission for cleansing the river and ditches, arrangements were made for the regular removal of all 'mukke and fylth' from the banks of the Wensum by a special 'dongebote'.[197] Partly funded by the draconian penalties imposed a few years later on those who got rid of waste by any other means, and partly by the toll of 4*d.* he was allowed to charge for every load, the boatman was himself under strict instructions to dispose of his noisome cargo with care.[198] Once again, though, it proved all too easy to lose momentum until the arrival of the next royal commission of inquiry or letter of complaint, an event that was often so well timed as to suggest that local officials actively solicited government intervention. In any event, the prospect of further censure from Westminster empowered the Norwich Assembly in February 1467 'to make, move and exhort' all residents to remove any rubbish from the streets and improve the free flow of water into the drains by the following May, upon pain of a 40*d.* fine. Householders who permitted rural deliverymen to leave a trail of 'putrefying matter' in their wake faced an additional penalty of 12*d.* for each offence. In keeping with initiatives that had already proved successful in Coventry and London, and as an earnest demonstration of their own commitment to change, the authorities arranged for the election of two inspectors in every ward who would henceforward be responsible for supervising the streets and cockeys. They also adopted the ingenious stratagem of threatening any future mayor who failed to protect the river with a personal fine of 100*s.*, thereby ensuring that responsibility began at the top.[199]

---

[196] Being similarly blessed with a natural supply of water, medieval Winchester had no public conduits either. The constant struggle to protect its river and many brooks from blockages is described by Keene, *Survey of Medieval Winchester*, I.63–5.

[197] Reiterating complaints voiced in the 1370s, the commission declared that 'the river of the said city and the ditches under the walls ... are both obstructed and filled by weeds ... and by muck, muck-heaps and other filth cast there': *RCN*, II.318. A boatman had previously been employed 'for carrying muck' in 1382, perhaps in emulation of measures introduced in London, but does not appear to have served for long: Sabine, 'City Cleaning in Mediaeval London', pp. 24–5; Riley, *Memorials of London*, p. 299; *RCN*, II.85. If the specifications of the 'muk bote' commissioned in the mid-sixteenth century are any guide, the vessel acquired in 1453 would have been able to transport 2½ tons of refuse: NRO, NCR, 22G/1, Lease Book A, fol. 40v.

[198] *RCN*, II.91; NRO, NCR, 16D/1, Assembly Proceedings, 1434–1491, fol. 41r. *Ad hoc* committees were also appointed from 1453 onwards to deal with noxious gutters: fol. 42v; 16D/2, Assembly Proceedings, 1491–1553, fol. 15r.

[199] *RCN*, II.96–8; NRO, NCR, 16D/1, Assembly Proceedings, 1434–1491, fols 69v–70r. The chamberlains' accounts confirm that strenuous efforts *were* made in this respect. For example, a water cistern built near the river in Conesford in 1472–3 was cleansed regularly 'lest the filth flowing into it from the streets should enter the river': NCR, 18A/2, Chamberlains' Accounts, 1470–1490, fols 48v, 73r, 85r. By the sixteenth century 'costes of the cokeys' and river cleansing merited a designated budget of up to £7 a year: NCR, 18A/5, Chamberlains' Accounts, 1531–1537, fols 29r–31r, 33v–34r, 58r–60v, 80r–81v, 97r–98v, 124v–125r, 127v, 143v–145r.

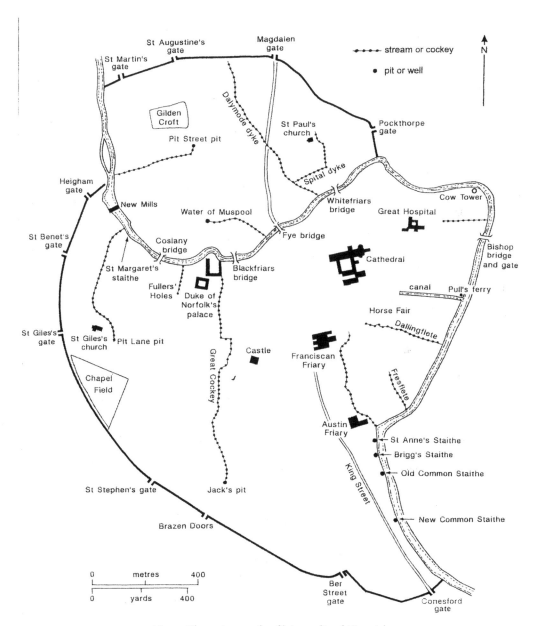

Map 4 The water supply of late medieval Norwich

The outcome was encouraging. One year later, a committee specifically concerned with the cleanliness of the Wensum and its immediate environs sprang into action, its first task being to report any major 'nuisances'.[200] Although we now know only the names of the two worst culprits, whose offences merited an official enquiry,[201] the original list may well have been similar to one made some forty years later. This was carefully preserved in the front of the Assembly Minute Book, which reflects the importance by then attached to monitoring all such misdemeanours. Since both sets of commissioners faced a penalty of 20*d.* a day for neglecting their duties, they were understandably meticulous, on the second occasion noting fifty-five separate complaints. These ranged from obstructions to the river and its banks, some of which constituted an impediment to navigability or a likely cause of flooding, to the actual pollution or endangerment of the water supply. Among the latter we may note the illicit washing of hides by local tanners; the keeping of 'noysfull' and 'very noysfull' privies, gutters and drains; the dumping of waste; the 'castyng up of muk'; and the diversion of water for industrial uses.[202] Whatever its findings, the commission of 1468 clearly made quite an impact, since over £16 was voted for a comprehensive programme of river cleansing, along with funds for the purchase of a large boat for this purpose.[203] The financial as well as logistical challenges posed by these developments should not be underestimated. But the stage was now set for further innovations, such as the levying of a communal rate of £40 in 1517 to improve the river and another of £10 for the weekly removal of 'muck' by 'common tumbrel', both of which helped to earn Norwich its nascent, if sometimes faltering, reputation as an orderly and hygienic city. It soon became a point of honour to boast that the thoroughfares and waterways were kept clean by means of 'dyvers good and *godly* actes and ordynaunces'.[204]

Measures of this kind were obviously a matter of civic pride and economic necessity as well as sanitary importance. Norwich expected a royal visit in 1469, and was anxious to create the right impression by eliminating any blots on the urban landscape.[205] The adverse effect of a dirty and sluggish water supply upon the production of one of its principal exports, finished cloth, must also have weighed heavily with the ruling elite. Crucially, too, the city depended for its survival upon the river-borne trade that conveyed merchandise to and from its out-port at Yarmouth; and, in this respect, the Wensum, 'beyng a thing very profitabyll to the hoole commynaltie', might be compared to the blood supply that nurtured the limbs and organs of commerce.[206] Such an analogy was, indeed, employed by

[200] NRO, NCR, 16D/1, Assembly Proceedings, 1434–1491, fol. 74r.

[201] NRO, NCR, 16D/1, Assembly Proceedings, 1434–1491, fol. 75v.

[202] NRO, NCR, 16C/2, Assembly Minute Book, 1510–1550, fol. 2r–v.

[203] NRO, NCR, 16D/1, Assembly Proceedings, 1434–1491, fols 75v, 76r. The money was voted in two separate grants of £6 13s. 4d. each.

[204] See p. 138 above; *RCN*, II.109–10, 127; Rawcliffe, 'Introduction' in Rawcliffe and Wilson, *Medieval Norwich*, pp. xxi–xxvi.

[205] NRO, NCR, 16D/1, Assembly Proceedings, 1434–1491, fols 78r, 79r–81v.

[206] NRO, NCR, 16D/2, Assembly Proceedings, 1491–1553, fol. 145v (pencil foliation 165). Blockages in the Fleet and Thames in London and the River Ouse in York

the Elizabethan traveller Fynes Moryson, who observed that 'channels of water' flowed through Venice just 'as the bloud passeth through the veines of mans body'.[207] And, as any health-conscious individual knew, the regular prophylaxis of phlebotomy was essential to prevent the entire system from becoming clogged with corrupt and dangerous matter.[208]

From this perspective, butchers, tanners, dyers, fullers and the practitioners of other noxious trades were similar to those less exalted or 'ignoble' parts of the human body that might perform an embarrassing function but were nonetheless essential for life. As the eminent French surgeon Henri de Mondeville explained, an inherently menial organ such as the bladder, anus or stomach demanded recognition 'not because it is noble ... or has an influence over the others, but because it does them services which they cannot do without'.[209] However, notwithstanding their vital importance, these 'servile' workers were best kept out of sight, and certainly far away from the sensitive nostrils of the 'better sort'. It was, indeed, for this very reason that the diaphragm served as a barricade to contain the 'malign fumes' and unpleasant waste generated by the digestive processes.[210] The problems occasioned by the concentration of tanners around the River Fleet in London are so well known to us because their neighbours were superior members of the body politic, whose complaints secured a ready hearing in parliament.[211] Few ordinary citizens could flex the well-developed legal muscles of the dean and chapter of Wells, who in 1439 simply banned a dyer from working near the cathedral 'on account of the corruption of the watercourses'.[212] Clearly aware of the need for compromise, Norwich's magistrates had begun by the early sixteenth century to favour what might today be regarded as an environmental tax, whereby 'barkers, dyers, calaundrers [cloth-pressers], parchementmakers, tewers [tawyers], sadelers, brewers, wasshers of shepe & all such gret noyers of the same rever' were to be 'ffurder charged than other persons' when rates were levied for cleansing the Wensum.[213] If, as the satirist Bernard Mandeville was later to maintain, the creation of wealth was a filthy business ('it is impossible *London* should be more cleanly before it is less flourishing ... dirty Streets are a necessary

were likewise seen as a threat to shipping as well as health: *RP*, I.200; *CPR, 1307–1313*, p. 38; *YMB*, II.70; *SR*, vol. 3, pp. 381–2; Riley, *Memorials of London*, pp. 367–8.

[207] Fynes Moryson, *An Itinerary*, 4 vols (Glasgow, 1907), I.163. This simile was further developed in the seventeenth century: Harris, 'This Is not a Pipe', pp. 203–28.

[208] See, for example, L. E. Voigts and M. R. McVaugh, eds, 'A Latin Technical Phlebotomy and its Middle English Translation', *Transactions of the American Philosophical Society* 74.2 (1984), pp. 1–69.

[209] Henri de Mondeville, *Chirurgie*, p. 369.

[210] Henri de Mondeville, *Chirurgie*, p. 64.

[211] *RP*, I.61, 200.

[212] HMC, *Calendar of the Manuscripts of the Dean and Chapter of Wells*, vol. 1, Royal Commission on Historical Manuscripts 12 (London, 1907), p. 134.

[213] NRO, NCR, 16D/2, Assembly Proceedings 1491–1553, fol. 145v (pencil foliation 165).

Evil'), it seemed entirely appropriate that some of the profits should be earmarked for civic improvement.[214]

4.6 Cleanliness and Godliness

We should also bear in mind that, although the preservation of health and prosperity remained paramount, other powerful considerations, less immediately apparent to a modern reader, inspired an interest in public works. Not for nothing were Norwich's efforts in this regard described as 'good and *godly*', since the provision of a reliable supply of clean and fresh water, suitable for drinking, cooking and a variety of hygienic purposes, resonated with spiritual overtones. In recognition of the generosity of his fellow-citizens, and no doubt in the hope of prompting further legacies, the mayor of Norwich proposed in 1456 that all 'benefactors of the community' who supported such schemes should be accorded a special memorial service to be held annually in the presence of the ruling elite and representatives from all the city's guilds.[215] There were, indeed, many individuals to remember and to speed on their way to paradise. 'Meved and inclyned to accomplissh a dede of charite', Alderman John Gilbert, who inspired the programme of river cleansing in mid-fifteenth-century Norwich, made generous testamentary provision for the realisation of his plans. He was assisted by the largesse of his principal executor, the master of St Giles' hospital, who contributed a further £20 out of his own coffers.[216] But Norwich was far from exceptional in this respect. The acquisition of a piped water supply by the burgesses of Southampton, described at the beginning of this chapter, was made possible by a munificent bequest from John Benet (d. 1420), a former mayor. He left enough money not only to restore the dilapidated conduit and construct a new stone water-house for the benefit of the townspeople, but also to re-cast the lead piping and lay it along a more convenient route.[217] Philanthropy on this scale was clearly beyond the means of all but the

[214] Bernard Mandeville, *The Fable of the Bees: Or, Private Vices, Public Benefits*, ed. F. B. Kaye, 2 vols (Oxford, 2001), I.12.

[215] *RCN*, II.92. Some benefactors took no chances, making their donations conditional upon commemoration. In 1375, for example, the executors of Thomas Legge, a former mayor of London, handed £100 to the City chamberlains for cleansing ditches, in return for a promise of prayers and masses at the Guildhall: Riley, *Memorials of London*, pp. 384–5. In 1476 a more modest offer of funding from the estate of William Burmond, for repairs to a conduit in Lynn, secured weekly intercession on his behalf for the next two years: KLBA, KL/C7/4, Hall Book, 1453–1497, pp. 363, 369.

[216] Rawcliffe, *Medicine for the Soul*, p. 36. His colleague on the aldermanic bench, 'that honourable man and special benefactor' Ralph Segrym (d. 1456), had already left £10 for cleansing the river: *RCN*, II.cvi–vii, 92.

[217] Platt, *Medieval Southampton*, p. 144: Southampton Record Office, SC4/2/238 (I am grateful to Dr L. S. Clark for this reference). In 1428–9 alone the stewards spent over £20 on this project: Gidden, *Stewards' Book of Southampton*, I.20–9. Some testators gave in kind rather than in cash. In 1441, for instance, the Bristol MP Thomas Blount left 500 lb of lead to the town for the construction of pipes to carry water from the Temple Gate to the cross: Roskell, Clark and Rawcliffe, *Commons, 1386–1421*, II.258.

wealthiest members of the mercantile elite, but ordinary men and women could club together in order to share the same celestial benefits. In 1371, for example, the religious fraternities of King's Lynn together raised the impressive sum of £163 for the construction and repair of watercourses; and in 1444 members of the Trinity Guild alone contributed £15 as a 'work of charity' towards the installation of new pipes.[218]

Historians of late medieval piety have documented a significant shift in the nature of the 'pious works' supported by urban oligarchs, who increasingly favoured useful projects, such as the upkeep of roads, bridges and conduits.[219] Since, as the authors of late medieval plague tracts invariably observed, 'gode dedes' were themselves a powerful prophylactic, we can readily appreciate why so many private individuals sank their capital into common utilities.[220] The practical value of this type of investment should not, however, lead us to ignore its spiritual merits, especially in a society notable for its 'unselfconscious linking of commerce and Christianity'.[221] Christ was, after all, described as a 'blessid brigge', over which the soul might cross the turbulent waters from this world to the next, while His mother, the Virgin Mary, seemed like an aqueduct, bearing a pure draught of grace from heaven.[222] Developing this metaphor, Henry of Lancaster (d. 1361) compared the heart of the Virgin with a cistern in which the rainwater from the roof of a house became 'good and wholesome for us to drink and use for all our worldly needs'. His own heart, by contrast, was like 'a foul cesspit that is made deep underground to receive the filth of the household', thereby concealing the unbearable stench within.[223] It was perhaps with similar thoughts in mind that in 1331 Bishop Burghersh of Lincoln offered an indulgence of forty days' remittance of penance to anyone who helped to pay for the conduit then being constructed by the Dominicans of Boston for the shared use of the townspeople.[224] In a more striking act of generosity Bishop Brown of Norwich promised £66 13s. 4d. to the chamberlains of Lynn, in 1444, so that they could pipe water from the east gate to the Tuesday market.[225] A learned man, he would have understood the appeal of aquatic similes to early Church fathers such as St Basil (d. *c.* 379), who sought

---

[218] Owen, *Making of King's Lynn*, pp. 324–30; KLBA, KL/C7/3, Hall Book, 1431–1450, fol. 189r. The executors of the former mayor John Asshenden gave £12 to the 1444 campaign in commemoration of the deceased (fol. 190r).

[219] J. A. F. Thomson, 'Piety and Charity in Late Medieval London', *Journal of Ecclesiastical History* 16 (1965), pp. 178–95, on pp. 187–8.

[220] See, for example, Pickett, 'Translation of the "Canutus" Plague Treatise', p. 273; Horrox, *Black Death*, p. 176.

[221] E. Duffy, *The Voices of Morebath* (New Haven, CT, 2003), p. 69.

[222] P. Hodgson and G. M. Liegey, eds, *The Orcherd of Syon*, vol. 1, EETS o.s. 258 (London, 1966), p. 68; Bernard of Clairvaux, 'In nativitate Beatae Virginis Mariae', in *Sermones de sanctis*, Patrologia Latina 183 (1854), cols 437–48.

[223] Henry of Lancaster, *Le Livre de seyntz medicines*, ed. E. J. Arnould (Oxford, 1940), pp. 226–7.

[224] Lincolnshire Archives Office, Register V (Burghersh), fol. 443r; Bond, 'Water Management', p. 57.

[225] Owen, *Making of King's Lynn*, p. 218. A third of this sum was later assigned for the repair of the south gates: KLBA, KL/C7/3, Hall Book, 1431–1450, fols 194v, 197r.

'to open the hearts of small town gentry so that the river of Christian charity might flow again from the doors of the rich into the hovels of the destitute'.[226]

The layout of London's earliest supply of piped water, which was carried from springs at Tyburn to an impressive 'great conduit' erected outside the hospital of St Thomas Acon in Cheapside during the second quarter of the thirteenth century, was certainly replete with spiritual symbolism. Dedicated to the martyred Thomas Becket and occupying the site of his birthplace, the hospital was an early manifestation of devotion to a rapidly burgeoning cult.[227] Pilgrims to Becket's shrine at Canterbury were, significantly, able to purchase *ampullae* of water allegedly containing droplets of his miraculous blood, and it may be that Londoners wished to harness some of this healing power by placing their own water supply under his protection.[228] Perhaps, too, they sought to create a model, however imperfect, of the celestial Jerusalem, where the river of the Holy Spirit issuing from God's throne

> Watz bryghter then bothe the sunne and mone.
> Sunne ne mone schon neuer so swete
> As that foysoun [copious] flode out of that flet;
> Swythe hit swange [swiftly it rushed] thurgh vch a strete
> Withouten fylthe other galle other glet [slime].[229]

Nor should we forget that giving drink to the thirsty figured among the seven fundamental acts of compassion, or Comfortable Works, which Christ expected his followers to perform in order to achieve salvation. During the later Middle Ages successful capitalists sought to evade – or at least shorten – their term in the fires of purgatory through the conspicuous discharge of these obligations. Attempts by the owners of certain Thames-side wharves to charge 'the poor common people' of London for the right to fetch water prompted a sharp response in 1417 from aldermen who were then investing heavily in civic amenities.[230] The contrast is remarkable. Having shortly afterwards commissioned a window depicting each of the Comfortable Works for St Bartholomew's hospital (whose impressive collection of relics was described as a 'welle of pyte ... and a streem and ryuer of helth and grace'), the executors of the celebrated London merchant Richard Whittington set about their systemic implementation for the benefit of ordinary citizens.[231] Prominent among the projects that were to secure his lasting reputation

---

[226] P. Brown, *The Body and Society: Men, Women and Sexual Renunciation in Early Christianity* (New York, 1988), p. 304.

[227] Keene suggests that, had convenience been the prime motive, the conduit would have been sited further west: 'Issues of Water', pp. 177–8.

[228] J. Alexander and P. Binski, eds, *Age of Chivalry: Art in Plantagenet England* (London, 1987), pp. 218–21.

[229] M. Andrew and R. Waldron, eds, *The Poems of the Pearl Manuscript: Pearl, Cleanness, Patience, Sir Gawain and the Green Knight* (London, 1978), p. 104.

[230] Riley, *Memorials of London*, p. 469.

[231] N. Kerling, ed., *The Cartulary of St Bartholomew's Hospital* (London, 1973), pp. 175–6. The hospital's relics are described in N. Moore, ed., *The Book of the Foundation of St Bartholomew's Church in London*, EETS o.s. 163 (London, 1923),

as a philanthropist were structural improvements designed to safeguard access to supplies of clean water at Paul's Wharf, Cripplegate and Billingsgate.[232] As we saw in the previous chapter, his executors also built a 'long house', or public privy, in Vintry ward with two rows of sixty-four seats (decently segregated by gender) for the use of Londoners. The gully over which it was constructed was flushed clean twice every day by the Thames, thus preventing the dangerous accumulation of miasmatic vapours.[233]

At about the same time Thomas Knolles (d. 1435), a wealthy grocer and sometime mayor of London, contracted with the master of St Bartholomew's hospital to convey surplus water from 'the cesterne nere to the common fountaine and chappell of Saint Nicholas (situate by the saide hospitall) to the gailes of Newgate, and Ludgate, for the reliefe of the prisoners'.[234] In spiritual as well as purely pragmatic terms this was a particularly effective form of charity, since, on the one hand, concern for those in prison was another of the Comfortable Works, while on the other, crowded, insanitary gaols were notorious breeding grounds for enteric disease. An analysis of coroners' certificates returned on prisoners who died in the Marshalsea, Southwark, between 1417 and 1509 reveals that a bare minimum of 375 individuals expired in custody during this period.[235] Although some verdicts are frustratingly imprecise, referring simply to 'divine visitation', at least sixty-seven of these unfortunates succumbed to pestilence, while no fewer than nineteen fell victim to an outbreak of 'flux' or dysentery between November 1468 and the following January. One is even said to have been shackled next to a cesspit, and thus to have been killed by constant exposure to corrupt air.[236] From the standpoint of its more affluent inmates, who could afford a few creature

pp. 12–14. Their power allegedly transformed the site of the hospital, which was initially 'right vncleene ... as a maryce [marsh], dunge and fenny, with water almost euerytyme habowndynge'.

[232] Stow, *Survey of London*, I.16, 208, 300–1; M. D. Lobel and W. H. Johns, *The City of London: From Prehistoric Times to c. 1520*, British Atlas of Historic Towns 3 (Oxford, 1989), p. 67. Whittington's other 'good works' are itemised in Stow, *Survey of London*, I.108–9.

[233] Jones, 'Whittington's Long House', pp. 27–34; and above p. 141.

[234] Stow, *Survey of London*, I.37; *CLB*, L, pp. 4, 130. Knolles laid the pipes at his own cost, that of repairs being assumed by the City after his death: N. J. Kerling, 'Notes on Newgate Prison', *TLMAS* 22 (1968–70), pp. 21–2. He also left £100 towards the discharge of debtors detained in these two prisons: Jacob, *Register of Henry Chichele*, p. 520.

[235] These figures derive from an unpublished paper on 'The Coroner of the King's Bench and Death in the Marshalsea of King's Bench', by Dr Hannes Kleineke, to whom I most grateful for sharing his research with me.

[236] According to *The Mirror of Justices*, it was illegal to house a prisoner who was awaiting trial 'among vermin or putrefaction', presumably because this seemed tantamount to a death sentence. In 1447, the keeper of Newgate was committed for nine days to his own goal for failing to remove the corpse of a prisoner, which would also have generated a lethal miasma: W. J. Whittaker, ed., *The Mirror of Justices*, Selden Society 7 (London, 1895), pp. 51–2; R. B. Pugh, *Imprisonment in Medieval England* (Cambridge, 1968), pp. 44, 331.

comforts, the Marshalsea was by no means the worst of London's prisons. Even the noisome environment of the Fleet seemed preferable to Newgate, which was so insalubrious that the justices of gaol delivery sometimes refused to hold sessions there for fear of infection.[237]

The deaths of sixty Newgate prisoners in 1315–16 may, in part, have been due to the desperate levels of famine and disease that blighted the entire country at this time, although it appears that the sewers were then badly in need of repair. Conditions had, if anything, deteriorated by 1414, when sixty-four inmates and the keeper expired.[238] The temporary closure of Ludgate, which housed debtors of higher status, and their removal in 1419 to 'the fetid and corrupt atmosphere that is the hateful gaol of Newgate', precipitated another epidemic. Perhaps because it killed their fellow citizens as well as hardened criminals, the rulers of London were finally spurred into action. Shocked by the 'sudden and terrible death that, on a daily basis', struck those incarcerated 'in the decaying and ruinous gate and gaol of Newgate, among the infected and corrupt air and other perils and horrible diseases', Richard Whittington left money to fund a complete rebuilding programme.[239] The new prison, which had opened its gates by 1432, was lighter, better ventilated, provided with an adequate number of privies and equipped with a drinking fountain, although it was Thomas Knolles who ensured that the water came from an uncontaminated source.[240]

Knolles and Whittington were not alone in their concern for London's water supply. The early sixteenth-century City's remarkable provision of fifteen conduits and cisterns, some elaborately crenellated with stone battlements, bears testimony to the importance of such works in the lexicon of civic fame, the names of their donors constituting a roll call of the late medieval elite and an even more effective means of commemorating the dead.[241] The most striking example of this quest for a lasting and useful memorial 'builded for the commoditie and honor of the citie' must surely relate to the aptly named mayor, John Wells (d. 1442), who orchestrated the campaign for the replacement and extension of London's ageing pipes, wellheads and conduit houses during the reign of Henry VI. The

---

[237] M. Bassett, 'Newgate Prison in the Middle Ages', *Speculum* 18 (1943), pp. 233–46, on p. 244. The problem was not confined to London. During the Cambridge assizes of 1522 several officials 'toke such an infeccion, whether it were of the savor of the prisoners, or of the filthe of the house, that manye gentle men … dyed, and all most all whiche were there present, were sore sicke': Cooper, *Annals of Cambridge*, p. 305.

[238] Bassett, 'Newgate Prison in the Middle Ages', p. 236; Pugh, *Imprisonment in Medieval England*, p. 331.

[239] Riley, *Memorials of London*, p. 677; H. Nicolas, ed., *Proceedings and Ordinances of the Privy Council of England*, 7 vols (London, 1834–7), III.79–80.

[240] Bassett, 'Newgate Prison in the Middle Ages', p. 239. Conditions soon deteriorated through lack of sustained investment.

[241] Lobel and Johns, *City of London*, pp. 67, 70, 74–5, 94, 97. Many Londoners left the residue of their estates, uncollected debts, or the reversion of property to the upkeep of the conduits. See, for example, *CEMCRL*, p. 112 (Katherine la Fraunceyse); *CWCHL*, II.218 (John Gille), 301 (John Clenhond), 307 (John Leycestre), 430 (William Est), 514 (John Costyn); and above p. 186 (John Walworth).

old 'standard', or wooden conduit house, in Cheapside was the site of one of the pageants staged in 1432 to welcome the young king on his formal entry into the City after being crowned in France. The aquatic theme of mercy, grace, and pity running as 'convenable welles moste holsom off saviour' was intended 'forto accorden with the meirys name', and no doubt to advertise his close personal involvement in schemes for urban improvement.[242] Following this very public triumph, the conduit was rebuilt in stone by his executors, its carved surround of 'wels imbraced by angels' and 'welles of paradys' clearly reflecting the testator's belief in the redemptive power of good works.[243] His example proved influential. When an assignment of £666 made in 1442 by the Common Council towards the cost of conveying water from 'diverse springes' in Paddington by 'pypes of leede' to a new conduit house in Fleet Street proved insufficient, Sir William Estfield (d. 1447) left enough money to complete this part of the project and to construct another conduit in Aldermanbury.[244] It has been estimated that, in all, the entire exercise must have entailed an expenditure of about £5,000, a significant part of which derived from private donors such as John Gedney (d. 1449), another former mayor, who alone promised over £130.[245]

However much we may speculate about the motives of these pious benefactors, there can be little doubt of their desire to protect and ameliorate the urban water supply. The inherent pragmatism of arrangements whose primary goal was the acquisition of spiritual merit is clearly apparent from a contract made in 1451 by Bishop Thomas Beckington of Bath with the burgesses of Wells. The latter were permitted to

> ... have a head for a water conduit with reservoirs, vents and other engines above and below ground, for taking and leading a portion of the bishop's water springing within the precinct of his palace at Wells ... upon a spot appointed by the said bishop, whereon he has built such a head at his own cost, sufficient for lead pipes 12 inches in circumference, with dikes, trenches, ponds, cisterns, etc, as well within the said precinct as in the public streets of the city, and power to repair the same, break ground and lay pipes, etc, so that the water may flow as far as the High Cross in the city market and other places as they shall think fit.[246]

The indenture specified in considerable detail the exact measurements and building materials of the new reservoir, or cistern, to be constructed by the bishop,

---

[242] Lydgate, *Minor Poems*, II.641–3; DeVries, 'And Away Go Troubles Down the Drain', pp. 401–18.

[243] Stow, *Survey of London*, I.17, 26, 265; II.251. Wells left £20 'ad renovacionem aqueductus et conductuum provisionem': Jacob, *Register of Henry Chichele*, p. 618.

[244] *CLB*, K, pp. l-li, 233, 355–7; Stow, *Survey of London*, I.109, 300; *CWCHL*, II.510.

[245] Barron, *London in the Later Middle Ages*, p. 256; Roskell, Clark and Rawcliffe, *Commons, 1386–1421*, III.172.

[246] HMC, *Dean and Chapter of Wells*, I.433 (I am grateful to Dr Christopher Bonfield for drawing this document to my attention). The burgesses had already begun to lay lead piping in 1448, perhaps in anticipation of the agreement: Shaw, *Creation of a Community*, pp. 132–3.

along with those of the other cisterns and pipes for which the burgesses undertook to pay. Arrangements for shared access to the conduit house were also ironed out, this being a matter of contention in some towns, such as Newcastle-upon-Tyne, where supplies were shared with the Franciscans.[247] Careful provision was also made for maintaining the reservoir, which was to be 'opened, inspected and cleansed every six months at least', so that any detritus could be flushed away in the bishop's mill stream. Being no less concerned about the environment in which he and his successors lived, Beckington claimed the right to divert all the water whenever the moat around his palace was being drained, scoured and refilled. In return, the burgesses promised that they would visit his tomb every year, in perpetuity, in order 'to render prayers for his soul', each of them being assured of forty days' remission of enjoined penance in return for his attendance. Notable for its preoccupation with the effective delivery of an essential public utility, this fascinating document also reflects the supernatural power of water – additionally blessed and protected by the High Cross – as an agent of spiritual cleansing and redemption.

We end, then, where we began, with a fruitful collaboration between secular and religious authorities for the provision of plentiful and readily accessible supplies of fresh water. Although arrangements of this kind sometimes proved unworkable, either because of technical problems or fraught relations, many laid the foundations for further investment and expansion on the part of the civic elite. That the purity as well as the availability of water mattered to the rulers and residents of late medieval English towns is apparent not only from the considerable sums of money expended on aqueducts, conduits, dikes, wells and gutters, but also the concerted efforts made to maintain them and keep them free from rubbish and pollution. And if, in the final resort, magistrates were all too often obliged to accept an uneasy compromise with the practitioners of noxious crafts and industries, they were, at least, generally determined to contain the worst offenders. In this regard, a combination of communal pride, economic necessity and religious belief went hand in hand with a steadily growing appreciation of the risks to health posed by contaminated water, which recurrent outbreaks of plague served graphically to reinforce. Similar considerations prompted a raft of measures concerning the food and alcoholic beverages on offer in markets, cook shops, alehouses and taverns, since it was here, in such potentially dangerous places, that further threats to both the human and the urban body so often lurked.

---

[247] Violence actually erupted over access to an enclosed well-head, whence the friars had permitted the townspeople to pipe their water: *CPR, 1340–1343*, p. 351; *CPR, 1343–1345*, pp. 412, 496.

✎ Chapter 5
Food and Drink

But it is not to be supposed that human constitutions in the Middle Ages were so unlike our own that men and women could with impunity go on for years devouring vast quantities of indigestible food without suffering serious consequences. Obviously, however, we cannot attribute every early death in the period we are discussing to immoderate indulgence in unwholesome food. There were innumerable unsuspected channels in the Middle Ages by which plague and fever and loathsome skin diseases could claim their victims among rich and poor. No one realized the dangers lurking in the feet of the common housefly, in dust, in over-kept food, in stale fish, and often even in clean water. The helplessness of our ancestors in the presence of diseases now almost entirely extirpated in civilized communities by means of intelligent sanitation is indeed one of the most striking differences between medieval times and our own.

William Edward Mead, *The English Medieval Feast* (1931)[1]

In chronicle, poem and legend the medieval city was characterised by its inexhaustible food supply and teeming markets. To a monastic author such as Lucianus of Chester, these very markets, strategically positioned at the centre of the urban landscape, symbolised the birth of Christ *in medio orbis* and the promise of an eternal, superabundant source of heavenly bread.[2] But it was hard to concentrate upon spiritual nourishment in the face of so much earthly temptation. William Fitz Stephen's celebrated description of London in the reign of Henry II dwells lovingly on the delights of 'a public cook-shop' (*publica coquina*), conveniently situated on the banks of the Thames near the vintners' cellars, where patrons could purchase a robust draught of wine to accompany a steaming joint or capon. Here, he boasts, 'you may find food according to the season, dishes of meat, roast, fried and boiled, large and small fish, coarser meats for the poor and more delicate for the rich, such as venison and big and small birds'.[3] However refined or fastidious one's palate, he adds, there will be plenty to satisfy it. Contemporary Paris likewise offered the traveller a mouth-watering selection of comestibles, from 'spiced pasties, filled with chopped pork, chicken or eel' to meltingly soft cheese tarts and crisp waffles.[4] Even Oswestry, according to a fifteenth-century panegyric, could rival London's Cheapside in the range, exoticism and luxury of the dainties on display, with spices such as cumin, jostling for space beside 'beer and sugar in a mulled-wine castle, comfits and pomegranates'.[5]

---

[1] W. E. Mead, *The English Medieval Feast* (London, 1931), p. 215.

[2] Lucanius of Chester, *Liber Luciani*, p. 47.

[3] Douglas and Greenway, *EHD, 1042–1189*, p. 1026. The Latin original may be found in Stow, *Survey of London*, II.222–3.

[4] Carlin, 'Fast Food', p. 29.

[5] T. Gwynn Jones, ed., *Gwaith Tudur Aled*, 2 vols (Cardiff, 1926), I, no. lxv, lines 61–4, 89–90.

Harsh reality was, of course, somewhat different. Recent research suggests that the Thames-side cook-shop or shops so eloquently described by Fitz Stephen catered for low-status travellers and boatmen rather than the City's wealthy gourmets.[6] And, however rough the clientele may have been, there were still many for whom any type of hot food represented an unusual and costly indulgence. In one late fourteenth-century satire a poor rustic trudging the streets of London is assailed at every turn by a tantalising variety of aromas and enticing foodstuffs, including 'hot peascods', 'strabery rype and chery in the ryse', 'hot shepes fete', 'ribes of befe and many a pie', none of which he can afford with his single penny.[7] It is clearly difficult, if not impossible, to generalise about urban diets, which ranged, at different times and in different places, from the extremes of privation apparent during the famine years of the early fourteenth century to the conspicuous excess of fifteenth-century guild feasts and civic ceremonies.[8]

The striking improvements in nutrition which Christopher Dyer has observed in England after the Black Death were, moreover, far from uniform, since in most towns and cities a significant – sometimes substantial – number of men and women, often elderly, sick or otherwise incapacitated, continued to live on or below the breadline. Although distressing events such as the death of fifty-one paupers in a stampede for alms at the London Blackfriars in 1322 were by then a distant memory, many people still teetered precariously on the brink of hunger.[9] It has been suggested that up to one fifth of the population of late medieval Wells may have been dependent upon handouts of food or cash at any given time, while approximately a quarter of households in Coventry faced considerable hardship by the second decade of the sixteenth century.[10] Such people relied upon the ruling elite not simply for charitable relief during periods of dearth, as occurred during the 1430s and 1520s, but also for the regulation of markets to prevent the rampant

---

[6] Carlin, 'Fast Food', pp. 29–30.

[7] 'London Lyckpenny', in X. Baron, ed., *London, 1066–1914: Literary Sources and Documents*, vol. 1: *Medieval, Tudor, Stuart and Georgian London, 1066–1800* (Mountfield, 1997), pp. 88–91.

[8] Phythian-Adams, *Desolation of a City*, pp. 110, 263–4; G. Rosser, 'Going to the Fraternity Feast: Commensality and Social Relations in Later Medieval England', *Journal of British Studies* 30 (1994), pp. 430–46; Schofield, *London, 1100–1600*, pp. 102–4. A typical 'breakfast' given in 1448 by the mayor and aldermen of Norwich for the justices of gaol delivery and the sheriff and escheator of Norfolk involved the purchase of, *inter alia*: nine gallons of red wine, twenty-seven gallons of ale, three swans, six cygnets, six geese, four suckling pigs, ten capons, twelve rabbits, a peacock, a calf, four quarters of lamb and five of mutton, six marrow bones, thirty-one chickens and 200 eggs. If it did not entirely accord with the recommendations of the *Regimen sanitatis*, it certainly constituted a powerful statement of civic pride: *RCN*, II.72.

[9] C. Dyer, *Standards of Living in the Later Middle Ages*, rev. edn (Cambridge, 1998), chap. 7; *CCRCL*, p. 61; W. Stubbs, ed., *Chronicles of the Reigns of Edward I and Edward II*, 2 vols, RS 76 (London, 1882–3), I.304.

[10] Shaw, *Creation of a Community*, pp. 228–48; Phythian-Adams, *Desolation of a City*, pp. 131–4.

profiteering and sale of inferior produce to which the underprivileged so often fell victim.

On the other hand, many town-dwellers achieved partial self-sufficiency by keeping gardens or suburban small-holdings for the cultivation of the herbs, fruit and vegetables that formed a significant part of their diet. In some provincial towns, such as Colchester, many residents pursued rural occupations involving livestock husbandry and the production of crops in the surrounding countryside.[11] And within the walls, a modest plot or backyard alone sufficed to accommodate the pigs and poultry whose impact upon the urban environment has already been explored. Yet even these more fortunate individuals depended heavily upon external suppliers for their food and drink, the delivery of which, often over long distances, not only posed a range of logistical and economic problems but also many potential threats to collective health.[12] The provision of adequate as well as wholesome food at prices that ordinary men and women could afford was essential for the survival and proper function of the entire community, it being the task of magistrates to maintain a careful balance between deprivation and gluttony. While ensuring that every limb and organ received appropriate sustenance, they had to prevent any from becoming overfed, bloated or suffused with malignant humours. In this respect, as in so many others, they were expected to devise and implement a regimen for the welfare of the urban body.

5.1 Medical beliefs

Although they strike a familiar note with today's readers, who are accustomed to a battery of measures relating to food safety, many of the earliest dietary regulations adopted in medieval England were more concerned with the avoidance of ritual pollution than the preservation of human health. Ecclesiastical prohibitions on the consumption of blood, of the flesh of 'unclean' animals and of beasts that had been found dead, along with anything that was either half-cooked or spoiled, constituted a reaction against pagan practices, as well as a reiteration of biblical taboos.[13] Whatever practical benefits may have derived from these rulings were incidental to their primary purpose, notwithstanding the fact that some probably helped to improve standards of hygiene, while also protecting against illness or even death. The conviction, explicitly stated in the Penitential of Archbishop Theodore (d. 690), that holy water would effectively disinfect food or drink contaminated by dung or other disgusting substances reflects this scale of values, as do the harsh penalties imposed on monks who consumed anything touched by a pregnant woman or sexually active man.[14] Mary Douglas's strictures concerning the 'medical materialists' who are inclined to regard Moses as 'an enlightened

---

[11] Britnell, *Growth and Decline in Colchester*, pp. 16–17.

[12] R. Britnell, 'The Economy of British Towns, 600–1300', and 'The Economy of British Towns, 1300–1540', both in *CUHB1*, pp. 116–17, and pp. 322–3, respectively.

[13] A. Hagen, *A Second Handbook of Anglo-Saxon Food and Drink* (Hockwold cum Wilton, 1995), pp. 187–94.

[14] J. T. McNeill and H. M. Gamer, eds, *Medieval Hand-Books of Penance* (New York, 1965), pp. 121, 191.

public health administrator, rather than a spiritual leader', seem particularly apt in this context, since, in accordance with the prescriptions set out in the Old Testament book of Leviticus, the aim of such rules was to preserve physical purity and prevent defilement.[15] The power of these beliefs remained strong, and traces of them may still be detected in some of the late medieval regulations discussed in the following pages.

Even so, an awareness of the *physiological* importance of diet and food hygiene became increasingly common from the twelfth century onwards. Reflecting this trend, the great rabbinical scholar and physician Moses Maimonides (d. 1204) sought to explain the numerous dietary prohibitions imposed by Mosaic Law in terms of the 'injurious character' and 'unwholesomeness' of the items in question. Being schooled in the work of Classical Greek and Islamic medical authorities, he thought in terms of humoral imbalance rather than bacterial infection, as we would today, but his approach was based upon the same 'rationalist' assumption that most foodstuffs must initially have been deemed taboo because of their propensity to cause sickness. Having first observed that pork was 'more humid than is proper' and replete with 'superfluous matter', he went on to stress that the pigs which rooted happily in the streets of European cities were filthy animals liable to spread disease:

> Now if swine were used [by the Hebrews] for food, market places and even houses would have been dirtier than their latrines, as may be seen in the present day in the country of the Franks ... The fat of the intestines, too, makes us full, spoils the digestion and produces cold and thick blood. It is more suitable to burn it. Blood ... and carcasses of beasts that have died ... are also difficult to digest and constitute a harmful nourishment.[16]

Occupying pride of place in medical texts from the Hippocratic corpus onwards, diet was not only regarded as 'the first instrument of medicine', but also as the principal means of preserving health.[17] It was, as we have seen, from food that humoral matter was created, and from it that the most potentially life-threatening imbalances arose.[18] The body's ability to withstand external assaults, most notably by the miasmatic vapours of pestilential air, was, moreover, dependent upon its internal equilibrium. For this reason many of the most popular medieval *regimina* concentrated heavily on the *ars diaetae*, providing lengthy guides to the cultivation of physical fitness through careful attention to the consumption of appropriate food and drink, often with specific regard to the age, gender and circumstances of the individual.[19]

---

[15] M. Douglas, *Purity and Danger: An Analysis of the Concepts of Pollution and Taboo* (London, 1994), p. 30.

[16] Moses Maimonides, *The Guide of the Perplexed*, ed. and trans. S. Pines (Chicago, 1963), p. 598.

[17] M. Grant, ed. and trans., *Galen on Food and Diet* (London, 2000), *passim*.

[18] See pp. 55–6 above.

[19] For the preponderance of advice about food in medieval *regimina*, see Nicoud, *Régimes de santé*, I, chap. 10; M. W. Adamson, *Medieval Dietetics: Food and Drink in the Regimen Sanitatis Literature, 800–1400* (Frankfurt, 1995). For a survey of the

The need to follow a carefully balanced diet (as understood at the time) was axiomatic in royal and aristocratic households, where cooks would routinely collaborate with resident medical staff when planning and preparing meals. The celebrated Middle English recipe collection known as *The Forme of Cury* was, for example, compiled by Richard II's 'chef maister cokes' with the specific 'assent and auysement' of his physicians.[20] One of the principal, and almost certainly most invidious, tasks of Edward IV's *medici* was likewise to recommend the 'metes or drinkes ... best according with the kynges dyet' and to ensure that the notoriously self-indulgent royal gourmand restricted his intake of rich and unsuitable foodstuffs.[21] Although advice of this kind, precisely tailored to suit the requirements of wealthy and powerful patrons, clearly lay beyond the reach of most people, by the early fifteenth century the Galenic equation of 'moderate diete' with health was sufficiently well known as to be noted by the compiler of Faversham's First Town Book alongside transcripts of charters and borough customs.[22] Short vernacular guides, based upon the principles of the *regimen sanitatis*, enjoyed growing popularity among the urban elite. One representative manual, authoritatively entitled the *Dieta Ypocras* (as personally devised by the great physician for 'kynge Cesar'), explained how best to temper one's diet in accordance with the seasonal changes that might so easily cause illness. In spring, for instance, the reader was urged to 'ete not the felsche of yonge swine, but ... moton, lambes & folwis that be norischid in drye & clene places' in order to purify the blood. By the same token, the consumption of heavy wine and hot food in summer seemed inadvisable, especially as it would open the pores to corrupt air.[23]

Another 'nobylle treatise of medysyns for mannys body' may be found in a commonplace book kept by the anonymous London citizen who completed the chronicle generally ascribed to the skinner William Gregory (d. 1467). He also chose to record poems on 'bloode latynge' and 'the wisdom of physicians', which, significantly, appear together with a list of the standard measures for bread and ale then enforced in the City.[24] Concentrating heavily on the need to adopt a sparing but wholesome diet, the 'nobylle treatise' warned against the long-term consequences of consuming 'euyll metes', which would eventually undermine even the strongest constitution:

> And soo euery day they ordayne hym selfe to the sekenys, or vnto soden deythe, as they that longe tyme vsyn beffe old saltyd as powdering [seasoning], as sum men vsyn ... for hyt kylle moo men in tyme of processe thenne I can vnterly determine, and bestely flesshe and rawe flesche ... and

period 1470 to 1650, see K. Alaba, *Eating Right in the Renaissance* (Berkeley, CA, 2002).

[20] C. B. Hieatt and S. Butler, eds, *Curye On Inglysch: English Culinary Manuscripts of the Fourteenth Century*, EETS s.s. 8 (London, 1985), p. 20. Nicoud stresses the attention to culinary matters in *regimina* produced for monarchs and aristocrats: *Régimes de santé*, I.126–35, 171–5.

[21] A. R. Myers, ed., *The Household of Edward IV* (Manchester, 1959), pp. 123–4.

[22] Harrington and Hyde, *Early Town Books of Faversham*, p. 60.

[23] Trinity College, Cambridge, MS R.14.32, fols 81r–82r.

[24] BL, MS Egerton 1995, fols 79r–81v.

many moo othyr suche. Hyt may be sayde but [unless] hyt ys lefte they schalle not a starte [escape] the stroke when hit comythe.[25]

The longstanding belief that medieval food was 'smothered in spices' to disguise the taste and smell of rotten meat or fish merits little serious consideration.[26] Writing about the cattle plague of 1319–20, when the market was glutted with cheap meat from infected animals, the chronicler John de Trokelowe reported that 'there was none among men who would dare to taste bovine flesh, lest perchance they might succumb, poisoned by their carrion'.[27] Contaminated foodstuffs, especially rancid oil or lard, fly-blown pork and rotten fish, seemed particularly dangerous because of their capacity to engender disease. Initially voiced by medical experts, the conviction that leprosy might develop in a vulnerable individual through the consumption of 'corrupt mete, and of mete that is sone corrupt, as of mesel [leprous] swynes fleische that hath pesen [eggs or lumps] therinne', was widespread by the fourteenth century.[28] The propensity of pork to exhibit the 'measly' spots and tubercules characteristic of leprosy was blamed upon the irregular reproductive cycle of mature sows, whose flesh was deemed unsafe for the table. As a further precaution the slaughtering of pigs and sale of their meat might be entirely prohibited in summer.[29] For this reason, the authors of medical texts and advice manuals cautioned anyone who suffered from skin problems to exercise particular care with regard to the risks posed by tainted pork ('ex carne porcina granulis infecta et superseminata').[30] Indeed, literature of this kind is suffused with more general warnings about 'malice of metes', 'quasy mettes', 'trypes & podynges & all inwards of bestes' and 'leprouse fyshes'.[31]

Comparatively few individuals were, however, able to pick and choose what they ate. Since the urban poor often had little alternative but to purchase the cheapest and most unsavoury items available, responsibility for policing markets and punishing unscrupulous traders lay squarely at the door of the ruling elite.

---

[25] BL, MS Egerton 1995, fol. 74r. The belief that a poor diet would cause problems in later life derives from Ibn-Sīna: Shah, *Avicenna's Canon of Medicine*, pp. 187, 313. Medieval physicians reiterated this warning: see, for example, H. P. Cholmeley, *John of Gaddesden and The Rosa Medicinae* (Oxford, 1912), p. 66.

[26] C. B. Hieatt, 'Making Sense of Medieval Culinary Records', in Carlin and Rosenthal, *Food and Eating*, pp. 101–2.

[27] Johannis de Trokelowe, *Chronica et annales*, ed. H. T. Riley, RS 28.3 (London, 1866), p. 105.

[28] *OPT*, I.426; Rawcliffe, *Leprosy in Medieval England*, pp. 78–80.

[29] C. Fabre-Vassas, *The Singular Beast: Jews, Christians and the Pig* (New York, 1997), pp. 55–6, 106; *BTD*, pp. 25, 129. In Yarmouth butchers were fined for selling pork out of season (NRO, Y/C4/116, rot. 17r), while in Northampton they had to obtain a warrant of 'clennes' from the producer (Markham, *Liber custumarum*, p. 35).

[30] BL, MS Sloane 282, fol. 129v. See also MS Sloane 5, fols 153r–155r; MS Harley 3, fol. 23.

[31] Guy de Chauliac, *The Cyrurgie of Guy de Chauliac*, ed. M. S. Ogden, EETS o.s. 265 (Oxford, 1971), p. 378; BL, MS Harley 1736, fol. 183r–v; Andrew Boorde, *A Compendyous Regyment or a Dyetary of Healthe* (London, 1547), sig. Iiir; Boorde, *Breviary of Helthe*, fols 10v–11r.

As we shall see, most late medieval borough courts made strenuous efforts to deal with the problem, threatening those victuallers who knowingly endangered public health with increasingly heavy fines and a variety of humiliating punishments. The imaginative rituals employed with telling effect in London, where a baker found guilty of fraudulent or insanitary practices might be 'drawn upon a hurdle from the Guildhall to his own house, through the great streets where there may be most people assembled, and through the midst of the great streets that are most dirty, with the faulty loaf hanging from his neck', both shamed the offender and warned the public to take its custom elsewhere.[32] In some cases the culprit would be subject to the further indignity of a paper crown, like that worn by the butcher John Pyntard in 1517. Spectators who could not read the legend inscribed on it – 'for puttyng to sale of mesell and stynkyn bacon' – would have been enlightened by the official who marched before him banging a bowl and, of course, by the maggot-ridden meat attached to his person.[33] Even an hour in the pillory could result in significant losses, as well as personal injury, for a dishonest fishmonger, butcher or dairywoman like Agnes Deyntee, whose carefully packaged churns concealed 'corrupte and olde butter not wholesome for mannys body'.[34] The fact that goods like these must also have seemed 'unclean' and 'polluted' served further to highlight the moral dimensions of the offence.[35]

From the thirteenth century onwards, the presentments made by urban juries reflect a desire to improve standards, prompted in part by royal intervention. In 1275 Edward I initiated a wide-ranging *Composicio*, or synthesis, of measures concerning the quality, inspection and availability of basic foodstuffs which, *inter alia*, imposed heavy penalties on the vendors of 'swines flesh meazled or flesh dead of the murrain'.[36] English provincial towns rapidly fell into line. Between 1287 and 1289 alone the leets of Norwich drew attention to four sellers of infected bacon ('baconem superseminatam') and two of 'measly' pork, four dealers in the flesh of dead animals passed off as sound, seven retailers of unwholesome veal, and 'all those Sprowston men', who sold contaminated pork, along with sausages and puddings unfit for human consumption ('non necessarias corporibus hominum'). They indicted two individuals for attempting to retail meat from beasts that had been ritually slaughtered by Jews and already condemned as unfit, and another

---

[32] *MGL*, III.83; G. Seabourne, 'Assize Matters: Regulation of the Price of Bread in Medieval London', *Journal of Legal History* 27 (2006), pp. 29–52, on pp. 43–51.

[33] Jones, *Butchers of London*, pp. 132–3.

[34] Agnes was sentenced by the mayor of London in 1476 to stand for an hour below the pillory with some of this rancid butter hanging round her neck, before being expelled from the City: *CLB*, L, p. 141; Kingsford, *Chronicles of London*, p. 187. Offenders were also punished with imprisonment and forfeiture; since confiscated bread was customarily sent to Newgate, a convicted baker might end up consuming his own loaves: Riley, *Memorials of London*, pp. 38–9, 122.

[35] Horden, 'Ritual and Public Health', p. 29.

[36] *SR*, vol. 1, 51 Henry III, p. 203. The *Composicio* has been convincingly dated by R. H. Britnell, '*Forstall*, Forestalling, and the Statute of Forestallers', *EHR* 102 (1987), pp. 89–102, on p. 94.

whose meat was putrid and badly salted ('putridas et male salsatas'). In addition, at least eighteen of the city's cooks and pasty-makers were fined 6*d.* each for reheating their wares for two or three days in succession, while a victualler named Adam de Cabel stood accused of mixing good and bad whelks together.[37] As time passed and the enormity of such offences became even more apparent, the penalties rose. In late fifteenth-century Yarmouth, butchers who sold 'leprous meat [*carnes leprositate infectas*] to the grave peril of the people' faced fines of 20*s.*, which was about fifteen times more than the current amercement for assault, and equivalent to the securities generally demanded of prostitutes and suspect lepers as an earnest of their readiness to leave the town.[38] It was at this time, too, that Leicester's 'flesh sayers', or inspectors of the shambles, were ordered to examine all meat 'that it be not takket [spotted] with pok, moreyn, mesell [leprosy] ne non other contagious syknes ne defaulte'.[39]

The disconcerting late medieval practice of donating substandard meat to the sick poor, and especially to the leprous, would have seemed perfectly humane in light of the belief that anyone who was already riddled with disease could eat it with impunity. From at least the early fourteenth century, the rulers of York allocated 'any measly meat' confiscated in the city markets to local *leprosaria*, while Scottish borough custom likewise decreed that 'corrupt pork and salmon' seized in similar circumstances should be assigned 'without any question' to lepers.[40] The inmates of St Giles's hospital, Maldon, traditionally claimed the right to all forfeitures of 'bread and ale and of unsound meat and fish' made in the town, and those of St John's, Oxford, to 'all flesh or fish that shall be putrid,

---

[37] Hudson, *Leet Jurisdiction*, pp. 6–32. In thirteenth-century Bristol buying meat from Jews ranked alongside the sale of 'measled pork or fish murrain' as an offence for which cooks and butchers incurred, successively, a fine, the pillory and imprisonment or expulsion, as specified in the *Composicio* of 1275. Sanitary considerations apart, *trepha* was considered inappropriate food for Christians: *LRBB*, II.218.

[38] NRO, Y/C4/186, rot. 15r. In York the fine for selling 'messyll swine' stood at 8*s.* in 1522, in contrast to sums of 6*d.* and 10*d.* paid in the previous year by butchers who sold veal that was unfit for human consumption: York City Archives, Chamberlains' Book 2, 1520–1525, fols 50v, 91r.

[39] *RBL*, II.321–2. Similar rules obtained in Sandwich from 1301 (BL, MS Cotton Julius B IV, fol. 75v), in Lynn from the 1460s (KLBA, KL/C7/4, Hall Book, 1453–1497, p. 169), and in Gloucester from 1500 (HMC, *Twelfth Report*, appendix 9, p. 433). The clerk of the market in Northampton was required to search for 'mesell hogges' and other substandard meat (*RBN*, I.373, and also 336–7). Salmon that was 'leper or ellys vnholsom for man is bodi' was specifically banned in fifteenth-century Bristol, alongside 'meselle porke': Veale, *Great Red Book of Bristol*, I.141, 143.

[40] *YCO*, p. 13; T. Thomson and C. Innes, eds, *The Acts of the Parliament of Scotland*, 12 vols (Edinburgh, 1844–75), II.729. Northampton butchers who sold 'sussemy flessh', the flesh of dead goats, the heads of sheep or calves, or 'suche manere of fowle thynges' risked the pillory; the confiscated meat was assigned to the 'seke men of seynt Leonardis', a suburban leper house: Markham, *Liber custumarum*, p. 36.

unclean, vicious or otherwise unfit'.[41] Similar regulations obtained in Ipswich, where arrangements were also made for the public display of unwholesome fish or meat on a table below the pillory, no doubt in order to allow hospital proctors the opportunity to acquire it for their charges. Any butcher, poulterer or fishmonger who offered such 'wikkid flessh' for sale elsewhere faced an escalating series of punishments culminating in the loss of trading rights for an entire year.[42]

As knowledge of the principles of contagion spread, people became increasingly nervous about the contamination of public displays of food and drink. In 1473, for example, the Norwich Assembly ruled that henceforward servants who bought supplies for the city's *leprosaria* should not touch any food in the markets with their hands, but only with a stick, those butchers or fishmongers who turned a blind eye being punishable at the discretion of the mayor.[43] Even greater concern arose over the health of the retailers themselves. An allegedly leprous married couple were ordered to leave Colchester in 1366 because they threatened public safety by roaming the marketplace, 'selling and buying victuals, and especially geese and capons'.[44] Unprecedented efforts by the rulers of London to expel a leper named John Mayn six years later cannot have been unconnected with the fact that he was a baker; far more explicit are the securities of £100 demanded from an Exeter merchant in 1428 as a guarantee that his diseased wife would remove herself within five weeks and immediately cease brewing and selling ale.[45] By then the merest suspicion of leprosy was enough to cause a dramatic loss of custom, with the result that smear tactics were sometimes deployed by unscrupulous victuallers to sabotage their competitors. A case of defamation brought in 1413 by Christine Colmere, an alewife from Canterbury, illustrates the devastating effects of such allegations on someone who was apparently 'healthy and clean ... without disfigurement', while also revealing the depth of anxieties that could so easily be exploited.[46]

An excessively rich, heavy or unwholesome diet not only exacerbated the type of acute humoral imbalance that led to leprosy and other chronic diseases, but also made the individual more vulnerable to the assault of miasmatic vapours. So too did extreme deprivation. That serious food shortages were often followed by

---

[41] *CIMisc, 1399–1402*, p. 102, no. 206; *CCR, 1402–1405*, pp. 17–18; G. G. Coulton, *Medieval Panorama* (Cambridge, 1939), pp. 455–6. Infected or 'unsesynable' fish confiscated in London markets was, like bread, dispatched to Newgate prison: *CLB*, D, p. 199.

[42] Twiss, *Black Book of the Admiralty*, II.104–5, 146–7.

[43] NRO, NCR, 16D/1, Assembly Proceedings, 1434–1491, fol. 95v. Previously, in 1430–1, a Yarmouth jury had insisted that Katherine Colkirke, the wife of a known leper, should not touch victuals in the marketplace; she was bound over in securities of 6s. 8d. to comply: NRO, Y/C4/139, rot. 12v.

[44] I. H. Jeayes, ed., *Court Rolls of the Borough of Colchester*, 3 vols (Colchester, 1938–41), II.185.

[45] Rawcliffe, *Leprosy in Medieval England*, pp. 22–3, 281.

[46] R. H. Helmholz, ed., *Select Cases on Defamation to 1600*, Selden Society 101 (London, 1985), pp. 5–6. J. M. Bennett argues that alewives were particularly vulnerable to such slurs: *Ale, Beer and Brewsters in England: Women's Work in a Changing World* (Oxford, 1996), pp. 135–6.

epidemics seemed axiomatic, since a starving body would more readily absorb, or even draw into itself, 'the stinking commixed vapours of the air'.[47] Responding in October 1348 to a royal command for an enquiry into the causes of the plague then raging throughout Europe, experts from the medical faculty of the University of Paris observed that 'major pestilential illnesses' were often caused by contaminated food, especially 'at times of famine and infertility'. And although the principal agent on this particular occasion was undoubtedly atmospheric, diet remained a key factor in determining levels of resistance. In short, anyone who overindulged or went hungry, rather than adopting 'a sensible and suitable regimen', was playing with fire, since he or she would be more susceptible to infection.[48] In the 'nedefull and necessarie' treatise 'ayenst the pestilens' that he produced specifically for a 'lewde' readership in about 1475, Friar Thomas Multon employed – or more accurately redeployed – this very metaphor to explain why some people fell sick while others, who breathed the very same air, escaped unscathed:

> Ye se wel and wete wel that the element of fire has non dominacion, ne wil not bren [burn] but in mater that is combustible and according to receyue fire. On the same wise, the element of the aier that is pestilence corrupt infecte nother man, nother woman, ne childe, but siche that hath venemes and corrupt humours within hemself.[49]

On the one hand, the 'vnkyndely hete' generated during such a volcanic digestive process would open the pores, thereby allowing 'venomous ayere' easy access to the veins and arteries, while on the other the noxious matter arising from so much unsuitable food and drink would make common cause with the invading miasmas as they surged towards the stronghold of the heart. Put more simply, in the words of another vernacular plague tract, 'full many for defaute of gud gouernance in dietynge falles in this sekenes, thare-fore that tyme vse none excesse nor surfete in mete & drynke'.[50]

In his aptly entitled *Dietary and Doctrine for Pestilence* John Lydgate also stressed the importance of consuming 'good wyn' and 'holsom metes', while taking care to avoid any 'gret flessh' or other unsavoury items.[51] As the self-proclaimed enemy of dishonest victuallers (who, in his opinion, deserved to be pelted with rotten eggs), he would certainly have approved of the sentence imposed on one Norwich butcher for selling beef and mutton that were pronounced 'measly, bad and putrid through age' in the aftermath of the Black Death. Having been sent

---

[47] Slack, *Impact of Plague*, p. 28.

[48] Horrox, *Black Death*, pp. 160–3.

[49] BL, MS Sloane 3489, fol. 45v. Multon is paraphrasing John of Burgundy, who in turn draws on the work of Galen: Keiser, 'Two Medieval Plague Treatises', pp. 209–311.

[50] Ogden, *Liber de diversis medicinis*, p. 51. For other versions of this text, see Keiser, *Works of Science and Information*, pp. 3662–5, 3856–7.

[51] Lydgate, *Minor Poems*, II.702. A few authorities maintained that 'hot food and fumous drink' offered the best defence against infection (Horrox, *Black Death*, pp. 101, 179), but the overwhelming weight of medical opinion favoured an abstemious and cooling diet: Arrizabalaga, 'Facing the Black Death', pp. 277–8.

first to prison and then the pillory, as the law required, he was obliged to inhale the fumes of his rancid wares as they were burnt beneath him.[52] The London cook who sold two pies containing 'putrid and stinking' capons to Henry Pecche and his friends shortly afterwards, 'to the scandal, contempt and disgrace of all the city and the manifest peril of the life of the same Henry and his companions', met a similar fate, the shameful evidence being ceremonially carried before him on his journey to the pillory, where the nature of his crime was loudly proclaimed to the jeering crowds. Unscrupulous hucksters found guilty of contravening new measures against the sale of 'poultry that is rotten or stinking or not proper for man's body', were likewise made into a common spectacle.[53] This type of exemplary punishment was not unprecedented, although it was, understandably, more often imposed in the aftermath of epidemics, as well as during periods of dearth, when good quality meat became scarce.[54] At such times the need for a powerful display of authority on the part of the ruling elite became especially important, with the result that the ritual of public humiliation served both a political and a sanitary purpose.[55]

Because the *smell* of food constituted such a reliable indicator of quality and freshness, it is hardly surprising that so many of these presentments, as well as the regulations that had been contravened, refer to the stench of suspect items.[56] But we should also bear in mind that the miasmatic odours arising from tainted food posed a serious threat to communal health long before it ever reached the table. One of the first decrees enacted in Venice when the Black Death struck in 1348 was for the incineration of infected pork, 'which creates a great stench and attendant putrefaction that corrupts the air'.[57] Ordinances passed by the mayor and aldermen of London in 1363 (not long after the second national outbreak of plague) specifically warned victuallers against retaining any goods until they became 'corrupt and stinking', upon pain of a spell in the pillory, with the additional threat of the evidence in question being burnt beneath them.[58]

[52] Hudson, *Leet Jurisdiction*, p. 80. For a similar case of 1348, involving the sale of meat from a sow found dead in a London ditch, see Riley, *Memorials of London*, pp. 240–1. For Lydgate's trenchant views, see Lydgate, *Minor Poems*, II.448–9.

[53] Riley, *Memorials of London*, pp. 270–1, 299–300, 328, 389, 448–9.

[54] As was the case throughout the famine years and murrains of the early fourteenth century: Sabine, 'Butchering in Mediaeval London', pp. 337–8; Riley, *Memorials of London*, pp. 132–3, 139–40.

[55] DeVries, 'And Away Go Troubles Down the Drain', pp. 407–8.

[56] See, for example, Riley, *Memorials of London*, p. 464 ('two pieces of cooked fish commonly called *congre*, rotten and stinking and unwholesome for man'); NRO, NCR, 16A/2, Mayor's Court Book, 1510–1532, p. 11 ('stynkyng makerelles', 'stynkyng saltforth herynges'); 16A/4, Mayor's Court Book, 1534–1549, fol. 51v (sausages 'corrupt & stynkyng & not holsom ffor mannes body'); Twiss, *Black Book of the Admiralty*, II.144–7 ('flessh of morreyn, stynkkyng').

[57] C. M. Cipolla, *Public Health and the Medical Profession in the Renaissance* (Cambridge, 1976), p. 11.

[58] Riley, *Memorials of London*, pp. 312–13. The authorities were also afraid that traders would stockpile goods in order to increase prices during food shortages: see section 5.9 below.

So anxious were 'certain reputable men of the trade of fishmongers' to protect 'their own good name and that of the said trade', that they reported one Solomon Salaman to the mayor of London in 1390 simply for warehousing several barrels of 'rotten and unwholesome' salted eels. Further inspection disclosed such a foul smell that the entire consignment had to be buried outside the walls 'lest the air might become infected from the stench arising there from'. Since Salaman had compounded his offence by dumping some of this 'stinking and rotten' fish down a well near Cripplegate, the fishmongers were understandably keen to distance themselves from the chorus of blame that ensued.[59]

Fish was one of the principal components of the national diet, along with meat, bread, ale and (increasingly) beer. As we shall see in the next four sections of this chapter (5.2–5), official attention focussed upon the victuallers who sold these essential commodities, and upon the many cooks who catered for the urban workforce. The proliferation of bye-laws relating to provenance, storage, cost and quality testifies to the dedication with which the authorities discharged their responsibilities.[60] Even in years of plenty, when harvests were good, flocks healthy and catches prolific, the scale of the challenge was daunting, given the problems of preserving perishable foodstuffs in an age before refrigeration, and of transporting heavy goods in sufficient quantities at a time when long distance carriage was slow, cumbersome and costly. The number of individuals, both resident and 'foreign', involved in the victualling trades further compounded the problem. It has, for instance, been estimated that up to a third of the men and women of known occupation in late fourteenth-century Exeter were employed in this capacity, over and above an indeterminate but considerable number of part-timers.[61] Moreover, the wholesomeness of the food and drink on sale in shops, taverns and markets was not simply a matter of public health, but also of collective *repute*, since the inability to safeguard denizens and visitors from the worst abuses reflected just as badly on a community as blocked drains and dirty streets.

The rulers of London were predictably keen to avoid the 'scandal and disgrace' caused by fraudulent victuallers whose unsavoury practices threatened to spread disorder as well as disease.[62] They, and other urban magistrates, were well aware that their sometimes tenuous hold on power depended upon the availability and fair pricing of basic necessities, the lack of which might easily prove a catalyst for discontent.[63] As the leading citizens of Norwich warned when petitioning the crown for an extension of their judicial powers in 1378, the lesser orders were likely

---

[59] Riley, *Memorials of London*, pp. 516–18.

[60] Kermode, 'Greater Towns, 1300–1540', p. 455.

[61] Swanson, *Medieval Artisans*, chap. 2; Kowaleski, *Local Markets*, pp. 129–32. In Norwich at least one quarter of the total trading population between 1275 and 1333 was engaged in provisioning as a primary occupation: Rutledge, 'Economic Life', p. 160.

[62] See, for example, Riley, *Memorials of London*, pp. 240–1.

[63] Most notably in the 1370s and 1380s, when hostility against the City's merchant capitalists focused upon the victualling guilds and especially the wealthy fishmongers: R. Bird, *The Turbulent London of Richard II* (London, 1949), *passim*; Thrupp, *Merchant Class of Medieval London*, pp. 95–6.

to remain 'moelt grauntement contrarious' (extremely fractious) unless better remedies could be provided 'pur le bone gouvernement du ville & de vitailles' (for the good government of the town and of [its] victuals).[64] Determined efforts by the mayor of Lynn to purchase subsidised grain during the slump of the 1430s are thrown into sharp relief by the imprisonment in March 1433 of various hot-heads for fomenting insurrection, and by several cases of 'malicious speech' impugning the honesty of officialdom in January 1439. Since, on the latter occasion, there had been a temporary failure to acquire emergency food supplies for 'common use', feelings may well have run extremely high.[65]

Because the more reputable butchers, cooks, bakers, fishmongers, brewers, and vintners had a vested interest in upholding high standards, and often occupied civic office themselves, they were expected to play their part in enforcing bye-laws and disciplining offenders (5.6). Attention was also paid to the physical conditions in which food was sold, it being clearly apparent that filthy, crowded and unsupervised markets would not only affect the health of individual consumers but might jeopardise the economic survival of the community as a whole (5.7). Both might be further undermined by a variety of commercial activities which, if not strictly illegal, appeared profoundly unethical in their search for personal gain at the expense of the poor. The regulation of weights, measures, monopolies and prices at both a national and local level has generated a substantial corpus of work by economic and legal historians, but rarely features in studies of public health in medieval England. Yet, since its avowed intent was to ensure that potentially vulnerable members of the urban body could afford the essentials of life and were protected from deceit and profiteering, it surely merits some consideration in the present context (5.8). As Sir Francis Bacon (d. 1626) was to observe, if '*Poverty, and Broken Estate, in the better sort, be joyned with a Want and Necessity, in the mean People, the danger is imminent, and great. For the Rebellions of the Belly are the worst.*'[66] His list of remedies for what he presciently regarded as a condition akin to the eruption of 'preternaturall Heat' and inflamed humours in a sick patient included several of the measures considered below. The penultimate section of this chapter examines the contribution that such controls might make to a collective *regimen sanitatis* (5.9), before concluding with an exploration of the religious imperative to provide food for the hungry and its impact upon the behaviour of the ruling elite (5.10).

5.2 Butchers

One of the most significant changes in the late medieval English diet was the steadily rising consumption of meat across most of the social spectrum. Although this development must have been welcome in towns such as Ipswich, where municipal rents from the flesh market doubled in value between 1345 and

---

[64] *RCN*, I.64–5.

[65] KLBA, KL/C7/3, Hall Book, 1431–1450, fols 33v, 101r, 102r–v; and section 5.9 below.

[66] Sir Francis Bacon, *The Essayes or Counsels Civill and Morall*, ed. M. Kiernan (Oxford, 1985), pp. 45–8.

1486,[67] it initially provoked alarm at the highest level. A widespread assumption that the robust digestive systems of 'labouryng men' functioned better on plain, simple fare, and would be weakened or inflamed by 'metys smale and sotyl in substaunce' of the kind consumed by the upper classes, served conveniently to justify the introduction of sumptuary measures from the early fourteenth century onwards.[68] In a critical letter of 1315 to the sheriffs of London, Edward II condemned the excessive amounts being spent on food ('trop outraiouses & desmesurables seruices des mees & viaundes') by the great lords of the realm, and the even more alarming propensity of lesser folk to follow suit. First among the many deplorable consequences of such extravagance, he noted damage to health ('empirement de bone saunte des corps des gentz'), followed by the general impoverishment of his subjects.[69] It is highly unlikely that he managed to limit the number of meat dishes that might be served by socially ambitious Londoners, but these concerns persisted. In 1336 they found expression in a statute promulgated by his son, Edward III, to redress 'the many evils' that had 'afflicted souls as well as bodies' because of the nation's growing appetite for flesh and fish.[70] On this occasion, the need to husband resources for a campaign against the French, rather than questions of wellbeing or status, clearly ranked uppermost. Twenty-seven years later, however, in the aftermath of the plague of 1361, fears that the labouring classes, who constituted the feet and legs of the body politic, might grow indolent, rebellious or sick through unaccustomed indulgence resurfaced with a vengeance. It was then formally enacted that agricultural workers and journeymen employed in crafts and manufacturing should be permitted only one meal of meat or fish a day, being otherwise obliged to eat food such as bread and cheese, that was more appropriate to their estate.[71]

There was, even so, no halting the march of the carnivores, as we can see from the spate of urban bye-laws that sought to guarantee the availability of a reasonably priced and wholesome meat supply for those with just a few pence to spare. Evidently in response to the demand for cheaper cuts, and also to prevent restrictive practices, the rulers of Coventry decreed in 1421 that 'foreign' butchers might trade freely within the walls; that no limit should be imposed on the number of beasts slaughtered; and that offal (which cost less) should be sold on every stall. The residents must already have developed the taste for beef so apparent a century later, when local butchers were again urged to 'kill & sell wekelie within the Citie asmoche beiff as they woll', being threatened with forfeiture should they have none to offer their customers, along with the usual joints of lamb, veal, pork and mutton.[72] The growing preference for beef may, perhaps, reflect an awareness of

---

[67] Amor, 'Trade and Industry of Late Medieval Ipswich', pp. 347–8. In Exeter, in 1380–1, an investment of £11 doubled the size of the covered meat market and created twelve additional stalls, which could be rented out: Kowaleski, *Local Markets*, p. 183.

[68] Lydgate, *Secrees of Old Philisoffres*, p. 58.

[69] BL, MS Cotton Claudius D II, fol. 135r.

[70] *SR*, vol. 1, 10 Edward III, statute 3, pp. 278–30.

[71] *SR*, vol. 1, 37 Edward III, cap. 8, p. 380.

[72] *Coventry Leet Book*, I.26, 32–3; III.715. An ordinance of 1463 required Nottingham butchers 'to stand in theyr shopps in weekeday shambles' for a specific time, and not to close early: Stevenson, *Records of the Borough of Nottingham*, II.425.

the medical concerns about pork discussed at the start of this chapter, as well as the improved circumstances of many working people. But whatever the reason, it was, predictably, accompanied by a corresponding increase in the number of presentments made against butchers for failing to bait bulls before slaughter, and thus selling what appeared to be less digestible, if not overtly 'poisonable', meat.[73] Whereas just two breaches of the relevant ordinance were reported by Ipswich jurors in 1438, the figure stood at five in 1465, eight in 1471 and no fewer than eighteen in 1484. Even allowing for the mounting vigilance of urban authorities throughout this period, patterns of consumption had clearly begun to change.[74]

Late medieval magistrates were well aware of the risks posed by contamination, and of the need to protect the public from fraudulent and potentially lethal practices. In November 1320, for example, three 'foreign' butchers were reprimanded by the London authorities for trading by candle-light after the curfew. Anxiety about the concealment of infected meat may have been intensified by recent outbreaks of murrain and rapidly rising cattle prices, although civic regulations had long forbidden the jointing of carcasses after a certain time in the afternoon, while insisting that dressed meat should never be held over for sale on the following morning or later.[75] York butchers had likewise been prohibited since the start of the century from selling any fresh meat left 'either in whole or in pieces, in the sun on their stall for more than one day', unless it had been either cleansed or salted.[76] As was the case in Beverley, many towns and cities not only punished the vendors of flesh that was 'maggoty [*superseminatas*], or kept beyond the proper time, or dead of murrain or carrion', but also demanded that butchers should be personally responsible for slaughtering their own animals and for disposing of the meat within a clearly defined 'safe' period (in this instance four days).[77] Coventry's butchers were warned 'that thei put no flesche to sale on

---

[73] Drawing upon Galenic concepts of physiology, contemporary medical opinion maintained that the 'violent heat and motion' of the baited animal would convert 'utterly unwholesome' flesh and 'gross blood' into tender and nutritious meat: C. A. Luttrell, 'Baiting of Bulls and Boars in the Middle English "Cleanness"', *Notes and Queries* 197 (1952), pp. 23–4, and 201 (1956), pp. 398–401. Whether out of real conviction or a desire to avoid unnecessary activity in plague time, some London butchers swore on oath in 1349 that unbaited flesh was more wholesome: *CPMRL, 1323–1364*, p. 228. For regulations about baiting, see section 3.6 above.

[74] SROI, C/2/8/1/11, C/2/8/1/13, C/2/8/1/20, C/2/10/1/2; Bacon, *Annalls of Ipswiche*, p. 128.

[75] Riley, *Memorials of London*, pp. 141–2, 426; Riley, *Liber albus*, p. 239; *CLB*, K, p. 10. D. L. Farmer provides a list of average annual cattle prices: 'Prices and Wages', in H. E. Hallam, ed., *The Agrarian History of England and Wales*, vol. 2: *1042–1350* (Cambridge, 1988), pp. 799–806. By 1443, if not before, the butchers of Lynn had to cease trading at 3 p.m. in winter and 4 p.m. in summer, on pain of heavy fines: KLBA, KL/C7/3, Hall Book, 1431–1450, fol. 172v. Nocturnal activities of any kind aroused the suspicions of urban authorities, especially in London; Rexroth, *Power and Deviance*, part 1.

[76] *YCO*, p. 13.

[77] *BTD*, pp. 28–9.

the Sonday that is left on the Thursday, but if hit be saltyd, and abull for mannys mette', on pain of an exemplary fine of 20s.[78] An even harsher penalty was adopted in Winchelsea, where the prospect of imprisonment awaited those who displayed 'vitaill vpon ther stalles lenger then it be good & holsom'.[79] In this way it was hoped to guarantee provenance and quality, as well as preventing any illicit trade in stolen beasts.

The infrequency of presentments for selling substandard meat made against fourteenth- and fifteenth-century London butchers outside the crisis years of 1314–18 and 1346–89 lends support to Ernest Sabine's contention that fear of prosecution and loss of trade generally served as an effective deterrent unless regular supplies were disrupted by pestilence or other natural disasters.[80] If the fine of £20 imposed on one London butcher in 1452 for attempting to sell the flesh of two diseased oxen is any guide, the financial consequences of such ill-advised activities could be crippling, even if (as often happened) the amount was eventually reduced.[81] Nor, despite their negligence in the matter of bull-baiting, did Ipswich's butchers encounter many complaints about the actual freshness of their wares. It can hardly be accidental that the first major exception occurred in the plague year of 1420–1, when seven of them allegedly brought 'corrupt, putrid and unwholesome' meat into the market, and eight were presented for overcharging, presumably because of shortages.[82] The second incident, during the 1480s, also coincided with severe outbreaks of epidemic disease and murrain, as well as the additional trauma of political upheaval.[83] The apparent failure of York butchers to sell 'good salted and fresh meat' during the early years of the fourteenth century probably reflects the unusually heavy demands made by an influx of hungry bureaucrats and soldiers,[84] but whatever the circumstances a

---

[78] *Coventry Leet Book*, I.26 (Friday was a fish day, when no meat was sold). In Leicester, from 1279, fresh meat was to be removed from sale after three days (*RBL*, I.180–1); Winchester adopted a similar rule by the fourteenth century (Keene, *Survey of Medieval Winchester*, I.258). Northampton followed, notably with regard to offal, which had to be sold on the day of slaughter (*RBN*, I.335–7).

[79] BL, MS Cotton Julius B IV, fol. 26r. By 1467 any butcher selling corrupt meat in Leicester faced imprisonment (*RBL*, II.288–9), while Londoners might be sent to Newgate for serious offences (Jones, *Butchers of London*, pp. 132–3).

[80] Sabine, 'Butchering in Mediaeval London', pp. 337–8. A similar concentration of presentments for the sale of 'measly' meat may be observed in Exeter: Kowaleski, *Local Markets*, p. 188 n. 47. As J. D. Blaisdell points out, the years between 1346 and 1389 were marked by cyclical rather than continuous outbreaks of murrain: 'To the Pillory for Putrid Poultry: Meat Hygiene and the Medieval London Butchers, Poulterers and Fishmongers Companies', *Veterinary History* 9 (1997), pp. 114–24, on p. 117. It was only in 1379, a plague year, that the sale of substandard meat and fish became an issue in Bridgwater. Eleven butchers and two fishmongers were then presented on this score: Dilks, *Bridgwater Borough Archives*, no. 330.

[81] Jones, *Butchers of London*, p. 132.

[82] SROI, C/2/8/1/5. For the plague of 1420, which hit East Anglia badly, see Appendix.

[83] SROI, C/2/8/1/20–21. At least eleven presentments for the sale of substandard meat are recorded between 1484 and 1487.

[84] *YCO*, p. 21.

hard core of dishonest victuallers was always determined to make a quick profit at any cost. The appropriately named Richard Bullock, who traded in Durham at the start of the sixteenth century, was certainly untroubled by any scruples about the health of his customers. The accusations levelled against him included keeping a dangerous dog, allowing his own pigs to roam but slaughtering those of a neighbour, and, more seriously, persistently selling diseased meat and rotten pork 'vocatum meseld'. He was also charged with killing and marketing male sheep out of season.[85]

To this list of insanitary practices may be added some potentially lethal attempts at deception. The rogues' gallery of crooked tradesmen depicted in John Gower's *Mirour de l'omme* (1376–9) includes butchers who disguise rotten or inferior meat, even stuffing carcasses with pieces of wood and other foreign bodies in order to make the flesh appear sound.[86] Although his exhaustive catalogue of human duplicity draws upon many conventional stereotypes, in this instance, at least, Gower can hardly be accused of poetic licence. Frustrated by a lack of action on the part of the ruling elite, a number of Londoners had petitioned the crown in 1341 about butchers who fraudulently attached 'the fat of fat oxen upon the flesh of lean oxen by thread and skewers of wood'.[87] Two centuries later, the Norwich Assembly showed less reluctance to condemn a similar trick of 'plumping up' lamb and veal carcasses with dangerous and unsavoury objects, when the court learned that several victuallers

> have heretoffore accustomably used ffor ther private lucre & advauntage not only to blowe [inflate] all suche veelles as thei have brought in to the market ... to be sold, but also have sette out the neres [kidneys], aswell of the seid veelles as off lambes, & stuffed them crastely with nylye [nails], ffoule cloutes & other vile stuffe to the gret disceyte of the kynges liege people, wherby the same veelles & lambes have appered outwardly the hyer & better fflessh & more pleasaunt to the byers theroff, wher off truthe the same veelles & lambes so blowen, sette out & stuffed is the more unhollesom ffor mans bodye; and also the same veelles & lambes ... have ben ... rosted & served at the tabill ffor mans sustenaunce, to the gret encresse off disseases, hinderaunse & detrement of the kynges subiectes & *to the grette slaunder off the hooll citie*.[88]

Monastic communities which purchased in bulk from local butchers were just as vulnerable to exploitation. During the 1440s the monks of St James's abbey, Northampton, accused their kitchener of buying infected flesh on the cheap in this way; and some decades later the meat served at Marton priory in Yorkshire seemed 'more lykly to poysen men then to noryshe them ... as stynkyng bief with

---

[85] *RBC*, nos 696, 699, 706, 709, 712, 714, 720.

[86] Gower, *Complete Works*, I.290–1.

[87] *CCR, 1339–1341*, p. 381.

[88] NRO, NCR, 16D/2, Assembly Proceedings, 1491–1553, fol. 175v (pencil 195v). The italics are mine.

maggotts in it'.[89] A heartfelt protest by the Durham Benedictines in 1455 that they had been obliged to subsist on a diet of 'pancakes and sausages for the most part made of flesh, very hurtful to the body … [and] were afflicted with diverse sicknesses, rendering them so ill that they were kept from the divine offices', can hardly have been unusual.[90] Yet butchers were not always to blame. The water used to cleanse the intestines that served as casing for sausages and black puddings might well be contaminated by the industrial waste discussed in the previous chapter. At York, for instance, the stretch of river known as the 'Piddynghole', where this activity took place, frequently became polluted. An ordinance of 1472 decreed that from henceforth no tanners or any other residents should 'lye, caste, or wesshe any manner of lymed skynnez or ledir or any inmetys or corrupcion of bestes' in the Ouse above this spot because of the risks involved.[91] The cooking process, too, could leave much to be desired. Along with pies and flans, sausages were one of the many comestibles sold in medieval England by a growing army of commercial cooks, who are recorded in towns and cities from the eleventh century onwards and soon became a familiar, indeed notorious, feature of urban life. Their tempting cry of 'Hote pyes hot! Good goos and grys!' was often best resisted by those who valued their health.[92]

5.3 Cooks and pie-bakers

Hot fast food was readily available in most late medieval towns, where it was eaten largely by the poor, or relatively poor, and particularly the unmarried who lived in shared lodgings. Artisans' dwellings of the type under construction in Norwich, Winchester and York during the first half of the fourteenth century represented the most basic form of urban housing, comprising two storeys with a single room in each. Such crowded places lacked even the most rudimentary cooking facilities, which would, in any event, have posed a serious fire risk. Even those members of the workforce who occupied more comfortable quarters tended to own comparatively few utensils and had little or no space for the storage of fuel.[93] This state of affairs was clearly recognised in a London ordinance of 1345, which assumed that only 'rich and middling persons' would need piped water 'for preparing their food', whereas the poor would rely upon it principally 'for their drink'.[94] Indeed, notwithstanding the marked improvement in the quality of rented accommodation apparent during the fifteenth century, as living conditions

---

[89] J. S. Purvis, 'Notes from the Diocesan Registry at York', *Yorkshire Archaeological Journal* 30 (1943), pp. 389–403, on p. 398.

[90] J. A. Twemlow, ed., *Calendar of Papal Letters*, vol. 11: *1455–1464* (London, 1921), pp. 5–6.

[91] *YMB*, II.247; Raine, *Mediaeval York*, pp. 224–5.

[92] William Langland, *Piers the Plowman in Three Parallel Texts*, ed. W. W. Skeat, 2 vols (Oxford, 1886), I.19.

[93] Rutledge, 'Landlords and Tenants', pp. 11–14; Carlin, 'Fast Food', pp. 27–51.

[94] Riley, *Memorials of London*, p. 225.

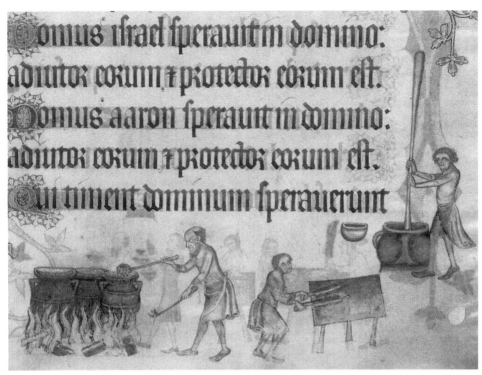

omnus ihrad ſperauit in domino:
adiutor corum ⁊ protector corum eſt.
Domus aaron ſperauit in domino:
adiutor corum ⁊ protector corum eſt.
Qui timent dominum ſperauerunt

18 A trio of rather grimy cooks preparing food, as depicted with remarkable verisimilitude in an illumination from the Luttrell Psalter of *c.* 1320–45

became less congested, a significant tranche of the population still remained dependent upon outside sources for all cooked meals (plate 18).[95]

The presence of a sizeable number of cooks and cook shops in a town or city can, therefore, reflect a preponderance of unattached workers and poor householders. Of the seventy-three cooks known to have worked in Norwich between 1275 and 1348, at least forty-two appear at the turn of the thirteenth century, when the population was rising dramatically and levels of overcrowding approached crisis proportions in some areas. Nonetheless, the city then employed even more bakers, which suggests that to a casual labourer surviving on 1*d.* a day 'a half penny pie would constitute a rare extravagance', and a diet of bread, cheese and water would generally have been the norm.[96] Householders with kitchens often preferred to buy bread direct from a baker or hand over their own dough for baking in his ovens, thereby accounting for the preponderance of bakers over cooks in towns with smaller and more affluent or settled populations.[97] But the economic and domestic circumstances of the proletariat were not the only factors likely to determine the number of outlets selling convenience food. In early fourteenth-century York, the

[95] Carlin, 'Fast Food', pp. 47–9.
[96] See Rutledge's two articles: 'Immigration and Population Growth', pp. 15–30; 'Economic Life', pp. 164, 171. An influx of casual labourers, earning a basic daily rate of 1*d.*, is known to have caused anxiety at this time: *RCN*, I.189–90.
[97] Carlin, 'Fast Food', p. 50.

major administrative centre and capital of the north, the balance was even, with thirty-five cooks and thirty-six bakers, who together catered for the demands of a constant stream of travellers as well as residents.[98] Visitors to London were, likewise, often reliant upon the city's numerous cook-shops, which earned an unenviable reputation for their cavalier disregard for hygiene.

The most celebrated portrait of a medieval cook appears in *The Canterbury Tales*, where Chaucer draws upon a long tradition of satirical verse linking dirt and gluttony with disease. Despite his apparent skill in producing a battery of dishes for wealthy gourmands, and, ironically, in making 'blank manger', a staple of the medieval *regimen sanitatis*, the cook himself inspires little confidence.[99] Almost certainly the result of a sexually transmitted infection, poor diet or lack of cleanliness, the chronic ulcer on his shin is as noxious as the reheated pies and fly-blown poultry he sells to the general public:

> For many a pastee hastow laten blood [drained of gravy],
> And many a Jakke of Dovere [pie] hastow soold
> That hath been twies hoot and twies coold.
> Of many a pilgrym hastow Cristes curs,
> For of thy percely [parsley] yet they fare the wors,
> That they han eten with thy stubble goos [fattened goose],
> For in thy shoppe is many a flye loos.[100]

By and large, those who were affluent enough to travel with their own kitchen staff and culinary supplies tended to shun the late medieval equivalent of the corner kebab house or greasy spoon, and cater for themselves. The well-known proverb that 'God may sende a man good meate but the devyll may sende an euyll coke to destrue it' resonated in the damning indictments levelled against filthy and dishonest cooks in cities such as York and Norwich, as well as in the measures taken elsewhere to curb their insanitary and deceitful habits.[101] These ranged from the use of contaminated or sub-standard meat to the reheating of wares that in today's parlance were long past their sell-by date. Chaucer's reference to pies that had been 'twies hoot and twies coold' would have struck a common chord in Coventry, where, in 1421, cooks were specifically forbidden from selling 'rechaufid meit' and buying dead pike or eels to make pasties. Standards had clearly slipped again by the 1470s, when they seem to have been endangering public health with 'flesshe and ffyshe' that was far from 'good, holsum & sesonnable' when cooked. As was then the case in Colchester and Yarmouth, fines of 40*d.*, along with the threat

---

[98] *YCO*, pp. 22–4.

[99] J. Mann, *Chaucer and Medieval Estates Satire* (Cambridge, 1973), pp. 168–70; W. C. Curry, *Chaucer and the Medieval Sciences*, 2nd edn (London, 1960), pp. 47–52. For *blanc manger*, a sanguine dish usually made of chicken and almonds, see T. Scully, 'The Sickdish in Early French Recipe Collections', in S. Campbell, B. Hall and D. Klausner, eds, *Health, Disease and Healing in Medieval Culture* (New York, 1992), p. 133.

[100] Chaucer, *Riverside Chaucer*, p. 29.

[101] Boorde, *Compendyous Regyment*, sig. Fiiir; Carlin, 'Fast Food', pp. 37–40.

of the pillory for a third offence, targeted the *recalcefactor* who boiled, roasted or baked meat more than once.[102]

Among the many dubious practices prompting civic intervention in the activities of the London pie-bakers in 1379 was their cost-cutting resort to rabbit, geese and offal 'not befitting, and sometimes stinking, in deceit of the people'. In some instances the offending wares had been purchased under dubious circumstances from the back doors of other cook shops or elite households, rather than fresh from the market. A draconian scale of fines, supported by the threat of imprisonment, was now introduced to contain such irresponsible behaviour, which also included the fraudulent substitution of beef for venison.[103] A century later, the mayor and corporation made all London cooks personally liable for any 'hurtes' arising from the sale of unwholesome or undercooked food, while also banning the practice of hawking hot pies around the streets, which constituted a particular source of irritation. Henceforward, street vendors, 'with their hands embrowed [greasy] and fowled', were forbidden 'to drawe and pluk other folk, as well gentilmen as other common people, by their slyves and clothes to bye of their vitailles', not least because their unwelcome attentions often provoked violence on the part of fastidious pedestrians.[104]

It is unlikely that an ordinance of 1212 for the prevention of fires in London had any significant effect on standards of hygiene in the more disreputable Thames-side cook shops, although regulations for the plastering and whitewashing of walls and the removal of internal partitions may have brought modest improvements.[105] Since some commercial cooks attempted to save money by illicitly keeping and slaughtering oxen, sheep and pigs on their own premises (a development to which the butchers of Norwich, for example, took serious exception), it is hardly surprising that so many people were wary of patronising them.[106] Others avoided such places because of poverty rather than prudence, for although standards of living rose appreciably during the late fourteenth century many of the urban

---

[102] *Coventry Leet Book*, I.26; II.398–9; *RPBC*, p. 19; NRO, Y/C18/1, fol. 21v. Complaints about the reheating of food were voiced in many towns, including Norwich in the late thirteenth century (see n. 37 above); Exeter in the fourteenth and fifteenth centuries (Kowaleski, *Local Markets*, p. 142); Winchester in 1370 (Furley, *Town Life*, pp. 142–3; Keene, *Survey of Medieval Winchester*, I.274); Nottingham in 1395 (Stevenson, *Records of the Borough of Nottingham*, I.271); Bristol in the mid-fifteenth century (Veale, *Great Red Book of Bristol*, I.142); Northampton at about the same time (*RBN*, I.317); Leicester in 1500 (*RBL*, II.321); and Rochester at some unspecified date (HMC, *Ninth Report*, part 1, appendix, p. 288). In 1475, the ordinances of the Company of Cooks of London stipulated that members were never to 'bake, rost nor seeth [boil] flessh nor fisshe ij tymes to sell': *CLB*, L, p. 129.

[103] Carlin, 'Fast Food', p. 40; Riley, *Memorials of London*, p. 438.

[104] *CLB*, L, pp. 129–30, 311. In Norwich from 1422 the sale of puddings and similar fare was confined to the marketplace: *RCN*, II.86.

[105] *MGL*, II.i.xxxii–xxxiii, 86.

[106] *RCN*, II.81. Four Bridgwater men were fined in 1387 for trading as both butchers and pie-makers: Dilks, *Bridgwater Borough Archives*, no. 429. In Winchester, too, 'cooks habitually sold fresh meats of all sorts', despite ordinances to the contrary: Keene, *Survey of Medieval Winchester*, I.273–4.

proletariat had still to survive on a subsistence diet. Families on a low or uncertain income with several mouths to feed were often forced to scrape by on bread and small beer; for them 'colde flessh and cold fyssh' seemed as good as baked venison, while 'a ferthyng-worth' of cockles or mussels made for a veritable feast on Fridays.[107] As the surviving evidence reveals, magistrates exercised particular surveillance with regard to the quality, as well as the regular availability, of each of these dietary staples.

5.4 Loaves and fishes

Bread, a major source of nourishment for almost all the late medieval English population, was baked, sold and devoured in enormous quantities. Concern generally focussed upon the weight, content and price of loaves, rather than any risks to physical health posed by contamination, although problems on the latter score inevitably arose from time to time. The assize, or regular testing, of bread made it easy to deal quickly and effectively with bakers such as the Londoner John de Strode, who was consigned to the pillory in 1323 for using sweepings and dirt from his boulting house to produce loaves in which the 'coppewebbes' were still clearly visible.[108] However, offences of this kind, involving 'putrid wheat', 'bad dough' and 'false, putrid and rotten materials', were generally confined to periods of dearth when good quality grain was in short supply.[109] The hyperbolic language employed in the Norwich records to describe the stench of loaves sold in 1441 by a local baker (who compounded his offence by dealing in short measure) confirms that such cases were rare and therefore particularly shocking.[110] High standards of production were clearly expected, not least by the authors of plague *regimina*. The dangers of consuming bread that was made from infected grain were stressed by the Italian physician Gentile de Foligno in his influential *Consilium contra pestilentiam* of 1348, while vernacular guides also warned the reader to exercise caution.[111] John Lydgate's *Dietary and Doctrine for Pestilence* dwells upon the importance of eating digestible 'lyht bred ... the past [dough] i-tempred cleene, and weel decoct of good whete flour'.[112] When, in 1495, London's bakers sought to

---

[107] Langland, *Piers the Plowman*, I.234.

[108] *MGL*, III.415–16. See also the 1330 case of a baker who mixed sand with his dough 'in deceptione populi': pp. 420–1.

[109] As, for example, in the famine years of 1311 and 1316: Riley, *Memorials of London*, pp. 90, 119–22.

[110] NRO, NCR, 16A/1, Mayor's Book, 1424–1449, p. 23. No other cases involving 'corrupt wheat' are recorded in this volume.

[111] Arrizabalaga, 'Facing the Black Death', p. 254. Durham bakers were warned that they should sell only bread that was 'well fermented, salted ... and fit for human use': Bonney, *Lordship and the Urban Community*, p. 221.

[112] Lydgate, *Minor Poems*, II.703. The optimum time for consumption was one day after baking, when bread was deemed to be easily digestible, an assumption reflected in mid-fifteenth-century Bristol ordinances: Veale, *Great Red Book of Bristol*, I.138.

restrict competition from the 'foreigners' of Stratford, they made much of the fact that their bread was 'unsesonable of past' and thus unsafe to eat.[113]

The relatively high level of attrition observed in medieval dental remains was in part due to poor milling, which left small particles of grit in the grain and damaged the teeth of the poor, who generally ate coarser bread made from less refined flour.[114] A growing demand for better-quality 'wastel' (white) loaves in late fourteenth-century London, and an attendant increase in the number of specialist bakers, gave rise to tighter regulation in order to protect consumers.[115] In 1378 the civic authorities ordered the *pestours blanks*, or bakers of wheaten loaves, to 'boult' their flour twice, through successively smaller sieves, and to knead their bread properly. Those who attempted to skimp on the quality of cheaper loaves or to mix 'bad meal with the good' faced the threat of expulsion from their craft and thus from trading privileges in the City.[116] To prevent the sale of stale bread, 'foreign' bakers who came into London each day from the suburbs were specifically forbidden from storing unsold merchandise overnight in 'hutches or selds or elsewhere in hiding places'.[117] Not surprisingly, given what we have already learned about the state of so many urban wells, streams and rivers, a far greater and more permanent risk to the urban bread supply came from the water that was used to mix yeast and flour.[118] Following complaints from the university authorities, Edward I intervened personally in 1293 to order an inspection of two particularly polluted places along the Thames where the bakers and brewers of Oxford had been drawing water, thereby endangering the health of scholars and residents alike. In the event of a negative report, the mayor and bailiffs were to provide an alternative source of clean water fit for human consumption.[119]

Bread often served as an accompaniment to fish, another staple for the elite as well as the masses. A combination of custom, price and ready availability accounted for its ubiquity in the average medieval diet, albeit with considerable variations according to class. The Church decreed that there should be two or three fast days every week, along with five continuous weeks in Lent and a number of major festivals, when meat should not be eaten. Given the wide variety of palatable alternatives, this restriction proved less of a hardship than might be supposed. Herring, 'the potato of the Middle Ages', was plentiful, nutritious and cheap, as were supplies of cod, smelt, sprats, eels and shellfish, such as oysters, whelks, cockles and mussels, which, as the archaeological evidence confirms, were

---

[113] *CLB*, L, pp. 305–6.

[114] Attrition was more pronounced when quernstones were used for grinding corn: Roberts and Cox, *Health and Disease*, p. 191.

[115] Dyer, *Standards of Living*, p. 199.

[116] *CLB*, H, pp. 106–7.

[117] Riley, *Liber albus*, pp. 322–3. In 1324 hucksters in Leicester were forbidden from keeping bread for more than a week: *RBL*, I.347–8.

[118] However, a ban on the use of piped spring water by bakers, introduced in London in 1378, was almost certainly to do with its perceived hardness rather than its impurity: *CLB*, H, pp. 106–7.

[119] *MCO*, pp. 291–2. In 1305 the brewers were again ordered to use pure water, because the ale being drunk by the scholars was contaminated (pp. 11–12).

hugely popular.[120] At Ipswich, the illicit disposal of shells and other waste from 'lez hoystere' (the place where oysters were sold) into the river occasioned such a serious nuisance by 1484 that seven culprits were threatened with substantial fines should they continue to offend.[121] Salted or smoked fish could be safely stored in barrels for weeks, or even months, but a wide range of marine and fresh-water fish was sold for immediate consumption in urban markets. By the fifteenth century, in particular, the opening up of new fishing grounds, some as far away as 'the costes colde' of Iceland, further increased the quantity and choice of marine stock on offer.[122]

The problem of ensuring that such perishable merchandise remained fresh was compounded by the fact that fish was frequently sold by hucksters, or intermediaries, who bought their supplies from fishermen and fishmongers. Most of the 141 sellers of fish active in Norwich between 1286 and 1305 fell into this category, while in York it appears that many residents regarded the trade as a secondary occupation to be pursued alongside other economic activities.[123] Such people were not only harder to police but also more likely to peddle wares that had begun to deteriorate.[124] It was, no doubt, partly for this reason that levels of regulation and surveillance in London were more stringent for fish-sellers than any other victuallers. Whatever their status, they were held personally responsible for the quality of the merchandise in their baskets, which had to be of one single kind, 'as good below as it is above, or better', upon pain of forfeiture, a spell in the pillory and even loss of trading rights for recidivists.[125] The need to maintain a rapid turnover of stock was recognised in most English towns. From 1301 any fresh fish remaining unsold in York for longer than a day had to be salted at once, although Londoners distrusted this practice on the ground that some might already be tainted.[126] Erring on the side of caution, in 1512 Canterbury magistrates imposed a blanket fine of 40*d.* on all hucksters and fishmongers who ignored these basic sanitary precautions.[127] With an eye on arrangements in London, the

---

[120] J. Campbell, 'Norwich before 1300', in Rawcliffe and Wilson, *Medieval Norwich*, p. 30; Rutledge, 'Economic Life', p. 174; *MGL*, I.lxxiv; Kowaleski, *Local Markets*, pp. 310–21.

[121] SROI, C/2/8/1/20. They were in trouble again four years later: C/2/8/1/22.

[122] D. Serjeantson and C. M. Woolgar, 'Fish Consumption in Medieval England', in D. Serjeantson, C. M. Woolgar and T. Waldron, eds, *Food in Medieval England: Diet and Nutrition* (Oxford, 2006), pp. 102–30; Kowaleski, *Local Markets*, pp. 310–21; E. M. Carus-Wilson, 'The Iceland Trade', in E. Power and M. M. Postan, eds, *Studies in English Trade in the Fifteenth Century* (London, 1933), pp. 159–65, 172–6.

[123] Rutledge, 'Economic Life', pp. 171–2; H. Swanson, 'Artisans in the Urban Economy: The Documentary Evidence from York', in Corfield and Keene, *Work in Towns*, p. 47. York was home to around sixty fishmongers and forestallers of fish at the start of the fourteenth century: *YCO*, pp. 24–5, 27.

[124] As, for example, at Colchester in 1311, when five female hucksters sold fish that 'stank by the time they could get it to market': Britnell, *Growth and Decline in Colchester*, p. 37.

[125] *MGL*, I.lxxiv–lxxix; *MGL*, III.149–50; Riley, *Liber albus*, p. 329.

[126] *YCO*, pp. 13, 24–5; Serjeantson and Woolgar, 'Fish Consumption', p. 123.

[127] HMC, *Ninth Report*, part 1, appendix, p. 172.

fourteenth-century borough customs of Ipswich not only insisted that every catch docking on the quays should be unloaded and sold in daylight, but also ordered traders to present any large fresh fish, such as salmon, conger and turbot, for inspection by the market officials upon arrival, and to prepare it in full public view on their stalls.[128] Yet even here potential threats lurked for the unwary. Conscious of the risk of contamination posed by the proximity of dried blood and similar waste products, the rulers of Coventry decreed in 1461 that no stallholder should 'cutte stokfysshe [dried cod] ne saltfyshe vppon such borde as he cutte fflesh the weke before'.[129]

Local juries generally kept a watchful eye upon the shifting population of hucksters, reporting those who, from time to time, dealt in goods that 'by reason of long custody had become foetid and stinking', had not been adequately watered or, conversely, had been made to appear fresh by over-frequent dowsing. Given the quantity of fish passing through the port of Ipswich, the number of indictments remained reassuringly low, usually hovering well below five a year, and only once rising to double figures.[130] In Yarmouth, too, presentments were infrequent, tending to focus, as in 1405–6, upon traders who not only attempted to corner the market but also sold 'corrupt' and 'unseasonable' shellfish.[131] In point of fact, the fishermen who supplied them were just as capable of deceit. Constant scrutiny was necessary to prevent the sort of fraud for which the captains of the ketches trading along the Thames were notorious. In order to preserve the freshness of whelks, oysters and mussels, the London authorities insisted that, with limited exceptions, all catches should be offered direct to the public on the riverside within 'two ebbs and one flood' after docking.[132] Reluctant to lose merchandise that remained on deck for longer, the captains would pull out to sea, cover their old wares 'with a freshening of new' and present them again to unsuspecting buyers. In 1422 the residents of Queenhithe complained that, because the assayer of oysters had sublet his office to women, such 'foul deceit' often went undetected, and the health of the citizenry was put at risk.[133] It is, of course, hardly surprising that consumers

---

[128] Twiss, *Black Book of the Admiralty*, II.102–3, 159–60; Riley, *Liber albus*, p. 329. Likewise in Southampton, from 1300 at the latest, fresh fish might only be sold between dawn and dusk, and solely by the person who had caught it: Studer, *Oak Book of Southampton*, I.64–7.

[129] *Coventry Leet Book*, II.312.

[130] In 1468 fourteen persons were presented for selling contaminated or 'badly watered' fish: SROI, C/2/10/1/5. Other notable years were 1482 (9 cases: C/2/8/1/18), 1416 (7 cases: C/2/8/1/3), and 1465, 1467 and 1488 (6 cases each: C/2/10/1/2, C/2/10/1/5, C/2/8/1/22). For similar complaints by leet courts, see Stevenson, *Records of the Borough of Nottingham*, I.271, 319.

[131] NRO, Y/C4/116, rot. 17r.

[132] *MGL*, I.lxxvi; *MGL*, III.253; Riley, *Liber albus*, p. 329.

[133] *CPMRL, 1413–1437*, pp. 138–9. Some physicians considered oysters inherently dangerous, however fresh they might be. One plague regimen warned readers to avoid eating them on a regular basis, 'for kind [the nature] off oystyrs is to geder to hym felones and corrupte maters as an adamant [magnet] draweth yren': Cambridge University Library, MS Ll.i.18, fol. 5r.

would be alive to the serious threat posed by bad fish and rancid meat. But their vigilance extended into other, less expected quarters.

5.5 Brewers, innkeepers and taverners

Irrespective of rank, most Englishmen, women and children regarded ale as their principal source of 'simple liquid refreshment', not least because the urban water supply might well be polluted and unsafe to drink. The process of boiling and sterilisation with alcohol rendered ale comparatively harmless in this respect, if not others. It has been estimated that adults may regularly have accounted for as much as one gallon a day on a *per capita* basis, thereby generating a continuous and heavy demand, although the less affluent tended to drink a weaker and correspondingly cheaper variety than the well-to-do.[134] Because of problems of preservation and transport, ale had to be brewed near the place of consumption and drunk fresh, within a matter of days, before it turned sour. These constraints account for the large number of brewers and, towards the end of the Middle Ages, the rapid proliferation of tipplers (retailers) and alehouses in towns. Moreover, despite a shift away from domestic to more overtly commercial production after the Black Death, the existing technology still did not permit brewing on an industrial scale or allow for long-term storage.[135]

Regimina repeatedly stressed the harmful effects of poor quality wine or ale and of excessive quantities of alcohol upon the human body, a theme developed with considerable eloquence by the Church. As preachers frequently observed, 'meen been enclynyd to synne, oon more than anothir, be excees of mete and drynk ... and for these same causys oon is enclynyd to bodyly sekenesse more than anothir'.[136] Pulling no punches, one homilist warned his readers that 'drunkenness takes away one's memory, blurs the senses, confuses the mind, stirs up lust, ties the tongue, poisons the blood, weakens all the limbs, and destroys one's health altogether'.[137] And, if this catalogue of misfortune were not enough to induce sobriety, the additional prospect of leprosy lay in wait for heavy drinkers, as well as gluttons, being held over their heads by moralists and medical experts alike. In his *Compendyous Regyment or a Dyetary of Healthe*, the Tudor physician Andrew Boorde drew on centuries of advice literature to caution those who were predisposed to chronic skin diseases that they should abstain from 'al maner of wynes & from new drynkes & stronge ale', as well as the 'ryot & surfetyng' that

---

[134] Holt, 'Water-Related Technologies', pp. 97–8; Bennett, *Ale, Beer and Brewsters*, pp. 9, 16–17.

[135] J. A. Galloway, 'Driven by Drink? Ale Consumption and the Agrarian Economy of the London Region, *c.* 1300–1400', in Carlin and Rosenthal, *Food and Eating*, p. 91; See also Dyer, *Standards of Living*, pp. 57–8; P. Clark, *The English Alehouse: A Social History, 1200–1830* (London, 1983), pp. 23–4, 31–4.

[136] P. Heath Barnum, ed., *Dives and Pauper*, vol. 1, 2 parts, EETS o.s. 275, 280 (Oxford: 1976, 1980), I.i.129.

[137] S. Wenzel, ed., *Fasciculus morum: A Fourteenth-Century Preacher's Handbook* (University Park, PA, 1989), pp. 638–9. For sermons on the theme of temperance, see Owst, *Literature and Pulpit*, pp. 425–41.

invariably followed.[138] Given the insalubrious company which often gathered there, alehouses and taverns were, indeed, as much sources of moral as of physical danger, fostering the sloth and dissipation that spread corruption from one limb or organ to another.

A celebrated passage in the poem *Piers Plowman* relates how Glutton, heading to church in the early morning to confess and attend mass, is soon lured into a disorderly alehouse. Egged on by a motley crowd of reprobates, he collapses insensible, and is carried home sick and filthy to sleep off the effects for the next two days.[139] As Duke Henry of Lancaster observed, crowded commercial centres offered particular temptations to the suggestible. Drawing upon scenes that would have been familiar to all his readers, he compared the human body to a city, whose open gates (or senses) freely admitted the seven deadly sins to ply their wares in the marketplace of the heart:

> Many folk are drunk, and the taverns are situated so close nearby that men eat and drink so much there that they can barely stagger out, they are so inebriated and their stomachs so bloated; and neither the cooks nor the inn-keepers cease from crying out their excellent dishes and good wines; but see, quite otherwise, they are not worth the price, for they boast that they are good, whereas they are most often really harmful ... and after visiting the tavern they must rest the stomach full of meat and the head full of wine, and fall asleep at a time when all manner of other things should be done, and consequently they are lost for ever ...[140]

By the later fifteenth century urban magistrates had begun to address the economic and social consequences of heavy drinking, although their principal concern lay with the essentially pragmatic questions of quality, pricing and basic hygiene.[141] As a rule, brewers were more likely to fall foul of the law for employing short measures, diluting their ale or flouting sanitary regulations than they were for encouraging misbehaviour. That boiling and fermentation would render any beverage safer to drink was clearly understood by medical authorities such as Ibn-Sīna, but did not preclude anxieties of the kind voiced by the chancellor of Oxford university in 1293, about the state of the water available for brewing as well as baking.[142] Indeed, the remarkably high level of alcohol consumption in Oxford (where at least 250 households were involved in supplying the market in 1311) encouraged an early trend towards commercialisation, as well as strict supervision by the eagle-eyed university authorities.[143] But across England attempts to reduce levels of water pollution along the lines explored in Chapter 4 often focussed upon the demands of cooks and brewers, as we can see from an

---

[138] Boorde, *Compendyous Regyment*, sig. Iiir.

[139] Langland, *Piers the Plowman*, I.158–65.

[140] Henry of Lancaster, *Livre de seyntz medicines*, pp. 119–20; see p. 59–60 above.

[141] McIntosh, *Controlling Misbehavior*, pp. 32, 76, 112. Unless it resulted in crime, drunkenness was generally a matter for the ecclesiastical rather than the secular courts.

[142] See n. 119 above.

[143] Bennett, *Ale, Beer and Brewsters*, pp. 111–20.

entry of about 1425 in The Red Paper Book of Colchester:

> Grevous compleynt ys made to the baillyfs ... that mochel peple of the same ton brewen hure ale and maken [cook] hure mete with water of ryver ... the which ... ther ben certeyn persones dwellyng upon, as barkers and white tawyers, that leyen many diverse hides ... in payryng [to the impairment] and corrupcion of the said water ... and in destruccion of the ffyssh therynne, to gret harmyng and noissaunce of the said poeple. Wherefore hit is ordeyned ... atte requeste of the comen poeple that no maner man of the craftes biforen said fro hennys forward ley ne put none swiche hides ne skynnes in the said ryver, but only in his owne water upon his owne ground, as in pettys [pits] made therefore, so that the water and the ordure ... have no cours into the said ryver; upon peyne of xxs.[144]

Dirty or careless brewers might themselves be responsible for the presence of unwelcome foreign bodies in beer and ale, at least if satirists such as John Skelton (d. 1529) are any guide. His 'scurvy and lowsy' ale-wife, Eleanor Rummyng, who thickens her yeast with 'hennes donge', was reputedly modelled upon an early sixteenth-century brewster of that name from Leatherhead.[145] Perhaps, as Judith Bennett suggests, his verses underscore the contrast between the quasi-domestic, often rural alehouses run by brewsters and the more businesslike and tightly regulated establishments increasingly to be found in towns and cities. On the other hand, attacks of this kind also reflect a general distrust of victuallers of both sexes, whose activities so often aroused suspicion.[146]

The introduction of hops on a commercial basis by Dutch aliens in the fifteenth century proved especially controversial, sparking a heated debate about the rival merits of beer and ale, in which medical opinion was eagerly enlisted by xenophobic English brewers, resentful of the growing competition. Notwithstanding the fact that hops possess both antiseptic and preservative qualities, thereby making it possible to produce a stronger, longer-lasting and cheaper beverage, physicians such as Andrew Boorde maintained that 'fresshe and cleane' ale was 'a naturall drynke', more suited to the national complexion. Beer, on the other hand, undermined it, proving fatal to those 'troubled with the colycke and the stone & the strangultion', while also causing obesity, 'as it doth appere by the Dutche mens faces & belyes'.[147] Persuaded by the force of such arguments,

---

[144] *RPBC*, p. 49. The editor erroneously transcribed 'barker' as 'barber', a mistake corrected here. A century later the rulers of Gloucester introduced a similar measure to remove pollution from the River Severn, 'where the bruars fett there water': HMC, *Twelfth Report*, appendix 9, p. 441.

[145] John Skelton, *The Complete English Poems*, ed. J. Scattergood (New Haven, CT, 1983), p. 219.

[146] Bennett, *Ale, Beer and Brewsters*, pp. 123–44; R. Hanna, 'Brewing Trouble: On Literature and History – and Ale-Wives', in B. Hanawalt and D. Wallace, eds, *Bodies and Disciplines: Intersections of Literature and History in Fifteenth-Century England* (Minneapolis, 1996), pp. 1–17.

[147] Boorde, *Compendyous Regyment*, sig. Fiiᵛ. However, ale could be 'unholsome for all men' if consumed too soon after brewing (sig. Fiiʳ). See also Bennett, *Ale, Beer and Brewsters*, pp. 79–80.

some urban authorities attempted to ban hops altogether. In 1471 the Norwich Assembly warned its brewers that they were henceforth to use neither 'hoppes, nor gawle [gall], nor noon othir thyng which may be found unholsom for mannes body, upon peyne of grevous punysshment', and elected two officials in each ward to enforce the decree. Early in the sixteenth century the rulers of Shrewsbury likewise outlawed 'that wicked and pernicious weed', while Coventry magistrates imposed a heavy fine of 20s. for brewing with 'hoppis'.[148]

They were, however, swimming against the tide. Then, as now, English drinkers displayed scant regard for the voice of authority, and increasingly voted for the stronger and more astringent option. With commendable foresight, in 1436 the sheriffs of London denounced rumours that beer was poisonous, pronouncing it 'a wholesome drink, especially in summer time'; five years later it was deemed necessary to introduce a national assize, or system of assay, for beer, similar to that already in place for bread and ale; and in 1443 specifications as to the quality of the ingredients were drawn up. In accordance with Continental practice, 'les hoppes' were to be 'perfect, sound and sweet', as well as plentiful, and the malt made of good corn that was 'not too dry, nor rotten, nor full of worms called "wiffles" [weevils]'.[149] North Sea ports, where the Dutch tended to settle, proved especially receptive; by the 1480s, for example, the Yarmouth leets were presenting brewers who refused to sell beer by the half-penny or penny measure so that less affluent consumers could also enjoy it.[150]

Chester audiences must have eagerly awaited the annual performance of 'The Harrowing of Hell', a mystery play staged, appropriately under the circumstances, by the city's cooks. The appearance of a condemned ale-wife with her escort of comic devils no doubt provoked stormy cheering (plate 19). Brewsters who served weak ale, dealt in short measures, or risked their customers' health by adding 'esshes and herbes' to the mash vat, clearly deserved to roast among the eternally damned. However, their torments were far from solitary, being shared by a crew of unscrupulous taverners:

> ... all mashers, mengers of wyne, in the night
> Bruynge so, blendinge against daylight:
> Syche newe-made claret ys cause full right
> Of sycknes and disease.[151]

---

[148] *RCN*, II.100; W. Page, ed., *VCH Shropshire*, vol. 1 (London, 1908), p. 422; Champion, *Everyday Life in Tudor Shrewsbury*, p. 80; *Coventry Leet Book*, III.683.

[149] *CLB*, K, p. 205; *CPR, 1436–1441*, p. 495; *CPR, 1441–1446*, pp. 184–5. The wording of the assize of beer was duly incorporated into borough ordinances, as, for example, at Colchester: *RPBC*, p. 20.

[150] NRO, Y/C4/189, rot. 13r. For Colchester, where beer soon began to overtake ale in popularity, see Britnell, *Growth and Decline in Colchester*, pp. 195–7; for Hull, see Evans, 'Infrastructure of Hull', p. 71; and for Ipswich, see section 4.3 above. At least four Dutch beer-brewers had settled in Southampton by 1488: Butler, *Book of Fines*, pp. xviii, 5.

[151] R. M. Lumiansky and D. Mills, eds, *The Chester Mystery Cycle*, vol. 1, EETS s.s. 3 (London, 1974), p. 388; Bennett, *Ale, Beer and Brewsters*, pp. 124–5. This entertaining image appealed to medieval artists as well as dramatists, appearing,

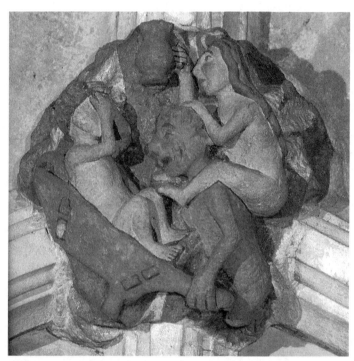

19 An early sixteenth-century roof boss from the north transept of Norwich cathedral on the popular theme of an ale wife being transported to hell, in this instance on the back of a devil, who pushes a tonsured monk in his wheelbarrow. The tankard in her hand would almost certainly have contained a short measure.

In common with other wines, claret was drunk by the wealthy, although the taverns which had become an established feature of the late medieval urban landscape increasingly catered for customers of 'middling' status with modest incomes. Whereas some establishments sold both wine and ale, others, often run by vintners, specialised in the former, providing a more select environment where reputable clientele could do business and even host official entertainments.[152] Prices, measures and quality were, in theory, tightly regulated in such places, but a variety of dubious practices alluded to by the Chester ale-wife might yet be employed to increase profits. In most cases patrons had simply to be on guard for the dilution of good wine with water or inferior vintages. But, as magistrates recognised, some activities were likely to prove as injurious to the body as they were to the pocket.

for example, on the doom of the parish church of Holy Trinity, Coventry, and in a celebrated misericord in St Lawrence's church, Ludlow: see, respectively, M. Gill, 'The Doom in Holy Trinity Church and Wall-Painting in Medieval Coventry', in L. Monckton and R. K. Morris, eds, *Coventry: Medieval Art, Architecture and Archaeology in the City and its Vicinity* (Leeds, 2011), pp. 211–12, 215–16 and plate 13A; C. Grössinger, *Picturing Women in Late Medieval and Renaissance Art* (Manchester, 1997), p. 101 fig. 36.

[152] Keene, *Survey of Medieval Winchester*, I.275.

John Gower's caustic observation that the unsuspecting drinker might well 'languish and suffer great infirmity, very often leading to death' after visiting a tavern may well reflect personal experience of Southwark's less salubrious hostelries.[153] Documentary evidence of concern at a national level certainly substantiates his complaint. In late thirteenth-century Oxford, for example, the sheriff himself had to inspect all the town's taverns following allegations that the sale of contaminated wine had caused fatalities as well as serious illness.[154] The practice of mixing spillages and lees with good wine, in order to avoid wastage, was both common and dangerous. Not long afterwards, in 1311, the vintners and taverners of London (which then boasted over 350 outlets for the sale of wine) were specifically forbidden from adulterating 'any drink that has to enter man's body' in this way.[155] Some forty years later a renewed campaign against the surreptitious addition of 'putrid and corrupt wine' to new vintages authorised customers freely to examine the cellars of any public tavern in order to ensure that all the vessels in use were clean and empty.[156] Since some landlords remained obdurate, the mayor and corporation imposed tougher penalties involving both imprisonment and incremental fines, rising by 6s. 8d. for each offence.[157]

Because wine was not at this date bottled, but drawn directly from the cask, the barrels and other vessels in which it was kept had to meet high standards, not only in terms of size but also with regard to the quality of the wood and the cleanliness of the interior.[158] Similar concerns obtained with regard to the storage of other perishable commodities, such as fish. Acting swiftly to protect their collective reputation and also to preserve a monopoly over production, the London coopers complained successfully in 1413 that a fishmonger named Richard Bartlot had taken delivery of some 260 vessels made of defective and unseasoned wood, which would contaminate whatever was placed in them. Following an inspection the entire consignment was burnt.[159] Yet not all members of the craft were themselves above suspicion. Six years later, the mayor and aldermen outlawed a variety of alarming practices, such as mixing the 'remenauntz of brokyn, sodyn, reboyllid and unthrifty wines' in vessels 'gummyd with picche, code [cobblers' wax] and

---

[153] Gower, *Complete Works*, I.288–9.

[154] *MCO*, p. 292.

[155] Riley, *Memorials of London*, p. 82; Clark, *The English Ale House*, p. 11. In 1330 a twice-yearly national assize of wine was introduced both for this reason and because of overpricing: *SR*, vol. 1, 4 Edward III, cap. 12, p. 264.

[156] Riley, *Memorials of London*, pp. 213–14.

[157] Riley, *Memorials of London*, p. 255. The fine was halved in 1370, perhaps because a new ruling that cellar doors should be kept open at all times made concealment harder. A group of vintners then undertook a tour of inspection to ensure that only 'good and proper' wine went on sale in City taverns (p. 341).

[158] At Southampton stringent rules obtained about the flushing out of barrels: Studer, *Oak Book of Southampton*, I.76–9. Medieval *regimina* stressed that vessels used for storing or cooking food and drink should be clean. See, for instance, H. Cameron Gillies, ed., *Regimen sanitatis: The Rule of Health* (Glasgow, 1911), p. 50.

[159] Riley, *Memorials of London*, pp. 596–7. In 1420 the London Coopers were ordered to inspect all the vessels in use by brewers and other victuallers: *CLB*, I, pp. 235–6.

othir horrible and unholsome thinges' in order to improve the colour, smell and taste.[160] One cooper who defied the ban by 'doctoring' his casks with gums and powders was immediately sent to the pillory, being fortunate to escape the fate of a taverner who had previously sold wine that was 'unsound and unwholesome for man, in deceit of the common people and to the shameful disgrace of the officers of the City'. Since many of his customers would have been far from 'common', it seemed advisable to make a particular spectacle of this miscreant. After a spell in prison he was obliged to consume some of the offensive brew in public, while the rest was poured ceremonially over his head. A less degrading but more serious punishment followed in the form of a prohibition on trading in the city until he secured a royal pardon, which took four years to materialise.[161]

The practice of adulterating new wine with the insalubrious remnants of the previous year's vintage was widespread in ports such as Ipswich, which boasted a flourishing wine trade in the fourteenth century. The borough authorities consequently instituted an annual search of all taverns and cellars just before the arrival of the fleet from Bordeaux. Accompanied by a group of 'good and trewe taverneres', whose probity could be relied upon, the bailiffs were to sample all the remaining stock, 'ony wyn that be corrupt and perlous to drynkyn for mannys body, or for to medelyn with newe wyn' being immediately flushed away in the gutters and the vessels confiscated.[162] The recruitment of expert assessors was widely adopted in English towns, not simply for inspecting ale, bread and eventually wine and beer, as required by the assize, but also for determining the quality of other merchandise, including leather, cloth and metalwork. As well as being best qualified to establish whether or not standards had been breached, senior practitioners of the relevant trades or crafts generally had a vested interest in retaining public confidence and driving out unscrupulous competitors. Given the serious, potentially lethal, consequences likely to arise from the sale of substandard food and drink, victuallers, in particular, were required by the authorities to adopt a system of self-policing and might well be enlisted as jurors to pass judgement upon the wares of others. However, delegation did not represent an abrogation of responsibility on the part of urban magistrates, since the inspectors were themselves monitored and, if necessary, held personally accountable for any lapses on their part.

---

[160] Riley, *Memorials of London*, pp. 670–2. The authorities intended to curb the production of 'counterfeit' Greek wine, which was very popular: *CLB*, G, p. 137.

[161] Riley, *Memorials of London*, pp. 318–19, 672. Despite the threat of exemplary punishment, *all* the taverners of Cheap Ward were indicted in 1422 for selling corrupt wine: *CPMRL, 1413–1437*, pp. 135–6. In 1454, a cooper's servant was accused of conspiring to adulterate six pipes of Rochelle wine, 'olde and feble of colour and tast', with eggs, alum, gums and 'othere horrible & unholsome thinges': *CLB*, K, p. 377.

[162] Twiss, *Black Book of the Admiralty*, II.176–7. Nicholas Bacon notes that from at least 1437 three official wine-drawers were assigned to supervise the assize of wine in Ipswich: *Annalls of Ipswiche*, p. 98.

5.6 Quality control

Most medieval craft and trade guilds made (or were obliged to make) provision for the inspection of the premises and merchandise of their members. When, after considerable economic vicissitudes, the pie-bakers of London finally formed their own company in 1495, the wardens were empowered to examine 'all manner of dressed victuals in open shops to see if they are wholesome' and to ensure that fair prices were being charged.[163] They had many models to choose from, most notably that offered by the City's butchers, whose complex regulatory system had long involved the supervision of three meat markets and their designated slaughterhouses. In 1484, the wardens of the mystery successfully petitioned the mayor to augment their already considerable powers of search to allow the examination of all swine entering the City or suburbs, on the ground that they could more easily detect 'measled' animals than anyone else. From this date onwards, any butcher, resident or 'foreign', who persisted in selling contaminated meat after an appropriate warning could expect even harsher treatment than before.[164] Although the wardens of London's guild of Butchers were unusual in both the extent of their authority and scale of their responsibilities, other towns and cities adopted similar practices as seemed appropriate.

From at least 1329, the butchers of Winchester chose two of their fellows 'to view the flesh slaughtered for sale within the city' before it reached the customer. Their attention initially focussed upon pork and the compulsory use of the town's scalding house for the preparation of carcasses. But because of the rising demand for beef, their remit soon expanded.[165] With its two bustling meat markets, Lynn required four such inspectors by the early 1460s, not least to collect the heavy fines then imposed on anyone who sold 'mesell' flesh. They also undertook to supervise the removal of whatever noisome waste remained behind after trading to 'le lawe water marke' in the River Ouse, but were soon obliged to delegate this task.[166] By 1488 their comprehensive oath was principally concerned with the quality of the meat on sale, which necessitated a daily tour of inspection to ensure that 'no bulle be slayne but with oute they be bated, nor porke slayne but in

---

[163] *CLB*, L, p. 311.

[164] Jones, *Butchers of London*, p. 132. Nevertheless, Blaisdell's observation that London's butchers rank as 'some of the first public health professionals' invites a measure of scepticism, especially as some members of the Company demonstrated scant respect for authority: 'To the Pillory for Putrid Poultry', p. 120. Others decamped to the less tightly regulated environment of Westminster: Rosser, *Medieval Westminster*, pp. 139–40.

[165] Keene, *Survey of Medieval Winchester*, I.258; Furley, *Town Life*, pp. 144–5. Even in Colchester, which was a smaller borough, meat inspectors are recorded from 1311 (Britnell, *Growth and Decline in Colchester*, p. 138). Sandwich had taken this step by the start of the fourteenth century, when four butchers' wardens oversaw slaughtering and sales (BL, MS Cotton Julius B IV, fol. 75v).

[166] KLBA, KL/C7/4, Hall Book, 1453–1497, pp. 169, 409. The butchers in the Tuesday Market had already been ordered to dispose of their refuse in 1453 (p. 32), but evidently required closer supervision.

sesonabyll tyme & that yt be flesh holsom for man is body'.[167] In order to spread the burden more fairly, the authorities decided soon afterwards to adopt a rota system whereby each butcher would, in turn, take charge of refuse collection for a fortnight, while two elected surveyors would continue to scrutinise the wares of both resident and 'country' butchers every day.[168] In many other towns and cities the powers of search exercised by guild officers extended far beyond their own ranks to encompass *all* sellers of meat, whether freemen or 'foreigners', in an arrangement which inevitably gave them a commercial edge when dealing with outsiders. Thus, in 1490, the mystery of butchers of Beverley was charged with examining any flesh sold by either residents or non-residents, of confiscating whatever appeared 'foule and not able' and of fining the vendor for each offence. As in Lynn, the overseers could themselves be fined for negligence, a penalty of 3s. 4d. being imposed for each dereliction of duty.[169] It was, no doubt, the prospect of financial loss (as well as insubordination and abuse) that made some of Exeter's butchers, who supervised the meat market from 1384 onwards, so reluctant to hold office.[170]

Although we know rather more about the inspection of meat supplies, butchers were by no means the only victuallers charged with safeguarding the quality of perishable food. Ordinances for the city of Worcester set down in about 1467 ruled that, on the arrival at the quayside or elsewhere of any consignment of fish, the alderman on duty was immediately to select 'ij of the ffysshmongers, to be indifferently chosen and sworn, to se that alle suche vytelle be able and sete for mannys body'.[171] Anyone dealing in rotten or substandard goods had to pay 13s. 4d., rising to 20s. in the case of freemen, who, it was assumed, should lead by example. Whether or not such hefty sums were actually collected is, of course, another matter, but the amounts involved suggest that food safety counted for a great deal. This was certainly the case in York, where, in 1418, the fishmongers were reminded that their overseers served 'to the honour and praise of the mayor and aldermen and the common community of this city and the people of our Lord King', and were therefore to be obeyed on all points, under the threat of serious retribution.[172]

---

[167] KLBA, KL/C7/4, Hall Book, 1453–1497, p. 547.

[168] KLBA, KL/C7/4, Hall Book, 1453–1497, p. 574; KL/C7/5, Hall Book, 1497–1544, fols 55v, 141r, 260v, 310r.

[169] *BTD*, p. 127.

[170] Kowaleski, *Local Markets*, pp. 188, 191. Attempts by the city's butchers in 1437 to sell meat in their own homes rather than in the shambles resulted in the imprisonment of the two ringleaders: DRO, ECA, book 51, fol. 305v.

[171] Smith, Smith and Brentano, *English Gilds*, pp. 396–7. In Norwich, the wardens of the fishmongers' guild assayed all the barrels of herring sold in the market, reporting any that were 'atteynt': NRO, NCR, 16A/2, Mayor's Court Book, 1510–1532, p. 160.

[172] *YMB*, I.197–8. One London butcher who refused to obey the wardens of his craft in 1365 was fined 10s. by the mayor and committed to Newgate for as many days: *CPMRL, 1364–1381*, p. 15.

Traders who slipped through the supervisory net might still find themselves in court as a result of prosecutions brought by civic officials or disgruntled customers. When hearing cases that involved the sale of questionable foodstuffs, the mayor and aldermen of London frequently assembled a jury of experts to pronounce upon the offending items. Such a system not only delivered a specialist opinion that was hard to gainsay, but was also extremely efficient, since a panel could generally be mobilised within a few hours, and before the goods in question deteriorated further. On 1 May 1383, for example, twelve bakers met on the very day that one of their craft was charged with selling half-penny loaves made of 'cinders, earth and other filth'. Unconvinced by his claims that they had been used to 'protect' white bread from the full heat of the oven and had gone on sale by mistake, they found him and his servant guilty.[173] Predictably, in light of what we have already learned about its fast food outlets, the City's more reputable cooks, some of whom kept superior premises on Bread Street, were in considerable demand as jury members. In 1351 eight of them passed judgement on the 'putrid and stinking' capon pies peddled at the Stocks Market by one Henry Passelewe, but they might just as often be required to inspect raw flesh and fish.[174] Two decades later 'divers cooks and good men of the City, as well cooks of Bread Street' were called upon to establish whether or not the meat sold by some London butchers was, indeed, 'unfit for human food'.[175] It was, perhaps, a point of honour that defendants should rarely be accorded the benefit of the doubt: a jury including five cooks and a fishmonger, 'having full knowledge of such victuals', roundly condemned one cargo of herring and mackerel shipped up the Thames in 1382 as 'putrid and corrupt, unwholesome as food for man and an *abomination*'.[176]

5.7 Policing the market

Well aware of the crucial role played by the digestive system in preserving health, medieval medical practitioners did their utmost to ensure that the culinary process begun in the stomach should produce a balanced mix of humoral matter, appropriate to the temperament and circumstances of the individual patient. While conceding that the stomach lacked the grace and dignity of the heart or brain, the surgeon Henri de Mondeville still accorded it a dominant position in the body's ruling hierarchy, since any malfunction on its part could result in starvation and was to be avoided at all costs.[177] As the stomach of the urban body, markets were likewise subject to intense regulation by the rulers of English towns and cities,

---

[173] *MGL*, III.426–8.

[174] Riley, *Memorials of London*, pp. 266–7.

[175] *CLB*, G, pp. 332–3.

[176] Riley, *Memorials of London*, pp. 471–2. Other victuallers were similarly employed. In 1377 a group of London vintners joined with certain Bordeaux merchants to pronounce a consignment of 'putrid' wine, 'unsound and unfit for human use': Riley, *Memorials of London*, pp. 408–9. Grocers and apothecaries were particularly active in assessing drugs and medicines: see section 6.4 below.

[177] Henri de Mondeville, *Chirurgie*, p. 67. For the relative status of organs and limbs, see pp. 78–80 above.

who employed salaried officials to enforce a steadily growing number of bye-laws regarding the quality and sale of provisions.[178] In 1473, when anxiety about the contamination of food by lepers was at its height, the Norwich Assembly retained a sergeant of the market specifically to inspect the stalls of victuallers.[179] Similarly, the Leicester 'fish sayers' were sworn in 1500 to 'take a lawfull asaye of all maner of fyshe and wekely [on] markett dais serche that it be salte and swete and able for mannys body', while also keeping a close eye upon the city's cooks.[180] Among the many duties assigned to these officers was the punishment of victuallers whose offences merited the pillory or some other public humiliation, invariably in the middle of a busy market. It was here, too, that contaminated produce would be burnt, as a warning to others and reassurance to the public.[181] And lest there should be any doubt about the ordinances that had been breached, a list of fines and penalties would be prominently displayed, as was the case at Lynn, upon a board or 'tabyll hangyng on the walle'.[182]

The supervisors' task was compounded by the fact that many markets, especially in older cities such as Chester, Dorchester, London and Lincoln, were held in streets, which created a raft of sanitary as well as logistical problems for those who shopped or lived there.[183] The press of crowds and livestock, and the detritus abandoned by stallholders may have been less of an issue when populations were small and fear of miasmatic air less pronounced, but urban expansion and epidemics brought a demand for higher standards including, if possible, the creation of specialist covered markets where particular commodities could be sold at fixed times. As early as 1301, Edward III's ministers had prepared for his arrival in York by insisting that 'the people of each trade' should 'remain in a specific place, so that no degrading business or unsuitable trade is carried out among those who sell food for humans'.[184] The tendency for existing markets to subdivide into 'rows', or clearly demarcated areas occupied by cooks, butchers, poulterers, fishmongers, apothecaries, cheesemongers and other victuallers, constituted one very obvious response to growth, prosperity and a desire for cleanliness and

---

[178] For the type of duties undertaken by these officials, see *RBN*, I.373–8. Because of their crucial role in the urban body, markets were occasionally also compared to the heart. See p. 255 above and p. 271 below.

[179] *RCN*, II.100–1.

[180] *RBL*, II.321. Supervisors of the fish market were active in Colchester from the 1440s (Britnell, *Growth and Decline in Colchester*, p. 245), and in Stamford from at least 1478, by which time all the town's food markets appear to have been tightly policed (Rogers, *William Browne's Town*, pp. 70–1). Even the small borough of Henley was employing 'tryers' of meat and fish from the 1440s onwards: Briers, *Henley Borough Records*, pp. 48, 56, 70, 80, 109, 122, 150, 163, 196–7.

[181] In 1445–6, for example, the treasurers of Norwich bought fuel for burning corrupt meat and fish in the open market: *RCN*, II.70. See also NRO, NCR, 16A/2, Mayor's Court Book, 1510–1532, pp. 11 (front of book), 169, 207. For similar purchases made in Dover in 1508–9, see BL, MS Egerton 2107, fol. 115v.

[182] KLBA, KL/C7/4, Hall Book, 1453–1497, p. 574.

[183] Schofield and Vince, *Medieval Towns*, pp. 49, 50; Mayo and Gould, *Records of the Borough of Dorchester*, pp. 104–12; Hill, *Medieval Lincoln*, pp. 153–4.

[184] *YCO*, p. 17.

order.[185] While presenting magistrates with a welcome opportunity to boost their rental income through the leasing of stalls, these developments also enabled them to exercise greater control and surveillance. The challenges involved were nonetheless still considerable, in part because the traders themselves were often resistant to change.

On the eve of Edward I's ceremonial entry into London in 1274, concern about the dirty and congested conditions along Cheapside prompted the mayor to order the removal of butchers' and fishmongers' stalls, 'lest any filth should remain in Cheap against the coming of the king'.[186] The alternative site provided at this time eventually became the covered Stocks Market, although it proved difficult to confine victuallers there. When, in 1321, the royal justices demanded that any butchers who had surreptitiously returned to Cheapside should be relocated, they were warned that such a step would encourage the illicit sale of meat in private houses, with potentially greater risks to the public.[187] However, action could not be postponed indefinitely. Shortly before the Black Death, in 1345, the rulers of London responded to renewed complaints about the 'crowded and impassable streets' between 'les Stokkes' and the great conduit in Cheapside, which were thronged on 'flesh days' with butchers and on 'fish days' with fishmongers, as well as a constant mêlée of poultry-sellers (map 2). By transferring all the butchers and fishmongers to the Stocks, and ordering the poultry-men to withdraw into adjoining shops or to the Leadenhall Market in Cornhill, it was hoped that a major source of aggravation would be eliminated.[188] By 1359 the Stocks boasted no fewer than seventy-one covered 'plots' arranged in four parallel rows for vendors of meat and fish, as well as twenty-seven more beneath the pentices on the outer walls. They, in turn, were replaced fifty years later by an even more imposing stone structure, which was easier to keep clean.[189] Meanwhile, the vendors of fruit and vegetables, who had hitherto caused such a tremendous din outside St Austin's church that they had drowned the celebration of mass, were relegated to a more

[185] See, for example, Cromarty, *Everyday Life in Medieval Shrewsbury*, pp. 41, 44; Lilley, *Urban Life in the Middle Ages*, pp. 228–9; U. Priestley, *The Great Market: A Survey of Nine Hundred Years of Norwich Provision Market* (Norwich, 1987), pp. 8–11; Tillott, *VCH York: The City of York*, pp. 484–5; Kowaleski, *Local Markets*, pp. 181–3. Spatially segregated markets might be found in towns as small as Loughborough and Newmarket: Dyer, 'Small Towns', p. 514.

[186] I. Archer, C. Barron and V. Harding, eds, *Hugh Alley's Caveat: The Markets of London in 1598*, London Topographical Society 137 (London, 1988), p. 4. Derek Keene suggests that the mayor wished to create 'a processional way' which would 'enhance the dignity of the city': *The Walbrook Study: A Summary Report* (London, 1987), p. 6.

[187] Jones, *Butchers of London*, pp. 72–4; Barron, *London in the Later Middle Ages*, p. 52.

[188] Riley, *Memorials of London*, pp. 222–3. A few recalcitrant butchers defied the ordinance by continuing to trade in the street (p. 226). The stalls and barrels in Old Fish Street were still annoying Londoners in 1422: *CPMRL, 1413–1437*, pp. 139, 152, 158–9.

[189] Keene, *Walbrook Study*, pp. 66, 23 fig. 2.

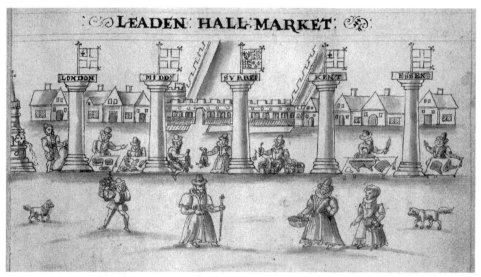

20 The Leadenhall building and outdoor market, London, from the north, as they appeared in Hugh Alley's *A Caveatt for the Citty of London* of 1598. In the foreground, 'country' produce, including meat, poultry and vegetables, is on sale in the open, while in the background stand the granary and covered market.

distant spot by St Paul's churchyard.[190] The rebuilding of the Leadenhall in the 1440s as a civic granary with a spacious courtyard where poultry, dairy produce and meat could be sold in more hygienic and sheltered conditions served further to clear the streets, while attracting traders from the countryside (plate 20).[191]

These problems were not confined to the capital. Their ranks and wallets swollen by the demand for meat from garrisons along the Welsh March, Chester's butchers were embroiled in the 1340s in an ongoing dispute with the authorities over their obstruction of the city centre and the risk to pedestrians occasioned by their penchant for hanging entire carcasses over their stalls.[192] It was then that the rulers of Bristol prohibited the erection of 'benches, stalls and pens' in the high street, where traffic was disrupted, and soon afterwards that Lynn juries began fining butchers who caused a similar nuisance.[193] There was little excuse for these practices in a town whose spacious markets had been improved through significant

[190] J. A. Galloway and M. Murphy, 'Feeding the City: Medieval London and its Hinterland', *The London Journal* 16 (1991), pp. 3–14, on p. 8.

[191] Schofield and Vince, *Medieval Towns*, pp. 48–50; Archer, Barron and Harding, *Hugh Alley's Caveat*, pp. 4–5, 9–10; A. H. Thomas, 'Notes on the History of the Leadenhall, AD 1195–1488', *London Topographical Record* 13 (1923), pp. 1–22; M. W. Samuel, 'The Fifteenth-Century Garner at Leadenhall, London', *Antiquaries Journal* 69 (1989), pp. 119–53; Barron, *London in the Later Middle Ages*, pp. 55–6.

[192] C. R. Lewis and A. T. Thacker, eds, *VCH Chester*, vol. 5: *The City of Chester*, 2 parts (London, 2003–5), I.50, 70. The problem persisted in 1504, when eighteen butchers were presented for slaughtering beasts in their shops, hanging the carcasses outside and fouling the streets: CCA, ZS/B/5b, Sheriffs' Book, 1504–1505, fol. 35r. See also ZS/B/5g, Sheriffs' Book, 1512–1513, fol. 137r.

[193] *LRBB*, I.34–5; KLBA, KL/C17/10, leet roll, 1379–80.

investment in paving and piped water since the 1320s.[194] Civic expenditure on the meat market in Exeter during the 1380s has likewise been regarded as evidence of the magistrates' 'eagerness to guarantee the sale of quality meat and to curb sanitation hazards' at a time of growing anxiety about virulent outbreaks of plague and substandard supplies.[195] Even more striking, major refurbishments at the start of the fifteenth century saw the raising, levelling, sanding and roofing of Reading's fish market so that it posed less of a threat to communal health.[196]

Another persuasive argument for restricting the sale of food to clearly designated places hinged upon the methods of waste disposal employed by victuallers, which could prove highly contentious. An extreme case in 1326 led to the murder of an itinerant eel-seller, who was beaten to death by two London apprentices for dumping refuse outside the shops where they worked.[197] Given their tendency to befoul the pavements and gutters with slops, it is hardly surprising that the fishmongers of Leicester were banned from setting up stalls in public thoroughfares and confined in 1335 to the market.[198] But, as the residents of Walbrook ward in London discovered, even the best-regulated system had its drawbacks, since the butchers and fishmongers of the Stocks were still polluting nearby streets during the 1420s, to the 'great nuisance and discomfort' of pedestrians.[199] The cooks of Bread Street ward seemed just as culpable, being then indicted for 'keeping their dung and garbage under their stalls and putting their spits too far out'.[200]

Coventry's fast-food sellers showed a similar disregard for the urban environment. An ordinance of 1421 insisted that 'no cook cast no maner of fylth vndur hur bordys [stall], ne in the hye stret, ne suffur hit ther to lye, that is to wit, fethurs, here [hair], ne entrails of pygges, ne of no othur bestes', on pain of a substantial fine for each offence. Two decades later the spotlight fell upon victuallers who contaminated the marketplace by washing entrails and bloodstained vessels, scalding hogs and performing other 'filthy operations' in full public view.[201] Nor were neighbouring householders exempt from censure: in 1509, for example, they were prohibited from depositing 'eny muk or swepynges' there until Friday night, ready for disposal by cart early the next morning.[202] A series of measures adopted in Leicester at the turn of the fifteenth century 'for making cleyne the markyt place' penalised all such nuisances, while appointing a salaried

---

[194] Owen, *Making of King's Lynn*, pp. 213–15.

[195] Kowaleski, *Local Markets*, p. 188.

[196] Slade, *Reading Gild Accounts*, pp. lxii–lxiii.

[197] *CCRCL*, pp. 169–70.

[198] *RBL*, II.21–2.

[199] *CPMRL, 1413–1437*, p. 135.

[200] *CPMRL, 1413–1437*, p. 137. In nearby Westminster, the cooks' stalls, with their outdoor benches, tables, spits, and jostling customers, constituted a permanent irritant: Rosser, *Medieval Westminster*, p. 129.

[201] *Coventry Leet Book*, I.26, 223. These ordinances suggest that the cooks were illicitly keeping and slaughtering animals: see section 5.3 above.

[202] *Coventry Leet Book*, III.624. Arrangements were also made for flushing clean the gutters in the fish market: Phythian-Adams, *Desolation of a City*, p. 78.

official to remove any rubbish on a weekly basis 'at vutter moste by Tewysday at nyght folowyng aftur the market day'.[203] In Dover a hired labourer performed this task, his work being greatly facilitated in 1505–6 by the decision to pave the entire area.[204]

The environs of markets had also to be kept clean, not least because piles of refuse, noxious drains and insalubrious activities might deter customers.[205] Conditions across the border in Edinburgh were so bad as to move the poet William Dunbar to verse, though it is unclear if his lament about the 'hurte and sclander', not to mention the lost profits, caused by the pungent aroma of rotting fish at the city gates was composed before or after orders were issued in 1505 for removing 'all maner of mwk, filth of fische and flesche' abandoned in the street on market days.[206] His concerns were clearly shared by the residents of far smaller towns. At Hythe in 1422, for example, jurors voiced particular objections to one noisome 'hoggisty' because it was 'abominable to all men coming to market, as well as to all dwelling in the town'.[207] Three Ipswich men were similarly amerced at this time for leaving dung 'in the common way of the merchants of the fish market', and thereby jeopardising trade as well as public health. However, the town's victuallers were themselves far from blameless, being charged between 1415 and 1424 with slaughtering sheep in the flesh market, dumping entrails in the road and failing to remove all manner of rubbish, including the guts of fish and dirty straw, from beneath their stalls.[208] The absence of further presentments on this score suggests that higher standards of hygiene subsequently prevailed, although the epidemic of 1420 may have prompted greater watchfulness. Colchester's butchers, who were castigated at this time for creating an unhealthy stench in the flesh market, had to

---

[203] 4*d.* was to be deducted from his pay for every instance of neglect: *RBL*, II.359. The salaried raker employed in Lynn from 1436 was responsible for cleansing the markets as well as the streets: KLBA, KL/C7/2, Hall Book, 1422–1429, p. 319 (later insert); C7/3, Hall Book, 1431–1450, fol. 60v.

[204] BL, MS Egerton 2107, fols 4v, 36v, 40r, 46r, 54r, 58r, 61r, 68v, 72v, 88r, 104v, 110r, 115r. One of York's principal markets, appropriately called The Pavement, was newly paved at this time: *YCR*, II.171.

[205] For example, a Winchester woman was presented in 1364 for permitting her drain to discharge filth into the market 'to the great peril and nuisance of the local people and merchants [*vicinorum & mercatorum*] being there': Furley, *Town Life*, pp. 132–3. In 1517, with similar concerns in mind, Basingstoke jurors demanded that all gutters 'about the market' should be fitted with grates to keep them free of dirt: Baigent and Millard, *History of the Town and Manor of Basingstoke*, p. 321. The antiquary John Kirkpatrick believed that Norwich's main market was sited on a steep slope because the gradient served to keep it clean in rainy weather, any waste being swept into the great cockey and thence into the river: *Streets and Lanes*, p. 24.

[206] William Dunbar, *The Poems of William Dunbar*, ed. J. Kinsley (Oxford, 1979), pp. 201–3; Marwick, *Records of the Burgh of Edinburgh*, p. 105. The provost then appointed an official with two servants and a covered cart to remove garbage. Significantly, plague was endemic at this time and had reached the city by October (pp. 106–7).

[207] HMC, *Fourth Report*, p. 432.

[208] SROI, C/2/8/1/2, 5–7.

provide a cart at their own expense for transporting miasmatic waste safely outside the walls.[209] Far more stringent regulations obtained in Cambridge, where traders were expected to remove 'all putrid flesh' from shops and stalls every morning and evening from 1376 onwards.[210] It is hard to see how such a demanding measure (which was probably devised by the university authorities) could have been enforced, but we might note that the burgesses of Salisbury opted to sink a deep pit in, or near, their market, so that ordure and noxious garbage could immediately be buried.[211]

In theory, the confinement of particular traders to separate markets, or at least to specific 'rows', also helped to curb fraud and blatant profiteering. Most English towns and cities recognised the need to impose such restrictions, especially in periods of dearth or uncertainty, when both the price and quality of foodstuffs were subject to dramatic fluctuations. Shortly after the Black Death, in 1351, four men from each London ward were appointed to prevent victuallers from trading covertly in unauthorised places, while hucksters were ordered to cease their customary practice of hawking fish in baskets round the streets.[212] Later, in 1388, all the City's fishmongers were obliged to swear on oath that they would only do business in 'pleyne market be fore the shoppis in the sight of people'.[213] The propensity of country poultry-sellers to wander about in search of a profitable deal, offering their wares 'in secret, to the great loss and grievance of the citizens and at extortionate prices', further justified their removal to Cornhill, while also necessitating a ban on out of hours purchases by cooks and retailers.[214] Similar regulations were enacted throughout England. In 1365, for example, the sale of meat in Beverley was confined to two designated markets; and in Leicester a century later to the common shambles or flesh market.[215] During the 1420s Lynn's butchers were told to set up their stalls in particular places on specific days and to stop using private premises or closed shops, especially at night, when contaminated meat might more easily be sold under cover of darkness. Two decades later the 'country' butchers, who lived outside the liberty, were assigned their own space near the guildhall, well away from the locals.[216]

[209] Britnell, *Growth and Decline in Colchester*, pp. 199–200.

[210] Cooper, *Annals of Cambridge*, p. 114.

[211] Carr, *First General Entry Book*, no. 335.

[212] Riley, *Memorials of London*, pp. 257, 267–8.

[213] *CLB*, D, pp. 198–9. The sale of fish caught in the Thames was restricted to Cornhill and Cheapside: Riley, *Memorials of London*, pp. 508–9. A century later the rulers of Bristol decreed that 'good and able' fresh fish was to be traded only in specific places: E. W. W. Veale, ed., *The Great Red Book of Bristol*, vol. 3, Bristol Record Society 16 (Bristol, 1951), p. 115. It is interesting that 'the women of Whitstable', who presumably sold oysters, had their own designated market in Canterbury, which was paved in 1480: HMC, *Ninth Report*, part 1, appendix, p. 137.

[214] Riley, *Memorials of London*, pp. 220–1.

[215] *BTD*, pp. 128–9; *RBL*, II.292. Norwich followed suit in 1441: NRO, NCR, 16D/1, Assembly Proceedings, 1434–1491, fol. 14v.

[216] KLBA, KL/C7/2, Hall Book, 1422–1429, pp. 224, 228, 232; C7/3, Hall Book, 1431–1450, fols 31v, 170v, 172v, 175v, 212r; C7/4, Hall Book, 1453–1497, p. 438. Bakers, too, had to trade in designated places: KL/C7/3, fol. 20v.

The potential for both conflict and collusion led many urban authorities to insist upon the physical separation of 'foreign' retailers, although such arrangements might be abandoned in times of shortage or pestilence.[217] At Beverley, from 1370 onwards, the fishmongers provided a convenient barrier between the stalls of the 'strange' and resident butchers, whose relations were far from cordial.[218] Commercial rivalry could certainly turn ugly. Following a fracas of 1382 involving a former alderman who had hurled abuse at 'foreign' fishmongers, the rulers of London threatened anyone who tried to prevent these 'strangers' from trading competitively in the City with imprisonment.[219] A similar attempt by locals to drive rival fishermen away from the official landing stage on the Ouse in 1418 led York's magistrates to provide an alternative quay, so that prices might be kept reasonably low and the poorer citizens adequately fed.[220] Their firm stand on this score also provoked some memorable confrontations with local bakers and butchers, as well as initiatives designed to attract less avaricious rural tradesmen. Regarding the excessive prices charged by resident butchers in 1425 as a serious threat to the community and its collective reputation, they urged 'foreigners' to attend the Thursday Market, guaranteeing them freedom from 'verbal impediments', or worse. This tactic was repeated in 1482; and in 1503 a general invitation was extended to the 'men of Thurn, Lincoln, Northfolk and all othir plasez that ar vitellers bryng[ing] good and holsome victale'.[221]

The very real possibility that some residents would buy up the outsiders' goods wholesale in order to secure a monopoly, or otherwise attempt to rig the market, had also to be prevented. In London 'foreign' poultry-men were not only instructed on pain of forfeiture and imprisonment to keep their distance from the stalls of the freemen, but were even prohibited from lodging with them or using their premises for storage. Nor could they do business with any of the City's other victuallers before the bells rang for prime, 'when the great and other the common people shall have bought what they need for their own use'.[222] Similar regulations are to be found in the custumals and ordinances of most English boroughs, such as the late thirteenth-century 'Usages of Winchester', which forbade the sale of fish and poultry until after nine o'clock.[223] Church and market bells, which constituted such a notable feature of the urban soundscape, were but one of the many controls employed in an attempt to ensure that the ordinary consumer could eat both cheaply and well.

---

[217] As, for example, at Salisbury (Carr, *First General Entry Book*, nos 145, 295, 298, 413), and York (Tillott, *VCH York: City of York*, p. 484).

[218] *BTD*, p. 29.

[219] Riley, *Memorials of London*, pp. 468–70, 473–4, 481–2. This particular controversy had wider political ramifications, for which see n. 63 above.

[220] *YMB*, I.198; *YMB*, II.72–3.

[221] *YMB*, I.57; Tillott, *VCH York: City of York*, p. 99; *YCR*, II.182.

[222] Riley, *Memorials of London*, pp. 299–300, 389.

[223] Rothwell, *EHD, 1189–1327*, p. 872.

5.8 Weights, measures, assizes and prices

In the marketplace of the human heart, described so eloquently by Henry of Lancaster, the weights and measures used to quantify good or bad behaviour were fixed and assayed by God, with the result that the penitent sinner who wished to have 'his merchandise truly weighed and sold, would lose nothing, gaining thereby more than three pence'.[224] Daily experience was often less reassuring, despite constant efforts on the part of both central and local authorities. Notwithstanding the prospect of their own suspension in St Michael's scales at the Last Judgement, traders could not always be trusted to deal fairly with their customers, while the perplexing lack of standardisation apparent throughout the realm made it difficult to establish consistency.[225] Edward I's insistence upon the twice-yearly inspection and authentication of weights and measures by urban magistrates constituted a basic requirement which was often exceeded, as we can see from the frequency with which assays and attendant prosecutions are noted in late medieval records.[226] In mid-fourteenth-century Bristol bushel and gallon measures stamped with the royal seal were kept under secure custody and used as a standard against which all others had to be checked and approved every six months, as the crown required.[227] But in Norwich inspections were held more often, being then conducted at least three, and sometimes four, times a year.[228] Sporadic bouts of activity in Exeter yielded spectacular results, as in 1390 when thirty fraudulent victuallers were fined and lost their equipment, but minor offenders generally escaped attention.[229] The rulers of London, in contrast, were predictably zealous. In 1310, for example, wood-turners, who made the vessels used for serving ale and wine, had to swear before the mayor that they would adhere solely to the three measures legally recognised in the City and produce nothing else. Even so, because of the 'manifold falsities and deceits' reported by angry drinkers, each turner was obliged, from 1347 onwards, to register his mark, and thus became personally accountable for every cup, bowl or jug that left his shop.[230] And from 1420 onwards, following the scandal about contaminated barrels described above, the coopers had to follow suit.[231]

---

[224] Henry of Lancaster, *Livre de seyntz medicines*, p. 122. Devils were notorious for attempting to tip St Michael's scales at the Last Judgement so that the soul being weighed would go to hell. See, for example, the late fifteenth-century doom at Wenhaston church in Suffolk.

[225] R. D. Connor provides a valuable survey: *The Weights and Measures of England* (London, 1987), chaps 8–10.

[226] *SR*, I.204–5; Keiser, *Works of Science and Information*, pp. 3687–8, 3900–1.

[227] *LRBB*, I.38; II.219. Infringements were prosecuted as forgery and punished with imprisonment.

[228] *RCN*, I.176–7.

[229] Kowaleski, *Local Markets*, p. 189.

[230] Riley, *Memorials of London*, pp. 78, 234–5.

[231] *CLB*, I, pp. 237–8. Because of the importance of the fish trade in Lynn, regulations for coopers were stringently enforced. The mayor conducted inspections in person, and punishments could be severe: KLBA, KL/C3, Hall Book, 1431–1450, fol. 214r; C7/4, Hall Book, 1453–1497, pp. 103–5.

The crown sought to curb other abuses on the part of dishonest bakers, brewers and hucksters. Developed in the reign of Henry II, and refined by Henry III, the *assisa panis et cervisae* (assize of bread and ale) imposed quality and price control on England's two basic dietary staples.[232] Its status as 'the most significant and long-lasting commercial law in medieval England' seems richly deserved, since it determined the strength and content of ale, as well as the size, weight and quality of up to nine different kinds of loaf, specifically in relation to the current price of grain.[233] Loaves were traditionally sold by farthing, half-penny and penny weights, although in practice both the amount and purity of the flour used in the baking process could fluctuate considerably according to the vagaries of the market. For this reason constant scrutiny was essential. In the words of the Norwich custumal of *c.* 1306, which themselves echo King Henry's statute, the assize of bread sought to ensure 'that the people be not deceived but rather that they be served ... rightly and faithfully without fraud'.[234] Fourteenth-century ordinances promulgated in Bristol against breaches of the assize of ale refer in similar terms to the exploitation of 'the poor people of the commonalty'.[235] Indeed, it was in 1347 that the city secured a grant by royal charter of the right to draw 'delinquents against the assize' through the streets on a hurdle, as was already the practice in London (plate 21).[236]

Because of the size of its population and its dependence on external grain supplies, London furnishes the most striking examples of strict and continuous enforcement of the assize, notably during the successive crises of the early fourteenth century. Praising the measures already adopted there to peg escalating ale prices, in January 1317 the royal council decreed that similar rates should be adopted throughout the realm, lest 'a great part of the lower and poor people [should] suffer from famine'.[237] Even when conditions improved, the authorities showed no sign of flagging. Although by the fifteenth century London's bakers had assumed greater powers of self-regulation, being required to hold twice-weekly

[232] Britnell, *Commercialisation of English Society*, pp. 94–6; Connor, *Weights and Measures*, pp. 194–205 (bread), 220–4 (ale); A. Ballard, ed., *British Borough Charters, 1042–1216* (Cambridge, 1913), pp. 157–9; *SR*, I.202–4.

[233] J. Davis, 'Baking for the Common Good: A Reassessment of the Assize of Bread in Medieval England', *EconHR*, 2nd series 57 (2004), pp. 465–502, on p. 465.

[234] *RCN*, I.175; Davis, 'Baking for the Common Good', p. 472; Bennett, *Ale, Beer and Brewsters*, p. 21.

[235] *LRBB*, II.38.

[236] N. Dermott Harding, ed., *Bristol Charters, 1155–1373*, Bristol Record Society 1 (Bristol, 1930), p. 109.

[237] *CCR, 1313–1318*, p. 449. On the assumption that London's population reached as many as 100,000 in 1300, it has been estimated that approximately 165,000 quarters of grain would have been needed every year to feed the human inhabitants alone: B. M. S. Campbell, *et al.*, *A Medieval Capital and its Grain Supply* (London, 1993), pp. 34–5. J. A. Galloway observes that, although the population had halved by 1400, *per capita* ale consumption rose significantly, thereby increasing the demand for malt: 'London's Grain Supply: Changes in Production, Distribution and Consumption during the Fourteenth Century', *Franco-British Studies* 20 (1995), pp. 23–34.

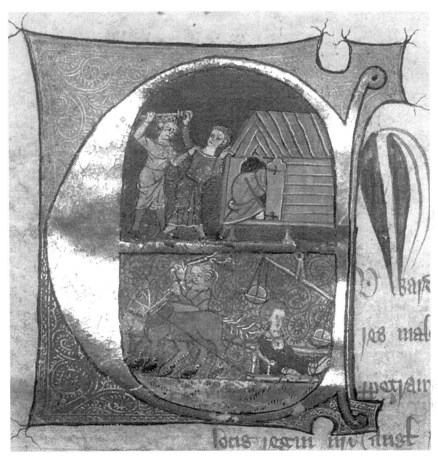

21 Bristol's royal charter of 1347 bestowed the right to draw 'delinquents against the assize' through the streets on a hurdle, and is decorated with an image of a dishonest baker (with his bread suspended in a pair of scales) undergoing this punishment.

searches for 'unseasonable' and under-weight loaves, the mayor and aldermen remained vigilant, when necessary throwing their formidable authority behind that of the inspectors.[238] The compulsory stamping of loaves with bakers' seals made it difficult to evade detection for long, though a few opportunists showed considerable ingenuity.[239] In 1327, for instance, a number of dishonest bakers were found to have placed false bottoms on their 'molding bordes' so that lumps of the dough brought to them by local people for baking could be surreptitiously cut away by an apprentice hiding under the table. A day in the pillory with the stolen

[238] Seabourne, 'Assize Matters'; *CLB*, L, pp. 170–1.

[239] For example, a piece of iron might be slipped into a loaf just before it was weighed: Riley, *Memorials of London*, p. 498; *CLB*, H, pp. 322–3. The use of seals was made compulsory by royal decree in the later thirteenth century (*SR*, I.203), and was immediately adopted in London (*CLB*, A, p. 216). Provincial cities such as Bristol followed soon afterwards: *LRBB*, II.224; Veale, *Great Red Book of Bristol*, I.138.

dough suspended around their necks was deemed appropriate retribution for 'a certain species of theft ... neither consonant with right nor pleasing to God'.[240] Since the victims of this clever trick included poor householders who lacked ovens, the crime must have seemed a blasphemous reversal of the Lord's Prayer, with its humble appeal for daily bread.

In some towns and cities information about current grain prices would be recorded in tabular form by the relevant office-holders and updated as the market rose or fell.[241] It proved necessary to modify the guidelines used in the Southampton assize of bread no fewer than six times between October 1482 and the following September to allow for these fluctuations.[242] In Norwich, too, magistrates were punctilious in monitoring any changes, sometimes imposing penalties of 30s. or more upon offenders who grossly overcharged their customers.[243] We should, however, bear in mind that the assize also presented magistrates with a lucrative form of licensing which enabled them to augment diminishing resources through the collection of standardised fines from brewers and bakers. As a result, the system tended to become more fiscal than supervisory or judicial, especially in smaller boroughs such as Colchester, where regulation was left to market forces and, in extreme cases, local juries.[244] More often, serious abuses would result either in private litigation or prosecution by the civic authorities, while the assize itself devolved into a welcome source of taxation.[245]

Once it had overcome the distaste with which it initially regarded commercial transactions, the medieval Church sought to temper the worst excesses of a free market by developing the doctrine of the 'just price'. As refined and qualified by late medieval theologians, the concept allowed producers and traders to charge proportionally more for their goods in times of dearth, but condemned any attempt to raise prices by collusion or to fleece the poor.[246] In matters of food supply, urban communities were among the most active exponents of the doctrine, notably during periods of crisis, when blatant profiteering flourished.[247] Their approach is exemplified in the oath demanded of fifteenth-century London fishmongers, that

---

[240] Riley, *Memorials of London*, pp. 162–5; *MGL*, III.416–19.

[241] Seabourne, 'Assize Matters', p. 33 n. 26; P. W. Hammond, *Food and Feast in Medieval England* (Stroud, 1993), p. 53. As we have seen, one such table survives in the commonplace book of a London citizen alongside a number of vernacular medical texts: BL, MS Egerton 1995, fols 80v–81v.

[242] A. S. C. Ross, 'The Assize of Bread', *EconHR*, 2nd series 9 (1956), pp. 332–42, on p. 332; Studer, *Oak Book of Southampton*, II.xii–xiii. The assize was strictly enforced in Southampton, where bakers were frequently amerced for selling 'light' loaves: Butler, *Book of Fines*, p. xvii.

[243] NRO, NCR, 16A/1, Mayor's Court Book, 1424–1449, *passim*. In 1427 William Barley, a recidivist, was fined the exemplary sum of 80s. (p. 7).

[244] Britnell, *Growth and Decline in Colchester*, pp. 89–90.

[245] Kowaleski, *Local Markets*, p. 187.

[246] J. L. Bolton, *The Medieval English Economy, 1150–1500* (London, 1980), pp. 335–6.

[247] R. de Roover stresses the civic aim 'to secure abundant supplies as cheaply as possible', especially during shortages: 'The Concept of the Just Price: Theory and Economic Policy', *Journal of Economic History* 18 (1958), pp. 418–38, on pp. 428–9.

they would 'retayle to the comyns for her propre use with owte takyng of excessif wynnyng'.[248] Since victuallers could not always be trusted to restrain their baser instincts, magistrates stepped in when necessary to impose price ceilings on basic commodities, supported after the Black Death by comprehensive national legislation.[249] That direct intervention had the ancillary benefit of privileging resident freemen over other retailers may have rendered it more acceptable, as it implicitly reinforced the social and economic status quo.[250]

Recognising the need for compromise in the case of minor infringements, the rulers of English towns and cities frequently opted for a thinly veiled tax, such as that levied upon brewers and bakers, which at least had the merit of replenishing communal coffers. By the 1420s, for instance, Ipswich taverners routinely paid an annual fine of a few pence for overcharging customers, and were thus effectively free to set their own prices within *reasonable* limits. Overt extortion would invite prosecution and the imposition of far heavier penalties.[251] Nor should we disregard the desire to protect less fortunate members of the urban body from exploitation. The rueful complaint of the poor peasant who wanders the streets bemused and hungry in verses known as 'London Lykpenny' may well reflect the experience of many, although the City's rulers did attempt from the 1270s to make cheap food and drink available to those on short commons.[252] Outbreaks of plague and other epidemics were often the catalyst for such measures. Thus, regulations of 1350 fixed the maximum amount to be charged by cooks for baking their customers' meat in pies or pasties at one penny, on pain of imprisonment.[253] Prices were similarly pegged thirteen years later as the cost of living rose after another pestilence; on this occasion victuallers were threatened with fines and the pillory for stockpiling their wares in order to increase profits.[254]

The quality of foodstuffs consumed by the labouring classes was also at issue, not least because traders tended to reserve inferior produce for their less affluent

---

[248] *CLB*, D, p. 199; Riley, *Memorials of London*, pp. 666–7.

[249] G. Seabourne provides a comprehensive survey of national and local controls: *Royal Regulation of Loans and Sales in Medieval England* (Woodbridge, 2003), chap. 3.

[250] R. H. Britnell, 'Price-Setting in English Borough Markets, 1349–1500', *Canadian Journal of History* 31 (1996), pp. 1–15; Britnell, *Growth and Decline in Colchester*, pp. 36–7.

[251] SROI, C/2/8/1/5–11, 13, 15–22; C/2/10/1/2, 3, 5.

[252] *MGL*, II.i.82–3 (poultry, 1273–4), 117–20 (fish, late thirteenth century), 192–3 (victuals generally, 1299–1300); *CLB*, A, p. 216 (ale, 1276–8). See also Jones, *Butchers of London*, pp. 106–9; Barron, *London in the Later Middle Ages*, pp. 57–60.

[253] Carlin, 'Fast Food', p. 21; Riley, *Memorials of London*, p. 257. By 1378 the ceiling had risen by 50 per cent: Riley, *Memorials of London*, p. 426. The prices to be charged by cooks and brewers were also fixed in fourteenth-century Bristol: *LRBB*, II.32, 227.

[254] Riley, *Memorials of London*, pp. 312–13. For the rising cost of a basket of consumables at this time, see D. L. Farmer, 'Prices and Wages, 1350–1500', in E. Miller, ed., *The Agrarian History of England and Wales*, vol. 3: *1348–1500* (Cambridge, 1991), p. 520.

customers. In order to resolve this problem, the pie-bakers of London were instructed in 1378 to produce half-penny 'pasties of beef' that were just as good as those selling at a penny, on pain of a significant fine of 3s. 4d. for each dereliction. Threats and reminders were often needed: from 1427 onwards any Coventry cooks who failed to bake nutritious 'halpeny pyes as other townes doth' stood to forfeit twice as much as the Londoners.[255] It was specifically to assist the victims of a long recession that, in 1467, Leicester magistrates instituted a comprehensive series of bye-laws for the more equitable distribution of wholesome food and drink. The brewers had to ensure that their cheaper ale was 'nother raw, red, nor roppie, but ... cleyn brweyd', and to provide half-penny measures for the benefit of 'pore peopyll'. Fishmongers and other victuallers were ordered to take no more than a 'reasonable encres' for their wares, while a directive to the bakers warned that the community should 'lak no maner of breed, wyght ne browne, ne non other kyndes of breed in payne of inpresonment'. The coarse farthing loaves bought by men and women on low wages were, in particular, to be 'of good paste, good bulture and well baken'.[256] One year later, the Norwich Assembly reprimanded local brewers for their callous neglect of an 'olde and laudable' civic custom which allowed anyone in need to purchase a modest quantity of food or drink for one farthing. Known locally as 'goddis good ... because it cometh of the grete grace of God', this concession was a cause of no little pride in a community that made much of its generosity to the deserving poor. Any victuallers who attempted 'by ffraude or subtilte' to ignore the practice and overcharge 'for their singular lucre and avayle' were henceforward to be named, shamed and heavily fined for each offence.[257]

Directives of this kind might well provoke a less than compliant response. From at least the 1380s, the bakers of Winchester were repeatedly fined for refusing to sell the cheap loaves which undercut their profits.[258] An extra minting of farthing coins was even undertaken in London in 1382–3 so that no brewer or baker could legitimately decline to serve anyone because he or she lacked change for a half-penny.[259] If all other evasive tactics failed it was always possible for bakers to ration, or even withhold altogether, supplies of the brown and black bread – as opposed to the more expensive 'wastel' made of wheat – that the poor consumed. In 1419, for instance, the bakers of Tamworth were ordered to make *all* kinds, sufficient to feed the *entire* town, on pain of a collective fine of 20s.[260] Following a standoff

---

[255] Riley, *Memorials of London*, pp. 157, 432; *Coventry Leet Book*, I.111.

[256] *RBL*, II.287–8; Davis, 'Baking for the Common Good', p. 487. Winchelsea bakers faced a fine of 12d. for failing to bake farthing loaves at least once a week (BL, MS Cotton Julius B IV, fol. 26v). In mid-fifteenth-century Bristol the sale of expensive 2d. loaves was forbidden: Veale, *Great Red Book of Bristol*, I.138.

[257] *RCN*, II.98–9. Reluctance on the part of Bristol's fishmongers to sell large fish such as salmon in small pieces likewise prompted legislation in 1451–2: Veale, *Great Red Book of Bristol*, I.141. For the same reason the rulers of London insisted in 1412 that eels should be sold by weight only, rather than size: Riley, *Memorials of London*, pp. 580–1.

[258] Furley, *Town Life*, p. 141; Keene, *Survey of Medieval Winchester*, I.254.

[259] *CLB*, H, p. 183; Galloway, 'Driven by Drink?', pp. 95–6.

[260] Davis, 'Baking for the Common Good', p. 487.

over the sale of loaves that were 'unhelefull and evill seissend and also not of weght according to the assise', the rulers of York employed similar tactics in 1486, by which time an artificial shortage of bread had inflicted 'grete hurt' upon 'the commons'.[261] Nine years later the city's butchers incurred a more substantial penalty of £5 'for that they had not flesche' on sale after Lent 'and other diverse tymez this yere past to serve the Kyngys people'.[262] Their characteristically stubborn refusal to pay up or reduce their prices led, in some cases, to imprisonment, and an impasse with the mayor that was only resolved when the bishop of Carlisle intervened on their behalf. This case reveals how hard it could be to face down well-organised resistance, which might even result in outright strikes. In Exeter such extreme steps were taken at least twice by the city's bakers, whose indignation over the measures deployed by the authorities in the difficult years of 1323–4 and 1362–3 boiled over into direct action.[263] However well-intentioned they may have been, magistrates often had to accept that the gap between enactment and enforcement could not always be bridged.

5.9 Forestalling and 'engrossing' the market

As Christopher Dyer observes, the ideal cherished by medieval elites of 'producers selling directly to the consumer, cutting out all middlemen, whose profit margins would raise the price' was rarely, if ever, realised. Nor, given fluctuations in the market and the demands of feeding so many people, was it easy to curb the mercenary behaviour of those involved in the supply chain.[264] Even so, the volume of evidence documenting this 'constant tussle' in both national and local archives testifies to the zeal, if not always the success, with which legislators approached their task. 'Forestalling', or the buying up of essential commodities such as grain and fish by intermediaries before they went on sale to the public, in order to maximise profits, appeared both antisocial and immoral, as did 'engrossing', which involved the purchase of excessive quantities of a particular item for the same purpose. Forestallers invited particular censure not only because their activities harmed the most vulnerable members of society, but also because valuable tolls were often lost to the authorities, whose attempts to control prices were, moreover, deliberately undermined.[265] Following precepts established in 1275 by the clerks of the Marshalsea (who were acting on behalf of the crown), first the mayor and aldermen of London and then provincial magistrates sought to penalise offenders, sometimes at the direct behest of the king or in conjunction with royal

---

[261] *YMB*, I.170–2; *YCR*, I.124.

[262] *YCR*, II.121; Swanson, *Medieval Artisans*, p. 15.

[263] DRO, ECA, Book 51, fol. 281r (and also fol. 303r for trouble in 1428); Kowaleski, *Local Markets*, pp. 140–1. See also *Coventry Leet Book*, II.518–19; and for problems in Canterbury, HMC, *Ninth Report*, part 1, appendix, p. 173.

[264] Dyer, *Standards of Living*, p. 198.

[265] Britnell, *Commercialisation of English Society*, pp. 92–3; Britnell, 'Price-Setting in English Borough Markets', p. 11.

commissions of inquiry.[266] As we have seen in the case of the assizes of bread and ale, minor infringements by petty traders might well provide a welcome source of cash in the form of a standard toll, but more serious offences merited condign punishment. Not surprisingly, one mayor of Exeter had the disgruntled citizen who accused him of forestalling herring and other victuals in 1396–7 thrown into prison for bringing both his office and person into disrepute.[267]

Forestalling prompted predictably harsh reactions when food was scarce, being described in the Norwich custumal of *c.* 1306 as a cause of great scandal and rebuke to the entire community.[268] A major offensive by the city's leet courts in 1374–5 against ninety or so individuals who had reputedly attempted to corner the market in oysters, eggs and grain, 'whereby there accrued great dearness of victuals', resulted in some draconian fines, rising to over £12 each. These inflated penalties served to underscore the seriousness of the offence, and were eventually reduced, the main aim being to deter others from following suit.[269] An overwhelming tendency to blame the trader for shortages, irrespective of wider economic factors, could sometimes prove counterproductive by penalising those who were scouring the countryside for much-needed supplies, and thus unwittingly exacerbate the problem.[270] But the authorities rarely tempered their opinions. Ordinances recorded in mid-fourteenth-century Bristol portray the forestaller in unequivocal terms as a social pariah, 'a manifest oppressor of the poor and a public enemy of the whole commonalty and country', whose crimes merited expulsion.[271] The borough customs of Ipswich, which were first recorded in the early fourteenth century and translated into English in the fifteenth, confirm that the regulation of markets and prevention of forestalling might be viewed in terms of a regimen for the benefit of the urban workforce. To this end, oysters and mussels, traditionally the food of less affluent residents, were to be sold only by the fishermen who had brought them to the quayside 'for the comoun profit of poure men as of ryche', rather than by

---

[266] For a comprehensive survey of the legislative framework, see Seabourne, *Royal Regulation of Loans and Sales*, chap. 4; Britnell, 'Forstall, Forestalling and the Statute of Forestallers', pp. 89–102. For the punishment of forestallers in London, see *MGL*, I.263–4; *CEMCRL*, pp. 50–2, 59, 157–8, 228–9, 231, 234, 241, 246; *CLB*, C, pp. 77, 156; *CLB*, D, p. 252; *CLB*, E, pp. 44, 113–14, 120; *CLB*, F, pp. 201, 208; *CPMRL*, *1323–1364*, p. 203.

[267] Kowaleski, *Local Markets*, pp. 117–18; Britnell, *Growth and Decline in Colchester*, pp. 131–4, 237–8.

[268] *RCN*, I.181–5. In 1304 a royal commission had been appointed to investigate allegations by 'the poor men of the community of Norwich' that 'certain rich men and forestallers of that city' had monopolised sales and driven up prices: *CPR*, *1301–1307*, p. 284.

[269] Hudson, *Leet Jurisdiction*, pp. 62–5. The price of wheat and consumables in general was then extremely high, and it rose further in the following year: Farmer, 'Prices and Wages, 1350–1500', pp. 503, 521.

[270] Britnell, *Commercialisation of English Society*, p. 174.

[271] *LRBB*, II.220 (the author is here paraphrasing *SR*, I.203). Over a century later, in 1472–3, a mayoral edict against forestalling imposed a minimum fine of 20s. for the first offence: Veale, *Great Red Book of Bristol*, III.96–7. For similar regulations in Winchester, see Rothwell, *EHD*, *1189–1327*, p. 872.

hucksters who pushed up the prices.[272] In a subsequent campaign during the early 1480s that reflects a notable improvement in the local diet, the mayor introduced stringent measures to prevent the illicit sale of meat to commercial buyers outside the flesh market in the homes or slaughterhouses of butchers.[273] It is unlikely that magistrates ever managed to eliminate such activities, or that they did not sometimes derive considerable personal benefit from them. Even so, legislation of this kind conveyed a powerful message designed to allay the understandable anxieties of ordinary consumers.

Some of the worst offenders were involved in the burgeoning fast-food business. Cooks not only contravened health regulations but were also notorious for cornering supplies, often for resale at excessive profits. Voicing a widely held opinion, William Langland accused them and other victuallers of lining their pockets when honest folk went hungry. For this reason he urged 'the comune'

> To punyschen on pillories and pynynge stoles
> Brewesteres and bakesteres, bocheres and cokes;
> For thise aren men on this molde that moste harme worcheth
> To the pore peple that parcel-mele buggen [can afford only small amounts].[274]

His concerns are mirrored in many contemporary bye-laws, such the above-mentioned ordinance of 1383 that prohibited London cooks and pie-bakers from buying poultry or fish before prime or attempting to engage in any type of retail trade.[275] The annual appointment in the 1440s of two aldermen, rather than lesser officials, specifically to oversee members of both crafts (along with other sellers of foodstuffs) sent an unambiguous warning to potential forestallers and unprincipled hucksters.[276] As we have already seen, traders throughout England were commonly forbidden from acquiring wholesale supplies when markets opened, thereby allowing one or two hours for individual shoppers to make their more modest purchases. In Bristol from the late 1320s, for instance, 'gross fish' such as salmon, herring and eels had to be offered at a fixed price 'to the profit of the commons', *before* itinerant retailers attempted to fill their baskets. Even more important, the city's bakers and brewers were categorically prohibited from

---

[272] Twiss, *Black Book of the Admiralty*, II.100–11, 160–1. In Berwick-upon-Tweed, purchases of herring, the food of the poor, had to be shared among all prospective buyers: Smith, Smith and Brentano, *English Gilds*, p. 345.

[273] Bacon, *Annalls of Ipswiche*, pp. 148–9. In 1488 fines of 3s. 4d. were imposed on fishmongers who attempted to trade outside the market.

[274] Langland, *Piers the Plowman*, I.68. He adds, for good measure, that such victuallers 'poysoun the peple priueliche and oft'. In Nottingham, just over a decade later, the city's cooks were presented *en masse* for forestalling poultry, eggs and other victuals: Stevenson, *Records of the Borough of Nottingham*, I.271.

[275] *CLB*, H, p. 214; see section 5.3 above. As the presentments made by London juries reveal, ordinary citizens eagerly reported infringements: *CPMRL, 1413–1437*, p. 122. Similar injunctions were approved in towns such as Beverley (*BTD*, pp. 29–30), Bristol (Veale, *Great Red Book of Bristol*, I.134–5), Canterbury (HMC, *Ninth Report*, part 1, appendix, p. 172), and York (*YMB*, I.221–3).

[276] Barron, *London in the Later Middle Ages*, pp. 58–9.

buying grain early in the morning, on pain of forfeiture, as, indeed, were all other victuallers.[277]

The success of these measures is hard to judge, although there can be little doubt that the urban grain market was subject to particularly close surveillance in order to maintain a regular, uncontaminated and affordable supply for both domestic and commercial use. From at least the early thirteenth century a plethora of rules determined how, when, where and at what price wheat, barley, oats, rye and malt should change hands in London, the penalties for disobedience reflecting the social and moral implications of the crime.[278] Various hucksters found guilty in 1300 of forestalling and selling corn (some of which was allegedly 'putrid') on the City's pavements 'in deception of the people' were immediately committed to prison to await sentencing.[279] During times of dearth convicted offenders could usually expect a spell in gaol even for relatively minor infractions. In 1347, for example, one small-time profiteer, who had attempted to charge 2*d.* over the fixed price for just a couple of bushels of wheat 'to the damage of the commonalty', earned a symbolic forty days' confinement, being fortunate to escape a session in the pillory as well.[280]

Elsewhere, patterns of enforcement appear to have been more sporadic. Suspecting that local juries had grown unduly lax when harvests were good, the mayor of Lynn insisted that they should report anyone responsible for driving up grain prices during the difficult autumn of 1457 '*as their consciences demanded*' (my italics).[281] The rulers of this busy North Sea port were, in fact, singularly well placed to take action during shortages because so many shipments of wheat and barley passed through the docks on their way to or from domestic and Continental markets. Their conduct during the agrarian crises of the late 1420s and 1430s reveals an effective deployment of existing legislation, together with a readiness to take independent action, sometimes in the face of opposition on the part of wealthy ship owners. Reserves had fallen dangerously low when, on 25 April 1429, the mayor placed an embargo upon all further exports of wheat, resident burgesses being threatened with the loss of trading privileges should they disobey. Between then and 25 June, as supplies dwindled even further, £60 was diverted from the treasury for the purchase of grain, and in early August the town's

---

[277] *LRBB*, I.38–9; II.73, 221–2, 225–6, 229. For York, see Swanson, *Medieval Artisans*, pp. 10–11. In Lynn the sale of grain was prohibited before nones (KLBA, KL/C7/3, Hall Book, 1431–1450, fol. 212r), and of fish before 8 a.m. (C7/4, Hall Book, 1453–1497, p. 574). Norwich food markets began trading two hours later (NRO, NCR, 16D/1, Assembly Proceedings, 1434–1491, fol. 24r). From 1467, Leicester's Saturday Market offered corn to *domestic* buyers only, once everyone was 'hool assembled' at 10 a.m., and not before. Stockpiling was strictly forbidden: *RBL*, II.291, 294.

[278] *MGL*, I.261–3; *CEMCRL*, p. 59; *CLB*, E, pp. 56–7; *CLB*, F, pp. 100–2, 165–7; *CLB*, G, pp. 33, 77, 103, 123, 138, 149, 167, 170–1, 225, 261, 330; *CLB*, H, pp. 13, 48, 147, 354; *CPMRL, 1323–1364*, p. 115.

[279] *CEMCRL*, p. 59.

[280] Riley, *Memorials of London*, pp. 235–6.

[281] KLBA, KL/C7/4, Hall Book, 1453–1497, p. 98. For the poor harvests and livestock mortality at this time, see Hatcher, 'The Great Slump', p. 246.

bakers attended an emergency meeting in the guildhall at which bread prices were fixed.[282]

The market briefly recovered, but worse lay ahead. Notwithstanding the royal council's refusal to sanction a second embargo in July 1431, the Lynn authorities were sufficiently concerned by the following summer to renew their appeal, which eventually proved successful. Indeed, by November 1432 they had already begun searching out and arresting cargoes of wheat, which were subject to compulsory purchase orders with 'reasonable' levels of compensation. It is impossible to tell how much was spent on providing the inhabitants with subsidised grain at this time, but the bill must have run to several hundred pounds, not least as a result of the legal costs involved.[283] Perhaps because of pre-emptive action, the poor harvests of 1437–9 prompted fewer such arrests. The mayor again moved rapidly to impose price ceilings and imprison anyone suspected of profiteering 'to the grave damage and nuisance of the community'. And although it proved necessary to replace the four officials who had initially been appointed 'to purchase victuals for the common use' because of their inertia, the populace did not starve. As before, the grain confiscated from offenders, together with supplies acquired at every opportunity from other sources, was sold by the constables to the residents of each ward at reduced rates.[284] Much-needed supplementary support came from the town's largest guild, whose distribution of charitable doles reached an unprecedented peak at this time.[285]

Members of the urban elite dug deep into their own pockets during periods of dearth. Recognising a personal obligation to supply their less affluent neighbours with daily bread, two Colchester aldermen undertook at considerable expense in 1489 to rebuild the town's dilapidated corn mill. Although they secured a preferential lease, it is unlikely that they ever recouped more than a fraction of the costs involved.[286] Others chose to offer cash for use in emergencies.[287] On his death in March 1519, following a run of poor yields and an outbreak of sweating sickness, John Haddon of Coventry left £20 'to by corne with at such tyme that corne risith, to brynge the market down, as farr as this said some ... will extend'. His bequest was timely, since devastating crop failures and an onslaught of plague

[282] KLBA, KL/C7/2, Hall Book, 1422–1429, pp. 246–7, 251, 252, 261.

[283] KLBA, KL/C7/3, Hall Book, 1431–1450, fols 11v, 25v, 30r–v, 31v–37r, 38r, 41r.

[284] KLBA, KL/C7/3, Hall Book, 1431–1450, fols 86r, 88v, 90r, 96v, 98v, 99v, 101r. Prices rocketed nationally at this time: Farmer, 'Prices and Wages, 1350–1500', p. 504. The author of one London chronicle noted the excessively high price of grain in 1438–9, observing that 'men ete moo benys, and pesyn, and barly that yere than euer whas etyn in Englond a c [100] winter beforn': Kingsford, *Chronicles of London*, p. 146. In Salisbury the hoarding of grain was then prohibited: Carr, *First General Entry Book*, no. 344.

[285] B. R. McRee, 'Charity and Guild Solidarity', *Journal of British Studies* 32 (1993), pp. 195–225, on p. 217. However, he does not connect these doles with current food shortages.

[286] Britnell, *Growth and Decline in Colchester*, pp. 228–9.

[287] For example, Mark William, sometime mayor of Bristol (d. *c.* 1434), who left £66 in his will to provide grain in times of dearth: Roskell, Clark and Rawcliffe, *Commons, 1386–1421*, IV.870.

later in that year created acute shortages throughout England.[288] So great were levels of distress in Norwich by March 1522 that every alderman was called upon to donate twenty combs of wheat 'to serve the people', only five from a list of twenty-two potential donors opting to pay a fine instead.[289] Meanwhile in Bristol, according to one chronicler:

> [The] Maire, of his gode disposition inclynyng his charitie towardes the comen wele and profite of this towne, auctorized Mr Ware and others, vndre the comon seale ... to provide whete, corn, and other graynys necessary and beneficiall for the comons of this same towne within the shire of Worcestre, or therabout ... by reason wherof greate abundaunce ... was so provided, that the inhabitauntes ... were greatly releved and comforted in mynysshing of the price of whete, corn and other graynys sold in the open markett.[290]

Fear of bread riots also served to loosen the purse strings.[291] In 1512, according to John Stow, barely 100 quarters of wheat remained in London's granaries, while the bread carts coming from Stratford were besieged by 'such presse about them that one man was readie to destroy an other'.[292] Prompt action by the mayor, Roger Achley, who purchased an abundant quantity of grain with his own funds, sufficed not only to feed the City but fully to replenish its reserves. The most important of them was stored in custom-built granaries at Leadenhall, whose construction provides a graphic illustration of civic philanthropy to rival the expenditure on pipes and conduits described in the previous chapter. Having experienced problems similar to those of Lynn during the late 1430s, the Corporation recognised the need for a specially designed building where supplies could be stockpiled in optimum conditions and, if necessary, protected from the mob (map 2). As we have seen, it also offered victuallers 'the largest and most imposing medieval market structure in the City and perhaps all England', outdoing the

---

[288] Pythian-Adams, *Desolation of a City*, pp. 55, 78. By October 1520 the crisis had reached such proportions that the mayor ordered a census of all grain supplies then in private hands: *Coventry Leet Book*, III.674–6.

[289] NRO, NCR, 16A/2, Mayor's Court Book, 1510–1532, p. 138. Although Norwich did not acquire a communal granary until the 1530s, the early fourteenth-century custumal provided for the purchase of grain and sale of subsidised bread to the populace before market trading began: *RCN*, I.174–6. In Lydd, too, the borough authorities occasionally funded the distribution of grain to 'poore people': A. Finn, ed., *Records of Lydd* (Ashford, 1911), pp. 194, 256, 297.

[290] Ricart, *Maire of Bristowe Is Kalendar*, p. 49. In Exeter at this time the mayor 'got him the love of the people, all the days of his life' by establishing a store house for grain, regulating the corn market, and strictly enforcing the assizes of bread and ale: S. Izacke, *Remarkable Antiquities of the City of Exeter* (London, 1723), pp. 111–12; DRO, ECA, Chamber Act Book 1, 1508–1538, fol. 94r; book 51, fol. 338r–v.

[291] As one Norwich chronicle reported in 1527, 'there was so great a scarceness of corn about Christmas that the commons of the city were ready to rise upon the rich men': Johnson, 'Chronological Memoranda', p. 144.

[292] Stow, *Survey of London*, I.156–7.

Parisian Halles in its elegant, hygienic and functional layout.[293] Just as aldermen such as Richard Whittington and John Wells had subscribed generously towards the provision of clean water, so the draper Simon Eyre agreed to advance most of the money needed to pay for the works at Leadenhall. Of particular note is the fact that he also built a chapel in the adjacent market from his own funds, an inscription being placed over the porch to record his alms deeds and solicit the intercessionary prayers of those who worshipped there.[294] Once again, the seamless connection between civic enterprise, public utilities and the quest for salvation had assumed concrete form.

5.10 Feeding the hungry

Despite the growing antagonism towards vagrant, able-bodied paupers apparent in England after the Black Death, the ritualised distribution of food and drink remained the most potent and emotive of the seven Comfortable Works.[295] As the translator of Archbishop Thoresby's Latin *Catechism* of 1357 explained:

> Furst, men schuld wilfully fede pore hungry men and thursty.
> For in that they fede Iesu Crist, as he hym self sayth in the gospel.
> And also Iesu crist gyfys body and sowle, lyf and catel to vs for this ende,
> And fedis vs wyth his flesch and his blod in the sacrament of the awter.[296]

Through a 'mysterious, superhuman form of nutrition' the consecrated Host appeared to promise both physical and spiritual health, protecting against earthly diseases, while dispensing a heavenly medicine, or *medicina sacramentalis*, to sick souls.[297] The first response of London's clergy to the onset of famine in 1315 was to process through the streets every Friday carrying just such a host in the hope of securing divine assistance.[298] There was, however, a price to pay for Christ's selfless generosity. In return for His sacrifice in shedding 'precious herte blod on the cros to bryng vs owt of mischef of synnys and paynys', an obligation to nurture the less fortunate fell heavily on all believers.[299] The reciprocity inherent

---

[293] Schofield, *London, 1100–1600*, p. 28.

[294] Samuel, 'The Fifteenth-Century Garner at Leadenhall', pp. 144–5; Thomas, 'History of the Leadenhall', pp. 16–20; Stow, *Survey of London*, I.153–4; Barron, *London in the Later Middle Ages*, pp. 55–6. One of the obligations of aldermanic office was to provide assistance at such times. During the shortage of 1390–1, for example, each of the twenty-four aldermen of London reputedly gave £20 to purchase grain: *CLB*, H, pp. 361–2.

[295] P. H. Cullum and P. J. P. Goldberg, 'Charitable Provision in Late Medieval York: "To the Praise of God and the Use of the Poor"', *Northern History* 29 (1993), pp. 24–39, on pp. 28–9.

[296] T. F. Simmons and H. E. Nolloth, eds, *The Lay Folk's Catechism*, EETS o.s. 118 (London, 1901), p. 72.

[297] P. Camporesi, *The Fear of Hell: Images of Damnation and Salvation in Early Modern Europe*, trans. L. Byatt (Oxford, 1991), pp. 146–65.

[298] Aberth, *From the Brink of the Apocalypse*, p. 27.

[299] Simmons and Nolloth, *Lay Folk's Catechism*, p. 73.

in this relationship constituted a powerful theme in the mystery plays beloved of late medieval urban audiences. In the 'Judgement Day' play that brought the East Anglian N-Town Cycle to a dramatic close, Christ berates the damned, to whom He has hitherto been 'so mercyfull and so gode', for their callous indifference towards the hungry.[300] The frequent depiction in word and image of dishonest victuallers burning in hell should be viewed in the context of their patent disregard for this uncompromising message (see plate 19).[301] Did a guilty conscience prompt the York butcher Richard Carlell (d. 1453) to arrange for five paupers to enjoy 'good food and drink' in his home every Sunday for a year after his death?[302] Among Norwich testators another butcher, Thomas Snellyng (d. 1506), is noteworthy for his bequests of 1*d.* and a square meal to each of the eighteen paupers who accompanied his body to burial, of a slap-up dinner for all his neighbours and fellow-parishioners, and of a half-penny loaf for every poor man, woman or child present at his funeral. He was clearly taking no chances.[303]

Their trading hours marked by the ringing of church bells, the stallholders who colonised urban markets could hardly forget the salutary lesson of the gospels. The mayor of Coventry's weekly inspection of the fish on sale in the Friday Market took place after his official attendance at the Jesus Mass in the nearby church of St Michael, to whom the task of weighing souls at the Last Judgement traditionally fell.[304] The Corpus Christi day procession of Norwich's medieval guilds around the city began, significantly, with a 'perambulation' of the great marketplace, which, from 1508 onwards was dominated by a new oratory and a cross standing almost 70 feet high (plate 22). It was here, too, that many of the mystery plays that celebrated the annual festival would have been performed.[305] Few markets, however small, lacked a cross, whose appearance reflected the wealth, as well as the piety, of a community. In 1421, for example, the widow of John Brathwayt, a former mayor of York, left over £13 for the erection of a new one in stone that would more effectively grace the Thursday Market.[306] Since civic pride clearly demanded that the surrounding area should remain free from 'mire & dong' at all times, magistrates made special arrangements for keeping their 'cross places' scrupulously clean.[307]

---

[300] S. Spector, ed., *The N-Town Play*, vol. 1: *Introduction and Text*, EETS s.s. 11 (Oxford, 1991), p. 412.

[301] See, for example, R. Morris, ed., *An Old English Miscellany*, EETS o.s. 49 (London, 1872), p. 189.

[302] P. H. Cullum, '"And Hir Name Was Charite": Charitable Giving by and for Women in Late Medieval Yorkshire', in P. J. P. Goldberg, ed., *Woman is a Worthy Wight: Women in English Society, c. 1200–1500* (Stroud, 1992), p. 191.

[303] NRO, Norwich Consistory Court, Register Ryxe, fols 383v–384r.

[304] Phythian-Adams, *Desolation of a City*, p. 77.

[305] Priestley, *The Great Market*, pp. 12–13.

[306] Tillott, *VCH York: City of York*, p. 485. The commissioning of a market cross was a matter of some debate, requiring the submission of an acceptable design: see, for example, KLBA, KL/C7/4, Hall Book, 1453–1497, p. 130.

[307] BL, MS Egerton 2107, fols 8v, 14v, 19v, 33r. Similar restrictions obtained in the far smaller borough of Henley, where the slaughtering of animals and drying of

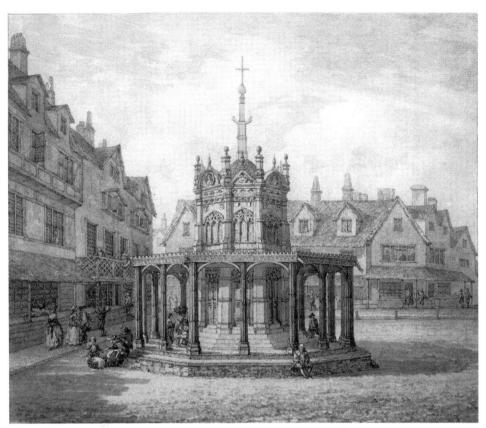

22 Norwich's spectacular early sixteenth-century market cross as depicted by Thomas Hearne shortly before its demolition in the 1730s

God's ominous warning to mankind that it held the earth and its fruits in stewardship only, and was therefore answerable to the landlord at the final reckoning, had profound implications for the wealthy. Rather than living like swine, their 'fowle flesche in fylthe to fede', and abandoning the poor to die 'in hunger and pyn', they were urged to save their souls before it was too late.[308] Not coincidentally, late medieval images of Dives, the rich sybarite who refused to assist a dying beggar and was condemned to roast eternally in hell as a result [Luke 16 vv. 19–31], often depict a dangerously choleric individual, whose disordered humours reflect years of overindulgence.[309] The association made between 'good diet & good gouernaunce' in contemporary advice literature is striking, it being clearly understood that a proper regimen would involve care for one's less fortunate neighbours as much as oneself. There can, indeed, be little doubt that the homiletic aspect of many vernacular *regimina* made an essentially pagan

bloodstained vessels was strictly prohibited anywhere near such a sacred space: Briers, *Henley Borough Records*, pp. 48, 124.

[308] Kail, *Twenty-Six Political and Other Poems*, p. 46.

[309] As in the Spinola Hours of *c.* 1515: J. Paul Getty Museum, Los Angeles, MS 83.ML.114.

text more acceptable to a Christian audience. Thus, for instance, a version of John Lydgate's *Dietary*, which appears under the title *Sapiencia phisicorum* (the Wisdom of Physicians) in the London commonplace book described at the start of this chapter, juxtaposes recommendations about restraint with an exhortation to care for the poor and needy:

> Thus in two thyngys stonde alle thy welthe,
> Of soule and of body, who lyste hym sewe:
> Moderate foode geuythe vnto a man hys helthe,
> And alle surfetys done from hym remeve;
> And charyte to the soule ys due.[310]

As in so many other aspects of late medieval life, the crown and aristocracy set a fashion that was enthusiastically followed by members of the urban elite, whose sense of social responsibility went hand in hand with a less altruistic desire to advertise their status and wealth through ostentatious philanthropy.[311] When reflecting upon the 'charitable almes in old times giuen' by 'men of honour and worship' in the City, John Stow recalled witnessing as a boy in the 1530s the throng of beggars at Thomas Cromwell's London house, where over two hundred people were served royally 'twise euery day with bread, meate and drinke sufficient'.[312] 'Doorstep' relief of this kind is rarely documented, but the formal distribution of bread among crowds of paupers constituted an important part of the funerals and anniversaries of wealthy townsmen and women throughout the later Middle Ages, being often undertaken on a scale destined to preclude selectivity. If few of them could afford the spectacular sum of £300 set aside by the London pewterer William Dere (d. *c.* 1464) to feed and clothe the multitude who mourned his passing, many still sought to demonstrate their compassion for the poor and hungry of Christ as effectively as funds allowed.[313]

Thomas Tanner of Wells (d. 1401), who left enough money for the annual distribution on 25 November of 1,440 half-penny loaves, or twice as many farthing ones, offers a less extravagant example of mercantile charity. As David Shaw points out, doles such as this, which were a regular feature of life in any cathedral city, would have attracted a potentially disorderly gang of beggars, 'conjuring up a scene of vagrant poor moving from town to town, on the circuit of poverty, looking for the large hand-outs'.[314] The ritual aspect of these occasions must have been

---

[310] BL, MS Egerton 1995, fols 77v–78v. For variants, see Furnivall, *Babees Book*, p. 58; and Wellcome Institute Library, Western MS 411, fol. 3v.

[311] M. Mollat, *The Poor in the Middle Ages*, trans. A. Goldhammer (New Haven, CT, 1986), p. 98; H. Johnstone, 'Poor Relief in the Royal Household of Thirteenth-Century England', *Speculum* 4 (1929), pp. 149–67.

[312] Stow, *Survey of London*, I.89.

[313] TNA, PROB11/5, fol. 20r.

[314] Shaw, *Creation of a Community*, pp. 235, 240. Despite its poverty, Carlisle was another magnet for indigents: Summerson, *Medieval Carlisle*, I.305. Tanner's bequest was actually quite generous; William Pownam of Bristol (d. 1454) made a more typical provision for the poor, arranging for 240 half-penny loaves to be handed out every year on his anniversary: Veale, *Great Red Book of Bristol*, III.107.

striking, as we can see from the will of the Bury St Edmunds merchant John Baret. Some of the 208 wheaten loaves that were to be given as alms every year on the date of his death were reserved for the sick, but the able-bodied recipients had to stand outside his former home patiently awaiting their portion.[315] An even more effective ceremony of commemoration took place every day at the gates of the hospital founded in Bristol by Maurice Gaunt (d. 1230), when the chaplains, 'each with a little knife in his hand to cut the bread for the weak and incapable', fed 100 paupers. Since the founder's livery (three white geese or 'gaunts') was prominently displayed on their habits, even the most casual bystanders would have recognised the source of this bounty.[316]

Yet, just as excess of any kind would harm the individual, so too indiscriminate almsgiving could inflict serious damage upon the body politic. From a canonical viewpoint, the charitable imperative was not only tempered by concern that assistance should be reserved for the truly deserving, but also by a conviction, based on the teachings of Galen, that the type of food on offer should accord with the social class and background of the recipient. Whereas the digestions of the poor were accustomed to a coarse and unrefined diet, and could not easily adjust to richer fare, the reverse held true of those who had once lived off the fat of the land. The assumption, already noted above, that rare delicacies would provoke lust and gluttony, propelling the lower orders into a downward spiral of sickness, indolence and vice, lent further weight to an argument that was supported as much by medical science as theology. On balance, it seemed advisable to adopt a system of rationing, based upon the moral worth and background of the recipient.[317] As the visionary and mystic Margery Kempe warned an open-handed priest of her acquaintance, it was far better to assist 'powyr neybowrys' who 'hadyn gret nede to ben holpyn and relevyd' than 'other strawngerys which thei knew not'.[318] Such entrenched ideas found expression in Juan Luis Vives' influential text on public charity, *De subventione pauperum*, which was composed in England during a stay at the royal court in 1526:

> Those who have ruined themselves in disgraceful and base ways, such as gambling, immorality, luxury, greed, must indeed be fed, since no one should die from starvation, but the more disagreeable tasks are to be assigned to them and harder fare, so that they may be an example to others and may themselves repent of their former life; they will thus not easily fall back into the same vices, restrained therefrom by their scanty food and hard labour, not dying of hunger, but being made lean withal.[319]

On the face of things, the desire for conspicuous displays of generosity to all comers sat uncomfortably both with national legislation against work-shy ruffians

---

[315] Tymms, *Wills and Inventories*, p. 28.

[316] C. Ross, ed., *The Cartulary of St Mark's Hospital, Bristol*, Bristol Record Society 21 (Bristol, 1959), pp. 8–9.

[317] B. Tierney, 'The Decretists and the "Deserving Poor"', *Comparative Studies in Society and History* 1 (1958–9), pp. 360–73, on p. 366.

[318] Margery Kempe, *Book of Margery Kempe*, p. 56.

[319] Salter, *Some Early Tracts on Poor Relief*, p. 13.

'giving themselves to Idleness and Vice' and with more localised attempts to tackle the perceived problem of vagrancy.[320] But it is apparent that, from a comparatively early date, the merchants and gentry who lived in late medieval towns and cities were also practising a more precisely targeted type of philanthropy. On 20 January 1337, for instance, the widow of Sir Walter de Norwich distributed 200 'gastellis', or loaves of coarse bread, among the poor of Norwich to mark the anniversary of his death; on the following day twenty-six paupers received one loaf and a red herring; and at other times she fed a symbolic number of thirteen hand-picked individuals in her household every day.[321] In a re-enactment of the parable of the rich man who invited 'the poor and the maimed and the halt and the blind ... from the streets and lanes of the city' to his feast [Luke 14, vv. 16–24], wealthy testators also provided *convivia*, or funeral repasts, for the poor, sometimes at considerable expense. The ceremony of remembrance held one month after the death of William Milett of Dartford (d. 1500) must have been a memorable affair, since it involved the provision of an ox, five sheep, two quarters wheat (for bread) and four of malt (for ale), specifically 'for the releff of pouere people'.[322] Contrary to the spirit of the gospel, however, these events were clearly intended for fellow parishioners, whose circumstances would be familiar to the organisers, and rarely extended to homeless vagrants.[323] Funerary and anniversary doles, too, could be earmarked for the men and women who had been chosen by relatives or executors to escort the body for burial or to bear candles in memory of the departed.[324] In other cases, bedridden or needy neighbours would be singled out for alms of the kind provided in 1476 by Richard Northern of the then flourishing sea port of Covehithe, in Suffolk, who left twenty-one cades of red herring to feed the *local* poor.[325]

Even more selective were the feasts held by pious fraternities and craft guilds, which customarily followed the celebration of a special mass dedicated to the patron saint. These convivial gatherings incorporated a highly ritualised element of almsgiving akin to the distribution of bread, blessed by the priest, among the assembled congregation after a parish mass. The brethren and sisters would often invite a group of paupers to share their meal or else to consume the leftovers

---

[320] *SR*, vol. 1, 23 Edward III, cap. 7, p. 308; *SR*, vol. 2, 12 Richard II, caps 7 and 8, p. 58; McIntosh, *Poor Relief in England*, pp. 43–5.

[321] C. Woolgar, ed., *Household Accounts from Medieval England*, vol. 1, Records of Social and Economic History n.s. 17 (Oxford, 1992), pp. 177–227, especially pp. 203–5.

[322] TNA, PROB 11/12, fol. 138r.

[323] Cullum and Goldberg, 'Charitable Provision in Late Medieval York', pp. 28–9; Cullum, 'And Hir Name Was Charite', pp. 189–90. John Baret's commemorative dinner was, for example, intended solely for deserving paupers 'suych as dwelle nexte myn place': Tymms, *Wills and Inventories*, pp. 29–30.

[324] For example, each of the twelve poor men who carried tapers on the anniversary of Alderman William Ramsey of Norwich (d. 1511) was to receive 'meat and drink': TNA, PROB 11/17, fols 183v–184r.

[325] SROI, IC/AA2/2, fol. 315. There were about 600 herring to one cade. Similarly, Henry Rudde of Bury (d. 1505) left a generous £10 'to pore folks *at hom at ther howses*, in bred and flessh' to mark his burial: Tymms, *Wills and Inventories*, p. 107.

afterwards.[326] Each married couple and single member of the guild of Corpus Christi at Grantham was, for example, expected to bring a poor friend or neighbour to the table, while several of the fraternities of Stratford-upon-Avon and Lincoln laid on extra supplies of ale for the needy.[327] As we shall see in the next chapter, the charitable relief offered by these organisations, even to their own members, was highly circumscribed, but food did play a significant part in the mutual support provided by several less affluent fraternities. Aware that some brethren might not be able to afford the commemorative doles described above, both the Fullers of Lincoln and guild of St John the Baptist, Lynn, organised special collections so that a decent number of loaves could be handed out at their funerals.[328] Also in Lincoln, members of the Smiths' guild undertook to welcome impoverished brethren 'courteously' into their homes for a square meal, while citizens who joined the fraternity of the Blessed Virgin were likewise expected to supply any sick, aged or disabled individuals in their ranks with 'needful food'.[329] Not surprisingly, the recipients were carefully vetted to exclude any idlers, drunkards, gamblers and other profligates whose misfortunes seemed to be of their own making.

By the close of the Middle Ages, a few urban parishes, such as Holy Trinity, Cambridge, and St Ewen's, Bristol, had begun to distribute modest amounts of food and drink among 'poor folk' at specific times of year. But hand-outs like these never provided more than 'symbolic assistance', and were certainly not for all.[330] Less formal, and sadly less well documented, local fundraising activities combined an element of self-help with communal support for deserving cases. Although their charitable purpose was sometimes overshadowed by rowdiness and inebriation, 'scot-ales' enabled any 'honest man decayed in his estate' to hold a kind of street party at which home-brewed ale could be purchased by friends and neighbours. Knowing well enough that they, too, might one day face destitution, they usually paid up, enabling the host to turn a useful profit. As well as fostering a sense of cohesion (at least among respectable householders) and making it possible to seek alms without the indignity of having to beg, events of this kind might also be staged to raise cash for group projects such as street cleaning, laying pavements and making good the effects of fire damage.[331] These *ad hoc* initiatives must have furnished many people with the wherewithal to feed their families when times were hard, although, as Marjorie McIntosh points out, they did not help the chronically poor or play any part in official relief before the Reformation.[332]

---

[326] At feasts of the Trinity Guild, Wisbech, a table was set aside for 'alle the pore people then there present', who received whatever food and drink remained: HMC, *Ninth Report*, part 1, appendix, p. 295.

[327] Rosser, 'Going to the Fraternity Feast', pp. 436–7; Smith, Smith and Brentano, *English Gilds*, pp. 173, 183, 217.

[328] Smith, Smith and Brentano, *English Gilds*, pp. 100–1, 180.

[329] Smith, Smith and Brentano, *English Gilds*, pp. 166, 169.

[330] McIntosh, *Poor Relief in Medieval England*, p. 110.

[331] J. M. Bennett, 'Conviviality and Charity in Medieval and Early Modern England', *P&P* 34 (1992), pp. 19–41.

[332] McIntosh, *Poor Relief in Medieval England*, pp. 106–7.

It has been argued that the 'selfish expectation of spiritual reward' so apparent in these rather haphazard acts of philanthropy militated against an 'efficient systematisation of social care' in later medieval and early Tudor England.[333] And in many respects the performance of the first of the Comfortable Works left much to be desired. Individual efforts, however generous, were at best short-term and uncoordinated, while the Church could not always fill the breach during periods of dearth. By the second and third decades of the sixteenth century, when a combination of population growth and rising prices hit the poor especially hard, not even the great urban monasteries such as Norwich cathedral priory and Westminster abbey were spending more than a minute fraction of their annual budgets on the distribution of bread, grain and other foodstuffs.[334] A broader definition of care, extending to the provision of cheap, wholesome food, sold in more hygienic conditions by reputable traders, would, however, suggest that significant improvements were being made. As we have seen, when it came to the enforcement of food standards, the creation of cleaner, better-organised markets and the stockpiling of grain, a combination of communal and individual effort *could* sometimes make an appreciable difference to the lives of less privileged members of the urban body. Hospitals and almshouses offer similar instances of collaborative endeavour, and it is to them, as well as to the provision of medical services for the sick and elderly in general, that we finally turn.

---

[333] Rosser, *Medieval Westminster*, p. 294.

[334] On average, the equivalent of 510 one-pound loaves was distributed every day by the almoner of Norwich cathedral priory during the difficult years between 1280 and 1330. Falling revenues and stringent economies meant that when food shortages and inflation struck during the 1520s the figure stood at just thirty-four loaves a day, to which would be added leftovers from the refectory table: C. Rawcliffe, *The Hospitals of Medieval Norwich* (Norwich, 1995), pp. 82–5. Notwithstanding Sir Thomas More's fulsome praise of monastic charity at Westminster on the eve of the Reformation, it seems that the abbey did no better, in part because of a shift towards more selective residential care: N. Rushton, 'Spatial Aspects of the Almonry Site and the Changing Priorities of Poor Relief at Westminster Abbey, c. 1290–1540', *Architectural History* 45 (2002), pp. 66–91; Rosser, *Medieval Westminster*, pp. 298–300.

Chapter 6
Sickness and Debility

If one-third of a town, or city, or state, is suffering from disease, there is cast upon the other two-thirds a proportionately greater amount of exertion than would otherwise be required of them, and there is exacted from them a proportionately greater contribution to the general expenditure, while there is less capacity both of work and contribution in the whole community. Time was when this obvious principle was unrecognised, and the state, which made paternal regulations to secure the health of men's souls ... wholly avoided any observation of those permanent and subtle causes of danger to the health of the citizens that were likely to exist wherever two or three were gathered together in community of houses or homes. Even in England, where every sort of ill or grievance has been searched out with keen anxiety ... the public health, a matter one would conceive of supereminent importance, was neglected.

Edward Jenkins, The Legal Aspects of Sanitary Reform (1867)[1]

The great Greek physician Galen is said to have advocated a welfare scheme whereby the state would provide free or heavily subsidised drugs and medical treatment for the needy. Although his surviving corpus of work is uncharacteristically silent on this point, he was well aware of 'the frightening anonymity of the great metropolis, where one can die unnoticed and unmourned, [and] where the charlatan and quack flourish at the expense of the ignorant'.[2] His repeated emphasis upon the importance of philanthropy and compassion in cementing the reputation of the individual practitioner was not, as we shall see, without an element of hard-headed calculation, but still reflects a real sense of professional obligation towards the urban proletariat. Far from knocking at a closed door, Galen was, in fact, writing at a time when the appointment of 'public' physicians and surgeons in the larger cities of the Roman world already boasted a long, if somewhat chequered history. They were remunerated in a variety of ways, including lucrative exemptions from office-holding and taxation, in return for what was, in theory, 'an honourable service to the poor'.[3]

After a long period of abeyance during the earlier Middle Ages, salaried physicians again became a feature of urban life, appearing in Bologna in the early thirteenth century and rapidly spreading to other Italian cities. By 1324, for example, the Great Council of Venice agreed as an economy measure to reduce the number of surgeons on its payroll from seventeen to twelve, while adding one

---

[1] E. Jenkins, *The Legal Aspects of Sanitary Reform* (London, 1867), p. 80.

[2] V. Nutton, 'Continuity or Rediscovery? The City Physician in Classical Antiquity and Medieval Italy', in A. W. Russell, ed., *The Town and State Physician in Europe from the Middle Ages to the Enlightenment* (Wolfenbuttel, 1981), p. 9.

[3] Nutton, 'Continuity or Rediscovery?', p. 19.

more physician to the existing roster of eleven.[4] Over the following century these *medici condotti* became ubiquitous, as even small communities began to boast the services of one or two hired personnel, whose terms of employment varied considerably according to the resources available and the status of the individual healer. Other European countries rapidly followed suit. Towns throughout the Crown of Aragon were soon well supplied with practitioners who offered advice about public health and preventative medicine, as well as more conventional treatment.[5] In France, too, a significant number of qualified professionals opted either for what might today be called general practice or to work in hospitals for the sick poor or in prisons. Allowing for the limitations of the evidence, it has been estimated that around 15 per cent of all the physicians and a slightly higher percentage of surgeons recorded in French sources between 1300 and 1500 accepted some type of municipal employment during their careers.[6]

As Vivian Nutton observes, this system was far from perfect. While recognising the need to retain 'an abundance of good doctors', magistrates were sometimes reluctant to foot the bill, especially if the 'doctors' in question took to their heels at the first sign of pestilence. For this reason some authorities, such as those of Parma and Urbino, eventually chose not to retain anyone, preferring instead to grant tax concessions to all practitioners on the clear understanding that they would provide free care for the 'poor and wretched' whenever required. Even without these inducements, many successful physicians and surgeons were ready to undertake charity work, offsetting their expenses against the substantial fees paid by wealthier patients.[7] We cannot, therefore, assume that communities without stipendiary medical staff were less well-equipped to care for the needy, or, indeed, showed less sympathy towards them. Nevertheless, the complete lack of officially funded medical services in the towns and cities of medieval England does highlight a striking divergence in approach from that of mainland Europe, where facilities for professional education and training were, in general, more highly developed. Nor, as often happened overseas, did the crown or aristocracy customarily step in with the promise of staff or funding. Henry IV's allocation of 6*d.* a day in 1400 for a tooth-drawer to assist the poor of London without charge constitutes a solitary example of royal intervention.[8]

---

[4] U. Stefanutti, ed., *Documentazioni cronologiche per la storia della medicina, chirurgia e farmacia in Venezia dal 1258 al 1332* (Venice, 1961), pp. 117–18. A typical contract obliged the practitioner to visit and treat the poor for nothing, to provide free consultations for all, and to charge the more affluent at a fixed rate, save in 'difficult' cases such as leprosy (pp. 107–8).

[5] M. McVaugh, *Medicine before the Plague: Practitioners and their Patients in the Crown of Aragon, 1285–1345* (Cambridge, 2002), p. 192.

[6] D. Jacquart, *Le Milieu médical en France du XIIe au XVe siécle*, Hautes Études Médiévales et Modernes, série 5, 46 (Geneva, 1981), pp. 121, 133–6.

[7] Nutton, 'Continuity or Rediscovery?', pp. 33–4; Park, *Doctors and Medicine*, p. 93; see section 6.2 below. On qualifying as masters of their craft, Parisian barber-surgeons had to tend the poor for six months free of charge: R. de Lespinasse, ed., *Les Métiers et corporations de la ville de Paris*, 3 vols (Paris, 1886–97), III.639–40.

[8] *CPR, 1399–1401*, p. 255.

The level of investment apparent in the great urban centres of continental Europe would have been both inappropriate and unfeasible in the far smaller provincial cities of late medieval England. That none ever employed the equivalent of a *medico condotto*, even on a part-time basis, is, however, less a reflection of demography or economics than of the nature of English medical practice, and particularly the limited involvement of academically trained physicians in civic life. The universities of Oxford and Cambridge lay some distance from London and other large towns, which placed them at a distinct disadvantage when compared to their European counterparts in cities such as Bologna, Montpellier, Paris and Vienna. To compound the problem, neither of the two faculties of medicine made much of a professional impact, in part because the number of graduates choosing to study there remained extremely small. In all, only ninety-four individuals are known to have obtained the degree of MB at Oxford between 1300 and 1500, and a mere fifty-nine at Cambridge during the same period.[9]

Notwithstanding the fact that many students began to practise without a formal qualification, university-educated physicians were rare birds, nesting in the sheltered confines of the royal court and the households of elite patrons. Since all but a few had also taken holy orders, this type of career seemed more fitting, not least because the conservative English syllabus, with its emphasis upon theory, was ill suited to the demands of ordinary working men and women. They wanted cheap, fast and effective cures, rather than the protracted and correspondingly expensive advice about lifestyle and regimen that English physicians were taught to provide.[10] Their needs were supplied in a teeming and only partially regulated medical marketplace where a wide range of healers, from surgeons, barbers and apothecaries, who were licensed and supervised by their respective guilds, to an irregular army of leeches, midwives, herbalists, charmers, bone-setters and other 'connynge' folk, plied their wares.[11] Relations between trained craftsmen and empirics were often fraught by professional jealousy and economic rivalry, while for most of our period the physicians were too numerically and politically weak to organise themselves, let alone others. Even in Oxford there could be problems, as happened in 1400 when the university enacted a measure against the multitude of 'lay and illiterate public practitioners' who worked under the very noses of the faculty but defied its jurisdiction. They were, significantly, to be punished as

---

[9] F. M. Getz, 'Medical Education in England', in V. Nutton and R. Porter, eds, *The History of Medical Education in Britain* (Amsterdam, 1995), pp. 76–93; Rawcliffe, *Medicine and Society*, pp. 108–9; J. M. Fletcher, 'Linacre's Lands and Lectureships', in F. Maddison, M. Pelling and C. Webster, eds, *Essays on the Life and Work of Thomas Linacre* (Oxford, 1977), pp. 110–20.

[10] F. M. Getz, 'The Faculty of Medicine before 1500', in Catto and Evans, *History of the University of Oxford*, II.396–9; Getz, *Healing and Society*, pp. xxii–xxiv. One eminent French physician complained that the masses preferred brutal but rapid cures, akin to horse-doctoring ('remèdes de cheval'), because they were cheaper and faster: J. Imbert, *Histoire des hôpitaux en France* (Toulouse, 1982), pp. 131–2.

[11] The term 'irregular' serves to define those whom the Royal College of Physicians deemed unqualified to practice, and embraces 'the rich variety of medical occupations' that flourished in urban society: Pelling, *Medical Conflicts*, pp. 4, 10.

disturbers of the peace ('pacis perturbatores').[12] In this respect, the situation in cities such as London, Norwich and York contrasts sharply with that in Florence, which lacked a university but nonetheless possessed a large and powerful guild to which *all* practitioners of medicine and surgery belonged, from graduates to wise-women. Closely integrated into the city's social and commercial fabric, it supplied a stream of well-qualified candidates for employment in a variety of public positions.[13]

This chapter begins by examining the two major initiatives for reform at a national level that occurred, respectively, during the early fifteenth and early sixteenth centuries (6.1). Although neither secured any appreciable benefits for the urban proletariat, even in London, the main focus of activity, the less affluent did enjoy greater access to medical treatment than is often supposed. As we shall see in the following sections, professional services might sometimes be subsidised or given freely (6.2), while more successful, if less ambitious, attempts at regulation and licensing were made jointly by urban magistrates and the various craft guilds to which surgeons, barbers and apothecaries belonged (6.3). Predictably, in view of what we learned in Chapter 5, apothecaries, who dealt in dangerous drugs as well as spices, were subject to particularly close surveillance (6.4). The sick and disabled poor needed other types of relief besides medicine and surgery, being often homeless and in want of shelter. Having examined the rather limited informal arrangements that might be made within the community (6.5), we move on to consider the changing face of institutional care in late medieval English towns. A general survey of the basic types of foundation available during this period and the important role that each might play in safeguarding spiritual as well as physical health (6.6), is followed by a more detailed examination of *leprosaria* (6.7), general or 'common' hospitals for the sick (6.8), and almshouses for the elderly and incapacitated (6.9). Although it sufficed when population levels remained low and the problem of vagrancy was less pressing, hospital provision became a matter of serious concern during the sixteenth century, again in tandem with the demand for improved medical services (6.10).

6.1 Attempts at reform

Sporadic efforts were made to adopt Continental practices, the first, in 1421, being almost certainly an indirect result of the war with France, which introduced English captains and their medical personnel to the more structured system of education and licensing that obtained in Paris.[14] Since, unlike their Parisian counterparts, English physicians lacked the authority to curb any unwelcome competition, it was necessary to enlist parliamentary support for reform.[15] Claiming an altruistic

---

[12] S. Gibson, ed., *Statvta antiqva vniversitatis Oxoniensis* (Oxford, 1931), p. 191.

[13] Park, *Doctors and Medicine*, pp. 17–41.

[14] C. O'Boyle, 'Surgical Texts and Social Contexts: Physicians and Surgeons in Paris, c. 1270 to 1430', in Arrizabalaga *et al.*, *Practical Medicine*, pp. 156–85, especially pp. 179–84.

[15] *PROME, 1413–1422*, pp. 267–8, 310.

desire to assist the common people of England, the petitioners described an alarming situation whereby

> every man, be he never so lewed, takyng upon hym practyse, [is] y suffred
> to use hit, to grete harme and slaughtre of men: where if no man practised
> theryn but al only connynge men and approved sufficieantly y lerned in art,
> filosofye, and fisyk, *as hit is kept in other londes and roialms* (my italics), ther
> shulde many man that dyeth, for defaute of help, lyve, and no man perysh by
> unconnyng.[16]

Although it secured the royal assent, the proposal that henceforth only graduates should practise medicine was doomed to failure at the outset. The suggested fine of £40 for non-compliance was a hollow threat, given that the number of qualified personnel emerging from the two universities barely served to fulfil the demands of the aristocracy, let alone those of the nation as a whole. Nor, as we shall see, were urban magistrates as tolerant of 'the charlatan and quack' as senior members of the medical profession cared to suggest. Having reconsidered their position, a small group of distinguished physicians made common cause with some of London's leading surgeons, in the hope of achieving a more workable solution that would win the support of the Corporation. Henry V's master surgeon Thomas Morstede, who had established close personal connections among the mercantile elite, was particularly well placed to lead the campaign for tighter regulation.[17]

The proposed College of Physicians and Surgeons of London marked a novel departure for the university-trained academics, whose readiness to submit to the jurisdiction of the mayor and aldermen signalled their acceptance of a more proactive role in urban society. Its attractions for the surgeons, who stood to gain both intellectual kudos and a long-awaited opportunity to restrict the activities of their commercial rivals, were self-evident. With the avowed intention of eliminating 'the disceites of vnkonnynge practisours in phisyk and cirurgy' and making affordable treatment available to all, the college set out in 1423 to impose a rigid system of inspection and licensing throughout the capital. It also sought to police the use of harmful drugs by subjecting the premises of apothecaries to regular searches for 'eny false medicyns, or sophisticate'. Mandatory consultation with colleagues in all cases likely to result in death or mutilation addressed another problem which greatly exercised the civic authorities.[18] Yet, despite its laudable motives, the college must have seemed remote from the needs of most Londoners, who rarely encountered a physician or master surgeon and traditionally turned elsewhere for assistance. The only item of business known to have been undertaken by the new 'Faculty of Physic' concerns a controversial award made in 1424 by its most distinguished members in a case of alleged mayhem involving three senior colleagues. Being conscious of the status of the defendants, and having perhaps themselves dealt with similar problems, the arbitrators not only found unanimously against the plaintiff (whose thumb had been mutilated during

---

[16] *RP*, IV.158.

[17] For details of his career, see R. T. Beck, *The Cutting Edge: Early History of the Surgeons of London* (London, 1974), pp. 76–82, 92–7.

[18] Beck, *Cutting Edge*, pp. 63–7.

surgery), but even accused him of defamation. Although it constituted a legitimate defence at law, the argument that a malign configuration of the heavens had further lengthened the odds against a successful outcome is unlikely to have carried much weight with the average citizen, and it is easy to see why there was so little popular enthusiasm for an organisation which apparently served to uphold the authority of the practitioner at the expense of his patient.[19]

An even more serious obstacle lay in the exposure of underlying tensions within the craft of surgery, which the Parisian Faculty of Medicine was sufficiently powerful to contain and even exploit to its own advantage, but which threatened to destabilise any English reforms from the start.[20] The London guild of Barbers, many of whose members offered a wide range of standard surgical procedures along with tonsorial services, resented any attempt to curtail their hard-won freedom.[21] From at least the early fourteenth century these men had let the blood, healed the fractures and drawn the teeth of the City's workforce, and were not prepared to accept a subordinate position. Being far superior in numbers to the small, select and more recently established guild of Surgeons, they had little difficulty in persuading the mayor and aldermen to confirm their independence from the college in November 1424, thereby effectively undercutting its authority.[22] Since neither the physicians nor master surgeons would countenance an equal partnership with the Barbers, whom they regarded as their social and professional inferiors, the project rapidly collapsed. The apothecaries, and by extension the powerful Grocers' Company to which they belonged, appear to have been equally intransigent. It seems likely, too, that the death of Henry V, who had taken an active interest in the welfare of his troops, removed an important source of support for the College, which looked in vain for new patrons.[23]

Not until the second decade of the sixteenth century, by which time several English physicians had observed at first hand the merits of the Italian system, was another attempt made to revive the campaign for inspection and licensing, this time at a national level. Circumstances certainly favoured any measure that

---

[19] *CPMRL, 1413–1437*, pp. 174–5. The long-term interests of guild members demanded a more even-handed approach, and there is sufficient evidence to suggest that most expert jurors and arbitrators recognised the need to win public confidence. In 1392, for instance, a panel of four York barber-surgeons awarded exemplary damages of £10 as compensation for 'une maheyme' inflicted upon a patient's jaw by one of their colleagues: *YMB*, II.25–7.

[20] Lespinasse, *Métiers et corporations de la ville de Paris*, III.622–9.

[21] Most of the observations made by Margaret Pelling on the early modern period also hold good for the later Middle Ages: 'Appearance and Reality: Barber-Surgeons, the Body and Disease', in A. L. Beier and R. Finlay, eds, *London, 1500–1700: The Making of the Metropolis* (London, 1986), pp. 82–112.

[22] *CLB*, K, p. 36. For the background to this struggle, see Barron, *London in the Later Middle Ages*, pp. 283–5; Beck, *Cutting Edge*, pp. 120–57; S. Young, *Annals of the Barber-Surgeons of London* (London, 1890), pp. 35–68. 'The wardens and other good folk of the fellowship of surgeons' were traditionally exempted from service as constables and jurors because there were so few of them: *CLB*, L, pp. 286–7.

[23] C. Rawcliffe, 'Master Surgeons at the Lancastrian Court', in J. Stratford, ed., *The Lancastrian Court* (Donington, 2003), pp. 192–210.

would increase the number and calibre of qualified physicians ready to work in towns. Henry VII's plans for the first London hospital to employ salaried medical personnel were well underway, while the combined onslaught of sweating sickness, the pox and repeated outbreaks of plague further highlighted the scale of the problem. Thomas Forestier's treatise on the epidemic of 1485 had begun with an attack upon the many 'vnexpart men', including carpenters and other artisans, who traded upon credulous and susceptible people. Claiming, by contrast, to be 'moved with very loue and charyte and not for no luker nor couetyse', he drew particular attention to the 'false lechys deceyuyng al the world', who advertised their remedies by posting 'letters vpon gatys and churche dores, as foles promysyng to help the peple of ther sykenesse withoute connyng'.[24] His concerns eventually found expression in a parliamentary statute 'Concerning Phesicions & Surgeons', which was enacted in 1512 just after another devastating pestilence. It, too, set out to combat the familiar threat posed by

> a grete multitude of ignoraunt persones of whom the grete partie have no maner of insight in [the science and connyng of physyke and surgerie] nor in any other kynde of lernyng. Some also can no lettres on the boke, soofarfurth that common artificers as smythes, wevers and women boldely and custumably take upon theim grete curis and thyngys of great difficultie. In the which they partely use socery and which crafte, partely applie such medicyne unto the disease as be verey noyous and nothyng metely therfore, to the high displeasoure of God, great infamye to the faculties and the grevous hurte, damage and distruccion of many of the Kynges liege people, most specally of them that cannot descerne the uncunnyng from the cunnyng.[25]

Adopting a more realistic approach than the previous attempt at legislation in 1421, the statute sought to weed out the worst offenders by insisting that all practitioners of physic and surgery should possess an episcopal licence (to be awarded in London after an examination by four qualified professionals and elsewhere at the bishop's discretion), or pay a fine of £5. A subsequent amendment in favour of herbalists and other empirics who gave their services freely 'to the poore people oonelie for neighbourhode and goddes sake and of pitie and charytie' suggests that it was strictly enforced.[26] It certainly offered aggrieved patients a stick with which to beat any unlicensed practitioner who failed to meet their

---

[24] BL, Add. MS 27582, fol. 70r; M. T. Walton, 'Thomas Forestier and the "false lechys" of London', *JHM* 37 (1982), pp. 71–3.

[25] *SR*, vol. 3, 3 Henry VIII, cap. 11. For the 1511 epidemic see Appendix. Norwich's decision to return the Cambridge-educated Robert Harydaunce, the first physician to represent an English borough, to this parliament suggests a keen interest in the legislation. Significantly, the wording of the statute was incorporated almost verbatim into regulations compiled in 1561 for a new company of physicians and surgeons in the city: Rawcliffe, 'Sickness and Health', pp. 319–20.

[26] *SR*, vol. 3, 34 and 35 Henry VIII, cap. 8. One of the posthumous miracles attributed to Henry VI concerned a blind man whose suffering had been compounded by the attentions of his friend, a weaver and part-time herbalist: R. Knox and S. Leslie, eds, *The Miracles of King Henry VI* (London, 1923), pp. 188–9.

expectations.[27] Yet, as its critics made plain, one did not need to study the more esoteric elements of medical theory in order to treat the ulcers, rashes, swellings, sprains, sore eyes, broken limbs and aching teeth that constituted the bread and butter of an urban practice. Nor had parliament addressed the underlying failure of the two universities to equip medical students for the type of *pro bono* work routinely undertaken by their French and Italian peers.

The impetus for change came initially from a small circle of humanist scholars at the royal court, led by Cardinal Wolsey's physician Thomas Linacre (d. 1524), who had studied in Padua as a young man and was scathing in his assessment of the English system. The glaring shortage of 'connyng and expert phisicions' constituted a national scandal, which, in his view, seemed especially pronounced in London. Indeed, he considered it essential that 'th'enhabitanntes in every cominaltie' should enjoy the benefits of a faculty of medicine for 'the comfort of the people and remedy of many maladies contynuelly channsyng'.[28] Having prudently dedicated his new translation of Galen's *De sanitate tuenda* to Henry VIII in 1517, Linacre set out to reform health provision in the City, a task greatly facilitated by the outbreak that year of widespread epidemics of sweating sickness and plague.[29] His personal knowledge of established Italian quarantine procedures clearly helped Wolsey to draft the first English regulations for the containment of 'contagious infections', which were introduced to the capital in January 1518. Although he was chiefly concerned about the health of the royal court and the enforcement of public order, the cardinal obviously understood the wider importance of such measures. Four months later they were adopted in Oxford on the insistence of Sir Thomas More, another of Linacre's friends, who was then approaching the end of his term as under-sheriff of London.[30]

It was against this background that the plans first mooted almost a century earlier for a faculty of medicine in the capital were revived. Soon afterwards, in September 1518, royal letters patent approved the incorporation of a college of physicians based upon the Florentine model, with powers to examine and license all practitioners of medicine in London and its environs who did not already possess a relevant degree. When confirming the foundation charter five years later, parliament extended these supervisory powers throughout the entire country, although, in practice, the college lacked any semblance of authority outside London. Here, by contrast, the readiness of the Common Council to sentence any unlicensed practitioner to twenty days' imprisonment made possible a series of test cases brought in the mayor's court against 'irregulars' whose 'speculacion

---

[27] See, for example, the suits brought against the surgeon Robert Peverel, in the Nottingham borough court in 1536. He was accused of negligence and practising without a licence: Stevenson, *Records of the Borough of Nottingham*, III.194–8.

[28] Fletcher, 'Linacre's Lands and Lectureships', p. 166.

[29] C. Webster, 'Thomas Linacre and the Foundation of the College of Physicians', in Maddison, Pelling and Webster, *Life and Work of Thomas Linacre*, pp. 207–8.

[30] Appendix, below; Slack, *Impact of Plague*, pp. 201–2; A. S. Macnalty, 'Sir Thomas More as a Student of Medicine and Public Health Reformer', in E. A. Underwood, ed., *Science, Medicine and History: Essays on the Evolution of Scientific Thought and Medical Practice*, 2 vols (Oxford, 1953), I.418–36.

and cunnyng' failed to satisfy the academic criteria laid down by the college.[31] Other initiatives targeted barber-surgeons and apothecaries who strayed into the forbidden realm of physic, however competent they might have been. When viewed from the perspective of the average citizen, Linacre's foundation must have seemed both remote and self-serving, its agenda driven by 'a cluster of self-conscious humanist intellectuals who were attempting to pursue a literary and legal project at the expense of the majority'.[32] Although it owed its origins to the disastrous epidemics of 1517–18 and Linacre's conviction that English physicians should play a more active role in the promotion of measures for urban health, the college rapidly developed into an elite organisation whose members identified with the royal court rather than the people of London. Indeed, their preoccupation with the more abstruse aspects of scholastic medicine, and hostility towards any potential competitors, made them intolerant of healers who supplied the needs of the wider public, while they themselves showed little enthusiasm for schemes to assist the less advantaged.

6.2 Access to treatment

In light of the failure of these sporadic attempts at reform, it is worth asking if the services of a competent *medicus* or surgeon really lay beyond the reach of all but the relatively prosperous. Was the rest of the population simply left to fend for itself, as some contemporary critics maintained? The greedy physician with a passion for gold belonged to the same literary stable as the crooked lawyer and lecherous monk; and it would be unwise to judge all late medieval practitioners on the basis of a few well-aimed gibes by satirists such as Chaucer and Gower, or, indeed, by the priests and friars who sought to equip their readers with the necessary skills to dispense with professional advice.[33] During the Tudor period the predicament of those who could not afford medical services did, however, begin to attract more widespread attention. Opponents of the Act of 1512 censured members of the Fellowship of Surgeons of London for 'mynding oonelie theyre owne lucres and nothing the profite or ease of the diseased', and for leaving the poor to 'rotte and perishe to deathe for lacke of helpe'.[34] Similar sentiments were echoed by Bishop Hugh Latimer (d. 1555), who observed ruefully that:

> physicians now-a-days seek only their own profits, how to get money, not how they might do good unto their poor neighbour. Whereby it appeareth, that they be for the most part without charity; and so, consequently, not the children of God. And no doubt but the heavy judgment of God hangeth over

---

[31] G. Clark, *A History of the Royal College of Physicians*, 2 vols (Oxford, 1964), I.54–61, 79–80.

[32] Pelling, *Medical Conflicts*, p. 11.

[33] C. H. Talbot, *Medicine in Medieval England* (London, 1967), pp. 136–41; Rawcliffe, *Medicine and Society*, pp. 115–18; Getz, *Medicine in the English Middle Ages*, pp. 49–53; P. Horton-Smith-Hartley and H. R. Aldridge, *Johannes de Mirfeld: His Life and Works* (Cambridge, 1936), pp. 48–51, 132–3.

[34] *SR*, vol. 3, 34 and 35 Henry VIII, cap. 8.

their heads: for they are commonly all wealthy, and ready to purchase lands: but to help their poor neighbour, that they cannot do.[35]

In reality, a number of factors made care more accessible than reformers like Latimer were prepared to allow. For a start, although the attentions of a physician, surgeon or even a barber-surgeon could prove extremely expensive, they were at least open to negotiation. Whereas elite *medici* were often retained at a fixed salary by aristocratic patrons who expected them to be constantly on call, it was more common for ordinary practitioners and patients to agree terms for each separate course of treatment. Not surprisingly, most of our evidence about these arrangements derives from lawsuits, since disgruntled patients frequently sued for debt, extortion, breach of contract, fraud and even trespass against the person.[36] The sums involved varied in accordance with the severity of the complaint, the length and complexity of the proposed cure and the cost of medicaments, which could be substantial.[37] In this respect, the relative wealth of the patient was clearly a determining factor; and the authors of medical text books would sometimes suggest cheaper alternatives that might be used when prescribing salves, pills and other remedies for poorer people.[38] The relative skill and reputation of the healer also affected the size of the bill, as the surgeon John of Arderne, who boasted a remarkable success rate in the cure of anal *fistulae*, explained. His sliding scale of fees, which rose from a cut-price £5 to £40 – along with robes and an annual pension of £5 – for treating 'a worthi man and a gret', was clearly beyond the means of most sufferers from this debilitating condition.[39] On the other hand, the more modest remuneration of 32s. 8d. promised by one patient to the London surgeon Nicholas Sax proved to be a false economy, since the latter's 'defaute and unkunnyng' in performing what was then a notoriously difficult procedure made matters worse, and it cost an additional 20s. to repair the damage.[40]

The cost of treatment might be cushioned in a variety of ways. Payment was customarily divided into instalments, either in kind or cash, according to a prearranged verbal or written contract; and it was by no means unusual for the patient to renege on at least part of the final settlement.[41] Practitioners were,

---

[35] G. E. Corrie, ed., *Sermons by Hugh Latimer* (Cambridge, 1844), p. 541.

[36] C. Rawcliffe, 'The Profits of Practice: The Wealth and Status of Medical Men in Later Medieval England', *Social History of Medicine* 1 (1988), pp. 61–78; M. Pelner Cosman, 'Medieval Medical Malpractice: The *Dicta* and the Dockets', *Bulletin of the New York Academy of Medicine* 49 (1973), pp. 22–47; R. C. Palmer, *English Law in the Age of the Black Death, 1348–1381: A Transformation of Governance and Law* (Chapel Hill, NC, 1993), pp. 185–96, 342–9.

[37] See, for example, BL, MS Sloane 428, fol. 18v; Rawcliffe, *Leprosy in Medieval England*, p. 206.

[38] Bodleian Library, MS Ashmole 1505, fol. 32r; Glasgow University Library Special Collections, MS Hunter 513, chap. 1; Getz, *Healing and Society*, p. 219. Plague *concilia*, in particular, recommend accessible substitutes for theriac, which was expensive: Aberth, *Black Death*, p. 49; see section 6.4 below.

[39] John of Arderne, *Treatises of Fistula in Ano*, ed. D. Power, EETS o.s. 139 (London, 1910), p. 6.

[40] TNA, C1/42/108. Sax was of German origin: TNA, E179/242/25, m. 8v.

[41] Rawcliffe, 'Profits of Practice', pp. 73–7.

moreover, expected to exercise restraint and avoid any hint of exploitation, a requirement enshrined in the oath taken by all master surgeons of London from the 1360s onwards and frequently noted by the mayor when he was called upon to determine cases of professional misconduct.[42] As advised by Galen, medical authorities urged their readers to shun excessive charges and to establish a reputation for generosity by tending freely to the poor. Confessors, too, were increasingly liable to ask probing questions about the amount of work being undertaken for the public good.[43] Compassion for others seemed particularly desirable in those who cared for kings and princes, since they provided a model for the monarch to follow as physician of the body politic.[44] But anyone fortunate enough to number 'riche men' among his patients could legitimately regard them as a means of subsidising assistance for the destitute.[45]

Aware that his own high fees might create the wrong impression, John of Arderne was at pains to list charity as one of the principal qualities necessary in a successful surgeon. The latter, he felt, should 'som tyme visite of his wynnyngis poure men aftir his myght, that thai by thair prayers may gete hym grace of the holy goste', although nothing is said about actually treating them.[46] Similar ambiguity surrounds the permits customarily granted by urban magistrates to barbers and surgeons which allowed them to evade the ban on Sunday trading if they set aside any profits for the benefit of those in need.[47] Some practitioners are certainly known to have provided free care, as we can see from the case of a small child who developed an infected ulcer and was driven to beg on the streets of London with her father. A surgeon dressed her sores twice, before pronouncing her condition incurable. Had she not then been miraculously healed by St Thomas Cantelupe, this act of kindness would have gone unrecorded, as no doubt did many others.[48]

According to its statutes, the short-lived Joint College of Physicians and Surgeons of London would have regularised such *ad hoc* activities by assigning 'a gode practisour' to 'euereche seke man, nedynge the practyk of phisyk or the workyng of cirurgy, fallen in such pouerte that he sufficeth nat to make good for the labours of his phisician, or of his cirurgean'. Although most patients would

---

[42] *CLB*, G, p. 337; Riley, *Memorials of London*, p. 337.

[43] D. W. Amundsen and G. B. Ferngren, 'Philanthropy and Medicine: Some Historical Perspectives', *Philosophy and Medicine* 11 (1982), pp. 1–31, on pp. 21–4.

[44] V. Nutton, 'Murders and Miracles: Lay Attitudes towards Medicine in Classical Antiquity', in R. Porter, ed., *Patients and Practitioners: Lay Perceptions of Medicine in Pre-Industrial Society* (Cambridge, 1985), pp. 28–9; Picherit, *Métaphore pathologique*, 55–6.

[45] Lanfrank, *Science of Cirurgie*, p. 9. Henri de Mondeville complained about wealthy patients who disguised themselves as paupers in order to obtain free treatment, or who protested when they found a surgeon assisting the poor that charity should be available for them, too. His response is revealing: 'pay me for yourself and for three paupers if I cure you and if I cure them; I'll pay for ... all the others myself and I will also heal them' (Henri de Mondeville, *Chirurgie*, pp. 112–13).

[46] John of Arderne, *Treatises of Fistula in Ano*, p. 4.

[47] *LRBB*, II.69–71.

[48] Finucane, *Rescue of the Innocents*, p. 122.

have been required to meet some basic costs, as determined by officials of the college, members were specifically forbidden from demanding 'ouer moche mone, or vnresonably ... bot after the power of the seke man, and mesurabely after the deseruyng of [their] labour'.[49] Despite the college's rapid demise, at least two of its founders took this message to heart. During the 1440s the royal physician John Somerset used a significant part of his personal fortune to establish an almshouse for elderly and disabled paupers in Brentford, while also dispensing relief to a stream of indigents each day from his home nearby.[50] In the following decade, his colleague Thomas Morstede followed suit by leaving at least £100 from the profits of a distinguished surgical career to 'the feeble poor' and other charitable projects.[51]

A few late medieval testators regarded the provision of expert care as an extension of the fifth Comfortable Work. Some bequests were specific, as in the case of one Norwich widow who left 10s. in 1516 to fund the cost of surgery for a poor relative;[52] others were more broadly philanthropic. For example, the London mercer John Donne (d. 1479) arranged for a young surgeon named Thomas Thornton to

> contynnewe in his daily besynes and comfort of the poure, sore and seke peple lakkyng helpe and money to pay for their lechecrafte in London and the subarbes of the same. In especiall, in the hospitalles of Saint Mary, Saint Bartholomewe, Saint Thomas, Newgate, Ludgate and in other places whereas peple shal have nede. And thus to contynnewe by this grace by the space of v [five] yere next ensuyng my decesse. For the which attendaunce and cost in medesines I wolle ther be paied for every yere of the v yere v *li.* in money ... And if it shall fortune him to be slouthfull and nott diligent to attende the pour peple, or and it shall fortune him to departe this life ... thenne my wille is that anothere able persone be provided.[53]

Yet however liberal they may have been with their own private resources, magistrates like Donne did not regard such expenditure as a legitimate claim upon the public purse. The few payments for surgery and medicaments that are recorded in civic archives generally concern individuals who became ill or sustained injuries when engaged on official business, rather than the sick poor.[54]

The rulers of English towns and cities showed far greater interest in matters

---

[49] Beck, *Cutting Edge*, pp. 65–6.

[50] G. J. Aungier, *The History and Antiquities of Syon Monastery* (London, 1840), pp. 215–20, 459–64; T. Hearne, ed., *Thomae de Elmham vita et gesta Henrici Quinti* (Oxford, 1727), p. 340; TNA, C1/19/65.

[51] Beck, *Cutting Edge*, p. 95.

[52] Rawcliffe, 'Sickness and Health', p. 322.

[53] TNA, PROB/11/7, fol. 11r. Thornton must have recently qualified, as he was still practising in 1517: Beck, *Cutting Edge*, pp. 129, 147–8.

[54] See, for instance, Butler, *Book of Fines*, p. 150. In 1520 and 1522 the corporation of Beverley distributed 'alms to divers poor' infected by plague, but no reference is made to medical treatment: HMC, *Report on the Manuscripts of the Corporation of Beverley*, Royal Commission on Historical Manuscripts 54 (London, 1900), pp. 173–4.

of regulation, not least because of the legal and commercial issues at stake. Since one of the manifold attractions of urban life was the ready availability of medical treatment at a price to suit most pockets, they had to ensure that residents and visitors alike received proper attention without being fleeced or mutilated in the process. London, in particular, was a magnet for those in search of professional help; the resentment felt by Nicholas Sax's disgruntled patient was undoubtedly compounded by the fact that he had travelled all the way from Southampton for surgery. Some, such as William Wattepas, who came up from Essex in 1300 'to be cured of a wound in his arm', did not survive the experience; yet more returned home disappointed and penniless. Having endured a long and painful journey by horse litter from his vicarage in Melbourne, Cambridgeshire, and spent six months 'at great costs' in London obtaining treatment for a stroke, John Dobson was left with nothing but the prospect of imprisonment for debt.[55] He, at least, was prepared to seek legal redress, but others had to be protected from exploitation and, if necessary, assured that official support would be readily forthcoming should problems arise.[56] In most communities of reasonable size, surgeons, barbers and apothecaries were subject to close supervision through the medium of their craft guilds, being answerable to the authorities for any breach of professional standards, just like other artisans. And, as a further safety net, national and local courts provided the machinery for investigating, and if necessary punishing, any cases of incompetence, dereliction or fraud reported to them.

6.3 The supervision and control of practitioners

As we have already seen, Edward I's decision to make York his administrative capital during the Scottish wars prompted a series of ordinances for the improvement of the environment in which crown servants were now obliged to live. Conspicuous among them were measures for the regulation of medical practitioners, including apothecaries, who were prohibited from making 'concoctions for human use' unless they possessed the necessary skill.[57] Highlighting the fundamental issues that were to preoccupy urban magistrates for centuries to come, the royal council and rulers of York also decreed that:

> No physician shall be called to that profession unless he is expert in the art of medicine, and he has been sworn to exercise his calling well and faithfully. He shall use only good, pure and clean drugs. No practitioner is to exercise his profession unless he has been instructed in the art of surgery at least so as to treat wounds and hurts. He is to swear not to treat anyone for any wound unless he first informs the mayor where the wounded man lodges, and of the nature of the wound.[58]

The additional requirement that neither fripperers (who dealt in second-hand clothes) nor *medici* should buy 'ripped or bloodstained' bandages in secret was

---

[55] TNA, C1/131/8.

[56] *CCRCL*, pp. 1–2.

[57] *YCO*, p. 18.

[58] *YCO*, p. 17.

less a hygienic precaution than another means of ensuring that violent crimes would not remain hidden. Similar concerns are apparent in Parisian regulations of this date, which were principally designed to assist the agents of law and order, and in the oath sworn before the mayor and aldermen by all master surgeons of London from at least 1369.[59]

Responsible practitioners favoured a mandatory process of consultation for professional reasons, too, emphasising the need for surgeons to confer with senior colleagues over the treatment of potentially 'desperate' cases, whatever their cause. In this way it was hoped to restrain the more reckless or mercenary brethren, as proved necessary in 1415 when a number of inexperienced London barber-surgeons were charged with endangering and even maiming their patients through lack of proper supervision. Condemning their desire for profit rather than 'honesty or a safe conscience', the mayor himself intervened to prevent further abuses. Henceforward, two respected masters were to oversee all guild members, to examine any problematic 'wounds, bruises, hurts and other infirmities' at the first opportunity, and to report cases of intransigence or malpractice to the civic authorities. As an additional safeguard, it was agreed shortly afterwards that all such inspections would take place within three days, under a fixed penalty of 6s. 8d.[60] The seriousness with which the Corporation viewed this requirement is apparent from an entry in the City Journal for 1417, recording the surrender of a bond in the substantial sum of 20 marks [£13 6s. 8d.] by the surgeon John Love, as security that he would present any cases likely to result in death or mutilation to the wardens of his guild within the requisite period.[61] When compiling their new ordinances in 1435, the Surgeons needed little persuasion to incorporate similar provisions, not least because they offered a degree of insurance against unwelcome litigation.[62]

All craft guilds were expected to guarantee an appropriate level of training and skill, but the pressure upon practitioners of surgery was especially acute in light of the potential risks to life and limb that accompanied even minor procedures in an age before antisepsis, anaesthesia and blood transfusion. Attention focussed in particular upon the calibre and education of apprentices, the expertise of those who went on to set up in business on their own account, and the inspection of 'foreyn' practitioners. Although, unlike many of their Continental peers, English surgeons did not enjoy the opportunity to study at university, considerable care was given to the choice and education of apprentices, who were indented to a

[59] R. de Lespinasse and F. Bonnardot, eds, *Les Métiers et corporations de la ville de Paris: XIIIe siècle: Le Livre des métiers d'Étienne Boileau* (Paris, 1879), pp. lxxix, xcii–xciii, 160, 208–9; *CLB*, G, p. 236; Riley, *Memorials of London*, p. 337.

[60] Young, *Annals of the Barber-Surgeons*, pp. 40–2; Riley, *Memorials of London*, pp. 606–9. Because of the risks attached to even minor procedures, surgeons were urged to be 'bold & hardy in sekyr thynges & fferfull & dowtfull in perelles', and above all 'to exchew from evyll currys': BL, MS Harley 1736, fol. 7r. Lanfrank of Milan warned of the 'perel of kuttynge', and attacked surgeons who 'for a litil money' risked the lives of their patients: *Science of Cirurgie*, pp. 271–2.

[61] If forfeit, the money would have been shared equally between the guild and the civic authorities: Riley, *Memorials of London*, p. 651.

[62] Beck, *Cutting Edge*, p. 132.

master for at least five or six years before submitting to an examination and, if successful, entering the guild as journeymen. A longer period might sometimes be required, as was the case from 1421 in Coventry and 1439 in Bristol, where any barber-surgeons who failed to train their charges for a full seven years faced fines of 10s. and 40s. respectively.[63]

In return, masters could demand a range of attributes that reflected the intimate and taxing nature of surgical practice: young recruits had not only to be physically strong, but also well groomed, with 'clene handes and wele shapen nailes & clensed fro all blaknes and filthe'.[64] Advice on this topic, which was readily available from a growing number of vernacular treatises, stressed the need for keen eyesight, 'stable handes noght quakynge', manual dexterity and 'a complexcioun weel proporciound and … temperat' that would reassure nervous patients.[65] In 1482 the London Barbers insisted upon a compulsory medical examination in order to eliminate any candidate who seemed 'avexed or disposed to be lepur or gowty, maiymed or disfigured in any parties of his body, whereby he shall fall in disdeyn or lothefulnesse'.[66] Although guild members derived considerable pride from the fact that surgery was a craft best learned through observation and practice, book ownership was becoming common, even among the lower ranks of provincial operatives. Acting upon the advice of authorities such as Guy de Chauliac that 'the cirurgien be a lettred man, noght onliche in the principles of cirurgie but also of phisique', by the 1470s the London Barbers had actually begun to assemble their own 'lyberary', to which many masters contributed. They may even have felt able, like their Scottish peers, to reject any potential recruit who could not 'baithe wryte and reid'.[67] The need for literacy is apparent from the list of topics upon which every Edinburgh apprentice was to be 'diligentlie and avysitilie' examined from at least 1505, if not before, in order to determine:

> that he knaw anotamell [anatomy], nature and complexion of euery member humanis bodie, and inlykewayes he knaw all the vaynis of the saymn, thatt he may mak flewbothomell in dew tyme, and als thatt he knaw in quhilk member the signe [of the zodiac] hes domination for the tyme, for euery man aucht to knaw the nature and substance of euery thing thatt he werkis, or ellis he is negligent.[68]

---

[63] *Coventry Leet Book*, I.225; *LRBB*, II.154. In York the basic requirement was five years (*YMB*, I.209–10), and in Norwich seven (*RCN*, II.279–80).

[64] John of Arderne, *Treatises of Fistula in Ano*, p. 6.

[65] Lanfrank, *Science of Cirurgie*, p. 8; Guy de Chauliac, *Cyrurgie*, p. 13. The case of the royal surgeon John Leche underscores the importance of these requirements. He obtained a pension from Richard II in 1383 because of his failing sight, but was accused by a Chester woman two years later of killing her husband through negligence: *CPR, 1381–1385*, pp. 283, 324, 527, 559.

[66] Young, *Annals of the Barber-Surgeons*, p. 62.

[67] Guy de Chauliac, *Cyrurgie*, p. 12; N. Ramsay and J. M. Willoughby, eds, *Hospitals, Towns and the Professions*, Corpus of British Medieval Library Catalogues 14 (London, 2009), pp. 165–8; Marwick, *Records of the Burgh of Edinburgh*, p. 103.

[68] Marwick, *Records of the Burgh of Edinburgh*, pp. 102–3. For the role of astrology in surgical practice, see Rawcliffe, *Medicine and Society*, pp. 87–9, 131.

The contents of a late fifteenth-century compilation of vernacular medical texts once owned by the York barber-surgeons suggest that their training corresponded to this model on every point, including tuition in the practical application of astrology and humoral theory (see plate 2).[69]

Apprentices were not alone in facing rigorous tests of theoretical knowledge and practical expertise. From the mid-fourteenth century, as opportunists sought to profit from the increasing demand for phlebotomy and other prophylactic procedures, the need arose for effective scrutiny at later stages in a practitioner's career. It was principally for this reason that in 1376 the mayor of London sanctioned the appointment of two wardens, one of whom was to be a barber-surgeon, to govern the Barbers' guild. Their principal task was to stem the tide of newcomers flooding into the City

> who are not instructed in their craft, and do take houses and intermeddle
> with barbery, surgery, and the cure of other maladies, while they know not
> how to do such things ... to the great damage, and in deceit, of the people,
> and to the great scandal of all good barbers of the said city.

The wardens were not only to examine and approve every new arrival, but also to inspect all 'the instruments of the said art' then being used in London, 'to see that they are good and proper for the service of the people, by reason of the great peril that might ensue thereupon'.[70]

It made sound commercial as well as professional sense to maintain a strict licensing system. In 1497, partly as a result of their rapprochement with the more prestigious guild of Surgeons and also because of their recent incorporation as an independent City company, the Barber-Surgeons of London sought to improve their credentials by appointing the university-trained physician John Smyth as an 'instructour & examiner'. Such a move also helped them to impose tighter controls upon the growing army of unqualified empirics who performed a variety of 'manwall operacions' on the unsuspecting public. The new examination (which Robert Anson, a leading surgeon, gamely volunteered to take) involved a long interrogation before 'a gret audiens of many right well expert men', during which the candidate had to prove himself 'abyll and discrete to ocopy & vse the practise

---

[69] BL, MS Egerton 2572, fols 50r–70r; I. Taavitsainen, 'A Zodiacal Lunary for Medical Professionals', in Matheson, *Popular and Practical Science*, pp. 283–300; Stell, *Medical Practice in Medieval York*, pp. 23–5.

[70] Young, *Annals of the Barber-Surgeons*, pp. 28, 35–6; Riley, *Memorials of London*, pp. 393–4. A overseer of the guild had been first appointed in 1308, with specific orders to make a monthly inspection of members' premises and to punish those who kept brothels – a reflection of the fact that barbers often superintended bath houses: Young, *Annals of the Barber-Surgeons*, p. 24; *CBL*, C, p. 165. That the rulers and senior practitioners of London 'were uncomfortable with the juxtaposition of sexual sin and the health professions' is apparent from their trenchant response in cases involving 'notorious behaviour' on the part of certain physicians and surgeons: McSheffrey, *Marriage, Sex and Civic Culture*, pp. 166–76. Both quotations are on p. 170.

of surgery, as well a bowte new woundis, as cansers, fystelis [*fistulae*], vlceracions & many other disessis'.[71]

Stringent regulations also obtained in York, where, in theory at least, all medical practitioners, from physicians to bone-setters and tooth-drawers, had to place themselves under the direction (*sub regimine*) of one of the city's master barber-surgeons, or pay a sizeable fine for each reported dereliction. In order to justify their monopoly, the guild members were themselves subject to close scrutiny by expert searchers whose authority was reinforced by the mayor and aldermen. Any newly appointed assistants or journeymen had to be assessed within a week, while every 'artificer' starting an independent practice faced a similar process of inspection 'to see if he is competent to work as a master or not'. Failure had serious economic as well as professional consequences:

> And if he shall be found wanting by the aforesaid searchers, he shall be warned by them to cease working as a master until such time as he shall be pronounced sufficiently learned in his art ... and approved as competent. And, if he refuses to desist upon the first warning, then on the second he shall forfeit 6s. 8d. to the chamber [of the city] and to his craft, payable by him in equal portions. If, however, after the third warning he will not desist, then his basins and other signs that he has hanging in the street to advertise his craft shall be seized by the searchers in office at that time and carried to the chamber on Ouse Bridge into the presence of the mayor, without impediment ... and then he will pay a fine to the mayor at his pleasure and that of the searchers, as they see fit.[72]

Swearing on oath 'to bee trustie and trewe vnto the kinge our soveraigne lord and to this Cittie of York and also to the Science of Barbars & Chyreurgions within the same', licensed masters played a similar role to their London counterparts in the policing of 'strangers and aliens' who intended 'to exercise any poynt of surgerie'. Their enthusiasm for this task is understandable, since they were authorised to charge a registration fee which everyone deemed competent had to pay. And because they also exercised the right to conduct spot checks whenever they wished upon 'all maner cures of surgerie which the said aliens and straungers shal have in hand' anywhere in the city or suburbs it was possible to steal a march on potential competitors.[73]

Although none of the surgeons and barber-surgeons who worked under this system can be described as municipal employees in the Continental sense, many assumed official duties that went far beyond the responsibilities of guild

[71] Young, *Annals of the Barber-Surgeons*, pp. 52–8, 69–70. The London Barber-Surgeons were probably influenced by their Parisian counterparts, who, from 1493 onwards, could attend lectures and study anatomy at the University: Lespinasse, *Métiers et corporations de la ville de Paris*, III.639.

[72] *YMB*, I.209.

[73] BL, MS Egerton 2572, fol. 1r; *YMB*, I.211. Economic considerations were clearly important. The barbers of Beverley seem to have been more concerned that any 'strange' physicians, surgeons, tooth-drawers or blood-letters who practised in the town for longer than a week should pay dues to the guild than they were about questions of expertise: *BTD*, pp. 112–13.

membership. In 1311, for example, one London barber-surgeon was commissioned to report on 'disturbances of filth' and similar health hazards in Langbourne ward.[74] Others were enlisted from then onwards to serve as keepers of the City's gates, largely because of their skill in identifying individuals who posed a threat to communal health and were therefore unwelcome in urban thoroughfares.[75] We know far less about their involvement in the examination of residents who appeared to have contracted dangerous diseases, such as leprosy. In France, Germany and the Low Countries it was common for salaried physicians and surgeons to undertake this task, while in the larger university towns, such as Cologne, Mainz and Paris, members of the faculty of medicine would provide a comprehensive service for the surrounding region.[76] Because they lacked such an accessible source of expertise, English magistrates could not usually request a formal *judicium*, or medical inspection, but relied instead upon juries of 'discreet persons' who were deemed capable of reaching an informed diagnosis.[77] It is hard to tell what role, if any, qualified practitioners played in these deliberations, but occasional scraps of evidence are suggestive. When equipping his readers with a comprehensive list of symptoms, the author of one vernacular text-book observed that surgeons were often expected 'to declar and judge lepurs', and should avoid making hasty decisions.[78] Physicians, too, may have been consulted from time to time: the expulsion from Yarmouth of a leper named Beatrice Easton in 1392 after a decade of complaints by her neighbours coincided not only with the first reference to miasmatic infection recorded in the leet rolls, but also a violent assault by her husband on a local *medicus*.[79]

6.4 Apothecaries and drugs

The development of trade with the Middle East from the twelfth century onwards facilitated the dissemination across Europe of works on pharmacy by Muslim scientists and physicians who had greatly augmented the basic *materia medica* of the Ancient Greeks, and pioneered important new techniques such as distillation. Since so many new imports (including almonds, cloves, cinnamon, cumin, ginger, nutmeg, pepper, saffron and sugar) were valued as much for their therapeutic as their culinary properties, some of the merchants who dealt in spices began to specialise in the preparation of compound remedies. The growing popularity of electuaries, which assisted digestion and therefore helped to maintain one's humoral balance, and of scented preparations designed to fortify the vital and animal spirits, both reflected and stimulated this

---

[74] *CLB*, D, p. 312.

[75] Riley, *Memorials of London*, p. 384; Young, *Annals of the Barber-Surgeons*, p. 25; *CLB*, D, p. 241; *CLB*, H, p. 9; *CLB*, L, pp. 102–3.

[76] Jacqaurt, *Milieu médical en France*, pp. 128, 231, 288–9; Demaitre, *Leprosy in Premodern Medicine*, pp. 34–71; G. B. Risse, *Mending Bodies, Saving Souls: A History of Hospitals* (New York, 1999), pp. 169–72.

[77] See sections 1.6 and 3.1 above.

[78] BL, MS Harley 1736, fols 133v–135r.

[79] NRO, Y/C4/104, rot. 11r–v.

trend.[80] Although the most exotic and costly wares were earmarked for royal and baronial households, by the late thirteenth century stalls selling a profusion of herbs and spices, as well as ready-made elixirs that could be bought cheaply over the counter, proliferated in urban marketplaces. A guild of apothecaries, whose wardens were required to ensure that its members dealt fairly with the public, had by then been established in London, the principal distribution centre for the country's burgeoning trade in spices and pharmaceuticals. But the provinces were catching up fast. Norwich even boasted its own *forum unguentorum* or *apothecaria* where most of the thirty-four apothecaries who appear in the civic records between 1288 and 1348 would have done business.[81]

As well as fostering a demand for bloodletting and the other types of purgation offered by barber-surgeons and empirics, the inescapable threat of pestilence created a lucrative market in the tonics, pills, potions, fumigants, unguents, oils and scented waters that were believed to protect against infection. Plague tracts and *regimina* did much to promote the innumerable prophylactics that might readily be purchased 'in th'appoticary shoppes' for a few pence or shillings.[82] As a result, the already brisk trade in drugs and medicaments increased exponentially, and many spicer-apothecaries, especially in major commercial centres, became very rich indeed. The prospect of wealth inevitably encouraged a number of abuses, which, as in the case of surgeons and barber-surgeons, were held in check by the combined vigilance of craft guilds and urban magistrates. Late medieval satirists, of whom John Gower furnishes the most vituperative example, tended to focus upon the unholy alliance between physicians and apothecaries, but municipal authorities were more concerned about the sale of over-priced, adulterated and potentially lethal merchandise. As we saw in Chapter 5, victuallers were expected to use officially approved weights and measures, a requirement that carried particular force in the case of apothecaries, who were widely believed to 'fix' their balances and sell expensive wares at short measure. In some cases, suspicion may have been unfairly aroused by their deployment of a different system of 'Troy' weights (with twelve rather than sixteen ounces to the pound), which had been sanctioned by Edward I. Uncertainty on this score probably explains why a Nottingham jury complained in 1395 that local apothecaries were selling merchandise 'by unusual and unfaithful weights, not adhering to the standard'. There was, however, no excuse for mixing old spices with new in order to dispose of unwanted stock, this being but one of many subterfuges employed to deceive the public.[83]

---

[80] Rawcliffe, *Medicine and Society*, pp. 148–51.

[81] P. Nightingale, *A Medieval Mercantile Community: The Grocers Company and the Politics and Trade of London, 1000–1485* (New Haven, CT, 1995), pp. 53, 61–80, 127–8; *CLB*, C, p. 17; Rawcliffe, 'Sickness and Health', p. 320.

[82] *Here Begynneth A Litill Boke*, fol. 5v. In April 1471 alone Edward IV spent £10 on medicines against the plague, provided by his apothecary: F. Devon, ed., *Issues of the Exchequer* (London, 1847), p. 493.

[83] Nightingale, *Medieval Mercantile Community*, pp. 108–9, 184, 272; Rawcliffe, *Medicine and Society*, pp. 155–62; Stevenson, *Records of the Borough of Nottingham*, I.281.

From the late thirteenth century onwards all spices and other pharmaceutical products entering the country were supposed to be cleansed of impurities, accurately weighed, 'as well for the poor as the rich', and stamped with an official seal of approval at the port of entry.[84] Yet deception remained common. London guild regulations of 1316 condemned the practice of soaking expensive goods such as cloves and saffron in water to make them heavier when weighed, and of placing a layer of high-quality merchandise on the top of bales and barrels filled with inferior wares or even sawdust.[85] Artificial colourings might also be used to render spices more attractive, while the sale of preparations that had remained too long on the shelf for safety posed a perennial problem. In 1415 the Company of Grocers (which had merged with the apothecaries' guild in the 1340s) set out to eliminate both hazards by instituting a search of all premises by expert surveyors. The results were sufficiently alarming to prompt the introduction of compulsory inspections of 'weyghtys, powdrez, confesciouns, plasters, oynementz and all othyr thynges that longyth to the same craft' by the wardens at least once a year, and more often if necessary.[86] Shrewdly, the Company decided to fine the entire membership rather than specific individuals, thereby exerting the most effective type of peer pressure upon potential offenders.

Attempts by the short-lived College of Physicians and Surgeons of London to take control of these procedures suggest that further regulation seemed necessary, and may well have prompted the Grocers to strengthen their position in 1425 by guaranteeing the quality of every consignment of 'sotil ware' and medicinal 'pouderes' sold to customers outside London. The adulteration of 'clene' merchandise with inferior goods and the lack of proper labelling caused concern a decade later, but in general the Grocers' desire to uphold their reputation and avoid outside intervention served to protect consumers from harm.[87] Not until 1525 did the Common Council of London see fit to intervene in the activities of apothecaries, and then only because the newly incorporated College of Physicians wished to prevent them from making up prescriptions on behalf of unlicensed 'irregulars'. The additional requirement that they should keep all documentation in a file, 'to th'entent that if the pacyent myscary it may be by the College considerid whether the bill were medecynall or hurtfull to the sickness' was ostensibly aimed at negligent practitioners, but it also curtailed the apothecaries' freedom to prescribe without professional supervision.[88]

Of all the exotic merchandise sold by apothecaries, theriac, or 'tryacle', was by far the most profitable. A compound drug initially devised by Greek and Roman physicians to counteract poison, by the later Middle Ages it was regarded as a universal panacea, whose unique properties accorded special protection against

---

[84] *CLB*, D, pp. 296–7; *CLB*, H, p. 400.

[85] Riley, *Memorials of London*, pp. 120–1.

[86] J. A. Kingdon, ed., *Ms. Archives of the Worshipful Company of Grocers of the City of London, 1345–1463*, 2 vols (London, 1886), I.111, 120.

[87] Kingdon, *Ms. Archives of the Worshipful Company of Grocers*, I.154; II.232.

[88] Beck, *Cutting Edge*, p. 151; Clark, *History of the Royal College of Physicians*, I.79. However, physicians were prohibited from selling any medicines that could be bought over the counter.

the venomous miasmas of pestilence. Plague tracts advised a regular, sometimes twice-daily, dose, with the result that demand rocketed and some apothecaries began to specialise as 'treacle-mongers'. No fewer than six were admitted to the freedom of York between 1412 and 1422, a decade notable for northern epidemics. The drug, which contained upwards of seventy separate ingredients, including the flesh of vipers, was produced in Italy under licence and shipped to England in carefully sealed pots.[89] The temptation to peddle 'fals triacle' at inflated prices could be hard to resist, especially during plague time, although the penalties were sufficiently daunting to deter all but the most foolhardy. In 1432, for example, the London Grocers fined one of their members 40s. for a second offence, warning him that he would 'be put owt of the craft for alle dayes' should he be caught again.[90] Incoming cargoes were searched as an added precaution, as happened in 1472 when the mayor commissioned two physicians and seventeen apothecaries to examine a consignment of theriac that had just arrived from Genoa under suspicious circumstances. Having been found 'unwholesome', the goods were consigned to three bonfires, one of which was in Cheapside where many apothecaries did business.[91] The need for a public spectacle may have seemed all the more pressing because pestilence had so recently ravaged the City; and it was, indeed, during the plague of 1475 that the authorities again saw fit to impose exemplary punishment (both the pillory and gaol) upon a dealer in 'counterfeit' sandalwood, a costly fumigant used to dispel miasmatic air.[92]

As noted above, physicians and surgeons had their own reasons for seeking to control the manufacture and sale of drugs. However limited its authority may have been elsewhere, the Oxford faculty of medicine was generally able to exercise close supervision over the more reputable practitioners, including apothecaries, who worked within the walls. By the 1520s, if not earlier, the latter were obliged to swear an oath to the effect that:

> I will always have in my shop all medicines, species of medicines and confections which concern the art and mystery of an apothecary, and are necessary for the health of man ... I shall be contented once a year (at least) that certain physicians practising in the University shall visit my shop upon the account of good and bad medicines, in the month of November, or any other time if occasion shall require it ... and these searchers and tryers of medicines ... shall have power to destroy and throw away all bad and

---

[89] Rawcliffe, *Medicine and Society*, pp. 152–5.

[90] Kingdon, *Ms. Archives of the Worshipful Company of Grocers*, II.225.

[91] *CLB*, L, p. 103. The import of dubious medicines appears to have been policed from an early date – at least if an intriguing case of 1300 involving the shipment of a cask containing the putrid flesh of four wolves is any guide. The owner, a clergyman, claimed that it was a cure for '*le lou*' (erysipelas or perhaps skin cancer), but an expert jury of 'all the physicians and surgeons of London' disagreed after consulting the relevant literature: *CEMCRL*, p. 51.

[92] *CLB*, L, p. 130. Prosecutions for falsifying spices were comparatively rare, although in 1394 William Whitman was sentenced to the pillory, where the 'divers false powders' and tansy seed that he had passed off as ginger and wormwood were burnt beneath him: *CLB*, H, p. 412.

unprofitable medicines and drugs ... I will sell all things appertaining to my trade at a low and reasonable price, and as sold in other places in England ... I will not make up any compound medicines without the presence and advice of some physician admitted to practice, who shall judge those samples fit to be made up into compositions.[93]

Alongside this commendable concern for public safety ran a less altruistic desire to corner the market in the face of some potentially daunting competition. Given their extensive knowledge of pharmaceutical preparations and humoral theory, many English apothecaries could easily hold their own among the medical elite. Although they were not formally required to attain the levels of expertise and literacy so often demanded in continental Europe, they underwent a lengthy apprenticeship and in some cases are known to have acquired the same text-books as their foreign peers.[94] Nor, however alarming it might sound, did their advance into the field of surgery necessarily pose a risk to others. Since medieval surgeons customarily treated conditions such as skin diseases and eye complaints that affected the outside of the human body, much of their work involved the use of plasters, ointments and salves rather than the lancet or cautery. Occasionally, however, apothecaries overstepped the mark by attempting invasive procedures without the necessary training. One such was the Norwich 'potycarye' George Hill, who faced imprisonment and then expulsion from the city in the 1530s for practising 'the science off surgerye, he nat beyng expert theryn, nor yet admytted therunto according to the lawe'.[95] His offence constituted a clear breach of the Act of 1512, but even before then allegations of ineptitude or fraud could have serious legal consequences.[96]

[93] R. T. Gunther, *Early Science in Oxford*, 14 vols (Oxford, 1925–45), III.8. But see also pp. 293–4 above.

[94] Rawcliffe, *Medicine and Society*, p. 165. Writing in about 1385, the Franciscan herbalist Henry Daniel maintained that English apothecaries were 'wel lewyd [ignorant] in here craft ... and wel defectif in her doynges': BL, MS Arundel 42, fol. 49v. Yet apprenticeships of up to ten years (including a grammar school education) are recorded in the fifteenth century, seven years being more common: TNA, C1/252/13–16, 309/43–4; *CLB*, D, p. 176. In Paris apprenticeships of just two years were the norm during the 1320s, and of four a century later, although greater familiarity with set texts was expected: F. Prevet, ed., *Les Statuts et règlements des apothicairès*, 15 vols (Paris, 1950), I.21–2, 44–59.

[95] *RCN*, II.168; NRO, NCR, 16A/4, Mayor's Court Book, 1534–1549, fol. 33v.

[96] For example, in 1354 the mayor and aldermen of London empanelled four surgeons to examine an 'enormous and horrible hurt' on the jaw of Thomas de Shene, a fishmonger. The surgeons accused John le Spicer, who was almost certainly an apothecary, of inflicting incurable injury through lack of skill and a failure to seek advice: Riley, *Memorials of London*, pp. 273–4; *CLB*, G, p. 21. For an exploration of similar cases, see Pelner Cosman, 'Medieval Medical Malpractice', pp. 22–47.

6.5 Care for the sick poor

Calculated deception certainly received short shrift from the London authorities, as is apparent from the case of Roger Clerk of Wandsworth, a confidence-trickster who pretended in the early 1380s to be 'experienced and skilled in the art of medicine'. Convinced that 'a straw beneath his foot' would have proved just as effective as the counterfeit charms against fever that Clerk had sold his victims, the mayor sentenced him to a humiliating punishment of the sort customarily inflicted upon the vendors of contaminated food. As a solemn warning to others, he was to be led on horseback through the City with an escort of trumpets and drums, the nature of his offence being apparent from the charm hung about his neck and the two glass urinals (denoting his medical pretensions) that were to be suspended before and behind him.[97] According to Thomas Walsingham, a similar fate awaited another impostor who spread panic through London at this time by forecasting an outbreak of plague.[98] Once they came to court, charlatans could expect a harsh and appropriate sentence that reflected their crime against gullible men and women who all too often lacked the resources to pay for professional treatment.[99]

Unless they posed a wider threat to the health or stability of the urban body, the sufferings of these people are rarely documented, and can best be understood through the analysis of skeletal remains rather than the written record.[100] As we have seen, a few would have been attended as charity cases by successful practitioners, while others would have turned to the Church for physical as well as spiritual care. Although the rector of St Leonard's, Aldgate, whom we encountered at the start of Chapter 2, was accused of laying claim to qualifications that he did not possess, some clergy pursued a serious interest in medicine and used their knowledge to assist needy parishioners.[101] We know, too, that members of the mendicant orders did not simply confine their expertise to the translation and abridgement of medical texts for lay readers, but were noted for their practical skills as herbalists, apothecaries, physicians and surgeons. The erosion of their earlier ideals of poverty and service to the urban poor, so often mocked by satirists and condemned by religious reformers, paved the way for the assiduous cultivation of high-status patients. Nonetheless, it seems likely that, despite the increasing restrictions placed upon them, *fraters medici* would often have dispensed advice and treatment among the destitute as well as the rich.[102]

---

[97] Young, *Annals of the Barber-Surgeons*, pp. 37–8; Riley, *Memorials of London*, pp. 464–6.

[98] Walsingham, *Historia Anglicana*, II.63.

[99] As, for instance, *CPMRL, 1381–1412*, p. 289.

[100] For the importance of 'osteobiography' as a means of illuminating the lives of particular groups of people, such as the elderly poor, see Gilchrist, *Medieval Life*, pp. 43–67.

[101] P. Horden, 'Small Beer? The Parish and the Poor and Sick in Later Medieval England', in C. Burgess and E. Duffy, eds, *The Parish in Late Medieval England* (Donington, 2006), pp. 161–2.

[102] Montford, *Health, Sickness, Medicine and the Friars*, pp. 113–27.

Meanwhile, informal and generally elusive networks based on kinship, gender, neighbourhood and parish helped the sick and disabled with *ad hoc* support, which, by its very nature, remains unquantifiable.[103] Archaeological evidence suggests that some of the most deprived communities accepted responsibility for the care of adults who had been incapacitated since childhood, but it would be unsafe to generalise on this score.[104] And, even though a significant proportion of late medieval wills contain bequests to the bedridden, lame, blind and needy, the practical impact of this sporadic and often ill-defined type of relief is just as hard to determine. Much was left to the discretion of executors, who might lack the resources for pious works once debts had been paid and other obligations met. Nor do testamentary records offer any guide to the 'doorstep' assistance which would have been readily forthcoming in a society so preoccupied with the spiritual merits of charity.[105] We are on slightly firmer ground with regard to the alms dispensed by late medieval religious fraternities and craft guilds, even though recent research suggests that the gap between intention and action may well have been far wider than was once believed. Their role as 'primitive insurance societies', so appealing to nineteenth-century historians, was in fact quite limited, as we can tell from an analysis of the returns submitted by 519 English guilds in response to a parliamentary inquiry of 1388–9. Only a third made any formal provision for members who could no longer fend for themselves, although in contrast to the more frugal rural guilds, which relied less upon the projection of a corporate image and were often poorer, just over half of those based in towns and cities felt able to promise – if not always deliver – some kind of financial relief.[106]

No English fraternity possessed the resources to fund the type of subsidised medical care that the wealthy *scuole* of Florence and Venice could offer their members, but several assigned a rudimentary type of sickness benefit, on the clear understanding that the recipient had not incurred his or her misfortune through reckless or sinful behaviour.[107] In theory, at least, arrangements were fairly elastic, being adjusted to the personal circumstances of each applicant. A few guilds, such as the Palmers of Ludlow and the votaries of St Mary, Hull, distinguished between 'grievous' but short-term illnesses that would merit temporary help, and incurable or chronic conditions such as leprosy and blindness, whose victims qualified for

---

[103] P. Horden, 'Household Care and Informal Networks: Comparisons and Continuities from Antiquity to the Present', in P. Horden and R. Smith, eds, *The Locus of Care: Families, Communities, Institutions and the Provision of Welfare since Antiquity* (London, 1998), pp. 21–67; Horden, 'Small Beer? The Parish and the Poor and Sick', pp. 339–64.

[104] A. Stirland, *Criminals and Paupers: The Graveyard of St Margaret Fyebriggate in Combusto, Norwich*, EAA 129 (Norwich, 2009), pp. 31–3, 35.

[105] For female networks of care in the community, see C. Hill, *Women and Religion in Late Medieval Norwich* (Woodbridge, 2010), chap. 5.

[106] McRee, 'Charity and Guild Solidarity', pp. 199–203.

[107] B. Pullan, *Rich and Poor in Renaissance Venice* (Oxford, 1971), pp. 64–5. Park considers that 'about a third of the Florentine population' may have benefited from this system: *Doctors and Medicine*, pp. 106–8.

permanent aid.[108] Cases were judged on their respective merits: the officers of St Mary's guild, Beverley, were empowered to visit 'poor, ailing or weak members' and assign relief of 8*d*., 6*d*. or 4*d*. a week on the basis of need.[109] Not surprisingly, some craft guilds prioritised the occupational injuries or ailments to which their members were especially prone. The Norwich Tailors, for example, favoured those who had lost their sight or become arthritic after years of sitting hunched over close work in poor light, while the London Goldsmiths were anxious to assist anyone who had 'been blinded by the fire and smoke of the glowing silver' or even rendered insane (*consternatus*) through the ingestion of mercury and other toxic substances.[110]

It was difficult to raise money on a regular basis for charitable purposes, as the statutes devised for the guild of St Clement, Cambridge, in 1431 clearly recognised. Accepting that the number of applicants might well exceed the available resources, they conceded that the modest 4*d*. a week promised to sick and indigent brethren would not always be forthcoming.[111] Not even the affluent fraternity of the Holy Trinity at Lynn could honour its undertaking to distribute £30 a year (a quarter of its income) among the local poor and members in need. On the contrary, its accounts suggest that annual disbursements never rose much above £18 and were sometimes far lower. As might be expected, most of the individual handouts were relatively small, the few larger awards being reserved for reputable brothers and sisters who had paid their dues in the past and therefore seemed especially deserving. Even so, the £15 17*s*. 6*d*. spent on relief in 1439 is still a considerable sum, and must have thrown a lifeline to many vulnerable people.[112] The quarterly inspections undertaken by guild officers enabled them to identify candidates for short-term support, which was then in particular demand as a result of dramatically escalating grain prices.[113] We should remember, too, that, like many other guilds, the confraternity ran its own 'house for the poor' from at least 1474, providing accommodation for brethren and other residents who needed full-time care.[114]

---

[108] Smith, Smith and Brentano, *English Gilds*, pp. 157, 194.

[109] Smith, Smith and Brentano, *English Gilds*, p. 150. The guild was supposed to maintain up to four 'bedridden poor folks' for life (pp. 148–9), presumably from the ranks of those initially awarded alms. Visiting the sick – a work of mercy – was also enshrined in the statutes of the guild of Holy Trinity, Coventry (p. 234).

[110] Smith, Smith and Brentano, *English Gilds*, p. 35; *CPR, 1340–1343*, p. 221; T. F. Reddaway, *The Early History of the Goldsmiths' Company* (London, 1975), pp. 6, 70, 103. For the striking incidence of occupational blindness, and the care available to its victims, see J. Hawkins, 'The Blind in Later Medieval England: Medical, Social and Religious Responses' (PhD thesis, University of East Anglia, 2011), chap. 6.

[111] Smith, Smith and Brentano, *English Gilds*, pp. 278–9.

[112] McRee, 'Charity and Guild Solidarity', pp. 214–19.

[113] See section 5.9 above.

[114] KLBA, KL/C50/451. The acquisition and cost of running this almshouse almost certainly explains the dramatic decline in disbursements to individuals made by the Trinity guild in the later fifteenth century. McRee seems unaware of this development: 'Charity and Guild Solidarity', p. 215.

On the face of things, the hospitals and almshouses that played such an important role in civic life should furnish a far better insight into the help available for diseased and debilitated paupers.[115] Yet here, too, we are dogged by the same lack of quantifiable evidence, largely because so many foundations were obscure, short-lived and poorly documented. Acknowledging the scale of the problem, Marjorie McIntosh has recently calculated that between 4,900 and 6,400 places may have been on offer throughout England during the 1520s, when the number of functioning institutions was at its height.[116] In theory, such apparently generous provision catered for at least one out of every 480 head of population, but in practice matters were rather different. Although the majority of these houses served urban communities, especially in the south, not all would by then have been operating at optimum capacity, especially since many of the larger hospitals had long since chosen to invest in liturgical spectacle at the expense of the poor, thereby abandoning some, if not all, of their original commitments.[117] Nor was most late medieval institutional care targeted at the truly destitute, being often sold to the highest bidder or reserved for those whom Bronislaw Geremek has aptly described as a 'begging aristocracy', deemed eligible by the authorities.[118] Nevertheless, even if the following assessment must remain impressionistic, it still helps to illuminate many of the ideas about communal health and the welfare of the civic body discussed in Chapter 2, notably with regard to the emphasis placed upon personal and collective responsibility for the less fortunate. In this respect, as in so many others, the study of medieval English hospitals presents a remarkably accurate picture of the changing demographic pressures of urban life. The challenge of providing succour for crowds of sick and destitute vagrants gave way from the Black Death onwards to a growing demand for sheltered accommodation on the part of the aged poor, before once again dominating the political agenda on the eve of the Reformation.[119]

6.6 The nature of institutional provision

In his *Utopia*, Thomas More envisaged a universal welfare system that accorded the sick free access to whatever medicines and professional services seemed appropriate, especially in the four spacious and well-equipped hospitals situated on the margins of every city. The skill of the physicians and outstanding level of care on offer meant that few people would choose to remain at home when they fell ill – a situation strikingly at odds with developments in contemporary England, where the Savoy, the only pre-Dissolution hospital to number trained medical personnel

---

[115] P. Horden, *Hospitals and Healing from Antiquity to the Later Middle Ages* (Aldershot, 2008), chap. 6.

[116] McIntosh, *Poor Relief in England*, pp. 74–5.

[117] At London's Elsyngspital, for example, numbers fell from at least one hundred to twelve: see n. 260 below.

[118] B. Geremek, *Poverty: A History* (Oxford, 1997), p. 45; McIntosh, *Poor Relief in England*, p. 94.

[119] M. K. McIntosh, 'Local Responses to the Poor in Late Medieval and Tudor England', *Continuity and Change* 3 (1988), pp. 209–45, especially pp. 213–17.

on its payroll, was then still being built.[120] In part an inevitable consequence of the wider failure to provide subsidised treatment for the urban poor, the complete absence of salaried practitioners from even the best-documented English medieval hospitals and *leprosaria* has prompted unfavourable comparisons with continental Europe.[121] And when viewed from this perspective, the contrast does, indeed, seem stark. By the fifteenth century most of the larger French, Italian and Spanish institutions retained at least one barber-surgeon, while some could boast a sizeable staff of physicians, surgeons and apothecaries.[122]

On a rough estimate, about 8 per cent of the surgeons and 10 per cent of the barber-surgeons known to have practised in late medieval France did some paid work in hospitals. This trend was encouraged by Charles IV's allocation in 1327 of 12*d.* a day to the two leading surgeons who served him in Paris in return for their regular attendance at France's largest hospital, the Hôtel Dieu.[123] Provincial authorities in cities such as Amiens, Lille, Marseilles and Nimes were just as keen to invest in the upkeep of a healthy workforce. In 1430, the rulers of Lyon complained that hospital patients were being treated by 'ignorant, superstitious monks, empirics or self-proclaimed sorcerers' rather than 'proper physicians [*véritables médecins*]', which suggests that their main priority was to secure a rapid turnover of acute cases.[124] In later medieval England, on the other hand, the great majority of institutions sought to provide residential support for a few chronically sick, elderly and disabled residents rather than medical facilities for short-stay patients or beds for more than a small number of transient paupers. With a few notable exceptions, such as St Leonard's, York, and St Bartholomew's, London, they can be directly compared with the many smaller, poorer and less 'advanced' Continental hospitals which tend to be overlooked by historians because of their apparent backwardness.[125]

Allowing for the fact that changes in function were far from unusual, we can identify three basic types of charitable foundation. Open-ward or 'common' hospitals, which often followed a religious rule, were initially designed to accommodate sick paupers, pilgrims and travellers, while frequently distributing food and other forms of outdoor relief as well. Few could rival the hospitality

[120] More, *Utopia*, p. 46; BL, MS Cotton Cleopatra C V, fol. 25v.

[121] See, for example, the 'dismal picture' painted by M. Carlin, 'Medieval English Hospitals', in L. Granshaw and R. Porter, eds, *The Hospital in History* (London, 1990), pp. 21–39.

[122] The Florentine hospital of Santa Maria Nuova, on which the Savoy was modelled, provides the most obvious example: Henderson, *The Renaissance Hospital*, chap. 7; J. Henderson and K. Park, '"The First Hospital among Christians": The Ospedale di Santa Maria Nuova in Early Sixteenth-Century Florence', *Medical History* 35 (1991), pp. 164–88.

[123] Jacquart, *Milieu médical en France*, pp. 121, 128–30; Lespinasse, *Métiers et corporations de la ville de Paris*, III.628.

[124] Imbert, *Histoire des hôpitaux*, p. 115. A. Saunier, *'Le Pauvre malade' dans le cadre hospitalier medieval: France du Nord, vers 1300–1500* (Paris, 1993), pp. 128–51.

[125] For the importance of these less conspicuous institutions, see P. Horden, '"A Discipline of Relevance": The Historiography of the Later Medieval Hospital', *Social History of Medicine* 1 (1988), pp. 359–74.

offered by St Cross's, Winchester, which every day gave a hot meal in the hall to 100 poor men, but many were required by their founders to dispense bread and ale to supplicants at the gates.[126] In all, about 250 such houses have been identified in pre-Reformation England.[127] The largest among them resembled monasteries and could support a hundred patients or more, but most were modest in size and might simply cater for an apostolic thirteen, or even fewer. Specialist 'lazar houses' for the long-term care of presumed lepers sometimes adopted this type of layout; others were informal, organic structures, comprising a few suburban cottages, perhaps with access to a small chapel. At least 300 *leprosaria* were founded in England between 1100 and 1300, when both the fashion and perceived need for endowments were at their height. By contrast, only about a score seem to have been established thereafter. Contrary to the enduring belief that they were banished to remote and isolated spots far from human habitation, most lepers lived very near centres of population. It has, indeed, been estimated that around 85 per cent of leper houses – accounting for about a quarter of *all* known English medieval hospitals – lay close to towns, but this trend may well have been even more pronounced.[128] Given the random nature of the surviving evidence, many such places must have escaped detection. For instance, our knowledge of Brichtiu's hospital in Norwich derives from a solitary reference in the twelfth-century *Vita* of St William, while a bequest in the will of Bishop Thomas Bitton (d. 1307) constitutes the only known source of information about a community of lepers outside the borough of Denbury in Devon.[129]

From the mid-fourteenth century onwards, both *leprosaria* and 'common' hospitals were overtaken in popularity by almshouses for the elderly, as urban communities began to adopt a very different scale of priorities. Most almshouses comprised a cluster of individual lodgings or single rooms, while those appropriating or inheriting a traditional open-ward plan erected screens or partitions to afford a degree of seclusion.[130] The creation of private quarters in the larger, custom-built foundations not only reflects the fact that residents came

---

[126] N. Orme and M. Webster, *The English Hospital, 1070–1570* (New Haven, CT, 1995), pp. 61–2. St Mark's, Bristol, was also supposed to feed a hundred paupers every day, but eventually abandoned its responsibilities: R. Price and M. Ponsford, *St Bartholomew's Hospital, Bristol: The Excavation of a Medieval Hospital*, CBA research report 110 (London, 1998), p. 226.

[127] That is 112 hospitals and 136 refuges that accommodated pilgrims and other travellers, both sick and healthy: R. Gilchrist, *Contemplation and Action: The Other Monasticism* (Leicester, 1995), pp. 10–11.

[128] Rawcliffe, *Leprosy in Medieval England*, pp. 106–8.

[129] Thomas of Monmouth, *The Life and Miracles of St William of Norwich*, ed. A. Jessopp and M. R. James (Cambridge, 1896), p. 148; Orme and Webster, *English Hospital*, pp. 172–7, 225–6.

[130] As, for example, William Browne's almshouse in Stamford, where the late-fifteenth-century dormitory hall was designed to reflect 'the prestige of antiquity': N. Hill and A. Rogers, *Guild, Hospital and Alderman: New Light on the Founding of Browne's Hospital, Stamford, 1475–1509* (Bury St Edmunds, 2013), pp. 34–7. For the conversion of an old infirmary ward into cells, see St Mary's Chichester: Orme and Webster, *English Hospital*, p. 102, plate 20.

from relatively comfortable backgrounds, but also testifies to growing levels of literacy and changes in devotional practice. A increasing number of almshouses, such as Pykenham's in Hadleigh, Whittington's in London and Wynard's in Exeter, assumed that at least some lay inmates would be able to read and even to master the psalter and other Latin texts. They would require space for study, prayer and meditation.[131] The circumstances of less affluent founders, who might only be able to offer a couple of cottages or a solitary tenement, likewise dictated the type of accommodation available. In this respect, many almshouses would have been indistinguishable from the dwellings occupied by extramural communities of lepers and, indeed, by ordinary working people.[132] Precise numbers remain elusive, but one estimate exceeds the seven hundred mark, over and above the older hospitals and *leprosaria* that changed their function in order to support the elderly, and a number of obscure houses described fleetingly in local records.[133] Their ubiquity reveals the extent to which institutional charity was becoming secularised, as members of the ruling elite stepped in to remodel or replace many long-established 'common' hospitals that had succumbed to the economic and demographic upheavals of the fourteenth century.[134] Although not always justified, the allegations of maladministration and incompetence levelled against the religious orders and secular clergy who traditionally ran these places further encouraged lay patrons to assume the initiative by setting up and managing houses of their own.

Leprosaria encountered particular problems, largely because so many were already under-funded and poorly managed, while changing fashions in piety attracted donors to newer and more prestigious projects, including the public works discussed in earlier chapters of this book. Improved standards of diagnosis also meant that far fewer people were actually being pronounced leprous. As a result, empty beds were occupied by the elderly or disabled, especially if they could afford to contribute towards their upkeep. We can document such a transition at the civic leper-house of St Mary Magdalen, Exeter, where the blind and aged were offering goods and property in return for support from at least the 1250s.[135] In several instances, the shift to what might anachronistically be termed

---

[131] Dean Spooner, 'The Almshouse Chapel, Hadleigh', *Proceedings of the Suffolk Institute of Archaeology* 7 (1891), pp. 379–80; Imray, *Charity of Richard Whittington*, p. 112; DRO, ED/WA/2.

[132] Rawcliffe, *Leprosy in Medieval England*, pp. 332–3.

[133] D. Knowles and R. N. Hadcock list a total of 742 almshouses, which together account for just over 55 per cent of *all* the medieval hospital foundations in their survey: *Medieval Religious Houses of England and Wales* (London, 1971), pp. 339–410. McIntosh's more sober figure of 138 almshouses and 55 hospitals which performed a similar function represents a 'minimal total' of more permanent foundations set up between 1350 and 1539: *Poor Relief in England*, p. 68 and appendix A.

[134] This trend is also discernible in continental Europe: M. Rubin, *Charity and Community in Medieval Cambridge* (Cambridge, 1987), pp. 123–4.

[135] DRO, ED/MAG/43. By the 1380s the hospital housed at least nine decrepit individuals (*decrepiti*): ED/MAG/50. New ordinances compiled in 1423 for the hospital of St Mary Magdalen, Colchester, are representative in their insistence that priority should be given to lepers 'if they are to be had', but otherwise to

'privatisation' caused friction between hospitals and the urban authorities who expected them to fulfil their original purpose by providing free care for the needy. A damning inquiry of 1291 into abuses at St Nicholas's hospital, York, found that the practice of admitting lepers and 'the old and feeble of the city' without charge had been abandoned by the master in favour of entry fees up to £15 payable by *all* newcomers, irrespective of their state of health. Even worse from the perspective of past and future benefactors, rampant commercialism was accompanied by a sharp decline in moral standards and religious observance, since the new residents felt no obligation to offer intercessionary prayers on behalf of others.[136]

Nonetheless, many suburban leper houses continued to receive support. Fears of infection in a society preoccupied by the miasmas of pestilence ensured that towns remained conscious of the need to maintain adequate provision for those whose presence seemed to threaten public safety. Having demolished at least one of their four *leprosaria* in 1331–2, presumably because there were so few patients, the burgesses of Lynn found it necessary to establish at least three new houses during the course of the later fourteenth century. Since from 1375 onwards they also began to employ panels of 'discreet persons' to sanction the removal of suspect lepers, the need for institutional care had clearly become a matter of some urgency.[137] Even greater nervousness on this score is apparent from a directive addressed by Edward IV to the rulers of London in 1472. He was shocked to discover that although several 'devout and weldiposed persones' had endowed hospitals outside the City 'for th'abitacion and dewllyng of people enfecte with the contagious and perilous siknes of lepour', their intended inmates remained at large,

> vagrant and walkyng contrarye to the will and entent of the edifiers and bilders of the same, aswel abought in this citee and suburbies of the same, comenyng and medlyng daily with other people which ben of clene compleccon and not enfecte with the said sykynes, which, if it shuld be suffered, shuld cause grete hurt, jerobardy and perell to persones of clene compleccon .... For it is certaynly undirstond that the said siknes daily growith and encresith by suche medlyng and comynycacion, more than it hath doon in daies passed.[138]

the 'infirm' poor. Significantly, all were to be admitted free of charge: J. L. Fisher, ed., 'The Leger Book of St John's Abbey, Colchester', *Transactions of the Essex Archaeological Society*, n.s. 24 (1951), pp. 77–127, on p. 120.

[136] Rawcliffe, *Leprosy in Medieval England*, p. 299. Similar complaints were voiced by the commissioners who inspected the hospital of Holy Innocents, Lincoln, in 1316: *CIMisc, 1307–1349*, pp. 72–3.

[137] Owen, *Making of King's Lynn*, p. 213; KLBA, KL/C7/2, Hall Book, 1422–1429, p. 242; KL/C10/1, fols 122r, 131r. It is impossible to date or properly identify all of Lynn's *leprosaria*, but testators itemised between five and seven after the Black Death: KL/C12/1/3; C12/5; C12/7; C12/11.

[138] Records of the Corporation of London, Journal 8, fol. 21r; *CLB*, L, p. 102. Outbreaks of plague in 1471–2 and the diagnosis of a case of leprosy in the royal household may explain why Edward threatened the Corporation with a massive fine of £500 should it fail to act: Rawcliffe, *Leprosy in Medieval England*, pp. 281–2.

That the Corporation took the supervision of its own leper houses (in Hackney and Southwark) more seriously than Edward's order implies is apparent from a readiness to exempt the wardens from all other civic responsibilities, 'considering their meritorious labour, their unpleasant and onerous occupation and the expenses and losses ... by them incurred'. Another round of exemptions issued between 1514 and 1518 may well reflect the admission of increasing numbers of patients suffering from the pox, who eventually colonised both hospitals.[139]

Whatever form they assumed, hospitals, *leprosaria* and almshouses played an important role as purveyors of spiritual medicine for the salvation of patrons as well as patients. Physical care was certainly not neglected, and it would be misleading to assume that nursing staff, in the larger houses at least, were any less skilled than trained professionals.[140] However, the emphasis upon a regimen that would heal sick souls as well as bodies, where possible through a constant round of prayer, masses and liturgical performance, meant that religious ritual tended to dictate most aspects of daily life – from the design of buildings to the routine of the inmates.[141] From the outset, the principal task of institutionalised lepers was to deploy their exalted spiritual status as intercessors on behalf of their benefactors. The elderly and disabled, too, had their part to play. The obligation to pray for members of the wider urban community obtained as much in the tiny almshouse for 'two or three poor persons' maintained by the commonalty of Scarborough in the 1390s as it had done in far earlier and larger foundations that followed a monastic rule.[142] Indeed, from the 1350s onwards, collective anxiety regarding the imminent threat of *mors improvisa* created an even greater desire to transmute hard cash into the grateful prayers of deserving paupers.[143] As the executors of Richard Whittington so clearly explained when founding the London almshouse that bore his name:

> The fervent desire and besy intension of a prudent wise and devoute man shold be to cast before & make seure the state and thende of his short lyff with dedes of mercy and pite. And namely to provide for suche pouer persones whiche grevous penurie and cruelle fortune have oppressed and

[139] *CLB*, I, p. 184; *CLB*, K, pp. 142–3; Riley, *Memorials of London*, pp. 510–11; Honeybourne, 'Leper Hospitals', pp. 8, 31–7, 44–54.

[140] C. Rawcliffe, 'Hospital Nurses and their Work', in R. Britnell, ed., *Daily Life in the Late Middle Ages* (Stroud, 1998), pp. 43–64.

[141] See, for example, Henderson, *The Renaissance Hospital*, chaps 4 and 5; C. Rawcliffe, 'Christ the Physician Walks the Wards: Celestial Therapeutics in the Medieval Hospital', in Davies and Prescott, *London and the Kingdom*, pp. 78–97; C. Rawcliffe, 'A Word from Our Sponsor: Advertising the Patron in the Medieval Hospital', in J. Henderson, P. Horden and A. Pastore, eds, *The Impact of Hospitals, 300–2000* (Oxford, 2007), pp. 169–93.

[142] Unless they were sick, the almsmen had to say fifty Aves and five Pater Nosters every day: Jeayes, *White Vellum Book of Scarborough*, p. 25.

[143] The reciprocal nature of this relationship was clearly understood, for 'according to the law of charity the rich are held to support the poor, just as the poor on the other hand are held to pray for their benefactors': Wenzel, *Fasciculus morum*, p. 541.

be not of power to gete their lyvyng either by craft or by eny other bodily labour, wherby that at ye day of the last Jugement he may take his part with hem that shalle be saved.[144]

As we shall see, some critics of the Church's mismanagement of established hospitals expressed indignation at the diversion of funds into costly religious ceremonies and lavish building schemes rather than patient care.[145] Yet in many instances this trend was driven by affluent laymen who dreaded the prospect of a long sojourn in purgatory. The foundation of the hospital and guild of the Holy Trinity at Salisbury was effected 'as part of a general movement to increase divine service in the city' in the aftermath of the second pestilence of 1361, and the rebuilding at great expense of St Giles's hospital, Norwich, in the 1380s served to provide liturgical space for the commemorative masses, private altars and elaborate funerals demanded by the civic elite.[146] In order to survive in a harsh economic climate, urban hospitals had to invest in such facilities, which, in turn, served to attract new patrons. Craft guilds and religious fraternities, for example, were constantly on the lookout for appropriate places to meet for the commemoration of deceased brothers and sisters, and, of course, to accommodate their own dependents. The Corpus Christi guilds of Canterbury and York, the guild of St George, Norwich, the Mariners of Bristol, the Tailors of Winchester, the Drapers, Mercers and Skinners of London and the Mercers of York each maintained close relations with local hospitals, sinking considerable funds into the fabric and furnishings of their chapels, and, on occasion, helping to balance the books.[147]

These institutions were a ubiquitous physical, as well as a spiritual, presence in the lives of medieval townspeople. Because of the devastating effects of the Dissolution and its aftermath, we can easily overlook their dominant position in the urban and suburban landscape, where they testified to the responsible stewardship of wealth and exercise of Christian compassion by the urban elite. The approaches to towns and cities were identifiable by the wayside chapels and collecting boxes of *leprosaria*, hospitals and almshouses. In Norwich, for example, leper houses stood immediately outside five of the city gates, exemplifying in bricks and mortar the

[144] Imray, *Charity of Richard Whittington*, p. 109.

[145] Elsyngspital, London, offers a classic example of ill-advised expenditure. Debts of over £425 in 1438 seem largely to have been incurred by the rebuilding of the church, no doubt in the hope of attracting more endowments: C. M. Barron and M. Davies, eds, *The Religious Houses of London and Middlesex* (London, 2007), pp. 166–7; A. Bowtell, 'A Medieval London Hospital: Elsyngspital, 1330–1536' (PhD thesis, Royal Holloway University of London, 2010), p. 117.

[146] A. D. Brown, *Popular Piety in Late Medieval England: The Diocese of Salisbury, 1250–1550* (Oxford, 1995), p. 192; Rawcliffe, *Medicine for the Soul*, chap. 4. For the 'cult of remembrance' that developed after the Black Death, see Aberth, *From the Brink of the Apocalypse*, pp. 210–13.

[147] C. Rawcliffe, 'Dives Redeemed? The Guild Almshouses of Later Medieval England', *The Fifteenth Century* 8 (2008), pp. 1–27, on p. 11; Rawcliffe, 'Christ the Physician', pp. 85, 87, 90.

salutary lesson of Christ's parable of Dives and Lazarus.[148] Well aware that eternal damnation had followed fast upon the rich man's brutal rejection of a diseased beggar 'full of sores', the citizens sought to demonstrate their generosity. A similar message was conveyed in the later Middle Ages by the strategic placement of almshouses next to the halls of prosperous guilds, as we can see in the case of London's Butchers, Cutlers, Drapers, Grocers, Haberdashers, Merchant Tailors, Parish Clerks, Salters and Vintners.[149] Not surprisingly, given the prominence accorded to Judgement Day in its annual mystery cycle, York's almshouses were equally conspicuous. One stood at the entrance to the common hall, and another where the London road passed through Micklegate Bar. The terrible sentence pronounced by Christ upon condemned sinners had demonstrably struck home:

> Whanne I had mistir [need] of mete and drynke,
> Caytiffs, ye cached me *fro youre gate*,
> Whanne ye were sette as sirs on a benke [bench],
> I stode ther-oute, werie and wette,
> Was none of yowe wolde on me thynke
> Pyte to haue of my poure state;
> Ther-fore till hell I schall you synke,
> Weele are ye worthy to go *to that gate.*[150]

Leper houses, in particular, offered a promise of redemption to the residents of English towns, and mark the emergence of a collective sense of responsibility for the sick that marched hand in hand with prosperity and growth.

6.7 Leprosaria

It is possible to distinguish three principal reasons for the suburban location of most leper houses, which can be summarised in terms of religious belief, practical necessity and political aspiration. As we have seen, medical assumptions about the alleged infectiousness of leprosy had little impact upon popular responses to the disease until at least the late thirteenth century.[151] The injunction that presumed lepers should live 'outside the camp' derived from the Old Testament book of Leviticus, and was designed to protect the tribes of Israel from ritual pollution rather than contagion. *Leprosi* were certainly not excluded from the Christian community, or initially prevented from entering towns to purchase food, visit healing shrines and beg for sustenance. The provision of appropriate physical and spiritual services for them as 'suffering members of the body of Christ' was enshrined from 1179 onwards in canon law, by which time their unique position was

---

[148] C. Rawcliffe, 'The Earthly and Spiritual Topography of Suburban Hospitals', in K. Giles and C. Dyer, eds, *Town and Country in the Middle Ages: Contrasts, Contacts and Interconnections, 1100–1500* (Leeds, 2005), pp. 251–74.

[149] Rawcliffe, 'Dives Redeemed?', pp. 4–9.

[150] L. Toulmin Smith, ed., *York Plays* (New York, 1963), pp. 510–11. The italics are mine.

[151] See section 3.1 above.

assured.[152] As the cautionary tale of Lazarus reveals, the New Testament furnished an altogether more positive image of their distressing symptoms, fostered by Christ himself. The identification of His own ordeal with that of the leper, which remained a constant *topos* in devotional writing and iconography throughout the Middle Ages, served as yet another powerful stimulus for compassion.[153]

Since Mosaic Law imposed a *ritual* rather than a sanitary prohibition, the actual distance of leper houses from urban boundaries was largely irrelevant, so long as physical exclusion could be maintained. Located immediately to the south of Lincoln next to the Augustinian priory of St Katherine, conveniently near a major road junction and the eventual site of an imposing Eleanor Cross, the hospital of Holy Innocents occupied a typically 'busy and cosmopolitan' site.[154] Extramural *leprosaria* often pre-dated the erection of boundary crosses, such as that constructed in marble by the burgesses of Lynn during the plague year of 1361 beside the hospital of St Mary Magdalen on the Gaywood causeway. As a result they formed an early bastion in the spiritual defences against disease already examined in Chapter 2.[155] If this supremely liminal situation reflected the leper's own transitory position between life and death, it certainly did not signal his relegation, forgotten and despised, to the outer margins of society.[156] On the contrary, as late as the fifteenth century the citizens of York used leper hospitals, as well as crosses, to mark the processional circuit that conferred divine protection upon those who lived within the walls.[157]

While demonstrating collective concern for the sick, the larger, more impressive institutions served also to advertise urban growth, independence and affluence. At the once prosperous port of Dunwich in Suffolk, for instance, the ruins of an imposing hospital chapel, positioned just outside the town ditch, still testify to lavish expenditure and an eye for display (plate 23). It is easy to forget that many extramural leper houses were prominent landmarks in their own right, whose chapels were frequented by the healthy as well as the sick. Matthew Paris's pen drawing in his *Chronica Majora* of St Giles's, Holborn, an early royal foundation on the main western approach to London, illustrates this point clearly.[158] Our preoccupation with exclusion and marginality, which have become recurrent themes in the historiography of leprosy, tends to obscure some persuasive evidence for integration into urban life. St Leonard's hospital, Northampton,

[152] J. Avril, 'Le IIIe Concile du Latran et les communautés de lepreux', *Revue Mabillon* 60 (1981), pp. 21–76, on pp. 27–8.

[153] Rawcliffe, *Leprosy in Medieval England*, chap. 3.

[154] D. Marcombe, *Leper Knights: The Order of St Lazarus of Jerusalem in England, c. 1150–1544* (Woodbridge, 2003), pp. 167–8.

[155] H. Harrod, *Report on the Deeds and Records of the Borough of King's Lynn* (King's Lynn, 1874), p. 79; Rawcliffe, *Leprosy in Medieval England*, p. 309 n. 32. For the devastating impact of this plague on Lynn, see Appendix.

[156] R. Gilchrist, 'Christian Bodies and Souls: The Archaeology of Life and Death in Later Medieval Hospitals', in Bassett, *Death in Towns*, p. 115.

[157] *YMB*, III.62–3, 230–1.

[158] Matthew Paris, *The Illustrated Chronicles of Matthew Paris: Observations of Thirteenth-Century Life*, ed. and trans. R. Vaughan (Stroud, 1993), p. 103.

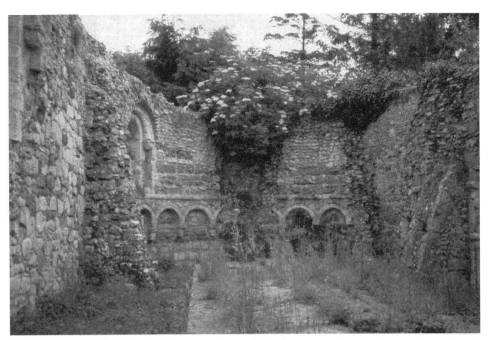

23 Ruins of the once imposing Norman chapel of the leper hospital of St James, which lay just outside bridge gate on one of the main approaches to the port of Dunwich in Suffolk

furnishes a particularly striking example of communal involvement, since its chapel served from the outset as a parish church, where local people worshipped alongside the patients. The advowson lay in the hands of the mayor and burgesses, whose misguided but short-lived decision to entrust the management of the house to a tenant during the 1470s led to the introduction of stringent controls for 'good governaunce' by the ruling elite.[159]

As was the case in France, many English towns and cities incorporated their *leprosaria* into civic ceremonies and guild festivities.[160] The spectacular procession staged annually in Norwich on the feast of Corpus Christi ended at the leper house of St Mary Magdalen in the fields to the north of the city, while a similar, if rather less ostentatious, event in Grimsby was marked by a service for the aldermen and burgesses at the 'spitalhous' chapel, just outside the bars.[161] In this way, the inmates of both establishments were confirmed in their continuing membership of the urban as well as the Christian body. Some occasions were more overtly

[159] R. M. Serjeantson and W. R. D. Adkins, eds, *VCH Northampton*, vol. 2 (London, 1906), pp. 159–60; *RBN*, II.329–33. Lepers were still accommodated there in 1472–3, when they were allocated 5*d.* a week from the borough, along with regular doles of bacon and oatmeal: *RBN*, I.401–5.

[160] For French examples, see Avril, 'Le IIIe Concile du Latran', p. 72; E. Thévenin, 'La Léproserie Saint-Ladre de Reims: un espace de festivités', in B. Tabuteau, ed., *Lépreux et sociabilité du moyen âge au temps modernes*, Cahiers du Groupe de Recherche d'Histoire 11 (Rouen, 2000), pp. 63–71.

[161] *RCN*, II.230; Rigby, *Medieval Grimsby*, p. 85.

secular and entertaining: Oxford's cooks began their yearly guild 'riding' at the leper hospital of St Bartholomew, before staging an entry into the town.[162] Further proof that lepers remained part of the wider community, even while sequestered beyond the walls, may be found in the Cornish town of Launceston, which forbade them from entering the gates, but welcomed them (and their laundress) into the town's principal religious guild of St Mary Magdalen. Several residents of the local leper house joined the fraternity, thereby sharing in – and no doubt augmenting – the benefits accrued through the prayers, masses and other intercessionary activities of the brethren.[163] Similarly, although the lepers of St Mary Magdalen, Southampton, could not attend the feasts held by the port's guild merchant, they were able to participate from a distance by drinking the ale that was set aside for them on these occasions.[164]

Healthy townsmen and women were particularly anxious to gain entry to the religious confraternities run by the more affluent *leprosaria*, not least because of the merits that association with the sick poor of Christ bestowed. The *mortilegium*, or obit book, of the Gaywood leper hospital records the names of hundreds of Lynn tradesmen and merchants for whom the residents undertook to pray, both in life and death, in return for modest donations (plate 24).[165] It now, unfortunately, constitutes a unique survival, since the archives of English medieval hospitals in general, and of *leprosaria* in particular, suffered terrible losses both before and during the Reformation.[166] However, we know from passing references that many other houses, such as St James's, Doncaster, St Bartholomew's, Dover, and St Giles's, Holborn, offered membership of a spiritual brotherhood to their patrons, whose support secured permanent commemoration and often the promise of a hefty remission of sins as well.[167]

The extramural situation of *leprosaria* was in many respects a pragmatic response to requirements that were shared by other hospitals and religious houses, a striking number of which gravitated towards the suburbs.[168] They needed land, as well as a regular supply of water for laundry, waste disposal, brewing, cooking, gardening, animal husbandry and the creation of fishponds. But self-sufficiency was rarely, if ever, achieved; and some institutions, including St Mary Magdalen, Yarmouth, and St Laurence, Bristol, lay within a stone's throw of the intramural

---

[162] Wood, *History and Antiquities of the University of Oxford*, I.636.

[163] *CIMisc, 1377–1388*, p. 147 (the customs were recorded in 1383, but allegedly dated 'from time immemorial'); M. I. Somerscales, 'Lazar Houses in Cornwall', *Journal of the Royal Institution of Cornwall*, n.s. 5 (1965), pp. 61–99, on pp. 71–2.

[164] Studer, *Oak Book of Southampton*, I.26–7, 87; C. Gross, ed., *The Gild Merchant*, 2 vols (Oxford, 1890), II.215.

[165] NRO, BL/R/8/1, fols 7r–27r. The town's brewers and bakers were singled out as special patrons.

[166] C. Rawcliffe, 'Passports to Paradise: How English Medieval Hospitals and Almshouses Kept their Archives', *Archives* 27 (2002), pp. 1–22, on pp. 8–10.

[167] BL, MS Cotton Tiberius C V, fols 263r–264v; Add. MS 37503, fols 16r–v, 27r–v; Add. Charter 19137; Bodleian Library, Oxford, MS Rawl. B.335, fols 1v, 4v; TNA, E135/38, no. 17.

[168] Rawcliffe, 'Earthly and Spiritual Topography of Suburban Hospitals', pp. 251–74.

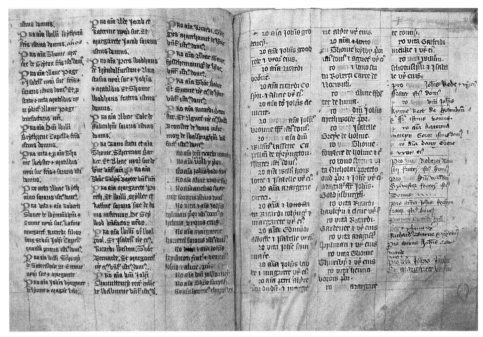

24 The last two pages of the obit book of the leper hospital of St Mary Magdalen, Gaywood, near King's Lynn, begun in the thirteenth century. The names of hundreds of local benefactors were assiduously recorded until just before the Dissolution, by which point the calligraphy had, significantly, begun to deteriorate.

marketplaces to which they turned for additional supplies.[169] Others could expect a share of local produce allocated to them without charge by borough custom. As we saw in Chapter 5, they might be given meat or fish that had been pronounced unfit for human consumption, but in general the food assigned to lepers was as fresh and palatable as anything on sale to the general public.[170]

Permission to stage a two or three-day fair on hospital property offered another useful way of boosting resources, both directly from market tolls and indirectly through the influx of visitors likely to give alms in cash or kind.[171] Indeed, whether or not leper houses were able to benefit from these lucrative annual gatherings, the proximity of major public thoroughfares remained vital. All but the richest relied heavily upon casual alms, which could more easily be solicited on busy roads. This was especially the case at stopping places, such as town gates, bars and bridges, where traffic was congested, and where obligatory tolls from local traders might more easily be collected. Hospital chapels presented an important port of call for

[169] Rawcliffe, 'Earthly and Spiritual Topography of Suburban Hospitals', figs 13.3, 13.8. Some houses, such as the Cowgate *leprosarium* next to the Tuesday market and common staithe at Lynn, were engulfed by urban development, having initially been sited at a distance from the town centre: Rawcliffe, *Leprosy in Medieval England*, p. 307.

[170] See section 5.1 above; Rawcliffe, *Leprosy in Medieval England*, pp. 311–14.

[171] Rawcliffe, *Leprosy in Medieval England*, pp. 314–15.

travellers wishing to give thanks for a safe journey or to enlist divine protection when they were setting out. As a security measure, the hospital of St Nicholas on the south-eastern outskirts to York was supposed to keep the alms-box in its chapel under three separate locks and to distribute the proceeds regularly among the inmates.[172] Measures of this kind became increasingly important as the financial exigencies faced by many late medieval *leprosaria* made begging a prerequisite of survival. An inquiry of 1316 found that the hospital of the Holy Innocents, Lincoln, which maintained a similar box, had come to depend almost entirely upon 'the devotion of the surrounding people' for its basic income.[173] The bustle of well-trodden routes was, therefore, a key factor in determining location, as also was the need to site institutions strategically in order to avoid unnecessary competition for finite resources. At Ipswich one leper house lay to the north of the borough on the Woodbridge road, the second to the south-east, on the way to Felixstowe, and the third on an ideal site by the Orwell bridge on the Manningtree road, heading due south.[174]

The involvement of *leprosaria* in the daily business of urban life is further underscored by the fact that the largest were property-holders of note, whose vested interests hardly differed from those of other *rentiers*. In their early days, at least, extramural houses such as St Giles's, Holborn, and St Mary Magdalen, Exeter, were liberally endowed with rents, tenements and market stalls in the very heart of English towns and cities.[175] They attracted a groundswell of support from members of the merchant elite, who not only hoped to secure both physical and spiritual health in return for their donations, but also to ape the fashionable piety of the crown and nobility. Although her gift was relatively modest in comparison with the largesse of an aristocrat, the widowed Scientia de la Gaye was clearly influenced by her social superiors: she left 10s. a year in the mid-thirteenth century to a leper house in Bury St Edmunds for the celebration of commemorative masses.[176] Nor should we disregard a very real sense of collective concern for the care of the sick on the part of affluent townsmen and women. The growing conviction that urban communities functioned in exactly the same way as human bodies had a powerful impact upon institutional philanthropy, since it was understood that the more robust limbs and organs would do their utmost to protect the 'sick and sore'.[177]

Although the first English leper houses were royal, aristocratic and ecclesiastical foundations, it did not take the bourgeoisie long to follow suit, first by sharing the management and financial support of existing institutions, and then by endowing

---

[172] W. Page, ed., *VCH York*, vol. 3 (London, 1913), p. 348.

[173] *CIMisc, 1307–1349*, pp. 72–3. By then years of mismanagement and the appropriation of resources by corrupt masters had caused popular support for the hospital to decline.

[174] R. Wear, 'Aspects of Institutional Provision for the Sick Poor in Medieval Ipswich c. 1305–1555' (MA thesis, University of East Anglia, 1997), pp. 32, 37–8, 40–1, 51–2. These three houses also strengthened the town's spiritual defences.

[175] BL, MS Harley 4015, fols 5r–214v; Orme and Webster, *English Hospital*, pp. 226–31.

[176] HMC, *Fourteenth Report*, appendix 8 (London, 1885), p. 156.

[177] See section 2.3 above.

their own. The sense of disillusionment they must have experienced when faced by the administrative laxity and corrupt practices that obtained in some established hospitals clearly prompted them to demand – if not always to achieve – higher standards. Having fought a long, but ultimately unsuccessful, battle to gain control of St Giles's, Holborn, during which they claimed (on the flimsiest of evidence) that it had actually been endowed by a citizen with leprosy rather than by Queen Matilda, the rulers of London had to content themselves with launching a constant battery of complaints to the crown. These focussed principally upon the many abuses perpetrated by the Order of St Lazarus, which assumed responsibility for the hospital at the end of the thirteenth century and promptly began stripping away its assets.[178] In 1354, not long after the Black Death, when fears of both infection and vagrancy were running high, the mayor and alderman forced the Order to make fourteen places permanently available for lepers from the City, but even after St Giles's changed hands protests about dereliction continued.[179] Under the circumstances, the Corporation felt justified in annexing two of the smaller suburban *leprosaria* that had been founded by lay people for the benefit of Londoners, namely the Lock in Southwark (to the south, just across the river) and a house at Kingsland in Hackney (to the north east). While imposing more stringent restrictions upon the entry of lepers through the city gates, they were anxious to provide decent lodgings and support for infected citizens who also faced exclusion.[180] Since they were obliged to visit their charges daily, the wardens of these two hospitals ranked from 1389 onwards as full-time municipal employees.[181]

The rulers of Exeter found it much easier to acquire the extramural hospital of St Mary Magdalen, for, although it was an episcopal foundation, they provided most of the funding and eventually took charge of the management as well. Their hands-on approach is apparent not only from the strict supervision exercised by the city's magistrates, who elected a warden from among their own ranks and examined his accounts annually, but also the attention lavished by local people upon the well-appointed chapel.[182] Matters were far less satisfactory in York, where the laity opted from an early date to establish their own independent leper houses, four of which were already described as 'ancient' on their first recorded appearance in 1364.[183] This course of action is easy to understand in light of the allegations of maladministration and embezzlement in which the royal hospital of St Nicholas became embroiled from the 1280s onwards. The new master's refusal to comply with rules about residence caused particular concern to the

---

[178] Honeybourne, 'Leper Hospitals', pp. 20–2; Marcombe, *Leper Knights*, pp. 161–6; Williams, *Early Holborn*, vol. 2, nos 1612, 1624–5.

[179] *CLB*, G, pp. 27–9; *CLB*, I, pp. 13–14; Williams, *Early Holborn*, vol. 2, nos 1626–54.

[180] Other houses in Knightsbridge and at Mile End were also under civic management by 1475, but little is known about them: Honeybourne, 'Leper Hospitals', pp. 7–8.

[181] See n. 139 above. They were also empowered to supervise the care of Londoners who had been admitted as patients to St Giles's in Holborn.

[182] Orme and Webster, *English Hospital*, pp. 226–31.

[183] P. H. Cullum, 'Hospitals and Charitable Provision in Medieval Yorkshire, 936–1547' (DPhil thesis, University of York, 1990), pp. 35–7.

citizens because the daily celebration of masses for them and their ancestors had suffered as a result of his absenteeism. They were also incensed by the practice of charging patients handsomely for admission, when they had previously paid nothing, and of selling much-needed accommodation to healthy individuals. Several prominent members of the ruling elite served on successive commissions of inquiry into abuses at the hospital and were involved in attempts to reform the recalcitrant brethren, an experience which can only have confirmed their distrust of organisations over which they had only limited authority.[184]

So far as we can tell, the hospital of St Mary Magdalen, Norwich, attracted little in the way of criticism, but relations between the Benedictine monks who ran it and the citizenry were often so strained that the latter chose to follow a similar path by providing more modest lodgings for local lepers immediately outside the gates. As was generally the case, none of these small, rather *ad hoc* settlements adopted a religious rule, which made them more attractive to inmates who wished to remain with their spouses or had little sense of vocation.[185] Nor would such people, at least some of whom retained close contact with friends and family and were actually buried alongside them in Norwich cemeteries, have necessarily been deemed eligible for admission to St Mary's, with its strict adherence to the *opus Dei*. The five civic *leprosaria* continued to attract donations until the mid-sixteenth century, by which time they had been placed under the direction of lay keepers or wardens, who were answerable to the corporation for a variety of disabled and pox-ridden inmates. It is worth noting that over 40 per cent of the wills of Norwich residents proved between 1370 and 1517 record specific, often quite generous, gifts to 'the syke lazare people' living at the gates, whereas few testators remembered those at St Mary's.[186]

Almost all of these later foundations were endowed by laymen such as the Cambridge burgess Henry Tangmere, who established the leper house of Saints Anthony and Eligius in the 1360s just outside the Trumpington gate. By 1526 the mayor and bailiffs had assumed a supervisory role, appointing the wardens and overseeing the production of proper accounts. A detailed inventory of possessions compiled at this time reveals both the punctiliousness of the authorities and the generosity of those who enriched its chapel with images, vestments and plate.[187] The importance placed upon religious observance in the wealthier suburban *leprosaria* is equally apparent from a contract made in 1521 between the mayor and burgesses of Nottingham and the chaplain newly appointed as master of St Leonard's hospital. Although due emphasis was given to 'sustaining and housing

[184] W. Brown, ed., *Yorkshire Inquisitions*, vol. 2, YASRS 23 (Worksop, 1898), pp. 30–1, 123–32; Page, *VCH York* III.346–8. Similar anxieties about absenteeism were voiced in 1316 with regard to the *leprosarium* of St Leonard, Lincoln: *CIMisc, 1307–1349*, p. 72.

[185] Some founders may have sought to provide for specific individuals, rather than contemplating a more permanent arrangement. This clearly happened in Beverley, where a 'lodge' for lepers, erected in 1402, had to be rebuilt for another inmate at the end of the century: *BTD*, p. 42.

[186] Rawcliffe, *Hospitals of Medieval Norwich*, pp. 33–59.

[187] W. M. Palmer, ed., *Cambridge Borough Documents*, vol. 1 (Cambridge, 1931), pp. 55–6; Rubin, *Charity and Community*, pp. 119–26.

the lepers', the greater part of the document comprises a minute rehearsal of the intercessionary round intended to assure the spiritual health of the townspeople.[188]

The creation of extramural *leprosaria* can also be viewed in political terms as the flexing of fast-developing urban muscle. Significantly, whereas over 50 per cent of the boroughs established in Yorkshire before 1200 boasted at least one leper house, *none* of the townships which failed to achieve borough status made such a conspicuous investment. In other words, the possession of a hospital not only reflects a significant level of population growth and economic prosperity, but also of nascent urban pride.[189] Along with this display of self-confidence went a very public demonstration that the community in question could succour and protect all its members, however sick and needy they might be.[190] As was later to prove the case with the foundation of almshouses, involvement in such enterprises gave ordinary men and women of limited means a sense of proprietorship and, of course, a welcome share in any attendant celestial benefits.[191] From this perspective, benefactor and patient were locked in a symbiotic relationship that endured far beyond the grave. The leper may, strictly speaking, have lived 'outside the camp', but he or she still had a crucial role to play within it.

6.8 'Common' hospitals

General hospitals for the sick and vagrant poor also proliferated from the late eleventh century, as England's rapidly expanding towns and cities attracted rising numbers of malnourished indigents. With a few notable exceptions, most of the larger and older houses were, in theory, answerable to royal, aristocratic or episcopal patrons, and remained under the direct management of religious orders or secular clergy rather than local magistrates. Urban communities gave enthusiastic support to this movement, but naturally sought to establish hospitals of their own. A second wave of smaller, less imposing foundations coincided with the award of liberties to towns and boroughs during the late twelfth and early thirteenth centuries, when the same combination of political and charitable motives that gave rise to the endowment of civic *leprosaria* prompted investment in institutions principally, but by no means exclusively, designed for the care of local people rather than outsiders.[192] Although the ritual of the mass remained

---

[188] Stevenson, *Records of the Borough of Nottingham*, III.150–5.

[189] A. E. M. Satchell, 'The Emergence of Leper Houses in Medieval England, 1100–1200' (DPhil thesis, University of Oxford, 1998), pp. 91–9; P. H. Cullum, 'Leper-Houses and Borough Status in the Thirteenth Century', *Thirteenth Century England* 3 (1991), pp. 37–46, p. 42.

[190] M. Rubin, 'Development and Change in English Hospitals, 1100–1500', in Granshaw and Porter, *Hospital in History*, pp. 42–3.

[191] S. Watson, 'The Origins of the English Hospital', *TRHS*, 6th series 16 (2006), pp. 75–94, on p. 93.

[192] S. Watson, 'City as Charter: Charity and the Lordship of English Towns, 1170–1250', in C. Goodson, A. E. Lester and C. Symes, eds, *Cities, Texts and Social Networks: Experiences and Perceptions of Urban Space* (Aldershot, 2010), pp. 235–63; S. Sweetinburgh, 'The Hospitals of Medieval Kent', in S. Sweetinburgh, ed., *Later Medieval Kent, 1220–1540* (Woodbridge, 2010), p. 115.

paramount, these hospitals were more often run by the laity, sometimes in the face of opposition from ecclesiastical authorities, who resented any potential loss of revenue.[193] There was, even so, considerable prestige to be had from a monastic or episcopal connection. William Elsyng, one of the few English merchants rich enough to contemplate an *elemosinaria* for 100 'poor, blind, needy and wretched people of either sex', entrusted the patronage of his eponymous London hospital jointly to the dean of St Paul's and the bishop, and staffed it from 1340 with Augustinian canons.[194] Yet, as he knew only too well, it could not survive without continuing patronage from his fellow citizens.

From the date of its foundation under royal protection in 1123, St Bartholomew's, Smithfield, one of London's oldest hospitals, had relied upon the alms of neighbouring householders and tradesmen, who donated supplies 'with maruellus deuocion ... that studied to fulfill the plenytude of the lawe that is charite'.[195] Later generations of Londoners were just as magnanimous, endowing the house with land, shops and rents that still generated an income of over £300 a year in the 1530s.[196] In Norwich, too, Bishop Walter Suffield's hospital of St Giles received most of its endowments from the laity, among whom the most notable, William Dunwich (d. 1272), ought properly to rank as co-founder. The close cooperation between hospital and city that marked its early years continued with only a few minor disruptions until the Dissolution, and probably explains the otherwise perplexing lack of almshouse foundations in late medieval Norwich. It also accounts for the speed with which the Corporation moved to acquire St Giles's after its surrender to the crown in 1547.[197] Despite the failure of their own claims to proprietorship, the people of Exeter proved just as open-handed towards the episcopal hospital of St John, as its surviving cartulary clearly attests. Well aware that donations might be diverted for other purposes, some benefactors nonetheless stipulated that their gifts should be reserved for the use of the poor alone, even threatening to anathematise anyone who ignored their wishes.[198]

There can be little doubt that initially, at least, donors were attracted by the

[193] See, for example, C. Rawcliffe, ed., 'The Cartulary of St Mary's Hospital, Yarmouth', in C. Rawcliffe, M. Bailey and M. Jurkowski, eds, *Poverty and Wealth: Sheep, Taxation and Charity in Late Medieval Norfolk*, Norfolk Record Society 71 (Norwich, 2007), pp. 166–71.

[194] Bowtell, 'Medieval London Hospital', appendices 1 and 2; William Dugdale, *Monasticon Anglicanum*, ed. J. Caley *et al.*, 6 vols (London, 1817–30), VI.ii.703–8. The change was effected in order to safeguard 'divine worship' and thus, implicitly, to ensure the donor's salvation.

[195] Moore, *Book of the Foundation of St Bartholomew's Church*, p. 26. The house was allegedly founded by Rahere, minstrel to Henry I, and followed the Augustinian rule.

[196] Kerling, *Cartulary of St Bartholomew's Hospital, passim*; J. Caley and J. Hunter, eds, *Valor ecclesiasticus, temp. Henrici VIII*, 6 vols (London, 1810–34), I.388.

[197] Rawcliffe, *Medicine for the Soul*, pp. 46–7, 94–5, 110, 154–8, 162–3, 198–210.

[198] Orme and Webster, *English Hospital*, pp. 233–9; DRO, ECA, book 53A, fols 57v–58r. Similarly, in 1382 one Norwich testator left 15s. to the poor rather than the rich (*non divitibus*) in the hospitals of St Giles and St Paul: NRO, Consistory Court Wills, Reg. Heydon, fols 183r–184r.

open door policy adopted by houses such as St James's, Northallerton, which not only supported thirteen of the town's bedridden paupers in its infirmary but also fed and, if necessary, accommodated up to thirty wayfarers every evening.[199] Yet, aside from a widespread refusal to receive suspect lepers and the victims of other 'intolerable' diseases (who would be dispatched to nearby *leprosaria*), such 'common' hospitals could in practice be surprisingly particular about admissions. Anyone with sufficient resources to contribute towards his or her care might well be accorded priority, whereas those who seemed likely to prove disruptive, to pose a drain on resources or to corrupt the moral environment of the house were frequently denied entry.[200] A professed readiness to shelter 'the wayfaring poor of Christ' could soon be tempered by harsh reality. Mid-thirteenth-century regulations for the reception of vagrants who sought overnight lodging at St Mary's, Chichester, suggest that pilfering, rowdy behaviour and disturbances on the sick-wards must have been common. Even greater anxiety arose over the need to house the sexes in separate quarters, and thus to avoid any risk of promiscuity. Either for this reason, or because of financial mismanagement, the hospital soon ceased to welcome vagrants and by the 1380s stood charged with neglecting its regular patients too.[201]

Poor 'lewd' women were often excluded, especially when pregnant, not least because, like victims of physical violence (*vulnerati*), they threatened to pollute the sacred space of an infirmary in which mass was regularly celebrated.[202] Notwithstanding his renowned compassion for the needy, Walter Suffield banned female patients and overnight visitors from St Giles's, while insisting as an added precaution that the nurses should be over fifty. Desperate cases were presumably directed to the nearby monastic hospital of St Paul, which accepted 'the sick, infirm and child-bearing poor' of Norwich, as well as offering a night's board and lodging to anyone 'seeking hospitality'.[203] In general, however, maternity services were confined to the wealthiest institutions, where it was possible to maintain separate facilities for mothers and infants, well away from the public wards.[204] St Leonard's,

---

[199] J. Raine, ed., *The Register of William Gray*, Surtees Society 56 (Durham, 1870), pp. 180–1. Despite such auspicious beginnings, by 1379 the house was so poor that it could only support three inmates: Page, *VCH York*, III.315–16.

[200] Rubin, *Charity and Community*, pp. 157–8.

[201] H. P. Wright, *The Story of the 'Domus Dei' of Chichester* (London, 1885), p. 16; W. Page, ed., *VCH Sussex*, vol. 2 (London, 1907), pp. 100–1.

[202] See, for instance, the ban upon lepers, lunatics, epileptics, people with contagious diseases, pregnant women, nursing infants and 'other intolerable persons, even though they be poor and infirm' in place from 1219 at St John's, Bridgwater: H. C. Maxwell-Lyte and M. C. B. Dawes, eds, *The Register of Thomas Bekyngton*, vol. 1, Somerset Record Society 49 (London, 1934), p. 289.

[203] NRO, DCN 2/5/8. The hospital was founded in about 1130.

[204] The best north-European example is the Hôtel Dieu, Paris, which provided a salaried midwife and assistant for the care of women in its maternity ward: E. Coyecque, *L'Hôtel Dieu de Paris au môyen âge*, 2 vols (Paris, 1889–91), I.100–1. More typical is the chamber at St John's hospital, Oxford, 'for the use of women labouring in childbirth'. It was built in 1240 with a royal grant of £16: Rawcliffe, *Hospitals of Medieval Norwich*, p. 69. Hospitals on pilgrimage routes may have

York, which could accommodate over 200 patients, made special provision for the care of foundlings and indigent children, although there was evidently room for improvement. Following a visitation in 1364, the master was told to place one of the sisters in charge of the nursery, and to ensure that a regular supply of fresh cow's milk was available for her charges. Further concern for their general health is apparent from orders for the construction of a new chimney, to provide better ventilation.[205]

When making additional bequests worth over £26 to 'the veray nedy, lakkyng frendeship, comfort and help' in London's three largest hospitals, the above-mentioned John Donne had specifically excluded 'commyn beggers going aboute alle the daie light and lying in thies places the nyght tyme', as well as any expectant mothers already in receipt of financial support, perhaps through immoral earnings.[206] Most of the pregnant women who sought refuge there seem, however, to have been destitute and friendless. Indeed, from at least 1344 at St Mary's, Bishopsgate, and from 1352 at St Bartholomew's, Smithfield, women who died in labour could rest assured that their orphaned offspring would be maintained and educated until the age of seven, when they might be found a respectable trade.[207] St Bartholomew's, in particular, enjoyed a reputation for its sensitive handling of single mothers: one fifteenth-century Londoner noted approvingly that it offered 'grete comforte to poore men as for hyr loggyng, and yn specyalle unto yong wymmen that have mysse done that ben wythe chylde'. The latter were not only accommodated for at least forty days after the birth (until the ceremony of purification), but also accorded the anonymity necessary to protect their reputations and thus become useful members of society.[208] St Thomas's, Southwark, was just as discreet, thanks to a bequest from 'that nobyl marchaunt' Richard Whittington, who constructed a separate chamber with eight beds for the reception of 'fallen women'.[209] Unfortunately, since both houses lay close to public brothels, such pious hopes of redemption may often have been disappointed.

Elsewhere, the exclusion of vagrants of both sexes became more pronounced during the fourteenth century as a result of hardening social attitudes towards the

---

been more accommodating, as we can see from evidence at Canterbury and Sandwich: Sweetinburgh, 'Hospitals of Medieval Kent', p. 122.

[205] TNA, C270/20.

[206] TNA, PROB 11/7, fol. 10v. He also left £13 6s. 8d. for repairs to the 'logyng, howsyng and kychin' set aside for the transient poor and 'wymmen with chylde and lying in childebedde' at St Mary's Bishopsgate (fol. 11r). Other testators preferred to assist those 'poor women in labour' who belonged to the parish and were known to be respectable: Sweetinburgh, *The Role of the Hospital*, p. 212.

[207] *CCR, 1343–1346*, p. 432; *CCR, 1349–1354*, pp. 414–15.

[208] Gairdner, *Historical Collections of a Citizen*, pp. viii–ix. John Mirfield, who lived in the precinct, included 'an especially detailed' section on childbirth and female complaints in his medical compilation known as the *Brevium Bartholomei*: Getz, *Medicine in the English Middle Ages*, p. 52.

[209] Gairdner, *Historical Collections of a Citizen*, p. ix. A catalogue of complaints made by local people against the master of St Thomas's in 1536 included the allegation that he had refused to admit a pregnant woman who had died in labour as a result: TNA, SP1/106, fol. 177r–v.

homeless and unemployed. Within two decades of the Black Death, for example, St Paul's, Norwich, had effectively become a home for twenty-four reputable 'sisters' rather than the sick paupers and pregnant women for whom it had been founded.[210] But there were other reasons for the selectivity shown by hospitals that had initially welcomed the indigent poor. In order to solve entrenched financial problems caused by theft, incompetence and worsening economic circumstances, or simply to line their own pockets, hospital managers increasingly resorted to the sale of places or 'corrodies' on the open market. In return for a substantial cash payment, usually based upon the cost of ten years' support, the purchaser could expect free board and lodging, often in agreeable private quarters, for life. Although, in theory, such transactions ought to have a garnered a handsome profit that could be used to provide facilities for the destitute, in practice they tended to monopolise accommodation intended for the needy, to consume valuable resources and to alienate potential benefactors. They were, moreover, a temporary expedient, which might raise cash in the short term, but could prove cripplingly expensive should the corrodian survive for longer than anticipated. The ubiquity of this practice is reflected in the frequent but ineffective complaints voiced by royal commissioners and ecclesiastical visitors about 'indiscreet sales and grantings of liveries' and the preference accorded to the idle rich in hospitals throughout England from Southwark to York and Bury St Edmunds to Bristol.[211]

The imposition of entry fees, a phenomenon already observed in *leprosaria*, could be deliberately employed by local authorities to target deserving individuals while discriminating against others. From at least the fourteenth century, applicants for admission to the hospitals of St Bartholomew and St John, Sandwich, which were both run by the ruling elite, had to pay for the privilege. Affluent residents who could afford between £10 and £19, and were presumably in search of a comfortable retirement home, went to St Bartholomew's, while poorer (but far from destitute) folk with up to 50s. to spare found more basic accommodation at St John's.[212] The rationale behind this policy is clearly apparent in other south coast ports, such as Rye, where hospital beds were reserved for reputable men and women who had 'competently borne their charges ... in their time for the welfare of the town', but had grown so 'impoverished and impotent, decayed of their goods and chattels' that they could no longer support themselves in an appropriate fashion at home. Here, as in Pevensey, however, suitable candidates were generally accepted without charge in return for a promise of good behaviour, which the bailiffs and wardens were expected to enforce. Hospitals in Hastings and Winchelsea, too, provided relief for any decrepit member of the community who had hitherto 'borne him or her well by all his or her lyffe'.[213] In Florence or

---

[210] Rawcliffe, *Hospitals of Medieval Norwich*, pp. 69–77.

[211] Rawcliffe, *Medicine for the Soul*, pp. 171–2; Price and Ponsford, *St Bartholomew's Hospital*, p. 227.

[212] Sweetinburgh, *The Role of the Hospital*, pp. 188–92.

[213] W. Holloway, *The History and Antiquities of the Ancient Town and Port of Rye* (London, 1847), pp. 156–7; E. Turner, 'The Statutes of the Marshes of Pevensey and Romney', *Sussex Archaeological Collections* 18 (1866), pp. 42–53, on p. 50; W. Durrant Cooper and T. Ross, 'Notices of Hastings', *Sussex Archaeological Collections* 14 (1862), pp. 65–118, on pp. 79–80; Page, *VCH Sussex* II.107.

Venice, such people would have ranked among the 'shamefaced poor' and have seemed especially worthy of help.[214]

In some respects the growing social problem posed by elderly paupers from the later fourteenth century onwards is testimony to the rising standards of living enjoyed by those fortunate enough to survive successive outbreaks of plague. Being better fed and better housed, and perhaps also benefiting from the sanitary reforms described in previous chapters of this book, more members of the urban workforce appear to have reached old age than before. Yet a significant proportion had to manage without the assistance of younger relatives who would traditionally have assumed a caring role, for many of them died in epidemics, while others had little choice but to seek work elsewhere, leaving behind them shrinking communities blighted by chronic underemployment and a rapidly ageing population.[215] It was in response to this challenge that in 1386 the rulers of Yarmouth decided to convert the near-moribund hospital of St Mary into an almshouse for the accommodation of sixteen respectable but destitute and decrepit residents. In line with developments elsewhere, the new rules, which were, significantly, devised in English for ease of comprehension, imposed a strict code of conduct upon the inmates.[216]

By this date the lack of facilities for the sick and disabled poor had already begun to exercise perceptive English clergy, such as the Dominican John Bromyard, who complained that hardly any other nation on earth possessed 'so few places of hospitality or God's Houses'.[217] His belief that most existing foundations had fallen victim to mismanagement and greed, if not overt corruption, was shared by other, more hostile critics of the Church, and gave rise to demands for a radical overhaul of the entire system. Legislation of 1388 for the maintenance of 'impotent' beggars, which required indigents who could not find accommodation where they were living to return to their place of birth, drew yet more unwelcome attention to the inadequacies of the existing infrastructure.[218] A manifesto circulated in London during the parliament of 1395 by followers of John Wycliffe attacked the diversion of hospital resources into extravagant liturgical display; and in turn inspired a plan for the creation of 100 new almshouses from confiscated ecclesiastical property.[219] By 1410, this inflammatory scheme had secured influential advocates in the House of Commons, who argued that 100,000 marks a year [£66,666] could easily be raised to fund refuges that would be run 'by oueresiht of goode and trewe

---

[214] Pullan, *Rich and Poor in Renaissance Venice*, pp. 229–30, 274–5. This point is developed at length by Frank Rexroth, who regards the almshouses of London, in particular, as a means of dividing 'the poverty milieu into desirable and undesirable persons': *Deviance and Power*, chap. 6, and p. 232 for the quotation.

[215] As was demonstrably the case in Wells: Shaw, *Creation of a Community*, pp. 230–2, 244–7.

[216] Rawcliffe, 'Cartulary of St Mary's Hospital', pp. 182–9.

[217] Owst, *Literature and Pulpit*, p. 177.

[218] *SR*, vol. 2, 12 Richard II, cap. 7, p. 58. The statute recognised that 'the people of cities or other towns' might well lack both the resources and the inclination to accept this burden.

[219] Orme and Webster, *English Hospital*, pp. 132, 134.

sekulers, because of preestes and clerkes that nowe haue full nygh destroyed alle the houses of almesse withinne the rewme'.[220] Not surprisingly, given its controversial content, this particular item of business was never entered in the official parliamentary record. But according to the Benedictine chronicler Thomas Walsingham, it enjoyed the overwhelming support of the county representatives, whom he predictably described as 'sons of Pilate' and a 'detestable gang of lollard knights'. Many of the burgesses, too, must have been enthusiastic, since urban communities had suffered most from the decline in hospital provision, and the plan was skilfully promoted as a way of helping them to look after all the 'poor men and beggars' for whom they were now legally responsible.[221]

Although the proposal was far too radical for open debate, it did inspire a more measured and pragmatic request for change that chimed with the newly crowned Henry V's zeal for religious reform.[222] Four years later, a bill lamenting current levels of decay and abuse in houses run by the laity as well as the clergy obtained the royal assent, and an official inquiry into the management of *all* English hospitals was set in train. Recognising that 'many men and women have died in great misery for default of aid, living and succour', the king agreed to appoint ecclesiastical commissioners with the authority to inspect royal foundations and 'make correction and reformation' of others, 'according to the laws of Holy Church'.[223] The topic of hospital reform was then added to a schedule allegedly compiled by the king himself as part of his personal drive to rid the Church of heresy and corruption.[224] Yet however promising this start, nothing was done to implement the terms of the new statute. A cynic might argue that the decision to entrust such a potentially damaging enquiry to senior clerics without some element of lay involvement doomed it from the start. Vociferous protests from the Commons in 1415 proved futile, and the campaign to revitalise institutional care – along with that for medical licensing – fell victim to Henry's preoccupation with conquests in France. His reluctance to court controversy at such a sensitive time effectively removed both issues from the parliamentary agenda. Such, indeed, were the vagaries of the political and economic climate that each remained dormant for almost a century.[225]

Despite these setbacks, the shire knights and burgesses who had pushed so hard for change did not abandon their quest, electing rather to take matters into their own hands by setting up and running almshouses themselves. Several of the MPs and other prominent members of the urban elite who did so, such as Thomas Elys

[220] A. Hudson, ed., *Selections from English Wycliffite Writings* (Cambridge, 1978), p. 135.

[221] D. Preest, trans., and J. G. Clark, *The Chronica Maiora of Thomas Walsingham, 1376–1422* (Woodbridge, 2005), pp. 376–9.

[222] See J. Catto, 'Religious Change under Henry V', in G. L. Harriss, ed., *Henry V: The Practice of Kingship* (Oxford, 1985), pp. 97–115. Catto does not explore Henry's short-lived interest in hospitals.

[223] *RP*, IV.19–20; *SR*, vol. 2, 2 Henry V, statute 1, cap. 1; Orme and Webster, *English Hospital*, pp. 132–6. Criticisms of this sort were not confined to England: Pullan, *Rich and Poor in Renaissance Venice*, pp. 204, 211.

[224] Orme and Webster, *English Hospital*, pp. 135–6.

[225] *RP*, IV.80–1.

(Sandwich), William Ford (Coventry), Joan Gregg (Hull), the brothers Robert and Thomas Holme (York), John Perfay (Ipswich), John Plumtree (Nottingham), Roger Thornton (Newcastle-upon-Tyne), Degory Watur (Shrewsbury) and Richard Whittington (London), were determined that their foundations should be managed by hard-headed businessmen rather than the Church. Many, being themselves aldermen, chose to vest authority in their fellow magistrates, while others turned to a craft guild or religious fraternity.[226] None were so naïve as to imagine that laymen were inherently more competent or principled. Indeed, the hospitals of Rye and Sandwich furnish some salutary examples of financial irregularity and mismanagement on the part of leading burgesses.[227] But it was widely, and often rightly, assumed that such abuses would not only be harder to conceal and easier to correct, but also less often tolerated. In some cases, distrust of ecclesiastical institutions and personnel was apparently born of personal experience. William Wynard's insistence in 1436 that the chaplain who served his foundation in Exeter should eschew any 'secular cares and offices', as well as avoiding 'all taverns and places whatsoever that may give occasion for his leaving or wandering from the house', was underscored by a ban upon 'fowlers, hunters, fornicators, adulterers and frequenters of brothels'.[228] His anxiety that regular and effective intercession should be made for his immortal soul was no doubt intensified by notorious scandals such as that concerning the warden of St Mary Bethlehem, London, whose vicious lifestyle had prompted an official inquiry at the start of the century and was still causing repercussions in the 1430s.[229]

Less scurrilous, but more representative, the long history of mismanagement at the hospital of St Leonard, York, which followed the Augustinian rule, exemplifies the various problems highlighted by the House of Commons. In 1399, the mayor was appointed to a royal commission of inquiry into 'the dissipation of ... lands, goods and possessions, and the burden of excessive pensions, maintenances and corrodies', which had plunged the house heavily into debt. The financial irresponsibility of successive masters, coupled with the widely reported cases of malfeasance at St Nicholas's, mentioned above, helps to explain why late medieval York boasted as many as eighteen privately run *maisons Dieu*.[230] From the early fourteenth century onwards, Bristol's *leprosaria* and older hospitals seem also to

---

[226] Sweetinburgh, *The Role of the Hospital*, pp. 200–1; Rawcliffe, 'Dives Redeemed?'; Roskell, Clark and Rawcliffe, *Commons, 1386–1421*, IV.93; P. H. Cullum, '"For Pore People Harberles": What was the Function of the *Maison Dieu*?', in D. J. Clayton, R. G. Davies and P. McNiven, eds, *Trade, Devotion and Governance: Papers in Later Medieval History* (Stroud, 1994), pp. 36–54; Tymms, *Wills and Inventories*, p. 111. For a striking example of tight managerial control, see the account book of William Browne's almshouse, Stamford: Bodleian Library, MS Rawl. B.352.

[227] Page, *VCH Sussex*, II.104; Sweetinburgh, *The Role of the Hospital*, pp. 230–1.

[228] DRO, ECA, ED/WA/2.

[229] *CPR, 1401–1405*, pp. 231, 273; *CPR, 1436–1441*, p. 87; TNA, C270/22.

[230] *CPR, 1399–1401*, pp. 131–2; P. M. King, *The York Mystery Cycle and the Worship of the City* (Cambridge, 2006), p. 187; P. H. Cullum, *Cremetts and Corrodies: Care of the Poor and Sick at St Leonard's Hospital, York, in the Middle Ages*, Borthwick Paper 79 (York, 1991), pp. 22–8. The irritation voiced by the commissioners was compounded by the current master's decision to dismiss the 'discretus vir' and

have succumbed to a lethal combination of incompetence, 'shady dealings' and an all too familiar inability to make ends meet. Dissatisfaction gave way to outright hostility, as attempts by the master of St John's to extract more money from his tenants led in 1399 to violent attacks upon the hospital and its archives by 'large numbers' of citizens 'in warlike array'.[231] Already by then involved in successive royal commissions for the reform of St Laurence's leper house, which had been reduced to penury through the ill-advised grant of corrodies, leading magistrates were called in to manage St John's a decade later, after attempts by the archbishop of Canterbury had failed.[232] It is hardly surprising that prominent local merchants and MPs such as John Barnstaple, William Canynges and his close friend William Spencer should establish institutions of their own, so that by the early sixteenth century Bristol possessed no fewer than twelve almshouses under municipal, guild or private management.[233]

6.9 Almshouses and *maisons Dieu*

The pious citizens who provided shelter for debilitated and elderly paupers were following a popular trend that appealed as much to artisans as aristocrats. Well over half the charitable institutions founded in pre-Reformation England, and almost all those established after the Black Death, can be classified as almshouses or providers of residential care.[234] At one end of the spectrum are to be found the imposing, often custom-built institutions favoured by members of the nobility and mercantile elite (plate 25), and at the other a host of temporary refuges for the vulnerable, comprising no more than a couple of cottages or a single tenement.[235] Like so many *leprosaria*, the great majority were small, short-lived and obscure, being designed from the outset to answer an individual need. Testators who wished to provide for elderly relatives or servants might set aside a dwelling or two for their accommodation, on the clear understanding that such property would eventually revert to their heirs or be sold for pious purposes. Others regarded their foundations as a type of chantry, which would function for a finite period until the money ran out or another benefactor stepped in to foot the

---

citizen Thomas Thurkill, who had previously offered financial advice: Page, *VCH York*, III.341.

[231] Price and Ponsford, *St Bartholomew's Hospital*, pp. 210–13. Hospitals were the inevitable casualties of conflict between monastic houses and urban communities. For example, St Saviour's, Bury St Edmunds, was looted during the riots of 1327: W. Page, ed., *VCH Suffolk*, vol. 2 (London, 1907), p. 136.

[232] *CPR, 1401–1405*, p. 413; *CPR, 1405–1408*, p. 419; *CPR, 1408–1413*, p. 320.

[233] Price and Ponsford, *St Bartholomew's Hospital*, pp. 201–2. Barnstaple's foundation of the Holy Trinity is here classed as a hospital, but it functioned from its inception in 1395–6 as an almshouse for twenty-four 'poor persons' supported by a fraternity. He entrusted its management to the mayor and corporation: *CPR, 1405–1408*, pp. 410–11; *CPR, 1416–1422*, pp. 68–9; W. Leighton, 'Trinity Hospital', *Transactions of the Bristol and Gloucestershire Archaeological Society* 36 (1913), pp. 251–87.

[234] Gilchrist, 'Christian Bodies and Souls', p. 102.

[235] For a general survey see Orme and Webster, *English Hospital*, pp. 136–46, 181–3.

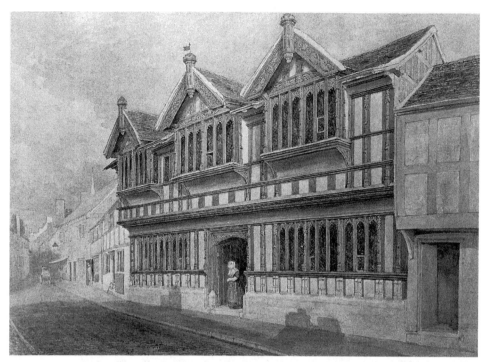

25 The striking frontage of William Ford's almshouse in Coventry, which was built in the early sixteenth century in the style of a merchant's house. It initially supported five aged men and one woman, but by 1529 was home to eleven elderly couples.

bill.[236] The costs and legal obstacles involved in endowing a more permanent establishment of any size were sufficiently great to deter all but the richest donors, and even then additional resources might well be required to maintain the fabric and support the residents. The London draper Sir John Milbourne (d. 1535) settled a generous rental income upon the fourteen brick and timber almshouses that he built for the use of his livery company, but its members had still to make up an annual shortfall of £20 because of inflation.[237]

Several of the better-known urban foundations owed their origins to a single wealthy benefactor working in partnership with the wider community in order to ensure long-term financial viability and high administrative standards. Some of these donors were clerics, who had first hand experience of urban poverty and may also have shared the laity's reservations about the management of monastic hospitals. Although the hospital of St John, Lichfield, had been established by one of his predecessors, Bishop William Smith was clearly dissatisfied with standards

---

[236] Cullum, 'For Pore People Harberles', pp. 36–54. For further examples, see E. M. Phillips, 'Charitable Institutions in Norfolk and Suffolk, *c.* 1350–1600' (PhD thesis, University of East Anglia, 2001), appendix.

[237] Rawcliffe, 'Dives Redeemed?', p. 3. The blurring of institutional and personal authority meant that relations between guilds and almshouses could deteriorate, as was notably the case at William Browne's foundation in Stamford: Hill and Rogers, *Guild, Hospital and Alderman*, pp. 46–51.

there and may even have expelled the remaining brethren for their 'ill living' before converting it into a home for thirteen bedesmen and a grammar school for local boys in 1495.[238] The almshouse of the Holy Saviour, Wells, was the outcome of a collaborative effort on the part of the dean and chapter and the townspeople, the latter being permitted to nominate two-thirds of the inmates in return for an annual subvention. This arrangement reflects far happier relations between Church and laity than those described earlier in this chapter, since the executors of Bishop Nicholas Bubwith (d. 1424) provided most of the initial funding.[239] During his time as rector of Hadleigh in Suffolk, William Pykenham (d. 1497) was likewise prompted to build twenty-four separate dwellings for the accommodation of poor men and women whose plight clearly evoked his compassion.[240]

It is easy to see why so many almshouses were collective ventures on the part of guilds, fraternities, parishes and corporations, since members could share the costs while reaping the social and spiritual benefits of charity to the poor. The original statutes of the Saffron Walden almshouses reveal a strong sense of communal involvement in both their foundation and ongoing financial support, describing how, in August 1400:

> the more worshipful men [*valenciores*] in the parish and town of Walden with the consent and support of all, in the presence of the whole assembly of the same, advantageously providing for the remedy and health [*remedio et salute*] of their souls, decided piously to erect certain well-built houses to the honour of God and his glorious mother for the refuge and support of thirteen paupers ... who are to comprise the more indigent individuals, namely such as are decrepit, blind [and] lame, whether from among the fifty-two poorer persons of the town or from elsewhere, as may seem most expedient to the ... custodians and governors. For the assistance of those thirteen paupers, the aforesaid parishioners have appointed two keepers, namely a man and a woman: so that the man [occupies himself] humbly seeking alms for the aforesaid paupers once a week at the homes of the worshipful [*valencium*], while the woman busies herself at the almshouse serving, washing and ministering all things necessary to the aforesaid paupers.[241]

The identification and precise enumeration of the town's neediest inhabitants presuppose an existing system of surveillance (and perhaps of outdoor relief) that

---

[238] M. W. Greenslade, ed., *VCH Stafford*, vol. 3 (Oxford, 1970), pp. 280–1. Soon afterwards, in 1502–4, Thomas Milley, a canon of Lichfield cathedral, completely rebuilt and re-endowed another hospital in the town as an almshouse for fifteen poor women (p. 276).

[239] Shaw, *Creation of a Community*, pp. 241–8.

[240] Spooner, 'Almshouse Chapel, Hadleigh'.

[241] F. W. Steer, ed., 'The Statutes of Saffron Walden Almshouses', *Transactions of the Essex Archaeological Society*, n.s. 25 (1955–60), pp. 161–221, on pp. 166–7, 172–3. Twenty-four leading residents formed what might be termed a management committee, which ran the almshouse, while the community as a whole constituted a guild of the Blessed Virgin 'in sustynounce of this forsayd dede of charyte' (pp. 174–7).

may have been deputed to churchwardens.[242] The almshouse was further absorbed into local networks of care by virtue of its responsibility for providing each of these designated paupers with a Christian burial, should one be needed, and for distributing alms every year among all the 'decrepit' and bedridden individuals resident in the area.[243]

As was the case at Saffron Walden, a fraternity might be formed to assist with management and fund-raising, while also promising spiritual and sometimes even physical security to less affluent benefactors who could never have contemplated such an ambitious venture on their own.[244] Thus, for example, the refoundation, re-endowment and complete rebuilding of St John's hospital, Sherborne, was undertaken by a specially constituted brotherhood of twenty leading residents, who raised £80 by individual subscription between September 1438 and June 1439 alone, largely to cover legal expenses.[245] The handsome new two-storey foundation cost at least £204 to build over a period of five years, and enjoyed a significantly higher income than the old, of well over £30 a year (plate 26). Significantly, the increased revenues sufficed to guarantee any member of the fraternity an income of 20*d.* a week (and half that sum for his widow) should he (or she) ever succumb to sickness and poverty.[246] Established organisations, too, could step in to share some of the burden. In 1424 the influential guild of St George, Salisbury, agreed to support the reconstituted hospital of Holy Trinity by making fixed annual contributions for its upkeep.[247]

What sort of care might these almsmen and women expect? Larger and better-funded houses like that at Sherborne could offer a weekly dole 'to be paied and disposed yn mete and drynke', an annual subvention for linen, shoes, hosiery and other essentials, a warm outer robe with a livery, adequate fuel, and the services of a 'hosewyfe' to cook, clean and perform rudimentary nursing duties. With 7½*d.* a week to spend on consumables and 3*s.* 4*d.* a year on clothing, as well as copious helpings of food and ale at major festivals, the residents would, theoretically, have

---

[242] C. Dyer, 'Did the Rich Really help the Poor in Medieval England?', in N. Salvador Miguel *et al.*, eds, *Ricos y pobres: opulencia y desarraigo en el occidente medieval*, Actas de la 36 semana de estudios medievales de Estella (Pamplona, 2009), p. 318.

[243] Steer, 'Statutes of Saffron Walden Almshouses', pp. 168–9, 174–5.

[244] Almshouses were often part of a 'package' of endowments, including a fraternity or college and chantry, established by a pious benefactor. See, for example, John Smythe's refuge for four poor men at Bury St Edmunds, Thomas Spring's house for ten paupers at Lavenham, and John Barnstaple's hospital of the Holy Trinity, Bristol: Phillips, 'Charitable Institutions', appendix, pp. vii, xxii; and n. 233 above.

[245] Dorset Record Office, D/SHA A11. Contributions are recorded street by street and came from almost all the townspeople. New brethren who joined the fraternity later paid handsomely for the privilege, offering between £4 and £6 on entry, above an annual subscription of 13*s.* 4*d.* or more: D/SHA A18; D/SHA A30.

[246] Dorset Record Office, D/SHA A14–18; C. H. Mayo, *A Historic Guide to the Almshouse of St John the Baptist and St John the Evangelist, Sherborne* (Oxford, 1933), pp. 13–27, 33, 35, 63–8. Mayo mistakenly assumes that the number of inmates doubled immediately from eight to sixteen, but the accounts confirm that twelve men and women was the norm between 1425 and 1447: D/SHA A1–19.

[247] Brown, *Popular Piety*, pp. 181, 192.

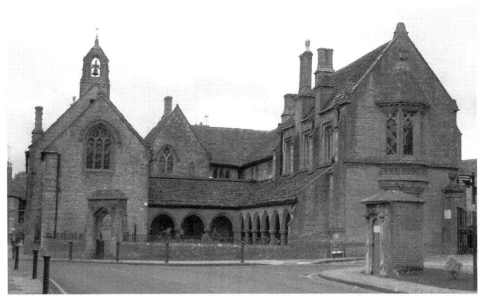

26 Now heavily restored, the almshouse of St John, Sherborne, represented a major investment – and assertion of collective independence – by the townspeople, who spent over £200 on rebuilding the old hospital in the early 1440s.

been able to observe the strict prohibition on begging, which was punishable by expulsion.[248] Garden produce and donations from local people would have provided a welcome supplement, and were vital for most other alms-folk, who could expect no more than basic lodgings and, perhaps, a token allowance of cash or fuel. Without further support, begging was essential for survival and formed part of the quotidian round in many institutions. A degree of coercion evidently obtained at the guild hospital of SS Giles and Julian, Lynn, whose inmates were locked out each day in order to solicit alms or work. One of them was even employed in dredging the town's ditches, which suggests that some, at least, must still have been quite active, if understandably reluctant to undertake such heavy labour.[249]

The medieval almshouse was never intended to relieve poverty on a broad scale or even to assist the truly destitute.[250] On the contrary, few accommodated more

[248] Mayo, *Historic Guide*, pp. 33–6. Initially, at least, they had to make do with less generous allowances, and would almost certainly have been obliged to beg (pp. 51–2).

[249] Phillips, 'Charitable Institutions', pp. 156–7.

[250] The common requirement that inmates should bring all their moveable possessions with them, and should leave them to the house when they died, underscores this assumption. It was expected at, for example, Gregg's almshouse, Hull: J. Tickell, *History of Kingston-upon-Hull*, pp. 757–8; at the almshouse for 'feble people' run by the leading parishioners of St Mary's, Lambeth: C. Drew, ed., *Lambeth Churchwardens' Accounts 1504–1645*, vol. 1, Surrey Record Society 40 (London, 1940), pp. 24–5; at the *domus Dei* in Newcastle-upon-Tyne: J. C. Hodgson, 'The "Domus Dei" of Newcastle: Otherwise St Katherine's Hospital of

than the symbolic number of thirteen inmates, as earthly representatives of Christ and his apostles.[251] Not surprisingly, establishments run by craft guilds and livery companies tended to admit only long-serving members and their dependents, while sometimes imposing further restrictions regarding status, reputation and financial circumstances.[252] When leaving a large messuage to his company for the use of its bedesmen, the London skinner Henry Barton (d. 1435) insisted that they must be respectable householders who had not disgraced the craft by becoming 'common beggars'.[253] With an eye on the mutability of fate, he, like many other benefactors, aimed to assist the 'shamefaced' poor who had known better times and whose neglect would reflect badly upon the entire community. Because of the emphasis placed upon religious observance and intercessionary prayer in so many institutions, the character and morality of applicants inevitably assumed particular importance, as did the need to discourage vagrants, 'strangers', the dissolute and the work-shy. The *maison Dieu* established by James de Kyngeston in mid-fourteenth-century Hull was typical in its requirement that the thirteen residents should be 'poor men and women broken by age, misfortune or toil, *who cannot gain their own livelihood*' (my italics).[254] Mindful of the risks and reversals faced by members of the mercantile elite, Joan Gregg gave priority to those who had previously 'been of most worship yn the town' when setting up another almshouse there in 1416.[255] The burgesses of Wells struck an ideal compromise by assigning half the twenty-four places in their almshouse to unfortunates of 'fallen status' who could no longer afford a home and would otherwise be thrown onto the streets, and half to decrepit paupers whose begging days were over.[256]

Gender and marital status also mattered to donors. The majority of houses seem to have accepted only reputable single men and/or women, although a few such as Holy Cross, Stratford on Avon, offered rooms to impoverished elderly couples.[257] Even in the larger establishments, such as Gregg's in Hull, St John's, Sherborne,

the Sandhill', *Archaeologia Aeliana*, 3rd series 14 (1917), pp. 191–220, on p. 206; at St John's, Sherborne: Mayo, *Historic Guide*, p. 36; at Holy Cross, Stratford-on-Avon: W. Page, ed., *VCH Warwickshire*, vol. 2 (London, 1908), p. 114; and at Holy Saviour, Wells, where modest payments might also be charged for admission: Shaw, *Creation of a Community*, pp. 244–6.

[251] Rawcliffe, 'Dives Redeemed?', p. 5; Cullum, 'For Pore People Harberles', p. 49; McIntosh, *Poor Relief in England*, p. 75.

[252] For instance, entry to the almshouse run by the Merchant Tailors of London was confined to those who had worn the livery for at least seven years (as opposed to journeymen and servants), and had paid all their dues: C. M. Clode, ed., *Memorials of the Guild of Merchant Taylors* (London, 1875), p. 207.

[253] Thomson, 'Piety and Charity', p. 182.

[254] *CPR, 1343–1345*, p. 239.

[255] Tickell, *History of Kingston-upon-Hull*, p. 757. The almshouse endowed by the executors of Roger Smith in Chester in 1509 gave priority to members of the ruling elite ('the twenty-four') and their widows 'fallen into poverty': HMC, *Eighth Report*, part 1, Royal Commission on Historical Manuscripts 7 (London, 1881), p. 371.

[256] Shaw, *Creation of a Community*, pp. 231–2.

[257] Page, *VCH Warwickshire*, II.114.

and St Mary's, Yarmouth, which received single people of both sexes, women were generally in the minority and might well be expected to perform domestic duties. This was certainly the case at William Browne's almshouse in Stamford, where two 'lowly, devout and poor' female pensioners had to cook and clean for ten men.[258] In some instances need was clearly subordinated to gender: despite the fact that the elderly widows of Wells suffered characteristically higher levels of deprivation, over three-quarters of the inmates of the civic almshouse were male. Such a striking imbalance may reflect the common assumption that men were more susceptible to the indignity of begging and generally more deserving of help.[259] Nevertheless, the contraction of employment opportunities for working women in the later fifteenth century seems to have prompted a steady rise in the number of *pauperes mulieres* who ended their days in care.[260] Often founded by women, less permanent and smaller urban refuges appear to have catered for them in growing numbers. In 1506, for example, Alice Neville of Leeds stipulated that, when either of the women she was supporting in 'ij howses' died, another should replace her, but 'no man'.[261] It was certainly unacceptable for the relics of leading burgesses to be left in want, and their neglect might provoke a scandal. The abbot of St John's, Reading, was reported to King Edward by the townspeople in 1479 for failing in his obligation to support an almshouse for the reception of 'onest mennys wyvys that had borne offyce in the towne before, and in age were fall in pouerte'.[262]

Some of the institutions that had developed out of older, open-ward hospitals for the sick and homeless poor continued to accept a few short-stay patients alongside the permanent residents. On acquiring the extramural hospital of St Thomas the Martyr, in 1478, the York guild of Corpus Christi agreed to retain seven 'almus beddes, convenyently clothed ... for the ease, refresshyng and herberyng of pore, indigent and travayling [labouring] people'.[263] After its

[258] H. P. Wright, *The Story of the 'Domus Dei' of Stamford* (London, 1890), pp. 37, 39.

[259] Orme and Webster, *English Hospital*, p. 109; Shaw, *Creation of a Community*, pp. 242–3. In Kent men were on average twice as likely to obtain a place as women: S. Sweetinburgh, 'Joining the Sisters: Female Inmates of Late Medieval Hospitals in East Kent', *Archaeologia Cantiana* 202 (2003), pp. 17–40, on pp. 20–4. However, some permanent foundations were reserved for women (see n. 238 above). John Plumtree's almshouse in Nottingham was intended for thirteen widows, 'broken by age and laid low by poverty', but subsequently accommodated just seven: *CPR, 1391–1396*, p. 116; W. Page, ed., *VCH Nottingham*, vol. 2 (London, 1910), pp. 174–5. Simon Grendon established a similar refuge for ten poor women in Exeter around the time of his mayoralty in 1405: DRO, ECA, book 51, fol. 296v.

[260] For example, Elsyngspital had originally been designed for one hundred blind and poor people of both sexes, but, by the early sixteenth century, had become an almshouse for just twelve sisters: Bowtell, 'Medieval London Hospital', p. 174.

[261] Cullum, 'For Pore People Harberles', pp. 48–9.

[262] BL, Add. MS 6214, fol. 22r. Successive abbots were also charged with stripping the assets from the monastic leper hospital of St Mary Magdalen, and allowing it to decay.

[263] As late as 1546 the house maintained eight beds for 'poore peeple beyng straungers', and an unspecified number for the 'beddrydden of the cytye': R. H.

conversion into an almshouse, the hospital of Holy Trinity, Salisbury, likewise maintained the tradition of welcoming needy travellers, although in 1456 and again in 1492 the civic assembly reversed this policy by excluding all 'but the pore pepull such as hath been dwelling in the cyte longe tyme'.[264] More typically, on its re-foundation in the 1430s St John's, Sherborne, shut its doors to outsiders and accepted only applicants from the ranks of 'contynuel householders', or, at the very least, 'other men and wymmen dwelling with yn the same towne'.[265] Yet hostility to vagrants was not universal. The founders of Saffron Walden's almshouse not only offered beds to sick paupers 'casuellyche come by the forseyd toun' until they recovered, but – quite exceptionally – undertook to help 'ony stronge [strange] poure woman with childe'.[266] Prompted by the acute social problems so visible on the streets, one Westminster guild turned the hospital of St Mary Rounceval into a hospice for sick and dying beggars, while another established a small refuge for homeless epileptics.[267] On balance, however, the transient poor had to look elsewhere for assistance, which may have been in increasingly short supply. A general, if by no means universal, suspicion of 'foreigners' was compounded by the fact that in many towns almshouses and other public works tended to attract the financial support previously earmarked for outdoor relief. In Wells, for example, it seems that the monetary value of funeral doles declined as donations to the new almshouse increased, even though it accommodated only twenty-four individuals.[268] From a fifteenth-century perspective, the spiritual return upon the second type of investment seemed appreciably higher than the first.

The urban almshouse offered other, more immediate attractions to patrons, not least being the opportunity to demonstrate the same sense of communal pride that had prompted the foundation of suburban *leprosaria*. The prospect of outdoing commercial rivals had obvious appeal at a time when 'the rich and successful set out to express the prestige and position of their families in buildings and memorials that were meant to last'.[269] The construction of London's first purpose-built guild almshouse by the Merchant Tailors in 1416 set a trend that many companies sought to emulate over the following decades, although few commanded the same resources.[270] Charitable institutions were so closely woven into the fabric of urban life that, as Kate Giles observes, the decision to found a

Skaife, ed., *The Register of the Guild of Corpus Christi of the City of York*, Surtees Society 57 (Durham, 1871), pp. 272, 285–6. A few of the city's other *maisons Dieu* offered limited facilities to pilgrims and poor visitors: Cullum, 'For Pore People Harberles', p. 49.

[264] Brown, *Popular Piety*, p. 184; J. A. F. Thomson, *The Early Tudor Church and Society* (London, 1993), p. 284.

[265] Mayo, *Historic Guide*, p. 30.

[266] Steer, 'Statutes of Saffron Walden Almshouses', pp. 168–9, 174–5.

[267] A. G. Rosser, 'The Essence of Medieval Urban Communities: The Vill of Westminster, 1200–1500', *TRHS*, 5th series 34 (1984), pp. 91–112, on pp. 108–9.

[268] Shaw, *Creation of a Community*, p. 238.

[269] Nightingale, *Medieval Mercantile Community*, p. 402.

[270] Rawcliffe, 'Dives Redeemed?', pp. 4–8.

new one, or remodel another, could mark a crucial step in the development of corporate identity.[271] The most striking example of this 'refashioning' or 'assertion of independence' is to be found at Sherborne, where the conversion of the hospital into an almshouse during the 1430s constituted an unambiguous expression of defiance on the part of the townspeople, who had recently quarrelled with their lord, the abbot (plate 27). Situated on the very doorstep of the abbey, the new building exemplified a collective *amour propre*, underscored by the fact that the almsmen and women wore white robes emblazoned with 'a skochen [escutcheon] of the armes of Seynt George made yn maner and fourme as the yonge men of the saide towne … yn tyme passed haue vsed'.[272]

As the acceptable and deserving face of poverty, these liveried bedesmen conveyed a stern message to the younger and more rebellious elements of urban society. Their presence served to reinforce a code of conduct predicated upon obedience, virtue and honest labour, without which there would be little hope of a secure old age. By refusing entry to anyone who had 'fallen into poverty … through ryott, wanton or lavish expences, his owne negligence or other misdemeanure' almshouses played a significant – and generally underrated – part in the campaign for moral rearmament which so preoccupied late medieval magistrates.[273] Nor did admission mark the end of close surveillance, since residents were expected to comport themselves in a suitably pious and deferential fashion. Recognising that not all the paupers who survived their careful vetting procedure would be 'of good and honest conversation', the managers of the Saffron Walden almshouse threatened anyone who proved violent, inebriated, greedy, ribald or quarrelsome with expulsion after three warnings. Quarterly inspections ensured that they kept up to the mark and attended all the necessary services.[274] The 'sundry good & godly orders and constitucons' drawn up in 1436 by William Wynard, sometime recorder of Exeter, for the *domus Dei* that he founded outside the south gate required the mayor and trustees to hold 'visitations' in person twice a year. As well as resolving any grievances voiced by the chaplain and twelve poor inmates, they were to ascertain that nobody had misbehaved, notably by begging or neglecting the strenuous round of devotions itemised at considerable length in the statutes. Since Wynard lived nearby, he would have been able to exercise the level of personal supervision characteristic of founders who owed their commercial success to hands-on business methods.[275]

---

[271] K. Giles, *An Archaeology of Social Identity: Guildhalls in York, c. 1350–1630*, BAR British Series 315 (2000), p. 59.

[272] They also wore the arms of Bishop Neville of Salisbury, their new patron: Brown, *Popular Piety*, pp. 192–4; Mayo, *Historic Guide*, pp. 34, 52–3.

[273] Clode, *Memorials of the Guild of Merchant Taylors*, p. 207.

[274] Steer, 'Statutes of Saffron Walden Almshouses', pp. 168–9, 174–5. A similar fate awaited ill-behaved residents of St John's, Lichfield (Bodleian Library, MS Ashmole 855, fols 150v–161r), and of Thornton's almshouse in Newcastle (Hodgson, ' The "Domus Dei" of Newcastle', p. 208).

[275] DRO, ECA, ED/WA/2. According to John Hooker, he actually 'lived the resydew of his lyff' among the poor: ECA, Book 51, fol. 303v. So too did Degory Watur, the founder of an almshouse in Shrewsbury: Rawcliffe, 'Dives Redeemed?', pp. 16–17, 26.

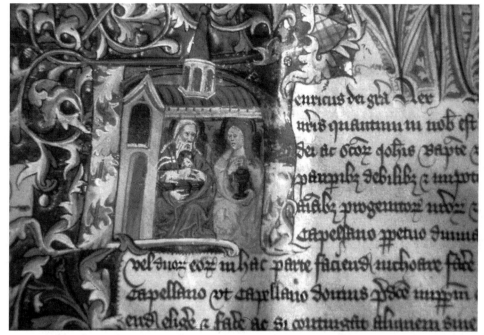

27 The richly illuminated foundation charter of the almshouse of St John the Baptist (and St John the Evangelist), Sherborne, drawn up in 1437, reflects the great pride taken by the townspeople in their achievement. It was most unusual for such documents to be embellished in this way.

The obligation to earn one's daily bread did not, of course, cease on entry. As we saw in Chapter 2, those who could do so were required to perform appropriate tasks, such as gardening, tending animals or spinning, while all except the senile and moribund could pray.[276] On the ground that 'idleness has taught much mischief and is likely to teach infinitely more evils', Wynard not only ensured that the chaplain of his almshouse would be occupied from dawn to dusk, but also expected the more mobile residents to attend a mass dedicated to his salvation each day in the nearby Franciscan friary. Nor were the bedridden excused from duty. John Stow's boyhood recollection of a row of almshouses in Houndsditch, 'a clean linnen cloth lying inn their window, and a payre of bedes to shew that there lay a bedred body, vnable but to pray onely', reminds us that the term 'bedesman' denoted a regular occupation.[277] Those who proved reluctant to intercede on behalf of their patrons were likely to be punished. Former parish clerks of London who secured a place in their guild almshouse stood to lose their weekly doles if they did not 'use themselves devoutely to prayer as they oughte to do', while inmates of the *domus Dei* in Newcastle would be made to fast or pray for twice as long.[278]

---

[276] Sweetinburgh, 'Joining the Sisters', pp. 28–9; see section 2.5 above.

[277] Stow, *Survey of London*, I.128.

[278] J. Christie, *Some Account of Parish Clerks, More Especially of the Ancient Fraternity of S. Nicholas* (London, 1893), p. 67; Hodgson, 'The "Domus Dei" of Newcastle', p. 208.

Should any of the 'nedy and devoute pore folke hable in conversacion and honest in lyving' who found refuge in Richard Whittington's almshouse be tempted to step out of line, the repercussions could prove far more serious. In 1482, for example, one inmate was expelled for being 'a grete brawler and chider amonge his brethern, and a comen & dayly dronken man, not wel-disposed to byde and here his seruice accordyng to his dutie and othe'.[279] Life in one of the City's most prestigious institutions was bound to be highly regimented, but even comparatively modest places, such as the guild almshouse established by Thomas Bond (d. 1506) in Coventry, allowed little time for idling. On paper, at least, the ten residents were expected to attend matins, mass and evensong every day, as well as reciting three psalters of the Virgin Mary, fifteen Pater Nosters, fifteen Aves and three creeds for the redemption of their benefactor's immortal soul and the spiritual health of all the guild membership.[280] It is, however, heartening to discover that not all founders were such hard task-masters. Convinced that carrots would prove more effective than sticks, John Craven of York (d. 1416) offered an extra 1*d.* a week to those of his almsmen who undertook to say morning and evening prayers on his behalf.[281]

6.10 The need for change

The patrons of *leprosaria*, hospitals and almshouses hoped that their generosity to the sick poor would be rewarded in this world as well as the next. These expectations were clearly defined in the concluding paragraph of the statutes of the Saffron Walden almshouse, where the pious wish that its many benefactors would 'leve longe in erthe wyth helthe and prosperyte of body' was accompanied by an appeal for salvation. When the last trumpet sounded 'at the dredful day at dome' they would surely find a place 'on the rygt hond of God in the nombre of hem that be savyd and chosyn to the endeles blysse of hevene'.[282] It would be unduly cynical to dismiss the charitable efforts of late medieval men and women as little more than pious window dressing, but there can be no doubt that most of the institutional support available between the Black Death and Dissolution was quite narrowly targeted at an acceptable type of pauper whose prayers served to validate the bearer's passport to paradise. The limitations of what was, at best, a highly selective response to hardship at a local level came to the fore in the early sixteenth century, as the combined impact of the pox, population growth and rising levels of urban deprivation led to renewed demands for reform. As the mayor of London pointed out, there were precious few facilities for the accommodation, much less the treatment, of all the 'myserable people lying in the streete,

---

[279] Imray, *Charity of Richard Whittington*, pp. 111–12; L. Lyell, ed., *Acts of Court of the Mercers' Company, 1453–1527* (Cambridge, 1936), pp. 286–7.

[280] William Dugdale, *The Antiquities of Warwickshire*, 2 vols (London, 1730), I.193–4. A similar devotional round obtained at St John's, Sherborne: Mayo, *Historic Guide*, pp. 37–8. That at Gregg's almshouse in Hull was even more onerous: Tickell, *History of Kingston-upon-Hull*, p. 758.

[281] Cullum, 'For Pore People Harberles', p. 46.

[282] Steer, 'Statutes of Saffron Walden Almshouses', pp. 182–3.

offending every clene person passyng by the way with theyre fylthye and nastye savors'.[283]

Exercised by the steadily mounting problems of vagrancy and epidemic disease, Henry VII reflected in his will of 1509 upon the continuing decline of the 'commune hospitall', as a result of which 'infinte nombre of pouer nedie people miserably dailly die, no man putting hande of helpe or remedie'.[284] With an eye upon posterity, he set aside over £6,000 for the completion of the Savoy, an Italianate showcase for Tudor philanthropy on the western approach to London that would accommodate and provide professional treatment for 100 sick and transient paupers.[285] His plans for the construction of 'two semblable commune hospitalls, aswel in fourme and faction' on the outskirts of Coventry and York came to nothing, but confirm that the dearth of hostels for the homeless in major urban centres had once again begun to preoccupy the ruling elite. Similar concerns about the 'ruyne & decaye' of institutions throughout England were articulated in a bill presented to the second session of the 1512 parliament by a group of petitioners purporting to represent the sick and mendicant poor. Along with eloquent expressions of compassion ran less altruistic fears about rising levels of disorder and the likelihood that 'infeccon and sekknes' would spread among 'cleyne and hole people'.[286]

Yet notwithstanding its manifestly humanist agenda, the bill commanded none of the official support accorded to the campaign for medical licensing that had come before the same parliament, and was effectively sidelined, almost certainly as a result of pressure by Convocation.[287] Although couched in impeccably orthodox

---

[283] *Memoranda, References and Documents Relating to the Royal Hospitals of the City of London* (London, 1863), appendix 1. However, some diseased beggars were already being treated at St Bartholomew's: Fabricus, *Syphilis in Shakespeare's England*, p. 60.

[284] T. Astle, ed., *The Will of King Henry VII* (London, 1785), pp. 15–19; M. Condon, 'The Last Will of Henry VII: Document and Text', in T. Tatton-Brown and R. Mortimer, eds, *Westminster Abbey: The Lady Chapel of Henry VII* (Woodbridge, 2003), pp. 99–140. His words echo Henry V's response to the parliamentary bill of 1414, with which he must have been familiar: see p. 337 above.

[285] Henderson and Park, 'The First Hospital among Christians'. David Thomson adopts a dismissive approach to contemporary ideas about institutional care: 'Henry VII and the Uses of Italy: The Savoy Hospital and Henry VII's Posterity', in B. Thompson, ed., *The Reign of Henry VII* (Stamford, 1995), pp. 104–16.

[286] The bill survives in a damaged manuscript copy, which lacks the opening address: TNA, E175/11/65. According to a transcription made by the antiquary Joseph Hunter (d. 1861), it was intended for submission 'to the king our soveraigne lord and to the lords sperituall & to the welldisposed and discrete comyns at this parliament assembled': BL, Add. MS 24459, fol. 157. I am most grateful to Dr Paul Cavill for this reference.

[287] A bill 'concerning masters and keepers of hospitals and of other almshouses' reached the Lords on the twenty-seventh day of the first session and was referred to Convocation by the lords spiritual on the thirty-second: *Journal of the House of Lords*, vol. 1: *1509–1577* (London, 1767), pp. 14–15. I am again indebted to Paul Cavill for this information. Thomas More, who was then under-sheriff of London, may well have helped to promote it. Although he was not returned to this parliament, he is known to have been engaged in business in the Lords: S. T. Bindoff, ed., *The History of Parliament: The House of Commons, 1509–1558*,

terms, its appeal for a national survey of all hospitals and almshouses and the forcible resumption of any deemed unsatisfactory was clearly still a step too far for the Church to contemplate. It is, therefore, hardly surprising that the 'lollard' manifesto of 1410 should be copied as a preface into a parliamentary petition of 1529 for the confiscation of ecclesiastical property,[288] or that Protestant polemicists should agitate for the creation of hospitals in every 'good towne, or city ... to lodge and kepe poore men in, such as be not able to labor, syck, sore, blynd, and lame'. The campaign for subsidised medical care was also revived, with a demand that 'phisicyans and surgens be found in euery such town or cyte, where such houses be, to loke vpon the pore in that towne and in all other ioyning vnto it'.[289] The expectation that they would 'lyue vpon their stipend only', eschewing all forms of private practice under threat of the pillory may have been wishful thinking (as well as a gibe aimed at the London College), but other, less radical reformers were equally convinced of the need for action.

The humanist Juan Luis Vives, who spent some time during the early 1520s at the court of Henry VIII, maintained that effective provision for the disabled and deserving poor should be the *raison d'être* of every community. His ideas found their most forceful expression in the tract *De subventione pauperum*, which was addressed in 1526 to the burgomasters of Bruges, but owed much to his earlier association with Thomas Linacre and other members of his circle.[290] They were taken up with enthusiasm by advocates of social change in the following decade, when new poor law legislation was being drafted.[291] Since, in his view, the ultimate purpose of civic life was to create an environment in which 'charity [could] be consolidated and human society strengthened', it was demonstrably the duty of every magistrate to foster 'concord of fellowship and association' between all social classes.[292] 'Those who care only for the rich and show disdain for the poor',

3 vols (London, 1982), II.620. More's celebrated attack upon Simon Fish in 1530 for grossly exaggerating the problem of destitution (and especially of pox-ridden paupers) in England was motivated by Fish's assault on the doctrine of purgatory and his revival of demands for the construction of hospitals from the assets of religious houses: Simon Fish, *A Supplicacyon for the Beggars*, ed. F. J. Furnivall, EETS e.s. 13 (London, 1871), pp. 13–14. More stressed his own commitment to less controversial forms of institutional relief, and tellingly observed that the number of diseased indigents had declined appreciably since the 1500s: Thomas More, *The Supplication of Souls*, in F. Manley *et al.*, eds, *The Complete Works of St. Thomas More*, vol. 7 (New Haven, CT, 1990), pp. 117–22.

[288] R. W. Hoyle, 'Origins of the Dissolution of the Monasteries', *Historical Journal* 38 (1995), pp. 275–305, on pp. 277–8, 301–5. On this occasion the need for more hospitals was not specifically mentioned.

[289] J. M. Cowper, ed., *Henry Brinklow's Complaynt of Roderyck Mors*, EETS e.s. 22 (London, 1874), p. 52.

[290] It is tempting to suggest that he may have known about the parliamentary petition of 1512. His strictures on idleness also prompt a strong sense of *déjà vu*: J. L. Vives, *De subventione pauperum*, ed. and trans C. Matheeussen and C. Fantazzi (Leiden, 2002), pp. 97, 103–9.

[291] Rawcliffe, *Medicine for the Soul*, pp. 216–17.

[292] Vives, *De subventione pauperum*, p. 3.

he warned, 'are just like a doctor [*medicus*] who would think that he did not have to provide much relief for the hands or feet because they are far removed from the heart'.[293] His sentiments were hardly new; as we saw in Chapter 2, John of Salisbury had argued three centuries earlier that:

> ... magistracies were instituted for the reason that injuries might be averted from subjects and the republic itself might put shoes, as it were, on its workers. For when they are exposed to injuries it is as if the republic is barefoot; there can be nothing more ignominious for those who administer magistracies. Indeed an afflicted people is like proof and irrefutable demonstration of the prince's gout. The health of the whole republic will only be secure and splendid if the superior members devote themselves to the inferiors and if the inferiors respond likewise ... so that each individual may be likened to a part of the others ...[294]

Both authors, however, were inclined to modify their strictures in the case of the feckless or otherwise undeserving poor, who appeared to feed like parasites upon the urban body. Support, whether from a single benefactor, a guild, a corporation or the State, was, as so many indigents discovered, rarely unconditional in its demands, or available to all.

[293] Vives, *De subventione pauperum*, p. 89.
[294] John of Salisbury, *Policraticus*, p. 126.

❧ Conclusion

If, therefore, we begin our history of English public health with the medical pioneers of the eighteenth century, this is not to ignore the work of the great epidemiologists and sanitarians of Grecian and Roman times, or to overlook the practice of quarantine and the steps taken to check the spread of diseases such as venereal disease and leprosy in Europe at least since the Middle Ages. But it serves as a convenient point of departure, because the centuries that had intervened had mainly been spent, so far as concerns public health, in the wilderness ... we hear little during these dark centuries, except the major explosive pandemics of infection.

C. Fraser Brockington, *A Short History of Public Health* (1956)[1]

Having flourished for so long in the pages of both popular and academic history, the belief that later medieval England entered 'a dark age' in the annals of public health is surely now due for revision. Driven in part by Victorian ideas about the march of scientific progress, along with a resilient strain of medical materialism, this dismissive attitude has been further encouraged by an assumption that the English trailed far behind their Continental (and especially Italian) peers in terms of sanitary regulation. Careful scrutiny of a wide range of primary sources reveals that the rulers of England's towns and cities were, in fact, just as anxious to remove recognised hazards, even if they lacked the wealth and technological infrastructure to implement more ostentatious schemes for urban improvement. The crown and central government played a leading role in identifying and legislating against persistent nuisances, but local magistrates and a significant proportion of ordinary citizens proved no less committed to change. As this book has clearly demonstrated, they were far from passive in the face of mortality, being all too aware of the risks posed by a filthy environment or polluted water supply. Measures for the implementation of better food standards and the policing of markets met with widespread approval, while the provision of reliable medical treatment, as well as care for the sick and aged poor, ranked high on the communal agenda. Not all these initiatives were as effective as their advocates might have hoped. Some encountered resistance; others proved too costly or ambitious; and many more were hampered by economic imperatives that made the close proximity of noxious trades and industries an unavoidable fact of life, even for the most affluent citizen. Yet all testify to a keen awareness that collective action was both necessary and desirable.

It was, of course, much harder to take any meaningful steps in this direction during periods of dearth and recession, but in the last resort the relative success or failure of sanitary regulation depended largely upon more specifically local factors. At one extreme, the case of Carlisle reminds us that, for a border town faced with endemic poverty and constant warfare, investment in the most basic

---

[1] C. Fraser Brockington, *A Short History of Public Health* (London, 1956), p. 3. Brockington was then Professor of Social and Preventative Medicine at the University of Manchester.

projects could be little more than a pipe dream. Yet a small borough like Ruthin on the Welsh March could embark on an effective campaign of fire prevention, while Newcastle, in the north-east, was proud of its clean and professionally paved streets and markets. On balance, although the richer and more populous south may have led the way in matters of public health (and perhaps have regarded the north as inherently less sophisticated in this respect), it would be unsafe to generalise. Durham's multiple jurisdictions and lack of one single source of authority may have proved a greater obstacle to progress than its location – at least if the comparable experience of Southwark is any guide. Problems such as loss of trade or of natural resources and the failure to replace skilled workers who died in epidemics could strike anywhere, with predictable consequences. Even in London, the replacement and extension of the thirteenth-century piped water system proceeded in fits and starts as funding became available. Given the many challenges faced by most late medieval towns, it is, indeed, remarkable that so much was actually accomplished.

Anthropologists disagree as to whether human beings possess an innate, biological sense of revulsion towards dirt and decay, or whether distaste is simply the result of cultural conditioning. Our desire to avoid such things as blood and excrement has, for example, been famously described by Mary Douglas as no more than 'the by-product of a systematic ordering and classification of matter'.[2] The present study confirms that historical circumstances will, at the very least, determine *how* particular communities conceptualise their fears and *why* they choose to act upon them as they do. The decision to target some threats rather than others is clearly dependent upon a wide range of external influences, which are neither immutable nor universal. During the three centuries covered here, the rulers of English towns and cities became more sensitive to contemporary medical ideas about the avoidance of polluted air and the dangers of substandard food, while tending increasingly to stigmatise certain types of 'unhygienic' behaviour – such as idleness and prostitution – that appeared to undermine spiritual wellbeing and to fragment the urban body. A complex combination of cultural, religious and political considerations affected the ways in which pre-Reformation society envisaged public health, not least with regard to those lapses in personal morality that might so easily incur divine retribution. The conviction that pestilence was sent as a scourge to punish towns, cities and entire nations 'mired in monstrous sin' meant, inevitably, that penitential processions and other conspicuous displays of collective contrition would head the list of essential prophylactics.[3]

It has for this reason often been assumed that English magistrates were either reluctant or unable to take a more proactive, 'rational' stance against the plague, as exemplified by their failure to adopt the travel restrictions and quarantine

---

[2] Douglas, *Purity and Danger*, p. 36. Against this view, Marvin Harris contends that food taboos reflect an inherent awareness of nutritional and ecological risk: *Good to Eat: Riddles of Food and Culture* (London, 1986), pp. 15–16, while V. A. Curtis argues forcibly that 'the proper domain of hygiene is biology': 'Dirt, Disgust and Disease: A Natural History of Hygiene', *Journal of Epidemiology and Community Health* 61.8 (2007), pp. 660–4.

[3] Horrox, *Black Death*, p. 120.

measures pioneered in southern Europe. Setting aside the fact that a few towns are known to have imposed *ad hoc* embargoes of this kind, such a view ignores the spate of initiatives mounted after 1350 in response to the successive epidemics that so dramatically compounded the 'urban penalty'. Some innovations, including the regulation of butchery and slaughterhouses and the introduction of weekly refuse collections, represented an obvious and immediate attempt to purify the environment. Others were shaped by longer-term demographic trends, which created a demand for very different types of institutional care under secular rather than ecclesiastical management. Discrimination against the vagrant and apparently undeserving poor, first articulated in statute law during the later fourteenth century, became increasingly pronounced from the 1460s onwards, gaining even greater momentum after the arrival of the pox and sweating sickness two decades later. Repeated exposure to localised but nonetheless serious epidemics at this time was a powerful catalyst in mobilising campaigns for piped water, better street paving and wholesome, reasonably priced food. It also made people more aware of the need to safeguard their immortal souls by supporting public works and providing accommodation for sick and elderly paupers of reputable life. But we should remember that many of these developments predated the Black Death and, in some instances, were contemporaneous with innovations in Spain and Italy which have hitherto been regarded as groundbreaking in their originality.

Political and social factors also played a significant role in generating financial support for major utilities and schemes for the amelioration of public spaces. Civic pride and the quest for economic health, which were inseparably connected, stimulated investment. That even quite small towns took pains to impress visitors with the salubrity of their streets, rivers and markets is apparent from the most cursory reading of local archives. In this context it is interesting to speculate how far cleanliness was regarded as an emblem of *civilisation*, thereby setting town-dwellers apart from their rustic cousins. Was the creation of urban identity as much a matter of drains, public conveniences and conduits as it was of strong defences, guildhalls and chartered liberties? The evidence presented here is persuasive. By the close of the Middle Ages, lice and other unpleasant signs of physical neglect were pejoratively associated with 'wild people' (*homines ferales*), while concern for personal and domestic hygiene had increasingly become a hallmark of bourgeois life.[4] It was certainly common for urbanites to regard the 'foreigners' who thronged their streets with mixed feelings, if not a hint of superiority.[5] We might recall, for instance, the wording of the bye-law introduced by Norwich magistrates in 1467, which specifically blamed *rural* deliverymen for leaving heaps of 'putrefying matter' in their wake, but charged *residents* with the task of clearing it up.[6] Pejorative assumptions about the raucous and insanitary habits of bucolic outsiders are just as apparent in a small town like Basingstoke, where in 1507 complaints were voiced about the 'market folks' who sold their wares along Oat Street, causing no little inconvenience, mess and congestion. Four years later, the allegations had grown more specific, singling out 'the men of the

---

[4] Demaitre, 'Skin and the City', p. 108.

[5] See, for example, Strohm, *Hochon's Arrow*, pp. 25–7.

[6] See p. 218 above.

country' who tethered horses there, destroying fences, 'making great soil' and endangering children's lives because of the heavy traffic.[7] Examples of this kind suggest that, however dependent they were upon rural tradesmen, town dwellers remained ambivalent about exposure to people who might be less scrupulous in matters of health and hygiene.[8]

These anxieties were fuelled by the spread of medical knowledge among the upper and middling ranks of urban society, which constitutes another important theme of this book.[9] Far from succumbing to a collective bout of stunned fatalism and 'awe-struck despair' after the Black Death,[10] leading practitioners chose to concentrate upon the best means of preserving health and avoiding infection. We know of only one tract specifically intended for the guidance of English magistrates (that sent by the 'masters and doctors' of Oxford to the mayor of London during the epidemic of 1407), but there may well have been others.[11] As we have seen in each of the preceding chapters, sanitary regulations, court records and even devotional literature demonstrate a growing familiarity with this type of material. Initially the preserve of the aristocracy, specialist texts such as *regimina* and plague *concilia* soon began to circulate in abridged English versions, providing a rationale for the management of nuisances and the prosecution of offenders.

At the same time, royal mandates for cleaning streets and rivers, expelling lepers and eliminating industrial pollution alerted urban populations to the dangers of miasmatic air, while statute law for the enforcement of food standards inspired a host of local initiatives. Attendance at parliament and membership of royal commissions helped to disseminate more sophisticated ideas among the ruling elite. It has been suggested that Sir Thomas More's service as a commissioner of sewers while he was under-sheriff of London inspired those passages in *Utopia* concerned with the public water supply.[12] If nothing else, the experience of assessing the condition of noisome streams, rivers and fleets in the environs of towns and cities must have alerted magistrates to the problems caused by the indiscriminate dumping of refuse (even though they maintained a notoriously cavalier attitude to the suburban environment). Lower down the social hierarchy, service on juries promoted a basic understanding of the risks

---

[7] Baigent and Millard, *History of the Town and Manor of Basingstoke*, p. 314.

[8] As, for example, the 'Sprowston men' who sold contaminated pork and sausages in Norwich market: see p. 235 above.

[9] However, it is important to note that, just as germ theory barely impinged upon the 'folk physiologies' of lower status men and women during the nineteenth century (Jenner, 'Follow your Nose?', p. 346), so too the more recondite aspects of humoral medicine would have escaped the great majority of late medieval town dwellers.

[10] For a particularly damning assessment of the medical profession's response to plague, see P. Ziegler, *The Black Death* (Stroud, 1991), pp. 51–2.

[11] See p. 67 above. On its arrival in London, the tract was allegedly praised by the City's physicians and apothecaries ('per fisicos, apotecarios et alios quamplures maxime erat laudata'), which suggests that it circulated widely, even though it was not original: BL, MS Sloane 3285, fol. 68r.

[12] Macnalty, 'Sir Thomas More as a Student of Medicine', pp. 425–6.

posed by insalubrious nuisances and infectious diseases, as did guild membership in a period when trade and craft organisations played an increasingly important part in sanitary policing. Urban communities also learned from each other. The desire to emulate, and sometimes to outdo, other towns and cities meant that a significant number of health measures were based on initiatives which had already proved successful elsewhere. London naturally served as the benchmark for what today would be termed 'best practice'. Copies of its customs were stored among the official muniments of Bristol and Exeter for ready consultation, while towns such as Lynn consciously modelled their arrangements for the disposal of butchers' waste and management of conduits upon the 'bonum regimen' employed in the capital. As we saw in Chapter 4, communities often shared expertise, especially in the matter of hydraulics, and consulted widely before committing themselves to costly, long-term projects, such as the provision of piped water.

Late medieval beliefs about the working of the urban body fostered a strong sense of mutual responsibility, whereby the rich were expected to support the sick and vulnerable, or at least those who seemed deserving of help. If, in many instances, the concept of physical interdependence remained an empty platitude, it nonetheless appears that a significant proportion of the ruling elite sought to discharge these obligations. By adopting too narrow a definition of charitable effort, we have almost certainly underestimated the extent to which schemes for public health and welfare depended upon contributions from individual donors, as well as fund-raising campaigns by guilds and fraternities. By the fifteenth century, if not earlier, notions of what might constitute a 'comfortable work' were sufficiently flexible to encompass the provision of a striking range of amenities, from latrines to refuse carts, and from wells to street paving. In Bronislaw Geremek's opinion, most late medieval almsgiving represented the 'mere trappings of piety, flaunted by the benefactors for the better external expression of their own social prestige'.[13] And, indeed, it is all too easy to mock the Gradgrindian mentality of wealthy merchants, who expected a handsome return on their spiritual capital.[14] Yet, in the last resort, however calculating and solipsistic their motives, their investment in public utilities and poor relief far exceeded that of today's Whittingtons and Wynards.

Not all were extravagantly or ostentatiously pious. John Donne, the London mercer whose provision of free surgery for the needy is noted in Chapter 6, insisted that there should be no 'pompous araie' at his funeral, 'nor att my monethes mynde, nor in lightes, clothing nor in no grete dyners', but that the money customarily lavished on religious ceremonies 'be doon and given among poure peple'. True to his word, he left £20 in food for the immediate succour of 1,000 paupers, 20*d.* to each of the sisters and 'poure wymmen' in six London hospitals, £13 6*s.* 8*d.* to be shared among the 'poure seke peple' in St Mary Bethlehem (one of the few medieval English hospitals to accommodate the insane) and £6 to the inmates of the City's various leper houses. Other legacies were more spectacular. Donne's executors were instructed to supply destitute prisoners with food and drink to the value of £100 over a period of five years, and to distribute £200 'among pour

---

[13] Geremek, *Poverty: A History*, p. 25.
[14] Dyer, 'Did the Rich Really Help the Poor in Medieval England?', p. 311.

householders, chamberholders, bedred peple and ... veray seke and feble persones' in London and the suburbs. A similar bequest of £60 was earmarked for the sick, poor and blind residents of Sherborne in Dorset and Kidwelly in Carmarthenshire, with which he had family connections. When taken together with endowments for the education of university students, the marriage of poor girls, the release of prisoners and similar good works, the value of his charitable bequests exceeded £750.[15]

Donne's largesse reminds us, once again, of the important role played by civic pride as well as personal piety in promoting both individual and collective schemes for communal welfare. People recognised that a city or town could be beautified or defiled by its occupants, just as a human body might display signs of cosseting or neglect.[16] This conceit found its way into the many royal directives stressing the *dishonour* occasioned by filthy streets and dilapidated buildings. An order of 1370 against the demolition of unoccupied houses and other buildings in Oxford actually describes the damage that would ensue in terms of physical mutilation: like a lost limb or missing tooth, the empty spaces would result 'in deformitatem ville'.[17] We are afforded an interesting glimpse into this mentality through the wills of men such as Robert Gardener (d. 1508), alderman and three times mayor of Norwich, whose bequest of £10 for glazing his parish church of St Andrew helped to pay for the spectacular Dance of Death depicted at the start of this book (see plate 1).[18] In return, he asked for his name to be inscribed in 'every wyndowe', although the grateful parishioners went even further by commissioning an impressive portrait which commemorated his role in the government of 'this most comely city [*hujus civitatis comodissime*]' (plate 28).[19] We cannot now tell how much money Gardener sank into projects for the benefit of his fellow citizens, but his will, which made generous provision for the poor of his parish, as well as other bedridden folk and paupers, reflects concern both for the quality and appearance of the urban environment. He insisted that the devastated properties he had bought after a recent fire were to be 'covered with tile and with no reede', gave £10 for repairs to Norwich's walls and gates, and took steps to ensure that the new market cross would match the aspirations of England's flourishing second city (see plate 22). Stipulating that his contribution of £10 would be withdrawn unless the entire structure were completed to a suitably impressive standard within the next two years, he reinvigorated a project that had begun to lose some of its initial momentum.[20] As we saw in Chapter 2, crosses offered front-line protection against the miasmas of disease, a fact that prompted Gardener's colleagues on

---

[15] TNA, PROB/11/7, fols 9r–11v.

[16] We might note, for example, the expectation voiced in 1452 that the newly paved streets and recently repaired gutters, privies and sewers of Salisbury would serve to 'the adornment of the city': see pp. 118–19 above.

[17] *MCO*, p. 146.

[18] NRO, NCC Spyltymber, fols 93r–95r, on fol. 94r.

[19] This precise inscription was recorded in the early seventeenth century: NRO, Notebook of John Kirkpatrick, on deposit from the Fitch Collection, p. 39. I am grateful to David King for this reference.

[20] NRO, NCC Spyltymber, fols 93v–94v.

the aldermanic bench to rank the 'makyng of the crosse in the merket' alongside schemes for cleansing the River Wensum when they drew up their wills.[21]

Gardener's handsome city was about to face the major challenges of popular rebellion, rising levels of poverty and inflation, devastating outbreaks of plague and the mass immigration of thousands of religious refugees from continental Europe, the combined impact of which took a heavy toll upon its existing infrastructure. Reflecting wistfully on 'the comely and decent order' and 'goodly bewtefyng' of the urban fabric that had previously excited the admiration of visitors, the mid-sixteenth-century Corporation recognised that complacency in these matters was clearly misplaced.[22] Perhaps, too, they had come to realise that, notwithstanding the manifold problems encountered by their predecessors, the fifteenth century had offered hitherto unparalleled opportunities for magistrates to implement schemes for public health in towns that had been spared the blight of chronic overcrowd-

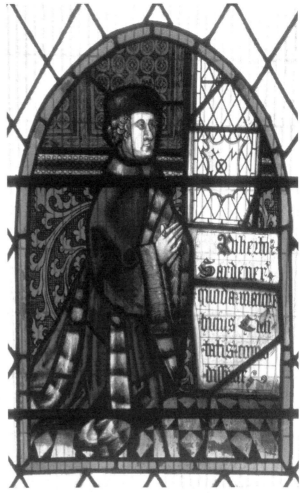

28 The stained-glass portrait of Robert Gardener (d. 1508), commissioned by his fellow parishioners at St Andrew's church, Norwich, reflects his achievements as 'mayor of this most comely city'.

ing and widespread unemployment. This perceptive attitude contrasts sharply with the condescension so often demonstrated by later generations of scholars, writers and reformers, whose opinions still exercise considerable influence today. The battle against debility and disease was a matter of pressing concern to the people whose struggles are documented here; and, although their beliefs and strategies can often seem alien to our own, they are no less deserving of study and respect.

---

[21] The words of Thomas Caus (d. 1506): TNA, PROB/11/16, fol. 166r.

[22] See p. 127 above.

Appendix

National and Urban Epidemics, 1257–1530

Documenting all but the most severe and widespread medieval epidemics is notoriously difficult; even in the case of national pandemics it can be hard to establish a precise chronology and to determine exactly what areas were affected. As J. M. W. Bean pointed out half a century ago, chroniclers were far from consistent in recording regional or local outbreaks of pestilence (especially in more distant parts of the country), while often noting those in London because they seemed more important.[1] Foreign visitors inevitably focussed upon the capital, as we can see from the latter part of this appendix. We should also bear in mind that many medieval authors were describing events that had occurred long before and may have been confused or uncertain about dating. It was also common for one chronicler to borrow wholesale from another, perhaps exaggerating mortality levels as he did so.[2] Urban historians are otherwise dependent upon the survival of private correspondence and of good local sources, such as probate records, university archives and monastic obituary rolls. Data compiled from debts registered under the Statute Merchant can also be used to trace patterns of mortality and pinpoint 'crisis years' when commercial activity was badly disrupted.[3] Inevitably, material of this kind tells us more about relatively prosperous adult male members of society than it does about the population as a whole, even though the poor and children were often far worse affected. The question of retrospective diagnosis is also highly contentious. A great deal of time and effort has been expended by scholars in an attempt to determine exactly how many of the 'pestilences' and 'sicknesses' listed below were actually bubonic, pneumonic or septicaemic plague, as opposed to typhus, smallpox, influenza or other, often famine-related, diseases.[4] However, since this book is less concerned with modern biomedical definitions than with the reactions of medieval men and women to the repeated onslaught of epidemic disease, the original terminology has been retained where possible.

---

[1] Bean, 'Plague, Population and Economic Decline', p. 427. On the other hand, as Sir Harris Nicolas observed in 1835, London chroniclers could be curiously reticent when it came to recording quite serious epidemics, such as those of 1433 and 1434, which are not mentioned by any of them: Nicolas, *Proceedings and Ordinances of the Privy Council*, IV.lxxx.

[2] P. J. P. Goldberg, 'Mortality and Economic Change in the Diocese of York, 1390–1514', *Northern History* 24 (1988), pp. 38–55, on p. 45 n. 18.

[3] Nightingale, 'Some New Evidence of Crises and Trends of Mortality', pp. 36–68.

[4] At least some answers are now being furnished by molecular biologists and geneticists: L. K. Little, 'Plague Historians in Lab Coats', *P&P* 213 (2011), pp. 267–90.

1257–8 Two years of famine caused by bad harvests led to an outbreak of 'lethal fevers' (*letales febres*). Matthew Paris provides an implausible figure of over 2,000 deaths in Bury St Edmunds alone by the end of the year: *Chronica majora*, ed. H. R. Luard, 7 vols, RS 57 (1872–84), V.660. Further shortages and high mortality followed in the spring of 1258 (p. 690).

1259 Paris describes an 'unexpected pestilence and mortality of men' that killed the bishop of London in May: *Chronica majora*, V.746–7. Other monastic chroniclers note the fatal impact of protracted famine, which had a devastating effect on the capital, in particular, at this time. Dearth and pestilence continued into the following year: Luard, *Annales monastici*, I.166; William Rishanger, *Chronica et annales, 1259–1307*, ed. H. T. Riley, RS 28.2 (London, 1865), p. 7.

1294 Many poor people succumbed both to hunger and an associated outbreak of diarrhoea (*lienteria*): Rishanger, *Chronica et annales*, p. 143.

1308–9 A striking fall in the number of debts registered under the Statute Merchant, and a corresponding rise in that of wills enrolled in the London Husting Court, point to 'a sudden epidemic with high mortality which shook commercial confidence': Nightingale, 'Some New Evidence of Crises and Trends of Mortality', pp. 43–4.

1316 Thomas Walsingham records a serious epidemic of dysentery (*dysentaria*) accompanied by acute and often terminal fever. He blamed the consumption of contaminated food after a long famine, which began in 1315, following years of rapidly escalating food prices, and continued to at least 1318: Walsingham, *Historia Anglicana*, I.146–7. An outbreak of what might have been scarlet fever (*pestis gutturosa*) is also reported: Johannes de Trokelowe, *Chronica et annales*, p. 94.

1320–4 Nightingale documents 'an unprecedented mortality' among creditors whose loans were registered under the Statute Merchant, and suggests that famine-related disease may have been the cause: 'Some New Evidence of Crises and Trends of Mortality', pp. 43–4.

1327 The 'virulent epidemic' evident in the countryside around Ely and Winchester may have reached London, where will enrolments rose and commerce was disrupted: Nightingale, 'Some New Evidence of Crises and Trends of Mortality', p. 45.

1337 Was notable for 'a grete moreyne off beestes and off men and a grete habundaunce off reynes': Kingsford, *Chronicles of London*, p. 10.

1340 Henry Knighton reports 'a repugnant and widespread sickness [*infirmitas*] almost everywhere in England, and especially in Leicestershire', where he lived, during which men barked like dogs and suffered paroxysms of intolerable pain: G. H. Martin, ed., *Knighton's Chronicle, 1337–1396* (Oxford, 1995), pp. 36–7. Martin believes that the epidemic may have been diphtheria, but Charles Creighton suggests ergotism: *History of Epidemics in Britain*, vol. 1: *From AD 64 to the Great Plague* (London, 1894), pp. 59–62.

1343 In August the rulers of London ordered all artisans, traders, servants and labourers to 'work as they used to do before the pestilence': *CPMRL, 1323–1364*, p. 164. We cannot tell if they were referring to the 1340 epidemic or an otherwise undocumented one.

1348–50 The Black Death

1355 Knighton describes the summer outbreak of 'a great sickness that was like some torment by evil spirits'. Throughout England 'people went out of their minds, and behaved like madmen in field and township', displaying the violent symptoms associated with ergotism: Martin, *Knighton's Chronicle*, pp. 132–3.

1361–2 A chronicler at King's Lynn dated the outbreak in London of 'the secounde pestilence', or 'Grey Death', to late September 1360, observing that first children and then large numbers of adults died. Sloane argues convincingly for its onset in April 1361: *Black Death in London*, p. 124. By the time that it reached East Anglia this plague seemed less virulent than the Black Death, but took a particular toll of children, adolescents and the affluent: A. Gransden, 'A Fourteenth-Century Chronicle from the Grey Friars at Lynn', *EHR* 72 (1957), pp. 270–8, on p. 275. Heavy child mortality is also noted by authors in the midlands and the north, where the epidemic persisted until 1362: V. H. Galbraith, ed., *The Anonimalle Chronicle, 1333 to 1381* (Manchester, 1927), p. 50; E. A. Bond, ed., *Chronicon monasterii de Melsa*, 3 vols, RS 43 (London, 1866–8), III.159; Martin, *Knighton's Chronicle*, pp. 184–5; Bean, 'Plague, Population and Economic Decline', p. 429. *The Brut*, on the other hand, retrospectively records 'a grete & houge pestilence of peple, and namely of men' (Brie, *The Brut*, p. 314).

1362 Walsingham observes that 'many died of the disease of lethargy' (*morbo litargiae*), while numerous women expired from dysentery (*per fluxum*): *Historia Anglicana*, I.298.

1368–9 There was a national epidemic, later known as 'the thyrde pestylaunce' and 'a great pestilence of nobles and children': Gairdner, *Historical Collections of a Citizen*, p. 88; Galbraith, *Anonimalle Chronicle*, p. 58; Bean, 'Plague, Population and Economic Decline', p. 429; Gransden, 'Fourteenth-Century Chronicle', p. 277. According to Walsingham, 'men and the larger animals' were worse affected: *Historia Anglicana*, I.309.

1374–5 One northern chronicler notes the onset in 1374 of 'the fourth pestilence in many towns in the south of England', adding that 'in the following year it killed a great number of citizens of London from among the best and richest of all the City', as well as several government officials: Galbraith, *Anonimalle Chronicle*, pp. 77, 79. Sloane suggests that London may, in fact, have escaped relatively lightly, with fewer than 2,000 deaths: *Black Death in London*, pp. 148–52. Others were less fortunate, as plague then spread north. Walsingham records a time of 'great pestilence' throughout England, which affected men and women alike, 'infinite numbers' being 'devoured by sudden death': *Historia Anglicana*, I.319; Bean, 'Plague, Population and Economic Decline', p. 429.

1377 Mortality among creditors whose loans were registered under the Statute Merchant rose to crisis levels: Nightingale, 'Some New Evidence of Crises and Trends of Mortality', p. 48.

1378–9 Walsingham describes the 'foule deth' that ravaged the north of England in summer 1379 as being worse than anything seen there before, killing almost all the ablest men, destroying whole families and depopulating villages and towns: *Historia Anglicana*, I.409–11; Bean, 'Plague, Population and Economic Decline', p. 428. According to one local chronicler, it began in York before Michaelmas 1378, lasted for an entire year and killed many children: Galbraith, *Anonimalle Chronicle*, p. 124. Its progress may have been even deadlier, as the Scots recorded what for them was the 'thryd pestilens' in 1380: Androw of Wyntoun, *The Orygynale Cronykil of Scotland*, ed. D. Laing, 3 vols (Edinburgh, 1872–9), III.15.

1380 There appears to have been an epidemic of some kind in Colchester: Britnell, *Growth and Decline in Colchester*, p. 96.

1382 One chronicler maintains that an outbreak of infectious disease in London was largely confined to 'boys and girls': Ranulph Higden, *Polychronicon Ranulphi Higden*, ed. J. R. Lumby, 9 vols, RS 41 (London, 1865–86), IX.14. Another describes it in more dramatic terms as the fifth major national epidemic since the Black Death, confirming that its many victims were generally under thirty: G. B. Stow, ed., *Historia vitae et regni Ricardi secundi* (Philadelphia, 1977), p. 74. The antiquary Francis Blomefield cites a reference in an unidentified local chronicle to 'very pestilential fever' in various parts of England, accompanied by 'very extraordinary inundations' in the Fens. However, either he or the chronicler may have misdated events which actually occurred one year later: Blomefield, *Topographical History of the County of Norfolk*, III.111.

1383 A 'great epidemic' broke out in parts of Norfolk, but allegedly killed only young people between the ages of seven and twenty-two. A second one occurred later in the year, around Christmas, in Kent 'and many other parts of England', this time respecting neither age or gender: Higden, *Polychronicon*, IX.21, 27. According to Walsingham, a large number of people contracted 'either lethal pestilence or serious illnesses and infirmities' through eating rotten fruit that had been infected by 'foetid fogs, exhalations and various corruptions of the air': *Historia Anglicana*, II.109.

1384 There may have been an epidemic in Colchester: Britnell, *Growth and Decline in Colchester*, p. 96. Death rates among creditors whose loans were registered under the Statute Merchant again reached crisis levels: Nightingale, 'Some New Evidence of Crises and Trends of Mortality', p. 48.

1387 Another epidemic seems to have broken out in Colchester: Britnell, *Growth and Decline in Colchester*, p. 96.

1389 Walsingham records a 'great and formidable pestilence' in Cambridge, during which many people succumbed to frenzy and died insensible without the last rites. The outbreak has been connected with 'the unclean keeping of the streets', about which the University authorities complained: *Historia Anglicana*, II.186; Cooper, *Annals of Cambridge*, pp. 136–7.

1390 An unusually hot summer gave rise to an epidemic that lasted until late September and spread through many parts of England, seizing the young rather than the old: Higden, *Polychronicon*, IX.237. Walsingham confirms that the 'great pestilence' carried off children and youngsters 'in incredible and excessive numbers' in town and country alike: *Historia Anglicana*, II.197; Bean, 'Plague, Population and Economic Decline', p. 429. For death rates among adult males, see Nightingale, 'Some New Evidence of Crises and Trends of Mortality', p. 48.

1391 From July onwards, according to Walsingham, the sun was obscured for several weeks and at the same time such a great mortality arose in Norfolk and many other counties as to rival 'the great pestilence' of 1348–50. In York alone, he reports, 11,000 bodies were buried in a short time: *Historia Anglicana*, II.203. Another chronicler claims that there were 12,000 deaths in the city, noting that this 'devastating pestilence' also spread to the west: Higden, *Polychronicon*, IX.259. Although these figures are wildly exaggerated, mortality rates did indeed rise sharply in the north, partly because of the 'flux and fever' occasioned by famine: Goldberg, 'Mortality and Economic Change', pp. 44–5.

1393 Walsingham records an attack of pestilence in Essex from which many died in September: *Historia Anglicana*, II.213. Colchester experienced unusually high mortality figures between the autumn of 1390 and that of 1394: Britnell, *Growth and Decline in Colchester*, pp. 96, 152–3.

1399–1400 Henry IV's first parliament, which sat in October and November, begged the king to avoid travelling to the north, because of the 'graunde pestilence' which was still raging there: *RP*, III.435. Nearer home, Westminster abbey was also affected: Harvey, *Living and Dying*, p. 122. This epidemic may have continued until 1400, since the chronicler Adam of Usk refers to a 'great pestilence' that then 'prevailed through all England, and specially among the young, swift in its attack and carried off many souls': *Chronicon Adae de Usk*, ed. E. M. Thompson (London, 1904), pp. 46, 207. The people of Hythe were probably referring to this outbreak when they petitioned parliament for relief in 1401: TNA, SC8/250/12465.

1407 In late October the Westminster law courts were adjourned because 'a deadly plague' had suddenly broken out in London and was 'newly spreading'. It proved to be a national epidemic, which Walsingham describes as being far worse than anything seen for many years, reputedly killing 30,000 people of both sexes in London alone and causing widespread depopulation in the countryside: *Historia Anglicana*, II.276; *CCR, 1405–1409*, p. 297; Bean, 'Plague, Population and Economic Decline', pp. 428–9. Nightingale documents rising death rates in the previous year, too: 'Some New Evidence of Crises and Trends of Mortality', p. 48.

1410 In late May the residents of Newcastle-upon-Tyne were excused taxes, in part because of 'the death of many of the inhabitants through pestilence in the past year': *CPR, 1408–1413*, p. 198.

1413 Walsingham reports outbreaks of pestilence in many parts of England (*Historia Anglicana*, II.297), evidently including Canterbury and Colchester: see, respectively, Hatcher, 'Mortality in the Fifteenth Century', p. 30; Britnell, *Growth and Decline in Colchester*, p. 202.

1417–18 Death rates among creditors whose loans were registered under the Statute Merchant rose to crisis level in both these years: Nightingale, 'Some New Evidence of Crises and Trends of Mortality', p. 48. A contemporary monastic chronicler describes cases of 'acute plague' at Canterbury in 1418: Connor, *John Stone's Chronicle*, p. 56.

1419 The records of Christ Church priory, Canterbury, suggest that there was another local epidemic this year: Hatcher, 'Mortality in the Fifteenth Century', p. 30; Connor, *John Stone's Chronicle*, p. 57. The death rate also rose dramatically at Westminster abbey between 1419 and 1421: Harvey, *Living and Dying*, p. 122.

1420 A pestilence occurred 'in parts of Norfolk': Luard, *Annales monastici*, III.485. Colchester and Canterbury may also have been affected at this time: see, respectively, Britnell, *Growth and Decline in Colchester*, p. 202; Hatcher, 'Mortality in the Fifteenth Century', p. 30.

1421 The residents of Northumberland, Cumberland and Westmorland petitioned the May parliament about the devastation occasioned by 'great mortality and pestilences which have reigned there for the last three years and still reign': *RP*, IV.14; see also Nightingale, 'Some New Evidence of Crises and Trends of Mortality', p. 48.

1423 The householders of Sutton in east Lincolnshire appealed to the steward of the Duchy of Lancaster for a rent rebate because of the 'utter destrucion' caused by flooding and plague. Their petition claims that, fearful of 'the grete pestilence that reignes in the said towne', 'the pepul is fled and flees dayly': L.G., 'Sutton in Holland', *Fenland Notes and Queries* 7 (1909), pp. 306–8, on p. 307.

1426–7 A letter sent in January [?] 1426 to William Paston I refers to a 'tyme of the pestelens' in Yarmouth (*PL*, II.3). It may perhaps have been written one year later, since at some point shortly before March 1427 a number of prominent Scottish hostages held under minimal surveillance in London died of a 'gret pestilence'. The ensuing correspondence reveals that the royal court promptly left the City, and the law courts at Westminster were suspended for fear of infection: Nicolas, *Proceedings and Ordinances of the Privy Council*, III.261–3. Colchester may also have experienced an epidemic, as mortality figures rose in 1426–7: Britnell, *Growth and Decline in Colchester*, p. 202.

1428 The Canterbury monk John Stone records an outbreak of 'epidemic plague' in his community: Connor, *John Stone's Chronicle*, p. 60.

1429 Unusually high mortality in the north suggests that bad harvests were followed by an epidemic of some kind: Goldberg, 'Mortality and Economic Change', p. 46.

1431 Deaths from pestilence occurred in Canterbury: Hatcher, 'Mortality in the Fifteenth Century', p. 30. The chronicles of St Albans abbey mention a local outbreak around Codicote: John of Amundesham, *Annales monasterii S. Albani*, ed. H. T. Riley, 2 vols, RS 28.5 (London, 1870–1), I.62.

1432 A tax rebate awarded to the people of Newcastle-upon-Tyne in May 1433 refers to 'the death of no small number of the inhabitants by pestilence in the preceding year' as one of many causes of financial hardship: R. Welford, *History of Newcastle and Gateshead in the Fourteenth and Fifteenth Centuries* (London, 1884), p. 294.

1433 The Westminster parliament was prorogued on 13 August 1433 because of a 'grave pestilence' then spreading through the City and suburbs: *RP*, IV.420. The *Brut* describes 'a grete pestilence in London, bothe of men, women and childern; and namely of worthy men, as aldermen and other worthi communiers', observing sadly that 'also thurgh England the peple deyed sore, bothe pore and riche, which was grete hevynesse to all peple': Brie, *The Brut*, p. 467; Nightingale, 'Some New Evidence of Crises and Trends of Mortality', p. 48.

1434 Legal staff had already abandoned the courts at Westminster when business was suspended on 28 October because 'mortal pestilence' was raging there and in London: Nicolas, *Proceedings and Ordinances of the Privy Council*, IV.282–3; Harvey, *Living and Dying*, p. 122. The death rate once again rose in Colchester, and exceeded previous levels in fifteenth-century Scarborough: Britnell, *Growth and Decline in Colchester*, p. 202; P. Heath, 'North Sea Fishing in the Fifteenth Century: The Scarborough Fleet', *Northern History* 3 (1968), pp. 53–69, appendix 3. Robert Gottfried's assumption that this particular epidemic continued until 1435–6 is based on the misdating of a London chronicle reference to 'a grete pestelens and a grete frost' in 12 Henry VI (the year ending September 1434): Gottfried, *Epidemic Disease*, p. 38; J. G. Nichols, ed., *Chronicles of the Grey Friars of London*, CS 53 (London, 1852), p. 16. Even so, death rates were high in the north in 1436: Goldberg, 'Mortality and Economic Change', p. 46.

1435 An *epidemia* of some kind occurred at Christ Church priory, Canterbury, and presumably in the town as well: Hatcher, 'Mortality in the Fifteenth Century', p. 30.

1437 The chief justice of the court of common pleas at Westminster withdrew to St Albans because of the plague ('propter epidemiae pestem') then raging in London: John of Amundesham, *Annales*, II.127.

1439–40 In November 1439 the Westminster parliament suspended the customary kiss of homage due to be exchanged between Henry VI and his feudal tenants because 'a sekeness called the pestilence, universelly thorough this youre roialme more comunely reyneth, than hath bien usuell bifore this tyme, the whiche is an infirmite most infectif'. A prorogation to Reading after Christmas suggests that further precautions seemed necessary: *RP*, V.4, 31. The Londoner William Gregory refers to 'a grete pestylaunce … in the northe contraye', which may have been typhus, dysentery or some other famine-related epidemic: Gairdner, *Historical Collections of a Citizen*, p. 181; Bean, 'Plague, Population and

Economic Decline', p. 429; Goldberg, 'Mortality and Economic Change', pp. 45–6. *The Brut* reports high mortality 'thurghout the ream, and principally at York and in the North Cuntre': Brie, *The Brut*, p. 473. The death rate in Scarborough reached unprecedented heights, unequalled during at least the first half of the fifteenth century: Heath, 'North Sea Fishing', appendix 3. Further south, Colchester appears also to have been affected: Britnell, *Growth and Decline in Colchester*, p. 202. Petitions to the crown from Wallingford in 1439, Richmond in 1440 and Winchester in both 1440 and 1442 refer to depopulation caused by 'pestilences and epidemics' which probably occurred at this time: TNA, C66/444, m. 11d; C66/446, m. 6; C66/447, m. 14d; C66/453, m. 31.

1442–3 The host of two Venetian merchants living in London informed the authorities that they had ceased trading and withdrawn to the country between April 1442 and late September 1443 'because of the pestilence': TNA, E101/128/30, m. 10r; Thrupp, *Merchant Class of Medieval London*, p. 227 n. 61.

1444 A letter from Henry VI to the abbot of Bury St Edmunds, almost certainly written in September of this year, refers to 'the aier and the pestilence' that had afflicted the University of Cambridge for some time and prevented a royal visit. Cooper dates this letter to 1447 (*Annals of Cambridge*, p. 199), but see J. P. C. Roach, ed., *VCH Cambridge and the Island of Ely*, vol. 3 (London, 1959), p. 378 n. 32.

1445 The Westminster parliament was prorogued on 5 June because of 'a grave pestilence' that had broken out in London and the suburbs: *RP*, V.67.

1446–7 A 'great pestilence which has continued there for a long time' is recorded in Lincoln, reinforcing the complaint that widespread depopulation, and especially 'the withdrawal of merchants', left the remaining citizens unable to pay their taxes: HMC, *Fourteenth Report*, appendix 8 (London, 1895), pp. 10–11; see also Nightingale, 'Some New Evidence of Crises and Trends of Mortality', p. 48. Plague deaths are also recorded in Canterbury in 1447: Hatcher, 'Mortality in the Fifteenth Century', p. 30.

1448 The antiquary Anthony à Wood records a pestilence in Oxford, which was allegedly caused by stagnant flood-water and the noxious air in student dormitories: *History and Antiquities of the University of Oxford*, I.596–7.

1449 On 30 May parliament was prorogued to assemble in Winchester on 16 June because of 'the corrupt air and pestilence' in various parts of London and Westminster: *RP*, V.143; see also Nightingale, 'Some New Evidence of Crises and Trends of Mortality', p. 48.

1450 The 'infection of the air' may have been a useful pretext for the prorogation of the Westminster parliament in December, and its eventual removal to the safe Lancastrian stronghold of Leicester in April 1451 (again reputedly because of 'insalubrious air'). Even so, a reference to 'this time of great pestilence' occurs in the Plympton area of Devon in late July 1450 and to 'vehement and sudden plague' in and around Chudleigh, some miles to the west, on 26 November following: Bean, 'Plague, Population and Economic Decline', p. 427; *RP*, V.172; G. R. Dunstan, ed.,

The Register of Edmund Lacy, Bishop of Exeter, 1420–1455: Registrum Commune, vol. 3, Devon and Cornwall Record Society n.s. 13 (Torquay, 1968), pp. 91, 272–3.

1453 The session of parliament that met in Reading on 12 November 1453 was immediately prorogued to 11 February following because 'the great mortality then reigning in the said town' had allegedly prompted Henry VI to stay away: *RP*, V.238. The king had, in fact, succumbed to a long period of mental illness, but we should note that fear of pestilence also disrupted studies not far away at Oxford: Wood, *History and Antiquities of the University of Oxford*, I.600.

1454 On 6 September William Paston proposed fleeing from London to the country because of the 'gret pestelens': *PL*, I.155–6.

1457 A 'great and serious plague' struck Canterbury and other parts of south-east England, causing the highest levels of mortality recorded at Christ Church priory in the fifteenth century: Hatcher, 'Mortality in the Fifteenth Century', pp. 28, 30; Connor, *John Stone's Chronicle*, p. 99. Westminster abbey was also affected (Harvey, *Living and Dying*, p. 122), while the port of Sandwich on the Kent coast virtually ceased trading (Clarke *et al.*, *Sandwich: A Study of the Town and Port*, p. 126).

1458–9 One Cambridge chronicler noted a 'virtually universal pestilence in many regions' in 1458 and a 'great and severe pestilence' in the following year: J. J. Smith, ed., *Abbreviata chronica ab anno 1377 usque ad annum 1469*, Cambridge Antiquarian Society 2 (Cambridge, 1840), p. 7. Levels of mortality were well above average in both East Anglia and the north: Gottfried, *Epidemic Disease*, pp. 37–8; Goldberg, 'Mortality and Economic Change', p. 46.

1463 The Shrewsbury chronicler who refers in this year to a 'greate pestelence with a dry soommer all England over', may perhaps have misdated the better-known epidemic of 1464: Leighton, 'Early Chronicles of Shrewsbury', p. 247. However, it was in 1463 that Edward IV was reputedly 'vysyted with the sykenesse of pockys', which may have been smallpox, while in the north: Robert Fabyan, *The New Chronicles of England and France*, ed. H. Ellis (London, 1811), p. 653. Death rates also rose sharply at Westminster abbey and in Colchester, remaining high in the following year: Harvey, *Living and Dying*, p. 122; Britnell, *Growth and Decline in Colchester*, p. 202.

1464 An anonymous chronicler describes 'a grete pestilence thorowe all the realme', although London seems to have been particularly badly affected; in early October a news letter from Bruges carried reports brought by Venetian merchants that there were 200 fatalities a day: J. Gairdner, ed., *Three Fifteenth-Century Chronicles*, CS n.s. 28 (London, 1880), p. 80; A. Hinds, ed., *Calendar of State Papers Milanese*, vol. 1 (London, 1912), p. 113.

1465 In mid-August Margaret Paston reported that 'they dyy right sore in Norwych', and that two of her relatives had left for the country because 'the pestylens' was 'so feruent' that they were afraid to remain: *PL*, I.315–16. Plague deaths are also recorded in Canterbury, and among the merchant class in general: Hatcher, 'Mortality in the Fifteenth Century', p. 30; Nightingale, 'Some New Evidence of Crises and Trends of Mortality', p. 48.

1467 On 1 July the Westminster parliament was prorogued to meet at Reading on 6 November because of the great heat and onset of an outbreak of plague ('pestilentie plagam regnare incipientem'), which had already struck some MPs: *RP*, V.618. At least two chroniclers report a 'great pestilence in England', one from Lincolnshire noting that 'an infection prevailed in the pestilential air over the dwellers in the land to such a degree that a sudden death consigned to a wretched doom many thousands of people of all ages, just like so many sheep destined for the slaughter': Smith, *Abbreviata chronica*, p. 10; H. T. Riley, ed., *Ingulf's Chronicle of the Abbey of Croyland* (London, 1854), p. 443. The mortality rate remained unusually high in the north between 1466 and 1468 (Goldberg, 'Mortality and Economic Change', p. 46), and there was plague in Canterbury (Hatcher, 'Mortality in the Fifteenth Century', p. 30).

1470 Plague deaths are again recorded in Canterbury: Hatcher, 'Mortality in the Fifteenth Century', p. 30.

1471 At the start of August the residential canons of Southwell minster took a month's absence on account of the 'morbi pestiferi' then in the town. The disease had tightened its grip by mid-September, when Sir John Paston wrote from Norfolk of 'the most vnyuersall dethe that euyre I wyst in Ingelonde', recording 'grete deth in Norwyche and in other borowghe townese': A. F. Leach, ed., *Visitations and Memorials of Southwell Minster*, CS n.s. 48 (London, 1891), p. 11; *PL*, I.440. Canterbury was so badly affected that the monks staged a procession with the relics of St Ouen, who reputedly protected against plague: Connor, *John Stone's Chronicle*, p. 131; Hatcher, 'Mortality in the Fifteenth Century', p. 30. Mortality rates in the north rose sharply throughout the autumn, only gradually subsiding in 1472: Goldberg, 'Mortality and Economic Change', p. 47.

1472 Plague attacked Oxford, causing considerable disruption: R. L. Storey, 'University and Government, 1430–1500', in Catto and Evans, *History of the University of Oxford*, II.734. According to a local antiquary, outbreaks of the 'most dreadful, fatal and contagious distemper, the plague' also occurred in Hull in 1472, and again in 1476 and 1478, on the last occasion killing 1,580 residents: Tickell, *History of Kingston-upon-Hull*, p. 132. Bean dismisses these claims, but Goldberg takes them more seriously in view of the convincing probate evidence for the north: Bean, 'Plague, Population and Economic Decline', pp. 429, 436–7; Goldberg, 'Mortality and Economic Change', p. 47 n. 29.

1473 The Yorkist chronicler John Warkworth describes a summer heatwave, 'by the whiche ther was gret dethe of menne and women, that … fylle downe sodanly, and unyversalle feveres, axes [agues or malaria], and the blody flyx [dysentery], in dyverse places of Englonde': J. O. Halliwell, ed., *A Chronicle of the First Thirteen Years of the Reign of King Edward the Fourth*, CS 10 (London, 1839), p. 23. R. S. Gottfried (*Epidemic Disease*, p. 43) argues that a reference in *The Brut* (p. 604) to a hitherto unknown disease called 'fflyx' that persisted for three years in the later 1470s must relate to this outbreak, though it may have been endemic throughout the decade. Certainly, death rates in the north rose in 1474: Goldberg, 'Mortality and Economic Change', pp. 41, 47.

1478 Some sixteenth-century chronicles record a serious epidemic in London, and there is indisputable evidence of a crisis at Westminster abbey, where the death rate in 1478–9 reached its highest point in the fifteenth century: Harvey, *Living and Dying*, p. 122. 'Great numbers of persons' are also said to have succumbed to plague in Newcastle-upon-Tyne: Welford, *History of Newcastle and Gateshead in the Fourteenth and Fifteenth Centuries*, p. 377.

1479 'Sekenese' was already ravaging London by late April, there being a general exodus from the City to avoid the 'greate deth, which continued all the yere': Kingsford, *Chronicles of London*, p. 188; Hanham, *Cely Letters*, pp. 47–8. The epidemic was national: it had reached Southwell by early July (Leach, *Visitations*, p. 40), and allegedly caused 3,300 deaths in Coventry (BL, MS Harley 6388, fol. 23v). On 6 November 1479, John Paston III reported that 'the pepyll dyeth sore in Norwyche, and specyally a-bought my house', adding that flight was out of the question because other areas were no safer. He wrote more cheerfully from London in December 1479 that 'the sykness is well seasyd [ceased] here': *PL*, I.616, 618; see also II.412. Both Richard Grafton – mistakenly under the year 1478 – and an anonymous Shrewsbury chronicler observe that it was 'so fyrse [fierce] and quycke a pestelence that there dyeed more therewith then xv yeres warrs before wastyd within the space of iiij moenthes': *Grafton's Chronicle*, 2 vols (London, 1809), I.742; Leighton, 'Early Chronicles of Shrewsbury', p. 249.

1485 The 'plague of pestilence' that was threatening York in early June may well have been the first outbreak of a new disease known as 'the English sweat', which struck with fearsome rapidity, singling out healthy males in the prime of life. It soon spread south, and on 26 September 'began the swetyng syknesse in London', killing two mayors, four aldermen and 'many worshipfull comoners': Kingsford, *Chronicles of London*, p. 193; *CLB, L*, p. v; J. A. H. Wylie and L. H. Collier, 'The English Sweating Sickness (*Sudor Anglicus*): A Reappraisal', *JHM* 36 (1981), pp. 425–45, on p. 428. Canterbury and Oxford were also badly affected: Hatcher, 'Mortality in the Fifteenth Century', p. 30; Wood, *History and Antiquities of the University of Oxford*, I.462.

1486 A note added to a late fifteenth-century copy of a plague tract records that 'pestilence infected many people' in August: BL, Add. MS 27329, fol. 238v. Meanwhile, 'another pestilential disease' in Oxford led the scholars of Magdalen College to decamp again to the country: Wood, *History and Antiquities of the University of Oxford*, I.642.

1487 On 14 April the business of the law courts in Westminster was postponed until the start of the Trinity term because of an epidemic there and in the London area: W. Campbell, ed., *Materials Illustrative of the Reign of Henry VII*, 2 vols, RS 60 (London, 1873–7), II.136. Plague also broke out in Canterbury: Hatcher, 'Mortality in the Fifteenth Century', p. 30. In Oxford it was reported in July that 'the sekenes of pestilens wych we trustyd to have been cessyd with us now at thys seson sharply begynnyd ayen': HMC, *Report on Manuscripts in Various Collections*, vol. 1, Royal Commission on Historical Manuscripts 55 (London, 1901), p. 224.

1490–1 The death rate rose appreciably at Westminster abbey: Harvey, *Living and Dying*, p. 122.

1493–4 York was visited by a 'lamentable plage of pestilence' in the summer, causing many deaths and the flight of other citizens, and lingering until the spring of 1494: Palliser, 'Epidemics in Tudor York', pp. 46–7; *YCR*, II.102, 104. Oxford, too, was badly affected between April and June: Wood, *History and Antiquities of the University of Oxford*, I.650–1.

1497 At about this time England first experienced 'the fowle scabbe and horryble sickness called the freanche pocks', which proved especially virulent during its early decades. Writing in 1529, Sir Thomas More maintained that 'of the french pokkys xxx yere a go went there about syk fyue agaynst one that beggeth with them now': Leighton, 'Early Chronicles of Shrewsbury', p. 250; More, *Supplication of Souls*, pp. 121–2.

1498 In April tenants of the borough of Crossgate in Durham were forbidden to offer hospitality to anyone from Bishop Auckland, where there was an outbreak of pestilence ('eo quod pestelencia est regnans ibidem'), under threat of a substantial 20s. fine: *RBC*, no. 140.

1499–1500 'The greate syknesse, wherof dyed within the Citie of London moch people of all maner of ages' (Kingsford, *Chronicles of London*, p. 232; Fabyan, *New Chronicles*, p. 687) is described by at least one chronicler as a national epidemic: Charles Wriothesley, *A Chronicle of England during the Reigns of the Tudors*, ed. W. D. Hamilton, vol. 1, CS n.s. 11 (London, 1875), p. 4. Death rates escalated in Westminster (Rosser, *Medieval Westminster*, p. 178), and many perished in Oxford (Wood, *History and Antiquities of the University of Oxford*, I.658–9). The epidemic also reached Bury St Edmunds: R. S. Gottfried, *Bury St. Edmunds and the Urban Crisis, 1290–1539* (Princeton, NJ, 1982), p. 64.

1501 A 'sekencz of pestilence' struck York, perhaps as a continuation of the previous year's epidemic: Palliser, 'Epidemics in Tudor York', p. 47. Plague was also recorded in Canterbury (Hatcher, 'Mortality in the Fifteenth Century', p. 30; HMC, *Ninth Report*, part 1, appendix, p. 147), and was still not 'clean purged' from Gravesend by October (Creighton, *History of Epidemics*, pp. 288–9).

1503 A serious outbreak of plague lasting from August to December prompted an exodus of Oxford students, and spread as far as Exeter: Wood, *History and Antiquities of the University of Oxford*, I.660–1. Mortality rates were also high in Norwich and the north: Slack, *Impact of Plague*, pp. 61, 84, 114; Goldberg, 'Mortality and Economic Change', p. 48.

1504–5 The poet and chronicler Bernard André left London for some time because of pestilence: Bernard André, *Historia regis Henrici septimi*, ed. J. Gairdner, RS 10 (London, 1858), p. 88.

1505–6 Death rates were unusually high in the north, a 'plague of pestilence' being recorded at Ripon: Goldberg, 'Mortality and Economic Change', p. 48; Palliser, 'Epidemics in Tudor York', p. 47; J. T. Fowler, ed., *Acts of the Chapter of the Collegiate Church of SS. Peter and Wilfrid, Ripon, 1452–1506*, Surtees Society

2 (Durham, 1875), part 1, p. 312. Parts of the south, including Canterbury, were similarly affected: Hatcher, 'Mortality in the Fifteenth Century', p. 30.

1506–7 In early October the mayor and aldermen of Chester explained that the city had been 'so visited with plague' as to prevent any of them from attending the council of the Marches. Either this epidemic or another one of sweating sickness reputedly killed ninety-one householders in three days, all but four of them male: G. Ormerod, *The History of the County Palatine and City of Chester*, vol. 1, 2 parts (London, 1882), p. 234. Pestilence is also recorded in Oxford: Wood, *History and Antiquities of the University of Oxford*, II.14.

1508 Death rates were high in the north between 1508 and 1510, perhaps as a result of an influenza epidemic: Goldberg, 'Mortality and Economic Change', p. 48. References by Wylie and Collier to outbreaks of sweating sickness in Oxford and Cambridge ('English Sweating Sickness', p. 430) are, however, based on a misdating of the 1517 evidence (see below).

1509 Bury St Edmunds was struck by an epidemic, as was Oxford: Gottfried, *Bury St. Edmunds*, p. 64; Wood, *History and Antiquities of the University of Oxford*, II.14.

1510 Studies at Oxford were once again suspended because of pestilence: Wood, *History and Antiquities of the University of Oxford*, II.2.

1511 In mid-September Erasmus noted that plague had broken out in London; it had grown 'violent' by early October, but had 'entirely gone' by 28 November, when Cambridge was still devoid of scholars because of fear of infection: *LPFD*, vol. 1, part 1, nos 865, 890–1, 905, 917, 933, 964. Oxford was likewise affected: Wood, *History and Antiquities of the University of Oxford*, II.14.

1513 Plague had reached London by September, and 'as war' was reputedly causing between three and four hundred deaths a day there within a month: *LPFD*, vol. 1, part 2, nos 2223, 2278, 2412; *CSP Venice, 1509–1519*, nos 333, 353, 360. Lectures were suspended at Cambridge during the Michaelmas term for fear of pestilence, and teaching at Oxford seems to have been similarly disrupted: Cooper, *Annals of Cambridge*, p. 295; Wood, *History and Antiquities of the University of Oxford*, II.6.

1514 A 'great sickness' led the royal court to leave London at Whitsuntide: *LPFD*, vol. 1, part 2, no. 2929. Lectures were again suspended at Oxford and Cambridge during the Michaelmas term as a precautionary measure: Wood, *History and Antiquities of the University of Oxford*, II.14; Cooper, *Annals of Cambridge*, p. 297. An epidemic also hit Nottingham: Stevenson, *Records of the Borough of Nottingham*, III.130–1.

1515 On 20 April a jittery Erasmus reported the return of pestilence to London, where especially heavy losses were sustained among the nuns of Aldgate: *LPFD*, vol. 2, part 1, no. 338; Nichols, *Chronicles of the Grey Friars*, p. 29.

1516 A 'contagious plague' in the earl of Shrewsbury's household prevented him from attending court in April, and in May Cardinal Wolsey's establishment succumbed. Thanks to prompt action, the epidemic appears to have been contained: *LPFD*, vol. 2, part 1, no. 1832; *CSP Venice, 1509–1519*, no. 737.

1517 Pestilence struck Chester with such a devastating effect on civic life 'that for want of trading the grass did grow a foot high at the cross and other streets in the city': Ormerod, *County Palatine and City of Chester*, I.i.234. In addition, an unusually deadly epidemic of the sweating sickness erupted in London in late summer, 'so cruell that it killed some within three houres', including several royal courtiers. On 19 August, Sir Thomas More reported that 'we are all in the greatest sorrow and danger; many are dying all around, almost everybody in Oxford, in Cambridge, in London has fallen ill over the last few days, and we have lost many of our best and most honoured friends': Desiderius Erasmus, *Opvs epistolarvm Des. Erasmi Roterdami*, ed. P. S. Allen, vol. 3 (Oxford, 1913), no. 623. Within a month people were also leaving the City because of a 'great plague', this being a year marked by 'generall famyn and pestelence', as well as 'the sweats': Wylie and Collier, 'English Sweating Sickness', p. 430; *CSPVenice, 1509–1519*, nos 944, 975, 975, 987, 990, 993, 996, 1000; *LPFD*, vol. 2, part 2, nos 3558, 3675, 3723, 3747. Oxford was predictably affected by both epidemics, 'to the dispersion and sweeping away of most, if not all of the students': Wood, *History and Antiquities of the University of Oxford*, II.13–14. By December 'pestilence' had reached the Scottish border: R. Welford, *History of Newcastle and Gateshead in the Sixteenth Century* (London, 1885), pp. 47–8.

1518 'The great death of pestilence, almost over all England in euery towne more or lesse' continued: John Stow, *Annales, or a Generall Chronicle of England* (London, 1631), p. 507. Plague struck the royal household in March, and in July the king left his refuge in Wallingford because of high mortality in the area, 'not only of the small pokkes and mezils, but also of the great sickness': *CSPVenice, 1509–1519*, nos 1015, 1046, 1057; *LPFD*, vol. 2, part 2, no. 4320. Measures devised by Cardinal Wolsey at the start of the year for quarantining 'the plague sick' in London were introduced to Oxford in April, but with limited success. It was reported in early November that the 'pestis inguinaria' had raged there for three months: *LPFD*, vol. 2, part 2, no. 4125, appendix no. 56.

1519 An outbreak of 'contageous sykkenesse' was evidently feared in the Cambridge area, as the queen wrote to enquire if it was safe to visit: Cooper, *Annals of Cambridge*, p. 302. Reports of a July epidemic in Coventry ('the plage rayneth sore') are supported by an increase in mortality rates: Phythian-Adams, *Desolation of a City*, p. 54.

1520 In September the Venetian ambassador reported that Henry VIII had left London, 'the plague being very rife': *CSPVenice, 1520–1526*, no. 123.

1521 Alarm was voiced in Basingstoke in April about vagrants who brought 'the reigning sickness' from other areas, placing the townspeople at risk of infection: Baigent and Millard, *History of the Town and Manor of Basingstoke*, p. 325. Not surprisingly, London again succumbed to 'a great pestilence and death', which lasted until November and spread to many other parts of England: Stow, *Annales*, p. 514; Grafton, *Grafton's Chronicle*, II.315; *LPFD Appendix*, vol. 1, no. 42. An outbreak of plague in Lincoln is noted on 16 July (HMC, *Fourteenth Report*, appendix 8, p. 29), and Lord Darcy was then informed that 'the sickness is somewhat quick in York and likely to be more' (*LPFD*, vol. 12, part 2, no. 186, p. 66).

In Cambridge, although surprisingly not in London, the start of the Michaelmas term was postponed for fear of infection: Cooper, *Annals of Cambridge*, p. 304; *LPFD Appendix*, vol. 1, no. 42, pp. 70–1.

1524 Cambridge University postponed the start of Easter term because of pestilence: Cooper, *Annals of Cambridge*, p. 310.

1525 In July it was reported that 'the plague is raging most violently in London', seizing upwards of fifty victims a day. A general exodus rapidly ensued. The Michaelmas law term was adjourned at Westminster because of the continuing 'great death', and Henry VIII, who had remained safely away from the capital, spent Christmas at Eltham 'for to eschue the plague': *CSP Venice, 1520–1526*, nos 1073, 1096, 1187, 1193; Grafton, *Grafton's Chronicle*, II.386. By mid-August 'the dethe' had reached Coventry (BL, MS Cotton Titus B I, fol. 81v), and yet again scholars left Oxford in droves because of 'a vehement plague': Wood, *History and Antiquities of the University of Oxford*, II.26.

1526 Many people fled London from May onwards in order to escape a serious epidemic, which caused so much panic that 'far greater caution than usual' was observed by the citizenry: *CSP Venice, 1520–1526*, no. 1294; *LPFD*, vol. 4, part 1, no. 2343. Easter term was again postponed at Cambridge for fear of infection (Cooper, *Annals of Cambridge*, p. 324), and 'plague' apparently reached as far as Shrewsbury (Leighton, 'Early Chronicles of Shrewsbury', p. 254).

1528 There was another major epidemic of sweating sickness, which took a particularly heavy toll in London before moving north. Forty-one people allegedly died of it in one night in Chester, and by December it had reached Sheriff Hutton: Wylie and Collier, 'English Sweating Sickness', p. 431; Lewis and Thacker, *VCH City of Chester*, II.71; Welford, *History of Newcastle and Gateshead in the Sixteenth Century*, p. 105. The Capital was also affected by plague, which brought government business to a halt in July: *CSP Venice, 1527–1533*, nos 320, 329.

1529 Easter term was dissolved at Cambridge for fear of plague (Cooper, *Annals of Cambridge*, p. 330), which afflicted London during the summer and early autumn. At the start of July the Imperial ambassador reported that 'the plague commences to rage vigorously and there is some fear of the sweating sickness': *CSP Venice, 1527–1533*, nos 504, 506; *LPFD*, vol. 4, part 3, no. 5636. The death rate remained high at Westminster abbey into the following year: Harvey, *Living and Dying*, p. 122.

1530 Parliament was prorogued on 26 April for two months 'on account of the pestilence in London and its suburbs'. It did not meet again until October because of the risks of infection: *LPFD*, vol. 4, part 3, no. 6356; *CSP Venice, 1527–1533*, no. 569. Bury St Edmunds was also affected: Gottfried, *Bury St Edmunds*, p. 64.

✒ Bibliography

✒ Manuscript Sources

Bodleian Library, Oxford
MSS Ashmole 855, 1505
MS Gough Norfolk 20
MSS Rawl. B.335, B.352

Borthwick Institute, York
York Registry Wills, iii

British Library, London
Add. Charter 19137
Add. MSS 6214, 6716, 24459, 27329, 27582, 37503
MS Arundel 42
MSS Cotton Claudius D II; Cleopatra C V; Julius B IV; Tiberius C V; Titus B I
MSS Egerton 1995, 2091, 2107, 2572
MSS Harley 3, 1736, 2378, 2390, 4015, 6388
MS Royal 7 F XI
MSS Sloane 5, 73, 122, 213, 282, 388, 398, 428, 983, 2435, 3285, 3489

Cambridge University Library
MS Ll.i.18

Chester City Archives
M/B/5k
ZS/B/4c, Sheriffs' Book, 1493; ZS/B/5a, Sheriffs' Book, 1502–1503; ZS/B/5b, Sheriffs' Book, 1504–1505; ZS/B/5d, Sheriffs' Book, 1508–1509; ZS/B/5f, Sheriffs' Book, 1510–1511; ZS/B/5g, Sheriffs' Book, 1512–1513

Corporation of London Records
Journal 8

Devon Record Office, Exeter
ECA, Book 51, Commonplace Book of John Hooker; Book 53A, Cartulary of St John's Hospital, Exeter
ECA, Chamber Act Book 1, 1508–1538
ECA, Mayor's Court Roll, 1421–1422
ED/MAG/43, 50, 62, 76, 168; ED/WA/2

Dorset Record Office
DC/LR B1/2 nos. 3, 8, 9, 13, 16, 19
D/SHA A1–19, A30

Glasgow University Library Special Collections

MSS Hunter 95, 117 (T.5.19), 307, 509, 513

J. Paul Getty Museum, Los Angeles

MS 83.ML.114

King's Lynn Borough Archives

KL/C7/2, Hall Book, 1422–1429; C7/3, Hall Book, 1431–1450; C7/4, Hall Book, 1453–1497; C7/5, Hall Book, 1497–1544
KL/C10/1
KL/C12/1/3, C/12/5, 7, 11
KL/C17/10, leet roll, 1379–80
KL/C39/39–45
KL/C50/63, 451

Lincolnshire Archives Office

Episcopal Register V (Burghersh)

The National Archives, Kew

C1/19/65, 42/108, 68/44, 131/8, 252/13–16, 309/43–4
C66/444, 446, 447
C270/20, 22
E101/128/30
E175/11/65; E179/242/25; E315/38
PROB 11/1, 5, 7, 16, 17
SC8/1/34; 3/103; 13/641; 23/1119, 1121; 27/1372; 76/3767; 90/4470, 4477; 99/4905; 100/4954; 129/6428; 130/6453; 142/7088; 223/11117; 250/12465; 259/12941; 269/13419; 299/14935, 14942
SP1/106

New College, Oxford

MS 3691

New York Public Library

MS Spencer 65

Norfolk Record Office

BL/R/8/1
DCN 2/5/8
NCR, 7C, Treasurers' Account, 1411–1412; 7D, Treasurers' Accounts, 1422–1423, 1426–1427; Chamberlains' Account, 1457–1458
NCR, 8A/1–2
NCR, 16A/1, Mayor's Book, 1424–1449; 16A/2, Mayor's Book, 1510–1532; 16A/4, Mayor's Court Book, 1534–1549
NCR, 16C/1, Assembly Minute Book, 1492–1550; 16C/2, Assembly Minute Book, 1510–1550
NCR, 16D/1, Assembly Proceedings, 1434–1491; 16D/2, Assembly Proceedings, 1491–1553; 16D/3, Assembly Proceedings, 1553–1583

NCR, 18A/2, Chamberlains' Accounts, 1470–1490; 18A/5, Chamberlains' Accounts, 1531–1537
NCR, 22G/1, Lease Book A
NCR, 24A, Great Hospital Accounts for Norwich Properties, 1415–1460, account for 1460–1461
NCR, 24B/25
Norwich Consistory Court, Registers Gyles, Heydon, Ryxe and Spyltymber
Notebook of John Kirkpatrick, on deposit from the Fitch Collection
Y/C4/93, 96, 103, 104, 105, 116, 139, 147, 149, 171, 186, 189, 190, 191, 202
Y/C18/1

Pierpont Morgan Library, New York

MS M.165

Suffolk Record Office, Ipswich

C/2/8/1/2–22; C/2/10/1/2–5, 7; C5/9
IC/AA2/2

Trinity College, Cambridge

MS R.14.32

Wellcome Institute Library, London

Western MSS 404, 408, 411, 564

Wiltshire Record Office

G23/1/2, Salisbury Ledger Book 2

York City Archives

Chamberlains' Account Book 2, 1520–1525

✒ Printed Primary Sources

Aberth, J., ed., *The Black Death: The Great Mortality of 1348–1350* (Boston, 2005)
Adam of Usk, *Chronicon Adae de Usk*, ed. E. M. Thompson (London, 1904)
Aldobrandino of Siena, *Le Régime du corps de Maître Aldebrandin de Sienne*, ed. L. Landouzy and R. Pépin (Paris, 1911)
Al-Majusi (Haly Abbas), *Liber Pantegni* (Lyon, 1515)
André, Bernard, *Historia regis Henrici septimi*, ed. J. Gairdner, RS 10 (London, 1858)
Andrew, M., and R. Waldron, eds, *The Poems of the Pearl Manuscript: Pearl, Cleanness, Patience, Sir Gawain and the Green Knight* (London, 1978)
Androw of Wyntoun, *The Orygynale Cronykil of Scotland*, ed. D. Laing, 3 vols (Edinburgh, 1872–9)
Archer, I., C. Barron and V. Harding, eds, *Hugh Alley's Caveat: The Markets of London in 1598*, London Topographical Society 137 (London, 1988)
Arnald de Villanova, *Arnaldi de Villanova opera medica omnia*, vol. 10.1: *Regimen sanitatis ad regem Aragonum*, ed. L. García-Ballester and M. R. McVaugh (Barcelona, 1996)

Arnold, M. S., ed., *Select Cases of Trespass from the King's Courts, 1307–1399*, vol. 2, Selden Society 103 (London, 1987)

Astle, T., ed., *The Will of King Henry VII* (London, 1785)

Attreed, L. C., ed., *York House Books, 1461–1490*, 2 vols (Stroud, 1991)

Augustine, *De ordine*, in *Contra academicos; De beata vita; De ordine; De magistro; De libero arbitrio*, ed. W. M. Green and K. D. Daur, Corpus Christianorum Series Latina 29 (Turnhout, 1970)

—— *Concerning the City of God against the Pagans*, ed. and trans. H. Bettenson (London, 1984)

Avicenna, *see* Ibn-Sīna

Bacon, Sir Francis, *The Essayes or Counsels Civill and Morall*, ed. M. Kiernan (Oxford, 1985)

Bacon, Nicholas, *Annalls of Ipswiche*, ed. W. H. Richardson (Ipswich, 1884)

Ballard, A., ed., *British Borough Charters, 1042–1216* (Cambridge, 1913)

Baron, X., ed., *London, 1066–1914: Literary Sources and Documents*, vol. 1: *Medieval, Tudor, Stuart and Georgian London, 1066–1800* (Mountfield, 1997)

Bartholomaeus Anglicus, *On the Properties of Things: John Trevisa's Translation of Bartholomaeus Anglicus De Proprietatis Rerum*, ed. M. C. Seymour, 3 vols (Oxford, 1975–88)

Bateson, M., ed., *Records of the Borough of Leicester*, vols 1 and 2 (London, 1899–1901)

——, ed., *Borough Customs*, vol. 1, Selden Society 18 (London, 1904; repr. 1972)

Benham, W. G., ed., *The Red Paper Book of Colchester* (Colchester, 1902)

Bernard of Clairvaux, 'In nativitate Beatae Virginis Mariae', in *Sermones de sanctis*, Patrologia Latina 183 (1854), cols 437–48

—— *Œuvres complètes*, vol. 21: *La conversion*, ed. J. Leclercq *et al.* (Paris, 2000)

Bickley, F. B., ed., *The Little Red Book of Bristol*, 2 vols (Bristol, 1900)

Bird, W. H. B., ed., *The Black Book of Winchester* (Winchester, 1925)

Blythe, J. M., ed. and trans., *On the Government of Rulers: De regimina principium: Ptolemy of Lucca with Portions attributed to Thomas Aquinas* (Philadelphia, 1997)

Bond, E. A., ed., *Chronicon monasterii de Melsa*, 3 vols, RS 43 (London, 1866–8)

Boorde, Andrew, *A Compendyous Regyment or a Dyetary of Healthe* (London, 1547)

—— *The Breviary of Helthe* (London, 1547)

Bradshaw, Henry, *The Life of Saint Werburge of Chester*, ed. C. Horstmann, EETS o.s. 88 (London, 1887)

Brain, P., ed., *Galen on Bloodletting* (Cambridge, 1986)

Brandeis, A., ed., *Jacob's Well*, EETS o.s. 115 (London, 1890)

Brewer, J. S., *et al.*, eds, *Letters and Papers, Foreign and Domestic, of the Reign of Henry VIII*, 21 vols, and *Addenda*, 2 vols (London, 1862–1932)

Bridget of Sweden, *The Liber Celestis*, ed. R. Ellis, vol. 1: *Text*, EETS o.s. 291 (Oxford, 1987)

Brie, F. W. D., ed., *The Brut*, vol. 1, EETS o.s. 131 (London, 1906)

Briers, P. M., ed., *Henley Borough Records: Assembly Books i–iv, 1395–1543*, Oxfordshire Record Society 41 (Banbury, 1960)

Britnell, R., ed., *Records of the Borough of Crossgate, Durham, 1312–1531*, Surtees Society 212 (Woodbridge, 2008)

Bromyard, John, *Summa praedicantium*, 2 vols (Venice, 1586)

Brown, R., ed., *Calendar of State Papers and Manuscripts Relating to English Affairs, Existing in the Archives and Collections of Venice, 1202–1554*, 5 vols (London, 1864–73)

Brown, W., ed., *Yorkshire Inquisitions*, vol. 2, YASRS 23 (Worksop, 1898)

Butler, C., ed., *The Book of Fines: The Annual Accounts of the Mayor of Southampton*, vol. 1: *1488–1540*, Southampton Record Society 41 (Southampton, 2008)

Caius, John, *A Boke, or Conseill against the Disease Commonly Called the Sweate, or Sweatyng Sicknesse* (London, 1552)

Calendar of Close Rolls, 1277–1509, 63 vols (London, 1892–1963)

Calendar of Inquisitions Miscellaneous, 1219–1485, 8 vols (London, 1916–2003)

Calendar of Liberate Rolls, 1251–1260 (London, 1960)

Calendar of Patent Rolls, 1216–1509, 54 vols (London, 1894–1916)

Caley, J., and J. Hunter, eds, *Valor ecclesiasticus, temp. Henrici VIII*, 6 vols (London, 1810–34)

Cameron Gillies, H., ed., *Regimen sanitatis: The Rule of Health* (Glasgow, 1911)

Cameron Gruner, O., ed., *A Treatise on the Canon of Medicine of Avicenna* (London, 1930)

Campbell, W., ed., *Materials Illustrative of the Reign of Henry VII*, 2 vols, RS 60 (London, 1873–7)

Carr, D. R., ed., *The First General Entry Book of the City of Salisbury 1387–1452*, Wiltshire Record Society 54 (Trowbridge, 2001)

Chaucer, Geoffrey, *The Riverside Chaucer*, ed. L. D. Benson (Oxford 1987)

Cheeke, Sir John, 'The Hurt of Sedition', in *Holinshed's Chronicles of England, Scotland and Ireland*, vol. 3 (London, 1808)

Chew, H. M., and W. Kellaway, eds, *The London Assize of Nuisance, 1301–1431*, LRS 10 (London, 1973)

Chew, H. M., and M. Weinbaum, eds, *London Eyre of 1244*, LRS 6 (London, 1970)

Cleese, J., *et al.*, *Monty Python and the Holy Grail: The Screenplay* (London, 2002)

Clode, C. M., ed., *Memorials of the Guild of Merchant Taylors* (London, 1875)

Cogan, Thomas, *The Haven of Health* (London, 1584)

Connor, M., ed., *John Stone's Chronicle, Christ Church Priory, Canterbury, 1417–1472* (Kalamazoo, MI, 2010)

Cooper, C. H., ed., *Annals of Cambridge*, vol. 1 (Cambridge, 1842)

Corrie, G. E., ed., *Sermons by Hugh Latimer* (Cambridge, 1844)

Cowper, J. M., ed., *Henry Brinklow's Complaynt of Roderyck Mors*, EETS e.s. 22 (London, 1874)

Dallaway, J., ed., *Antiquities of Bristow* (Bristol, 1834)

Davies, M., ed., *The Merchant Taylors' Company of London: Court Minutes, 1486–1493* (Stamford, 2000)

Davis, N., ed., *Paston Letters and Papers of the Fifteenth Century*, 2 vols (Oxford, 1971–6)

Dawson, W. R., ed., *A Leechbook, or Collection of Medical Recipes of the Fifteenth Century* (London, 1934)

Dermott Harding, N., ed., *Bristol Charters, 1155–1373*, Bristol Record Society 1 (Bristol, 1930)

Devon, F., ed., *Issues of the Exchequer* (London, 1847)

Dickens, Charles, *Dombey and Son* (Harmondsworth, 1985)

—— *Master Humphrey's Clock* (Oxford, 1958)

Diepgen, P., and J. Ruska, eds, *Quellen und Studien zur Geschichte der Naturwissenschaften und der Medizin*, vol. 5 (Berlin, 1936)

Dilks, T. B., ed., *Bridgwater Borough Archives, 1377–1399*, Somerset Record Society 53 (Bridgwater, 1938)

Dobson, R. B., ed., *York City Chamberlains' Account Rolls, 1396–1500*, Surtees Society 192 (Gateshead, 1980)

——, ed., *The Peasants' Revolt of 1381*, 2nd edn (London, 1983)

Dormer Harris, M., ed., *The Coventry Leet Book 1420–1555*, 4 parts, EETS o.s. 134, 135, 138, 146 (London, 1907–13)

Douglas, D. C., and G. W. Greenaway, eds, *English Historical Documents*, vol. 2: *1042–1189* (Oxford, 1981)

Drew, C., ed., *Lambeth Churchwardens' Accounts, 1504–1645*, vol. 1, Surrey Record Society 40 (London, 1940)

Dugdale, William, *The Antiquities of Warwickshire*, 2 vols (London, 1730)

—— *Monasticon Anglicanum*, ed. J. Caley *et al.*, 6 vols (London, 1817–30)

Dunbar, William, *The Poems of William Dunbar*, ed. J. Kinsley (Oxford, 1979)

Dunstan, G. R., ed., *The Register of Edmund Lacy, Bishop of Exeter, 1420–1455: Registrum Commune*, vol. 3, Devon and Cornwall Record Society n.s. 13 (Torquay, 1968)

Easting, R., ed., *The Revelation of the Monk of Eynsham*, EETS o.s. 318 (Oxford, 2002)

Eiximenis, Francesc, *Regiment de la Cosa Publica*, ed. P. D. de Molins de Rei (Barcelona, 1927)

Elyot, Sir Thomas, *The Castel of Helthe* (London, 1539)

—— *The Boke Named the Gouernour*, ed. H. H. S. Croft, 2 vols (New York, 1967)

Erasmus, Desiderius, *Opvs epistolarvm Des. Erasmi Roterodami*, ed. P. S. Allen, vol. 3 (Oxford, 1913)

—— *Enchiridion militis Christiani*, ed. A. M. O'Donnell, EETS o.s. 282 (Oxford, 1981)

Evelyn, John, *Fumifugium: Or, the Inconvenience of the Aer and Smoak of London Dissipated* (London, 1661)

Fabyan, Robert, *The New Chronicles of England and France*, ed. H. Ellis (London, 1811)

Finn, A., ed., *Records of Lydd* (Ashford, 1911)

Fish, Simon, *A Supplicacyon for the Beggars*, ed. F. J. Furnivall, EETS e.s. 13 (London, 1871)

Fisher, John, *The English Works of John Fisher*, ed. J. E. B. Mayor, EETS e.s. 27 (London, 1876)

Fisher, J. L., ed., 'The Leger Book of St John's Abbey, Colchester', *Transactions of the Essex Archaeological Society* n.s. 24 (1951), pp. 77–127

Fitzherbert, Anthony, *The New Natura Brevium* (London, 1677)

Flower, C. T., ed., *Public Works in Medieval Law*, 2 vols, Selden Society 32, 40 (London, 1915, 1923)

Fortescue, Sir John, *De natura legis naturae*, ed. T. Clermont (London, 1869)

—— *The Governance of England*, ed. C. Plummer (Oxford, 1875)

Fowler, J. T., ed., *Acts of the Chapter of the Collegiate Church of SS. Peter and Wilfrid, Ripon, 1452–1506*, Surtees Society 2 (Durham, 1875)

Fraser, C. M., ed., *The Accounts of the Chamberlains of Newcastle upon Tyne, 1508–1511*, The Society of Antiquaries of Newcastle upon Tyne Records Series 3 (Newcastle, 1987)

Furley, J. S., ed., *Town Life in the XIV Century as Seen in the Court Rolls of Winchester* (Winchester, 1946)

Furnivall, F. J., ed., *The Babees Book*, EETS o.s. 32 (London, 1868)

Gairdner, J., ed., *The Historical Collections of a Citizen of London*, CS n.s. 17 (London, 1876)

——, ed., *Three Fifteenth-Century Chronicles*, CS n.s. 28 (London, 1880)

Galbraith, V. H., ed., *The Anonimalle Chronicle, 1333 to 1381* (Manchester, 1927)

Getz, F. M., ed., *Healing and Society in Medieval England* (Madison, WI, 1991)

Gibson, S., ed., *Statvta antiqva vniversitatis Oxoniensis* (Oxford, 1931)

Gidden, H. W., ed., *The Book of Remembrance of Southampton*, vol. 2, Southampton Record Society 28 (Southampton, 1928)

——, ed., *The Stewards' Books of Southampton, from 1428*, 2 vols, Southampton Record Society 35, 39 (Southampton, 1935, 1939)

Gilbertus Anglicus, *Compendium medicine* (Lyon, 1510)

Given-Wilson, C., *et al.*, eds, *The Parliament Rolls of Medieval England, 1275–1504*, 16 vols (Woodbridge, 2005)

Gower, John, *The Complete Works*, ed. G. C. Macaulay, vol. 1 (Oxford, 1899)

Grafton, Richard, *Grafton's Chronicle*, 2 vols (London, 1809)

Grant, E., ed., *A Source Book in Medieval Sciences* (Cambridge, MA, 1974)

Grant, M., ed. and trans., *Galen on Food and Diet* (London, 2000)

Griffiths, J., ed., *The Two Books of Homilies Appointed to be Read in Churches*, 2 vols (Oxford, 1859)

Gross, C., ed., *The Gild Merchant*, 2 vols (Oxford, 1890)

Guilding, J. M., ed., *Reading Records: Diary of the Corporation*, vol. 1 (London, 1892)

Guy de Chauliac, *The Cyrurgie of Guy de Chauliac*, ed. M. S. Ogden, EETS o.s. 265 (Oxford, 1971)

Gwynn Jones, T., ed., *Gwaith Tudur Aled*, 2 vols (Cardiff, 1926)

Haas, E. de, and G. D. G. Hall, eds, *Early Registers of Writs*, Selden Society 87 (London, 1970)

Halliwell, J. O., ed., *A Chronicle of the First Thirteen Years of the Reign of King Edward the Fourth*, CS 10 (London, 1839)

Hanham, A., ed., *The Cely Letters, 1472–1488*, EETS o.s. 273 (Oxford, 1975)

Harding, V., and L. Wright, eds, *London Bridge: Selected Accounts and Rentals, 1381–1538*, LRS 31 (London, 1995)

Harington, Sir John, *The School of Salernum: Regimen sanitatis salernitanum* (London, 1922)

Harrington, D., and P. Hyde, eds, *The Early Town Books of Faversham, c. 1215–1581* (Chippenham, 2008)

Hearne, T., ed., *Thomae de Elmham vita et gesta Henrici Quinti* (Oxford, 1727)

Heath Barnum, P., ed., *Dives and Pauper*, vol. 1, 2 parts, EETS o.s. 275, 280 (Oxford, 1976, 1980)

Helmholz, R. H., ed., *Select Cases on Defamation to 1600*, Selden Society 101 (London, 1985)

Henderson, W. G., ed., *Missale ad usum insignis ecclesiae Eboracensis*, vol. 2, Surtees Society 60 (Durham, 1872)

Henri de Mondeville, *Chirurgie de Maitre Henri de Mondeville*, ed. E. Nicaise (Paris, 1893)

Henry of Lancaster, *Le Livre de seyntz medicines*, ed. E. J. Arnould (Oxford, 1940)

Here Begynneth A Litill Boke Necessarye & Behouefull agenst the Pestilence (London, 1485)

Hieatt, C. B., and S. Butler, eds, *Curye On Inglysch: English Culinary Manuscripts of the Fourteenth Century*, EETS s.s. 8 (London, 1985)

Higden, Ranulph, *Polychronicon Ranulphi Higden*, ed. J. R. Lumby, 9 vols, RS 41 (London, 1865–86)

Hinds, A., ed., *Calendar of State Papers Milanese*, vol. 1 (London, 1912)

Hippocrates, *The Medical Works of Hippocrates*, ed. J. Chadwick and W. N. Mann (Oxford, 1950)

HMC, *Fourth Report*, Royal Commission on Historical Manuscripts 3 (London, 1874)

—— *Sixth Report*, Royal Commission on Historical Manuscripts 5 (London, 1877)

—— *Eighth Report*, part 1, Royal Commission on Historical Manuscripts 7 (London, 1881)

—— *Ninth Report*, part 1, Royal Commission on Historical Manuscripts 8 (London, 1883)

—— *Eleventh Report*, appendix 7: *Supplementary report on the manuscripts of the Duke of Leeds, the Bridgewater trust, Reading corporation, the Inner Temple, etc.*, Royal Commission on Historical Manuscripts 22 (London, 1888)

—— *Twelfth Report*, appendix 9: *The manuscripts of the Duke of Beaufort, K. G., the Earl of Donoughmore, and others*, Royal Commission on Historical Manuscripts 27 (London, 1891)

—— *Fourteenth Report*, appendix 8: *The manuscripts of Lincoln, Bury St. Edmund's, and Great Grimsby corporations; and of the deans and chapters of Worcester and Lichfield*, Royal Commission on Historical Manuscripts 37 (London, 1895)

—— *Report on the Manuscripts of the Corporation of Beverley*, Royal Commission on Historical Manuscripts 54 (London, 1900)

—— *Report on Manuscripts in Various Collections*, vol. 1, Royal Commission on Historical Manuscripts 55 (London, 1901)

—— *Calendar of the Manuscripts of the Dean and Chapter of Wells*, vol. 1, Royal Commission on Historical Manuscripts 12 (London, 1907)

—— *Report on Records of the City of Exeter*, Royal Commission on Historical Manuscripts 73 (London, 1916)

Hodgson, P., and G. M. Liegey, eds, *The Orcherd of Syon*, vol. 1, EETS o.s. 258 (London, 1966)

Horrox, R., ed., *Selected Rentals and Accounts of Medieval Hull, 1293–1528*, YASRS 141 (Leeds, 1983)

——, ed., *The Black Death* (Manchester, 1995)

Hudson, A., ed., *Selections from English Wycliffite Writings* (Cambridge, 1978)

Hudson, N., ed., *Hortus sanitatis* (London, 1954)

Hudson, W., ed., *Leet Jurisdiction in the City of Norwich during the Thirteenth and Fourteenth Centuries*, Selden Society 5 (London, 1892)

Hudson, W., and J. C. Tingey, eds, *Records of the City of Norwich*, 2 vols (Norwich, 1906–10)

Hunt, T., ed., *Popular Medicine in Thirteenth-Century England* (Woodbridge, 1990)

Ibn-Sīna (Avicenna), *Liber canonis medicine* (Lyon, 1522)

Isaacson, R. F., and H. Ingleby, eds, *The Red Register of King's Lynn*, 2 vols (King's Lynn, n.d.)

Jacme d'Agramont, *Regiment de preservació de pestilència*, ed. J. Veny (Lerida, 1998)

Jacob, E. F., ed., *The Register of Henry Chichele, Archbishop of Canterbury, 1414–1443*, vol. 2 (Oxford, 1937)

Jeayes, I. H., ed., *Description of Documents Contained in the White Vellum Book of Scarborough* (Scarborough, 1914)

——, ed., *Court Rolls of the Borough of Colchester*, 3 vols (Colchester, 1938–41)

Johannes de Trokelowe, *Chronica et annales*, ed. H. T. Riley, RS 28.3 (London, 1866)

John of Amundesham (Amersham), *Annales monasterii S. Albani*, ed. H. T. Riley, 2 vols, RS 28.5 (London, 1870–1)

John of Arderne, *Treatises of Fistula in Ano*, ed. D. Power, EETS o.s. 139 (London, 1910)

John of Fordun, *John of Fordun's Chronicle of the Scottish Nation*, ed. W. F. Skene (Edinburgh, 1872)

John of Gaddesden, *Rosa Anglica practica medicine a capite ad pedes* (Pavia, 1492)

John of Salisbury, *The Letters of John of Salisbury*, vol. 1: *The Early Letters, 1153–1161*, ed. W. J. Millor, H. E. Butler and C. N. L. Brooke (London, 1955)

—— *Policraticus: Of the Frivolities of Courtiers and the Footprints of Philosophers*, ed. and trans. C. J. Nederman (Cambridge, 1990)

Johnson, G., ed., 'Chronological Memoranda Touching the City of Norwich', *NA* 1 (1847), pp. 140–66

Journal of the House of Lords, vol. 1: *1509–1557* (London, 1767)

Juvenal, *The Sixteen Satires*, trans. P. Green, rev. edn (Harmondsworth, 1974)

Kail, J., ed., *Twenty-Six Political and Other Poems*, EETS o.s. 124 (London, 1904)

Kempe, Margery, *The Book of Margery Kempe*, ed. S. B. Meech, EETS o.s. 212 (London, 1940)

Kerling, N., ed., *The Cartulary of St Bartholomew's Hospital* (London, 1973)

Khol, B. G., and R. G. Witt, eds, *The Early Republic: Italian Humanists on Government and Society* (Manchester, 1978)

Kingdon, J. A., ed., *Ms. Archives of the Worshipful Company of Grocers of the City of London, 1345–1463*, 2 vols (London, 1886)

Kingsford, C. L., ed., *Chronicles of London* (Oxford, 1905; repr. Stroud, 1977)

Knox, R., and S. Leslie, eds, *The Miracles of King Henry VI* (London, 1923)

Lanfrank of Milan, *Lanfrank's 'Science of Cirurgie'*, ed. R. von Fleischhacker, EETS o.s. 102 (London, 1894)

Langland, William, *Piers the Plowman in Three Parallel Texts*, ed. W. W. Skeat, 2 vols (Oxford, 1886)

Latini, Brunetto, *Li Livres dou tresor*, ed. P. Barrette and S. Baldwin (New York, 1993)

Lawrence, Edward, *Christs Power over Bodily Diseases* (London, 1672)

Leach, A. F., ed., *Visitations and Memorials of Southwell Minster*, CS n.s. 48 (London, 1891)

——, ed., *Beverley Town Documents*, Selden Society 14 (London, 1900)

Lee, W., *Report to the General Board of Health on a Preliminary Inquiry into the Sewerage, Drainage and Supply of Water, and the Sanitary Conditions of the Inhabitants of the City of Norwich* (London, 1851)

Leighton, W. A., ed., 'Early Chronicles of Shrewsbury, 1372–1603', *Transactions of the Shropshire Archaeological and Natural History Society*, 1st series 3 (1880), pp. 239–352

Leland, John, *Itinerary*, ed. L. T. Smith, 5 vols (London, 1907–10)

Lespinasse, R. de, ed., *Les Métiers et corporations de la ville de Paris*, 3 vols (Paris, 1886–97)

Lespinasse, R. de, and F. Bonnardot, eds, *Les Métiers et corporations de la ville de Paris: XIIIe siècle: Le Livre des métiers d'Étienne Boileau* (Paris, 1879)

Luard, H. R., ed., *Annales monastici*, 5 vols, RS 36 (London, 1866)

Lucianus of Chester, *Liber Luciani de laude Cestrie*, ed. M. V. Taylor, Lancashire and Cheshire Record Society 64 (London, 1912)

Luders, A., *et al.*, eds, *Statutes of the Realm*, 11 vols (London, 1810–28)

Lumiansky, R. M., and D. Mills, eds, *The Chester Mystery Cycle*, vol. 1, EETS s.s. 3 (London, 1974)

Lydgate, John, *Lydgate and Burgh's 'Secrees of Old Philisoffres'*, ed. R. Steele, EETS e.s. 66 (London, 1894)

—— *Lydgate's Troy Book*, ed. H. Bergen, vol. 1, EETS e.s. 97 (London, 1906)

—— *The Minor Poems of John Lydgate*, ed. H. N. MacCracken, 2 vols, EETS e.s. 107, o.s. 192 (London, 1911, 1934; vol. 2 repr. 1961)

Lyell, L., ed., *Acts of Court of the Mercers' Company, 1453–1527* (Cambridge, 1936)

Maimonides, Moses, *The Guide of the Perplexed*, ed. and trans. S. Pines (Chicago, 1963)

Maitland, F. W., ed., *Memoranda de Parliamento*, RS 98 (London, 1893)

Maitland, F. W., and M. Bateson, eds, *The Charters of the Borough of Cambridge* (Cambridge, 1901)

Mallock, W. H., *The New Republic: or Culture, Faith and Philosophy in an English Country House* (London, 1878)

Mandeville, Bernard, *The Fable of the Bees: Or, Private Vices, Public Benefits*, ed. F. B. Kaye, 2 vols (Oxford, 2001)

Manship, Henry, *The History of Great Yarmouth*, ed. C. J. Palmer (Yarmouth, 1854)

Markham, C. A., ed., *The Liber custumarum* (Northampton, 1895)

Markham, C. A., and J. C. Cox, eds, *Records of the Borough of Northampton*, 2 vols (Northampton, 1898)

Martin, G. H., ed., *Knighton's Chronicle, 1337–1396* (Oxford, 1995)

Marwick, J. D., ed., *Extracts from the Records of the Burgh of Edinburgh, 1403–1528* (Edinburgh, 1869)

Maxwell-Lyte, H. C., and M. B. C. Dawes, eds, *The Register of Thomas Bekington*, vol. 1, Somerset Record Society 49 (London, 1934)

Mayo, C. H., and A. W. Gould, eds, *The Municipal Records of the Borough of Dorchester, Dorset* (Exeter, 1908)

McNeill, J. T., and H. M. Gamer, eds, *Medieval Hand-Books of Penance* (New York, 1965)

Memoranda, References and Documents Relating to the Royal Hospitals of the City of London (London, 1863)

Merson, A. L., ed., *The Third Book of Remembrance of Southampton* vol. 2, Southampton Records Series 3 (Southampton, 1955)

Monson, Robert, *A Briefe Declaration for What manner of Speciall Nusance concerning dwelling Houses, a man may have his remedy by Assize* (London, 1639)

Moore, N., ed., *The Book of the Foundation of St Bartholomew's Church in London*, EETS o.s. 163 (London, 1923)

Moore, S. A., ed., *Letters and Papers of John Shillingford*, CS n.s. 2 (London, 1871)

More, Thomas, *Utopia*, ed. and trans. R. M. Adams (New York, 1975)

—— *The Supplication of Souls*, in F. Manley *et al.*, eds, *The Complete Works of St. Thomas More*, vol. 7 (New Haven, CT, 1990)

Morris, R., ed., *An Old English Miscellany*, EETS o.s. 49 (London, 1872)

——, ed., *Old English Homilies of the Twelfth Century*, EETS o.s. 53 (London, 1873)

Moryson, Fynes, *An Itinerary*, 4 vols (Glasgow, 1907)

Myers, A. R., ed., *The Household of Edward IV* (Manchester, 1959)

Nederman, C. J., and K. Langdon Forhan, eds, *Medieval Political Theory: A Reader: The Quest for the Body Politic, 1100–1400* (London, 1993)

Nicholas of Cusa, *The Catholic Concordance*, ed. and trans. P. E. Sigmund (Cambridge, 1995)

Nichols, J. G., ed., *Chronicles of the Grey Friars of London*, CS 53 (London, 1852)

Nicolas, H., ed., *Proceedings and Ordinances of the Privy Council of England*, 7 vols (London, 1834–7)

Northeast, P., and H. Falvey, eds, *Wills of the Archdeaconry of Sudbury, 1439–1474: Wills from the Register 'Baldwyne'*, part 2, Suffolk Records Society 53 (Woodbridge, 2010)

Ogden, M. S., ed., *The liber de diversis medicinis*, EETS o.s. 207 (London, 1938)

Ovid, *Metamorphoses*, ed. A. D. Melville (Oxford, 1986)

Owen, D. M., ed., *The Making of King's Lynn: A Documentary Survey*, Records of Social and Economic History n.s. 9 (Oxford, 1984)

Palmer, W. M., ed., *Cambridge Borough Documents*, vol. 1 (Cambridge, 1931)

Paris, Matthew, *Chronica majora*, ed. H. R. Luard, 7 vols, RS 57 (London, 1872–84)

—— *The Illustrated Chronicles of Matthew Paris: Observations of Thirteenth-Century Life*, ed. and trans. R. Vaughan (Stroud, 1993)

Paynell, Thomas, *A Moche Profitable Treatise against the Pestilence* (London, 1534)

Percy, J. W., ed., *York Memorandum Book*, vol. 3, Surtees Society 186 (Gateshead, 1973)

Phaer, Thomas, *A Treatyse of the Pestylence* (London, 1544)

Powell Harley, M., ed., *A Revelation of Purgatory by an Unknown, Fifteenth-Century Woman Visionary*, Studies in Women and Religion 18 (New York, 1985)

Power, E., ed., *The Goodman of Paris* (London, 1928)

Preest, D., trans., and J. G. Clark, *The Chronica Maiora of Thomas Walsingham, 1376–1422* (Woodbridge, 2005)

Prestwich, M., ed., *York Civic Ordinances, 1301*, Borthwick Paper 49 (York, 1976)

Prevet, F., ed., *Les Statuts et règlements des apothicairès*, 15 vols (Paris, 1950)

Raine, A., ed., *York Civic Records*, vols 1–4, YASRS 98, 103, 106, 108 (Wakefield, 1939–45)

Raine, J., ed., *Testamenta Eboracensia*, vol. 3, Surtees Society 44 (Durham, 1865)
——, ed., *The Register of William Gray*, Surtees Society 56 (Durham, 1870)
Ramsay, N., and J. M. Willoughby, eds, *Hospitals, Towns and the Professions*, Corpus of British Medieval Library Catalogues 14 (London, 2009)
Rawcliffe, C., ed., 'The Cartulary of St Mary's Hospital, Yarmouth', in C. Rawcliffe, M. Bailey and M. Jurkowski, eds, *Poverty and Wealth: Sheep, Taxation and Charity in Late Medieval Norfolk*, Norfolk Record Society 71 (Norwich, 2007)
Ricart, Richard, *The Maire of Bristowe Is Kalendar*, ed. L. T. Smith, CS n.s. 5 (London, 1872)
Riley, H. T., ed., *Ingulf's Chronicle of the Abbey of Croyland* (London, 1854)
——, ed., *Munimenta Gildhallae Londoniensis*, 3 vols, RS 12 (London, 1859–62)
——, ed., *Liber albus: The White Book of the City of London* (London, 1861)
——, ed., *Chronicles of the Mayors and Sheriffs of London* (London, 1863)
——, ed. and trans., *Memorials of London and London Life in the XIIIth, XIVth and XVth Centuries* (London, 1868)
Rishanger, William, *Chronica et annales, 1259–1307*, ed. H. T. Riley, RS 28.2 (London, 1865)
Robert of Brunne, *Robert of Brunne's 'Handlyng Synne'*, ed. F. J. Furnivall, 2 vols, EETS o.s. 119, 123 (London, 1901, 1903; repr. in 1 vol., 1973)
Rogers, A., ed., *William Browne's Town: The Stamford Hall Book*, vol. 1: *1465–1492* (Stamford, 2005)
Ross, C., ed., *The Cartulary of St Mark's Hospital, Bristol*, Bristol Record Society 21 (Bristol, 1959)
Ross, W. O., ed., *Middle English Sermons Edited from British Museum MS Royal 18 B XXIII*, EETS o.s. 209 (London, 1940)
Rothwell, H., ed., *English Historical Documents*, vol. 3: *1189–1327* (London, 1975)
Salter, F. R., ed., *Some Early Tracts on Poor Relief* (London, 1926)
Salter, H. E., ed., *Records of Medieval Oxford: Coroners' Inquests* (Oxford, 1912)
——, ed., *Mediaeval Archives of the University of Oxford*, vol. 1, Oxford Historical Society 70 (Oxford, 1920)
——, ed., *Munimenta civitatis Oxonie*, Oxford Historical Society 71 (Oxford, 1920)
Schopp, J. W., ed., *The Anglo-Norman Custumal of Exeter* (Oxford, 1925)
Second Report of the Royal Commission for Inquiring into the State of Large Towns and Populous Districts (London, 1845)
Sellars, M., ed., *York Memorandum Book*, vols 1 and 2, Surtees Society, 120, 125 (Durham, 1912, 1915)
Shah, M. H., ed. and trans., *The General Principles of Avicenna's Canon of Medicine* (Karachi, 1966)
Sharpe, R. R., ed., *Calendar of Letters from the Mayor and Corporation of the City of London, 1350–1370* (London, 1885)
——, ed., *Calendar of Wills Proved and Enrolled in the Court of Husting of London, 1258–1668*, 2 vols (London, 1889–90)
——, ed., *Calendar of Letter-Books Preserved among the Archives of the Corporation of the City of London, 1275–1498*, 11 vols, A–L (London, 1899–1912)
——, ed., *Calendar of Coroners' Rolls of the City of London, 1300–1378* (London, 1913)
Simmons, T. F., and H. E. Nolloth, eds, *The Lay Folk's Catechism*, EETS o.s. 118 (London, 1901)
Skaife, R. H., ed., *The Register of the Guild of Corpus Christi of the City of York*, Surtees Society 57 (Durham, 1871)
Skelton, John, *The Complete English Poems*, ed. J. Scattergood (New Haven, CT, 1983)

Slade, C., ed., *Reading Gild Accounts 1357–1516*, part 1, Berkshire Record Society 6 (Reading, 2002)

Smith, J. J., ed., *Abbreviata chronica ab anno 1377 usque ad annum 1469*, Cambridge Antiquarian Society 2 (Cambridge, 1840)

Smith, T., L. T. Smith and L. Brentano, eds, *English Gilds*, EETS o.s. 40 (London, 1892)

Sneyd, C. A., ed., *A Relation of the Island of England*, CS 37 (London, 1847)

Spector, S., ed., *The N-Town Play*, vol. 1: *Introduction and Text*, EETS s.s. 11 (Oxford, 1991)

Starkey, Thomas, *A Dialogue between Pole and Lupset*, ed. T. F. Mayer, CS 4th series 37 (London, 1989)

Steele, R., ed., *Three Prose Versions of the 'Secreta Secretorum'*, EETS e.s. 74 (London, 1898)

Steer, F. W., ed., 'The Statutes of Saffron Walden Almshouses', *Transactions of the Essex Archaeological Society*, n.s. 25 (1955–60), pp. 161–221

Stefanutti, U., ed., *Documentazioni cronologiche per la storia della medicina, chirurgia e farmacia in Venezia dal 1258 al 1332* (Venice, 1961)

Stell, P., trans., *The York Bridgemasters' Accounts* (York, 2003)

Stell, P., and L. Hampson, eds, *Probate Inventories of the York Diocese, 1350–1500* (York, 2006)

Stevenson, W. H., ed., *Records of the Borough of Nottingham*, vols 1–3 (London, 1882–5)

——, ed., *Calendar of the Records of the Corporation of Gloucester* (Gloucester, 1893)

Stow, G. B., ed., *Historia vitae et regni Ricardi secundi* (Philadelphia, 1977)

Stow, John, *Annales, or a Generall Chronicle of England* (London, 1631)

—— *Survey of London*, ed. C. L. Kingsford, 2 vols (Oxford, 1908)

Strachey, J., ed., *Rotuli Parliamentorum*, 6 vols (London, 1783–1832)

Stuart, J., ed., *Extracts from the Council Register of the Burgh of Aberdeen, 1398–1570* (Aberdeen, 1844)

Stubbs, W., ed., *Chronicles of the Reigns of Edward I and Edward II*, 2 vols, RS 76 (London, 1882–3)

Studer, P., ed., *The Oak Book of Southampton of c. AD 1300*, 3 vols, Southampton Record Society 10, 11 (Southampton, 1910–11)

Thomas, A. H., ed., *Calendar of the Early Mayors' Court Rolls of the City of London, 1298–1307* (Cambridge, 1924)

——, ed., *Calendars of Plea and Memoranda Rolls Preserved among the Archives of the Corporation of the City of London, 1298–1482*, 6 vols (Cambridge, 1926–61)

Thomas of Monmouth, *The Life and Miracles of St William of Norwich*, ed. A. Jessopp and M. R. James (Cambridge, 1896)

Thomson, T., and C. Innes, eds, *The Acts of the Parliament of Scotland*, 12 vols (Edinburgh, 1844–75)

Thorne, S. E., ed., *Bracton on the Laws and Customs of England*, 4 vols (Cambridge, MA, 1968–77)

Toulmin Smith, L., ed., *York Plays* (New York, 1963)

Trampe Bödtker, A. F., ed., *The Middle English Versions of 'Partonope of Blois'*, EETS e.s. 109 (London, 1911)

Twemlow, J. A., ed., *Calendar of Papal Letters*, vols 8, 11, 12 (London, 1909–33)

Twiss, T., ed., *The Black Book of the Admiralty*, 4 vols, RS 55 (London, 1871–6)

Tymms, S., ed., *Wills and Inventories from the Registers of the Commissary of Bury St. Edmund's*, CS 49 (London, 1850)

Veale, E. W. W., ed., *The Great Red Book of Bristol*, vols 1 and 3, Bristol Record Society 4, 16 (Bristol, 1933, 1951)

Vives, Juan Luis, *De subventione pauperum*, ed. and trans C. Matheeussen and C. Fantazzi (Leiden, 2002)

Voigts, L. E., and M. R. McVaugh, eds, 'A Latin Technical Phlebotomy and its Middle English Translation', *Transactions of the American Philosophical Society* 74.2 (1984), pp. 1–69

Vowell, John, *alias* Hooker, *Description of the Citie of Excester*, vol. 3, Devon and Cornwall Record Society o.s. 14 (Exeter, 1919)

Walsingham, Thomas, *Historia Anglicana*, ed. H. T. Riley, 2 vols, RS 28.1 (London, 1863–4)

Weinbaum, M., ed., *The London Eyre of 1276*, LRS 12 (London, 1976)

Wenzel, S., ed., *Fasciculus morum: A Fourteenth-Century Preacher's Handbook* (University Park, PA, 1989)

Whitaker, Tobias, *Peri ydroposias: or, a discourse of waters their qualities, and effects diaeteticall, pathologicall, and pharmacaiticall* (London, 1634)

Whittaker, W. J., ed. *The Mirror of Justices*, Selden Society 7 (London, 1895)

Wilkins, D., ed., *Concilia Magnae Britanniae*, 3 vols (London, 1737)

Williams, C. H., ed., *English Historical Documents*, vol. 5: *1485–1558* (London, 1967)

Williams, E., ed., *Early Holborn and the Legal Quarter of London*, 2 vols (London, 1927)

Woolgar, C., ed., *Household Accounts from Medieval England*, vol. 1, Records of Social and Economic History n.s. 17 (Oxford, 1992)

Worcestre, William, *Itineraries*, ed. J. H. Harvey (Oxford, 1969)

Wright, T., ed., *Political Poems and Songs*, 2 vols, RS 14 (London, 1859)

Wriothesley, Charles, *A Chronicle of England During the Reigns of the Tudors*, ed. W. D. Hamilton, vol. 1, CS n.s. 11 (London, 1875)

❧ Printed Secondary Sources

Aberth, J., *From the Brink of the Apocalypse: Confronting Famine, War, Plague, and Death in the Later Middle Ages*, 2nd edn (London, 2010)

Adamson, M. W., *Medieval Dietetics: Food and Drink in the Regimen Sanitatis Literature, 800–1400* (Frankfurt, 1995)

Addyman, P. V., 'The Archaeology of Public Health at York, England', *World Archaeology* 21 (1989), pp. 244–64

Alaba, K., *Eating Right in the Renaissance* (Berkeley, CA, 2002)

Alexander, J., and P. Binski, eds, *Age of Chivalry: Art in Plantagenet England* (London, 1987)

Allen, D., 'The Public Water Supply of Ipswich before the Municipal Corporation Act', *Proceedings of the Suffolk Institute of Archaeology* 40 (2001), pp. 31–54

Allison, K. J., ed., *VCH York: East Riding*, vols. 1 and 6 (London, 1969; Oxford, 1989)

Amor, N. R., *Late Medieval Ipswich: Trade and Industry* (Woodbridge, 2011)

Amundsen, D. W., and G. B. Ferngren, 'Philanthropy and Medicine: Some Historical Perspectives', *Philosophy and Medicine* 11 (1982), pp. 1–31

Armstrong, A., 'Population, 1700–1950', in C. Rawcliffe and R. Wilson, eds, *Norwich since 1550* (London, 2004)

Arrizabalaga, J., 'Facing the Black Death: Perceptions and Reactions of University Medical Practitioners', in J. Arrizabalaga *et al.*, eds, *Practical Medicine from Salerno to the Black Death* (Cambridge, 1994)

Arrizabalaga, J., J. Henderson and R. French, *The Great Pox: The French Disease in Renaissance Europe* (New Haven, CT, 1997)

Ashenburg, K., *Clean: An Unsanitised History of Washing* (London, 2007)

Atkin, M., 'Medieval Clay-Walled Building in Norwich', *NA* 41 (1991), pp. 171–85

Atkin, M., and D. H. Evans, *Excavations in Norwich, 1971–1978*, part 3, EAA 100 (Norwich, 2002)

Attreed, L., *The King's Towns: Identity and Survival in Late Medieval English Boroughs* (New York, 2001)

Aungier, G. J., *The History and Antiquities of Syon Monastery* (London, 1840)

Avril, J., 'Le IIIe Concile du Latran et les communautés de lepreux', *Revue Mabillon* 60 (1981), pp. 21–76

Ayers, B., *Digging Deeper: Recent Archaeology in Norwich* (Norwich, 1987)

——, ed., *Excavations at Fishergate, Norwich, 1985*, EAA 68 (Norwich, 1994)

—— 'The Infrastructure of Norwich from the Twelfth to the Seventeenth Centuries', in M. Gläser, ed., *Lübecker Kolloquium zur Stadtarchäologie im Hanseraum IV: Die Infrastruktur* (Lübeck, 2004)

—— *Norwich: Archaeology of a Fine City* (Stroud, 2009)

Baigent, F. J., and J. E. Millard, *A History of the Town and Manor of Basingstoke* (Basingstoke, 1889)

Bailey, M., 'Demographic Decline in Late Medieval England: Some Thoughts on Recent Research', *EconHR*, 2nd series 49 (1996), pp. 1–19

Baker, J. H., *An Introduction to English Legal History*, 2nd edn (London, 1979)

Barkan, L., *Nature's Work of Art: The Human Body in the Image of the World* (New Haven, CT, 1975)

Barron, C., 'London, 1300–1540', in D. M. Palliser, ed., *The Cambridge Urban History of Britain*, vol. 1: *600–1540* (Cambridge, 2000)

—— *London in the Later Middle Ages: Government and People, 1200–1500* (Oxford, 2004)

Barron, C. M., C. Coleman, and C. Gobbi, 'The London Journal of Alessandro Magno 1562', *London Journal* 9 (1983), pp. 136–52

Barron, C. M., and M. Davies, eds, *The Religious Houses of London and Middlesex* (London, 2007)

Bartlett, N., 'Lay Poll Tax Returns for the City of York in 1381', *Transactions of the East Riding Antiquarian Society* 30 (1953), pp. 1–91

Bassett, M., 'Newgate Prison in the Middle Ages', *Speculum* 18 (1943), pp. 233–46

Bean, J. M. W., 'Plague, Population and Economic Decline in England during the Later Middle Ages', *EconHR*, 2nd series 15 (1963), pp. 423–37

Beard, M., *Pompeii: The Life of a Roman Town* (London, 2008)

Beck, R. T., *The Cutting Edge: Early History of the Surgeons of London* (London, 1974)

Beckwith, S., *Signifying God: Social Relation and Symbolic Act in the York Corpus Christi Plays* (Chicago, 2001)

Bennett, J. M., 'Conviviality and Charity in Medieval and Early Modern England', *P&P* 34 (1992), pp. 19–41

—— *Ale, Beer and Brewsters in England: Women's Work in a Changing World* (Oxford, 1996)

Berger, P., 'Mice, Arrows and Tumours: Medieval Plague Iconography North of the Alps', in F. Mormando and T. Worcester, eds, *Piety and the Plague from Byzantium to the Baroque* (Kirksville, MO, 2007)

Besant, W., *Mediaeval London*, vol. 1: *Historical and Social* (London, 1906)

Biddle, M., ed., *Winchester in the Early Middle Ages* (Oxford, 1976)

Biddle, M., and R. N. Quirk, 'Excavations near Winchester Cathedral, 1961', *Archaeological Journal* 119 (1962), pp. 150–94

Bindoff, S. T., ed., *The History of Parliament: The House of Commons, 1509–1558*, 3 vols (London, 1982)

Biow, D., *The Culture of Cleanliness in Renaissance Italy* (Ithaca, NY, 2006)

Bird, R., *The Turbulent London of Richard II* (London, 1949)

Blaisdell, J. D., 'Rabies in Shakespeare's England', *Historia medicinae veterinariae* 16 (1991), pp. 1–48

—— 'To the Pillory for Putrid Poultry: Meat Hygiene and the Medieval London Butchers, Poulterers and Fishmongers Companies', *Veterinary History* 9 (1997), pp. 114–24

Blaxland Stubbs, S. G., and E. W. Bligh, *Sixty Centuries of Health and Physic: The Progress of Ideas from Primitive Magic to Modern Medicine* (London, 1931)

Blomefield, F., *An Essay towards a Topographical History of the County of Norfolk*, 11 vols (London, 1805–10)

Bocchi, F., 'Regulation of the Urban Environment by the Italian Communes from the Twelfth to the Fourteenth Century', *Bulletin of the John Rylands Library* 72 (1990), pp. 63–78

Bolton, J. L., *The Medieval English Economy, 1150–1500* (London, 1980)

—— '"The World Upside Down": Plague as an Agent of Economic and Social Change', in W. M. Ormrod and P. G. Lindley, eds, *The Black Death in England* (Stamford, 1996)

Bond, C. J., 'Water Management in the Urban Monastery', in R. Gilchrist and H. Mytum, eds, *Advances in Monastic Archaeology*, BAR British series 227 (Oxford, 1993)

Bonfield, C., 'Medical Advice and Public Health: Contextualising the Supply and Regulation of Water in Medieval London and King's Lynn', *Poetica* 72 (2009), pp. 1–20

Bonney, M., *Lordship and the Urban Community: Durham and its Overlords, 1250–1540* (Cambridge, 1990)

Bossy, J., 'The Mass as a Social Institution, 1200–1700', *P&P* 100 (1983), pp. 29–61

Boucheron, P., 'Water and Power in Milan, *c.* 1200–1500', *Urban History* 28 (2000), pp. 180–93

Bowers, J. M., 'Piers Plowman and the Unwillingness to Work', *Mediaevalia* 9 (1983), pp. 239–49

Bowers, K. W., 'Balancing Industrial and Communal Needs: Plague and Public Health in Early Modern Seville', *BHM* 81 (2007), pp. 335–58

Boys, W., *Collections for a History of Sandwich*, 2 vols (Canterbury, 1792)

Brennand, M., and K. J. Stringer, *The Making of Carlisle: From Romans to Railways*, Cumberland and Westmorland Antiquarian and Archaeological Society e.s. 35 (Kendal, 2011)

Brimblecombe, P., 'Early Urban Climate and Atmosphere', in A. R. Hall and H. K. Kenward, eds, *Environmental Archaeology in the Urban Context*, CBA research report 43 (London, 1982)

—— *The Big Smoke: A History of Air Pollution in London since Medieval Times* (London, 1987)

Britnell, R. H., *Growth and Decline in Colchester, 1300–1525* (Cambridge, 1986)

—— 'Forstall, Forestalling, and the Statute of Forestallers', *EHR* 102 (1987), pp. 89–102

—— *The Commercialisation of English Society, 1000–1500* (Cambridge, 1993)

—— 'The Black Death in English Towns', *Urban History* 21 (1994), pp. 195–210

—— 'Price-Setting in English Borough Markets, 1349–1500', *Canadian Journal of History* 31 (1996), pp. 1–15

—— 'The Economy of British Towns, 600–1300', in D. M. Palliser, ed., *The Cambridge Urban History of Britain*, vol. 1: *600–1540* (Cambridge, 2000)

—— 'The Economy of British Towns, 1300–1540', in D. M. Palliser, ed., *The Cambridge Urban History of Britain*, vol. 1: *600–1540* (Cambridge, 2000)

—— 'Town Life', in R. Horrox and W. M. Ormrod, eds, *A Social History of England, 1200–1500* (Cambridge, 2006)

Brown, A., ed., *The Rows of Chester*, English Heritage Archaeological Report 16 (London, 1999)

Brown, A. D., *Popular Piety in Late Medieval England: The Diocese of Salisbury, 1250–1550* (Oxford, 1995)

Brown, P., *The Body and Society: Men, Women and Sexual Renunciation in Early Christianity* (New York, 1988)

Bullough, V., and C. Campbell, 'Female Longevity and Diet in the Middle Ages', *Speculum* 55 (1980), pp. 317–25

Butcher, A. F., 'Rent, Population and Economic Change in Late-Medieval Newcastle', *Northern History* 14 (1978), pp. 67–77

Campbell, B. M. S., *et al.*, *A Medieval Capital and its Grain Supply* (London, 1993)

Campbell, J., 'Power and Authority, 600–1300', in D. M. Palliser, ed., *The Cambridge Urban History of Britain*, vol. 1: *600–1540* (Cambridge, 2000)

—— 'Norwich before 1300', in C. Rawcliffe and R. Wilson, eds, *Medieval Norwich* (London, 2004)

Camporesi, P., *The Fear of Hell: Images of Damnation and Salvation in Early Modern Europe*, trans. L. Byatt (Oxford, 1991)

Carlin, M., 'Medieval English Hospitals', in L. Granshaw and R. Porter, eds, *The Hospital in History* (London, 1990)

—— *Medieval Southwark* (London, 1996)

—— 'Fast Food and Urban Living Standards in Medieval England', in M. Carlin and J. T. Rosenthal, eds, *Food and Eating in Medieval Europe* (London, 1998)

Carmichael, A., 'Plague Legislation in the Italian Renaissance', *BHM* 57 (1983), pp. 508–25

—— *Plague and the Poor in Renaissance Florence* (Cambridge, 1986)

Carr, D. R., 'From Pollution to Prostitution: Supervising the Citizens of Fifteenth-Century Salisbury', *Southern History* 19 (1997), pp. 24–41

—— 'Controlling the Butchers in Late Medieval English Towns', *The Historian* 70 (2008), pp. 450–61

Carter, A., and J. P. Roberts, 'Excavations in Norwich – 1972', *NA* 35 (1970–2), pp. 443–68

—— 'Excavations in Norwich, 1973', *NA* 36 (1973–77), pp. 39–71

Carus-Wilson, E. M., 'The Iceland Trade', in E. Power and M. M. Postan, eds, *Studies in English Trade in the Fifteenth Century* (London, 1933)

Carver, M. O. H., 'Early Shrewsbury: An Archaeological Definition in 1975', *Transactions of the Shropshire Archaeological Society* 59 (1973–4), pp. 225–63

Catto, J., 'Andrew Horn: Law and History in Fourteenth-Century England', in R. H. C. Davis and J. M. Wallace-Hadrill, eds, *The Writing of History in the Middle Ages* (Oxford, 1981)

—— 'Religious Change under Henry V', in G. L. Harriss, ed., *Henry V: The Practice of Kingship* (Oxford, 1985)

—— 'Wyclif and Wycliffism at Oxford, 1356–1430', in J. Catto and R. Evans, eds, *The History of the University of Oxford*, vol. 2: *Late Medieval Oxford* (Oxford, 1992)

Champion, B., *Everyday Life in Tudor Shrewsbury* (Shrewsbury, 1994)

Cherry, J., 'Leather', in J. Blair and N. Ramsay, eds, *English Medieval Industries* (London, 1991)

Choay, F., 'La Ville et le domaine bâti comme corps dans les textes des architectes-théoriciens de la première Renaissance italienne', *Nouvelle Revue de psychanalyse* 9 (1974), pp. 239–51

Cholmeley, H. P., *John of Gaddesden and The Rosa Medicinae* (Oxford, 1912)

Chrimes, S. B., *English Constitutional Ideas in the Fifteenth Century* (Cambridge, 1936)

Christie, J., *Some Account of Parish Clerks, More Especially of the Ancient Fraternity of S. Nicholas* (London, 1893)

Cipolla, C. M., *Public Health and the Medical Profession in the Renaissance* (Cambridge, 1976)

—— *Miasmas and Disease: Public Health and the Environment in the Pre-Industrial Age* (London, 1992)

Clanchy, M. T., *From Memory to Written Record: England, 1066–1307* (Oxford, 1993)

Clark, G., *A History of the Royal College of Physicians*, 2 vols (Oxford, 1964)

Clark, P., *The English Alehouse: A Social History, 1200–1830* (London, 1983)

Clarke, H., *et al.*, *Sandwich: A Study of the Town and Port from its Origins to 1600* (Oxford, 2010)

Classen, C., D. Howes and A. Synnott, *Aroma: The Cultural History of Smell* (London, 1994)

Cockayne, E., *Hubbub: Filth, Noise and Stench in England, 1600–1770* (New Haven, CT, 2007)

Cohn, S., *The Black Death Transformed: Disease and Culture in Early Renaissance Europe* (London, 2001)

—— 'Triumph over Plague: Culture and Memory after the Black Death', in T. van Bueren, ed., *Care for the Here and the Hereafter: Memoria, Art and Ritual in the Middle Ages* (Turnhout, 2005)

Condon, M., 'The Last Will of Henry VII: Document and Text', in T. Tatton-Brown and R. Mortimer, eds, *Westminster Abbey: The Lady Chapel of Henry VII* (Woodbridge, 2003)

Connor, R. D., *The Weights and Measures of England* (London, 1987)

Cooper, T. P., 'The Mediaeval Highways, Streets, Open Ditches, and Sanitary Conditions of the City of York', *Yorkshire Archaeological Journal* 22 (1912), pp. 270–86

Coote, H. C., 'The Ordinances of Some Secular Guilds of London', *TLMAS* 4 (1871), pp. 1–59

Coulton, G. G., *Medieval Panorama* (Cambridge, 1939)

Cox, R., 'Dishing the Dirt', in R. Cox *et al.*, *Dirt: The Filthy Reality of Everyday Life* (London, 2011)

Coyecque, E., *L'Hôtel Dieu de Paris au môyen âge*, 2 vols (Paris, 1889–91)

Crawford, D. H., *Deadly Companions: How Microbes Shaped Our History* (Oxford, 2007)

Creighton, C., *History of Epidemics in Britain*, vol. 1: *From AD 664 to the Great Plague* (London, 1894)

Cromarty, D., *Everyday Life in Medieval Shrewsbury* (Shrewsbury, 1991)

Cullum, P. H., *Cremetts and Corrodies: Care of the Poor and Sick at St Leonard's Hospital, York, in the Middle Ages*, Borthwick Paper 79 (York, 1991)

—— 'Leper-Houses and Borough Status in the Thirteenth Century', *Thirteenth Century England* 3 (1991), pp. 37–46

—— '"And Hir Name Was Charite": Charitable Giving by and for Women in Late Medieval Yorkshire', in P. J. P. Goldberg, ed., *Woman is a Worthy Wight: Women in English Society, c. 1200–1500* (Stroud, 1992)

—— '"For Pore People Harberles": What was the Function of the *Maison Dieu*?', in D. J. Clayton, R. G. Davies and P. McNiven, eds, *Trade, Devotion and Governance: Papers in Later Medieval History* (Stroud, 1994)

Cullum, P. H., and P. J. P. Goldberg, 'Charitable Provision in Late Medieval York: "To the Praise of God and the Use of the Poor"', *Northern History* 29 (1993), pp. 24–39

Curry, W. C., *Chaucer and the Medieval Sciences*, 2nd edn (London, 1960)

Curtis, V. A., 'Dirt, Disgust and Disease: A Natural History of Hygiene', *Journal of Epidemiology and Community Health* 61.8 (2007), pp. 660–4

Davis, J., 'Baking for the Common Good: A Reassessment of the Assize of Bread in Medieval England', *EconHR*, 2nd series 57 (2004), pp. 465–502

Dawes, J. D., and J. R. Magilton, *The Archaeology of York*, vol. 12.1: *The Cemetery of St Helen-on-the-Walls, Aldwark* (London, 1980)

De Rouffignac, C., 'Parasite Remains from Excavations at St Mary Spital, London', Museum of London report 102 (London, 1992)

De Windt, A. R., 'Local Government in a Small Town: A Medieval Leet Jury and its Constituents', *Albion* 23 (1991), pp. 627–54

Demaitre, L., *Doctor Bernard Gordon: Professor and Practitioner* (Toronto, 1980)

—— *Leprosy in Pre-Modern Medicine: A Disease of the Whole Body* (Baltimore, 2007)

—— 'Skin and the City: Cosmetic Medicine as an Urban Concern', in F. E. Glaze and B. K. Nance, eds, *Between Text and Patient: The Medical Enterprise in Medieval and Early-Modern Europe*, Micrologus' Library 39 (Florence, 2011)

Denery, D. G., *Seeing and Being in the Later Medieval World* (Cambridge, 2005)

DeVries, D. N., 'And Away Go Troubles Down the Drain: Late Medieval London and the Poetics of Urban Renewal', *Exemplaria* 8 (1996), pp. 401–18

Dobson, B., 'Urban Decline in Late Medieval England', *TRHS*, 5th series 27 (1977), pp. 1–22

Dobson, M. J., *Contours of Death and Disease in Early Modern England* (Cambridge, 1997)

Dohar, W. J., *The Black Death and Pastoral Leadership: The Diocese of Hereford in the Fourteenth Century* (Philadelphia, 1995)

Douglas, M., *Purity and Danger: An Analysis of the Concepts of Pollution and Taboo* (London, 1994)

Drummond-Murray, J., and J. Liddle, 'Medieval Industry in the Walbrook Valley', *London Archaeologist* 10.4 (2003), pp. 87–94

Duffy, E., *The Stripping of the Altars: Traditional Religion in England, c. 1400–c. 1580* (New Haven, CT, 1992)

—— *The Voices of Morebath* (New Haven, CT, 2003)

Durrant Cooper, W., and T. Ross, 'Notices of Hastings', *Sussex Archaeological Collections* 14 (1862), pp. 65–118

Dutton, P. E., '*Illvstre civitatis et popvli exemplvm*': Plato's *Timaevs* and the Transmission from Calcidius to the End of the Twelfth Century of a Tripartite Scheme of Society', *Mediaeval Studies* 45 (1983), pp. 79–119

Dyer, A., '"Urban Decline" in England, 1377–1525', in T. R. Slater, ed., *Towns in Decline, AD 100–1600* (Aldershot, 2000)

Dyer, C., *Standards of Living in the Later Middle Ages*, rev. edn (Cambridge, 1998)

—— 'Small Towns, 1270–1540', in D. M. Palliser, ed., *The Cambridge Urban History of Britain*, vol. 1: *600–1540* (Cambridge, 2000)

—— 'Did the Rich Really Help the Poor in Medieval England?', in N. Salvador Miguel *et al.*, eds, *Ricos y pobres: opulencia y desarraigo en el occidente medieval*, Actas de la 36 semana de estudios medievales de Estella (Pamplona, 2009)

Elkwall, E., *Street-Names of the City of London* (Oxford, 1954)

Emery, P. A., 'The Franciscan Friary', *Current Archaeology*, 170 (2000), pp. 72–8

—— *Norwich Greyfriars: Pre-Conquest Town and Medieval Friary*, EAA 120 (Dereham, 2007)

Evans, D. H., 'The Infrastructure of Hull between 1270 and 1700', in M. Gläser, ed., *Lübecker Kolloquium zur Stadtarchäologie im Hanseraum IV: Die Infrastruktur* (Lübeck, 2004)

—— 'A Good Riddance to Bad Rubbish? Scatological Musings on Rubbish Disposal and the Handling of "Filth" in Medieval and Early Post-Medieval Towns', in K. de Groote, D. Tys and M. Pieters, eds, *Exchanging Medieval Material Culture*, Relicta Monografiëen 4 (Brussels, 2010)

Evans, T. A. R., 'The Number, Origins and Careers of Scholars', in J. I. Catto and R. Evans, eds, *The History of the University of Oxford*, vol. 2: *Late Medieval Oxford* (Oxford, 1992)

Fabre-Vassas, C., *The Singular Beast: Jews, Christians and the Pig* (New York, 1997)

Fabricus, J., *Syphilis in Shakespeare's England* (London, 1994)

Farmer, D. L., 'Prices and Wages', in H. E. Hallam, ed., *The Agrarian History of England and Wales*, vol. 2: *1042–1350* (Cambridge, 1988)

—— 'Prices and Wages, 1350–1500', in E. Miller, ed., *The Agrarian History of England and Wales*, vol. 3: *1348–1500* (Cambridge, 1991)

Fay, I. H. H., 'English Hygiene', in M. Carver and K. Klapste, eds, *The Archaeology of Medieval Europe: Twelfth to Sixteenth Centuries AD* (Aarhus, 2011)

—— *Health and the City: Environment and Politics in Norwich, 1200–1600* (York, forthcoming)

Finucane, R. C., *The Rescue of the Innocents: Endangered Children in Medieval Miracles* (New York, 1997)

Fisher, F. J., *A Short History of the Worshipful Company of Horners* (London, 1936)

Flaxman, T., and T. Jackson, *Sweet and Wholesome Water: Five Centuries of History of Water-Bearers in the City of London* (Cottisford, 2004)

Fleming, M. L., and E. Parker, *Introduction to Public Health*, 2nd edn (Sydney, 2012)

Fletcher, J. M., 'Linacre's Lands and Lectureships', in F. Maddison, M. Pelling and C. Webster, eds, *Essays on the Life and Work of Thomas Linacre* (Oxford, 1977)

Fraser Brockington, C., *A Short History of Public Health* (London, 1956)

Friedman, J. B., '"He Hath a Thousand Slain in this Pestilence": The Iconography of the Plague in the Late Middle Ages', in F. X. Newman, ed., *Social Unrest in the Late Middle Ages* (London, 1985)

Friedrichs, C. R., *The Early Modern City, 1450–1750* (London, 1995)

Frost, R., 'The Urban Elite', in C. Rawcliffe and R. Wilson, eds, *Medieval Norwich* (London, 2004)

Gairdner, W. T., *Public Health in Relation to Air and Water* (Edinburgh, 1862)

Galloway, J. A., 'London's Grain Supply: Changes in Production, Distribution and Consumption during the Fourteenth Century', *Franco-British Studies* 20 (1995), pp. 23–34

—— 'Driven by Drink? Ale Consumption and the Agrarian Economy of the London Region, *c.* 1300–1400', in M. Carlin and J. T. Rosenthal, eds, *Food and Eating in Medieval Europe* (London, 1998)

Galloway, J. A., D. Keene and M. Murphy, 'Fuelling the City: Production and Distribution of Firewood and Fuel in London's Region, 1290–1400', *EconHR*, 2nd series 49 (1996), pp. 447–72

Galloway, J. A., and M. Murphy, 'Feeding the City: Medieval London and its Hinterland', *The London Journal* 16 (1991), pp. 3–14

García-Ballester, L., 'The Construction of a New Form of Learning and Practising Medicine in Medieval Latin Europe', *Science in Context* 8.1 (1995), pp. 75–102

Gatrell, V., *City of Laughter: Sex and Satire in Eighteenth-Century London* (London, 2007)

Geltner, G., 'Public Health and the Pre-Modern City: A Research Agenda', *History Compass* 10.3 (2012), pp. 231–45

George, M. D., *London Life in the XVIIIth Century* (London, 1925)

Geremek, B., *Poverty: A History* (Oxford, 1997)

Gertsman, E., 'Visualising Death: Medieval Plagues and the Macabre', in F. Mormando and T. Worcester, eds, *Piety and the Plague from Byzantium to the Baroque* (Kirksville, MO, 2007)

Getz, F. M., 'Charity, Translation and the Language of Medical Learning in Medieval England, *BHM* 64 (1990), pp. 1–15

—— 'The Faculty of Medicine before 1500', in J. I. Catto and R. Evans, eds, *The History of the University of Oxford*, vol. 2: *Late Medieval Oxford* (Oxford, 1992)

—— 'Medical Education in England', in V. Nutton and R. Porter, eds, *The History of Medical Education in Britain* (Amsterdam, 1995)

—— *Medicine in the English Middle Ages* (Princeton, NJ, 1998)

Gil-Sotres, P., 'Derivation and Revulsion: The Theory and Practice of Medieval Phlebotomy', in J. Arrizabalaga *et al.*, eds, *Practical Medicine from Salerno to the Black Death* (Cambridge, 1994)

—— 'Els regimina sanitatis', in Arnald de Villanova, *Arnaldi de Villanova opera medica omnia*, vol. 10.1: *Regimen sanitatis ad regem Aragonum*, ed. L. García-Ballester and M. R. McVaugh (Barcelona, 1996)

—— 'The Regimens of Health', in M. D. Grmek, ed., *Western Medical Thought from Antiquity to the Middle Ages* (Cambridge, MA, 1998)

Gilbert, P. K., *Cholera and Nation: Doctoring the Social Body in Victorian England* (Albany, NY, 2008)

Gilchrist, R., 'Christian Bodies and Souls: The Archaeology of Life and Death in Later Medieval Hospitals', in S. Bassett, ed., *Death in Towns: Urban Responses to the Dying and the Dead, 100–1600* (Leicester, 1992)

—— *Contemplation and Action: The Other Monasticism* (Leicester, 1995)

—— *Medieval Life: Archaeology and the Life Course* (Woodbridge, 2012)

Giles, K., *An Archaeology of Social Identity: Guildhalls in York, c. 1350–1630*, BAR British series 315 (Oxford, 2000)

Gill, M., 'The Doom in Holy Trinity Church and Wall-Painting in Medieval Coventry', in L. Monckton and R. K. Morris, eds, *Coventry: Medieval Art, Architecture and Archaeology in the City and its Vicinity* (Leeds, 2011)

Gläser, M., ed., *Lübecker Kolloquium zur Stadtarchäologie im Hanseraum IV: Die Infrastruktur* (Lübeck, 2004)

Goldberg, P. J. P., 'Mortality and Economic Change in the Diocese of York, 1390–1514', *Northern History* 24 (1988), pp. 38–55

—— 'Pigs and Prostitutes: Streetwalking in Comparative Perspective', in K. J. Lewis, N. J. Menuge and K. M. Phillips, eds, *Young Medieval Women* (Stroud, 1999)

—— 'Coventry's "Lollard" Programme of 1492 and the Making of Utopia', in R. Horrox and S. Rees-Jones, eds, *Pragmatic Utopias: Ideals and Communities, 1200–1630* (Cambridge, 2001)

Goldberg, P. J. P., and M. Kowaleski, 'Introduction', in P. J. P. Goldberg and M. Kowaleski, eds, *Medieval Domesticity: Home, Housing and Household in Medieval England* (Cambridge, 2008)

Gottfried, R. S., *Epidemic Disease in Fifteenth Century England* (Brunswick, NJ, 1978)

—— *Bury St. Edmunds and the Urban Crisis, 1290–1539* (Princeton, NJ, 1982)

—— *The Black Death: Natural and Human Disaster in Medieval Europe* (London, 1983)

Gransden, A., 'A Fourteenth-Century Chronicle from the Grey Friars at Lynn', *EHR* 72 (1957), pp. 270–8

Greenslade, M. W., ed., *VCH Stafford*, vol. 3 (Oxford, 1970)

Greenslade, M. W., and D. A. Johnson, eds, *VCH Stafford*, vol. 6 (Oxford, 1979)

Greig, J., 'The Investigation of a Medieval Barrel-Latrine from Worcester', *Journal of Archaeological Science* 8 (1981), pp. 265–82

Grössinger, C., *Picturing Women in Late Medieval and Renaissance Art* (Manchester, 1997)

Guillerme, A., *The Age of Water: The Urban Environment in the North of France,*
  AD 800–1800 (College Station, TX, 1988)
Gunther, R. T., *Early Science in Oxford*, 14 vols (Oxford, 1925–45)
Hagen, A., *A Second Handbook of Anglo-Saxon Food and Drink* (Hockwold cum Wilton,
  1995)
Hale, D. G., *The Body Politic: A Political Metaphor in Renaissance English Literature* (The
  Hague, 1971)
Hammond, P. W., *Food and Feast in Medieval England* (Stroud, 1993)
Hanawalt, B. A., 'Childrearing among the Lower Classes in Late Medieval England',
  Journal of Interdisciplinary History 8 (1977–78), pp. 1–22
—— *Growing Up in Medieval London: The Experience of Childhood in History* (Oxford,
  1993)
Hanna, R., 'Brewing Trouble: On Literature and History – and Ale-Wives', in B. Hanawalt
  and D. Wallace, eds, *Bodies and Disciplines: Intersections of Literature and History in
  Fifteenth-Century England* (Minneapolis, 1996)
Harbottle, B., and M. Ellison, 'An Excavation in the Castle Ditch, Newcastle upon Tyne,
  1974–6', *Archaeologia Aeliana*, 5th series 9 (1981), pp. 75–250
Harris, J. G., 'This Is Not a Pipe: Water, Supply, Incontinent Sources, and the Leaky
  Body Politic', in R. Burt and J. M. Archer, eds, *Enclosure Acts: Sexuality, Property and
  Culture in Early Modern England* (Ithaca, NY, 1994)
—— *Foreign Bodies and the Body Politic: Discourses of Social Pathology in Early Modern
  England* (Cambridge, 1998)
Harris, M., *Good to Eat: Riddles of Food and Culture* (London, 1986)
Harrod, H., *Report on the Deeds and Records of the Borough of King's Lynn* (King's Lynn,
  1874)
Harvey, B. F., 'Introduction: The 'Crisis' of the Early Fourteenth Century', in B. M. S.
  Campbell, ed., *Before the Black Death: Studies in the 'Crisis' of the Early Fourteenth
  Century* (Manchester, 1991)
—— *Living and Dying in England, 1100–1540: The Monastic Experience* (Oxford, 1993)
Harvey, R. E., *The Inward Wits: Psychological Theory in the Middle Ages and Renaissance*
  (London, 1975)
Hastead, E., *The History and Topographical Survey of the County of Kent*, 12 vols
  (Canterbury, 1797–1801)
Hatcher, J., 'Mortality in the Fifteenth Century: Some New Evidence', *EconHR*, 2nd series
  39 (1986), pp. 19–38
—— *The History of the British Coal Industry*, vol. 1 (Oxford, 1993)
—— 'The Great Slump of the Mid-Fifteenth Century', in J. Hatcher and R. Britnell, eds,
  Progress and Problems in Medieval England (Cambridge, 1996)
Hatcher, J., A. J. Piper and D. Stone, 'Monastic Mortality: Durham Priory, 1395–1529',
  EconHR, 2nd series 59 (2006), pp. 667–87
Hawkins, D., 'The Black Death and the New London Cemeteries of 1348', *Antiquity* 64
  (1990), pp. 637–42
Healy, M., '"Seeing" Contagious Bodies in Early Modern London', in D. Grantley and N.
  Taunton, eds, *The Body in Late Medieval and Early Modern Culture* (Aldershot, 2000)
Hearnshaw, F. J. C., *Leet Jurisdiction in England* (London, 1908)
Heath, P., 'North Sea Fishing in the Fifteenth Century: The Scarborough Fleet', *Northern
  History* 3 (1968), pp. 53–69
Henderson, C. G., 'The City of Exeter from AD 50 to the Early Nineteenth Century', in R.
  Kain and W. Ravenhill, eds, *Historical Atlas of South-West England* (Exeter, 2000)

Henderson, J., 'The Black Death in Florence: Medical and Communal Responses', in S. Bassett, ed., *Death in Towns: Urban Responses to the Dying and the Dead, 100–1600* (Leicester, 1992)

—— *The Renaissance Hospital: Healing the Body and Healing the Soul* (New Haven, CT, 2006)

—— 'Public Health, Pollution and the Problem of Waste Disposal in Early Modern Tuscany', in S. Cavaciocchi, ed., *Le interazioni fra economia e ambiente biologico nell'Europa preindustriale, Secc. XIII–XVIII* (Florence, 2010)

Henderson, J., and K. Park, '"The First Hospital among Christians": The Ospedale di Santa Maria Nuova in Early Sixteenth-Century Florence', *Medical History* 35 (1991), pp. 164–88

Hieatt, C. B., 'Making Sense of Medieval Culinary Records', in M. Carlin and J. T. Rosenthal, eds, *Food and Eating in Medieval Europe* (London, 1998)

Higgins, A., 'Streets and Markets', in J. D. Cox and D. S. Kastan, eds, *A New History of Early English Drama* (New York, 1997)

Hill, C., *Women and Religion in Late Medieval Norwich* (Woodbridge, 2010)

Hill, J. M. F., *Medieval Lincoln* (Cambridge, 1948)

Hill, N., and A. Rogers, *Guild, Hospital and Alderman: New Light on the Founding of Browne's Hospital, Stamford, 1475–1509* (Bury St Edmunds, 2013)

Hilton, R. H., *English and French Towns in Feudal Society* (Cambridge, 1992)

Hobley, B., 'The London Waterfront – The Exception or the Rule?', in B. Hobley and G. Milne, eds, *Waterfront Archaeology in Britain and Northern Europe*, CBA research report 41 (London, 1981)

Hodgson, J. C., 'The "Domus Dei" of Newcastle: Otherwise St Katherine's Hospital of the Sandhill', *Archaeologia Aeliana*, 3rd series 14 (1917), pp. 191–220

Holloway, W., *The History and Antiquities of the Ancient Town and Port of Rye* (London, 1847)

Holt, R., 'Medieval England's Water-Related Technologies', in P. Squatriti, ed., *Working with Water in Medieval Europe* (Leiden, 2000)

Honeybourne, M., 'The Fleet and its Neighbourhood in Early Medieval Times', *London Topographical Record* 19 (1947), pp. 13–87

—— 'The Leper Hospitals of the London Area', *TLMAS* 21 (1967), pp. 4–54

Horden, P., '"A Discipline of Relevance": The Historiography of the Later Medieval Hospital', *Social History of Medicine* 1 (1988), pp. 359–74

—— 'Disease, Dragons and Saints: The Management of Epidemics in the Dark Ages', in T. Ranger and P. Slack, eds, *Epidemics and Ideas: Essays on the Historical Perception of Pestilence* (Cambridge, 1992)

—— 'Household Care and Informal Networks: Comparisons and Continuities from Antiquity to the Present', in P. Horden and R. Smith, eds, *The Locus of Care: Families, Communities, Institutions and the Provision of Welfare since Antiquity* (London, 1998)

—— 'Ritual and Public Health in the Early Medieval City', in S. Sheard and H. Power, eds, *Body and City: Histories of Urban Public Health* (Aldershot, 2000)

—— 'Small Beer? The Parish and the Poor and Sick in Later Medieval England', in C. Burgess and E. Duffy, eds, *The Parish in Late Medieval England* (Donington, 2006)

—— *Hospitals and Healing from Antiquity to the Later Middle Ages* (Aldershot, 2008)

Horrox, R., 'Introduction', in R. Horrox, ed., *Fifteenth-Century Attitudes: Perceptions of Society in Late Medieval England* (Cambridge, 1994)

Horton-Smith-Hartley, P., and H. R. Aldridge, *Johannes de Mirfeld: His Life and Works* (Cambridge, 1936)

Hoyle, R. W., 'Origins of the Dissolution of the Monasteries', *Historical Journal* 38 (1995), pp. 275–305

Hunnisett, R. F., *The Medieval Coroner* (Cambridge, 1961)

Hunt, T., *Building Jerusalem: The Rise and Fall of the Victorian City* (London, 2004)

Hutton, D., 'Women in Fourteenth-Century Shrewsbury', in L. Charles and L. Duffin, eds, *Women and Work in Pre-Industrial England* (London, 1985)

Hyde, J. K., 'Medieval Descriptions of Cities', *Bulletin of the John Rylands Library* 48 (1965–6), pp. 308–40

Imbert, J., *Histoire des hôpitaux en France* (Toulouse, 1982)

Imray, J., *The Charity of Richard Whittington* (London, 1968)

Izacke, S., *Remarkable Antiquities of the City of Exeter* (London, 1723)

Jack, R. I., 'The Fire Ordinances of Ruthin, 1364', *Transactions of the Denbighshire Historical Society* 28 (1979), pp. 5–17

Jacquart, D., *Le Milieu médical en France du XIIe au XVe siécle*, Hautes Études Médiévales et Modernes, série 5, 46 (Geneva, 1981)

Jacquart, D., and C. Thomasset, *Sexuality and Medicine in the Middle Ages* (Oxford, 1985)

James, M., 'Ritual, Drama and Social Body in the Later Middle Ages', *P&P* 98 (1983), pp. 3–29

Jenkins, E., *The Legal Aspects of Sanitary Reform* (London, 1867)

Jenner, M. S. R., 'The Great Dog Massacre', in W. G. Naphy and P. Roberts, eds, *Fear in Early Modern Society* (Manchester, 1997)

—— 'Underground, Overground: Pollution and Place in Urban History', *Journal of Urban History* 24 (1997), pp. 97–110

—— 'Civilisation and Deodorization? Smell in Early Modern English Culture', in P. Burke, B. Harrison and P. Slack, eds, *Civil Histories: Essays Presented to Sir Keith Thomas* (Oxford, 2000)

—— 'From Conduit Community to Commercial Network? Water in London, 1500–1725', in M. S. R. Jenner and P. Griffiths, eds, *Londinopolis: Essays in the Cultural and Social History of Early Modern London* (Manchester, 2000)

—— 'Follow your Nose? Smell, Smelling, and their Histories', *American Historical Review* 116 (2011), pp. 335–51

Jessopp, A., *The Coming of the Friars and other Historic Essays* (London, 1890)

Johnstone, H., 'Poor Relief in the Royal Household of Thirteenth-Century England', *Speculum* 4 (1929), pp. 149–67

Jones, C., 'Discourse Communities and Medical Texts', in I. Taavitsainen and P. Pahata, eds, *Medical and Scientific Writing in Late Medieval English* (Cambridge, 2004)

Jones, P. E., 'Whittington's Long House', *London Topographical Record* 23 (1974 for 1972), pp. 27–34

—— *The Butchers of London* (London, 1976)

Jones, R. H., *Medieval Houses at Flaxengate, Lincoln*, The Archaeology of Lincoln 11.1 (London, 1980)

Jones, W. R. D., *The Tudor Commonwealth, 1529–1559* (London, 1970)

Jørgensen, D., 'Co-operative Sanitation: Managing Streets and Gutters in Late Medieval England', *Technology and Culture* 49 (2008), pp. 547–67

—— '"All Good Rule of the Citee": Sanitation and Civic Government in England, 1400–1600', *Journal of Urban History* 36 (2010), pp. 300–15

Karras, R. M., *Common Women: Prostitution and Sexuality in Medieval England* (Oxford, 1996)

Kearns, G., 'The Urban Penalty and the Population History of England', in A. Brändström and L. Tedebrand, eds, *Society, Health and Population during the Demographic Transition* (Stockholm, 1988)

Keene, D., 'Rubbish in Medieval Towns', in A. R. Hall and H. K. Kenward, eds, *Environmental Archaeology in the Urban Context*, CBA research report 43 (London, 1982)

—— 'The Medieval Urban Environment in Documentary Records', *Archives* 16 (1983), pp. 137–44

—— *Survey of Medieval Winchester*, 2 vols (Oxford, 1985)

—— *The Walbrook Study: A Summary Report* (London, 1987)

—— 'Suburban Growth', in R. Holt and G. Rosser, eds, *The Medieval Town: A Reader in English Urban History, 1200–1540* (London, 1990)

—— 'Tanners' Widows', in C. M. Barron and A. F. Sutton, eds, *Medieval London Widows, 1300–1500* (London, 1994)

—— 'Issues of Water in Medieval London to *c.* 1300', *Urban History* 28 (2001), pp. 161–79

Keiser, G., ed., *A Manual of the Writings in Middle English, 1050–1500*, vol. 10: *Works of Science and Information* (New Haven, CT, 1998)

—— 'Two Medieval Plague Treatises and their Afterlife in Early Modern England', *JHM* 58 (2003), pp. 292–324

—— 'Scientific, Medical and Utilitarian Prose', in A. S. G. Edwards, ed., *A Companion to Middle English Prose* (Cambridge, 2004)

Kemp, S., 'A Medieval Controversy about Odor', *Journal of the History of the Behavioral Sciences* 33 (1997), pp. 211–19

Kerling, N. J., 'Notes on Newgate Prison', *TLMAS* 22 (1968–70), pp. 21–2

Kermode, J. I., 'Urban Decline? The Flight from Office in Late-Medieval York', *EconHR*, 2nd series 35 (1982), pp. 179–98

—— 'The Greater Towns, 1300–1540', in D. M. Palliser, ed., *The Cambridge Urban History of Britain*, vol. 1: *600–1540* (Cambridge, 2000)

King, P. M., *The York Mystery Cycle and the Worship of the City* (Cambridge, 2006)

King, W., 'How High is too High? The Disposal of Dung in Seventeenth-Century Prescot', *Sixteenth-Century Journal* 23 (1992), pp. 443–57

Kingsley, C., *Sanitary and Social Lectures and Essays* (London, 1889)

Kinzelbach, A., 'Infection, Contagion, and Public Health in Late Medieval and Early Modern German Imperial Towns', *Journal of the History of Medicine and Allied Sciences* 61 (2006), pp. 369–89

Kirkpatrick, J., *The Streets and Lanes of the City of Norwich*, ed. W. Hudson (Norwich, 1889)

Knowles, D., and R. N. Hadcock, *Medieval Religious Houses of England and Wales* (London, 1971)

Kowaleski, M., 'Town and Country in Late Medieval England: The Hide and Leather Trade', in P. Corfield and D. Keene, eds, *Work in Towns, 850–1850* (Leicester, 1990)

—— *Local Markets and Regional Trade in Medieval Exeter* (Cambridge, 1995)

Kucher, M., 'The Use of Water and its Regulation in Medieval Siena', *Journal of Urban History* 31 (2005), pp. 504–36

Labisch, A., 'History of Public Health: History in Public Health Looking Back and Looking Forward', *Social History of Medicine* 11 (1998), pp. 1–13

Laughton, J., *Life in a Late Medieval City: Chester 1275–1520* (Oxford, 2008)

Lawrence, C. H., 'The University in State and Church', in J. I. Catto, ed., *The History of the University of Oxford*, vol. 1: *The Early Oxford Schools* (Oxford, 1984)

Le Corbusier, *The City of Tomorrow and its Planning*, trans F. Etchells (London, 1947)

Le Goff, J., 'Head or Heart? The Political Use of Body Metaphors in the Middle Ages', in M. Feher, R. Naddaff and N. Tazi, eds, *Fragments for a History of the Human Body*, part 3 (New York, 1989)

Leguay, J.-P., *La Rue au Moyen Âge* (Rennes, 1984)

—— *La Pollution au Moyen Âge* (Paris, 1999)

—— *L'Eau dans la ville au Moyen Âge* (Rennes, 2002)

Leighton, W., 'Trinity Hospital', *Transactions of the Bristol and Gloucestershire Archaeological Society* 36 (1913), pp. 251–87

Lewis, C. R., and A. T. Thacker, eds, *VCH Chester*, vol. 5: *The City of Chester*, 2 parts (London, 2003–5)

Lewis, M., *Urbanisation and Child Health in Medieval and Post Medieval England*, BAR British series 339 (Oxford, 2002)

L.G., 'Sutton in Holland', *Fenland Notes and Queries* 7 (1909), pp. 306–8

Liddy, C. D., 'Urban Conflict in Late Fourteenth-Century England: The Case of York in 1380–1', *EHR* 118 (2003), pp. 1–32

—— *War, Politics and Finance in Late Medieval English Towns* (Woodbridge, 2005)

Lilley, K. D., *Urban Life in the Middle Ages, 1000–1450* (Basingstoke, 2002)

—— 'Cities of God? Medieval Urban Forms and their Christian Symbolism', *Transactions of the Institute of British Geographers*, n.s. 24 (2004), pp. 296–313

—— *City and Cosmos: The Medieval World in Urban Form* (London, 2009)

Little, A. G., and R. C. Easterling, *The Franciscans and Dominicans in Exeter* (Exeter, 1927)

Little, L. K., 'Plague Historians in Lab Coats', *P&P* 213 (2011), pp. 267–90

Lobel, M. D., and W. H. Johns, *The City of London: From Prehistoric Times to c. 1520*, British Atlas of Historic Towns 3 (Oxford, 1989)

Loewe, R., 'Handwashing and the Eyesight in the *Regimen sanitatis*', *BHM* 30 (1956), pp. 100–8

Lorcin, M.-T., 'Humeurs, bains et tisanes: l'eau dans la médecine médiévale', in *L'Eau au moyen âge*, Senefiance 15 (Aix-en-Provence, 1985)

Luff, R. M., and M. Garcia, 'Killing Cats in the Medieval Period: An Unusual Episode in the History of Cambridge', *Archaeofauna* 4 (1995), pp. 93–114

Luttrell, C. A., 'Baiting of Bulls and Boars in the Middle English "Cleanness"', *Notes and Queries* 197 (1952), pp. 23–4, and 201 (1956), pp. 398–401

Macnalty, A. S., 'Sir Thomas More as a Student of Medicine and Public Health Reformer', in E. A. Underwood, ed., *Science, Medicine and History: Essays on the Evolution of Scientific Thought and Medical Practice*, 2 vols (Oxford, 1953)

Maddern, P., 'Order and Disorder', in C. Rawcliffe and R. Wilson, eds, *Medieval Norwich* (London, 2004)

Magilton, J., et al., *'Lepers Outside the Gate': Excavations at the Cemetery of the Hospital of St James and St Mary Magdalen, Chichester, 1986–87 and 1993*, CBA research report 158 (London, 2008)

Magnusson, R. J., *Water Technology in the Middle Ages* (Baltimore, 2001)

Malden, H. E., ed., *VCH Surrey*, vol. 2 (London, 1905)

Manchester, K., 'Tuberculosis and Leprosy in Antiquity: An Interpretation', *Medical History* 28 (1984), pp. 162–73

Mann, J., *Chaucer and Medieval Estates Satire* (Cambridge, 1973)

Marcombe, D., 'The Late Medieval Town, 1149–1560', in J. Beckett, ed., *A Centenary History of Nottingham* (Manchester, 1997)

—— *Leper Knights: The Order of St Lazarus of Jerusalem in England, c. 1150–1544* (Woodbridge, 2003)

Martin, A. R., *Franciscan Architecture in England* (Manchester, 1937)

Marx, C. F. H., and R. Willis, *On the Decrease of Disease Effected by the Progress of Civilization* (London, 1844)

Marx, C. W., 'British Library Harley MS 1740 and Popular Devotion', in N. Rogers, ed., *England in the Fifteenth Century* (Stamford, 1994)

Mayo, C. H., *A Historic Guide to the Almshouse of St John the Baptist and St John the Evangelist, Sherborne* (Oxford, 1933)

McConchie, R. W., *Lexicography and Physicke: The Record of Sixteenth-Century English Medical Terminology* (Oxford, 1997)

McIntosh, M. K., 'Local Responses to the Poor in Late Medieval and Tudor England', *Continuity and Change* 3 (1988), pp. 209–45

—— *Controlling Misbehavior in England, 1370–1600* (Cambridge, 1998)

—— *Poor Relief in England, 1300–1600* (Cambridge, 2012)

McLaren, M.-R., 'Reading, Writing and Recording: Literacy and the London Chronicles in the Fifteenth Century', in M. Davies and A. Prescott, eds, *London and the Kingdom: Essays in Honour of Caroline M. Barron* (Donington, 2008)

McRee, B. R., 'Religious Guilds and Civic Order: The Case of Norwich in the Late Middle Ages', *Speculum* 67 (1992), pp. 69–97

—— 'Charity and Guild Solidarity', *Journal of British Studies* 32 (1993), pp. 195–225

—— 'Peacemaking and its Limits in Late Medieval Norwich', *EHR* 109 (1994), pp. 831–66

—— 'Unity or Division? The Social Meaning of Guild Ceremony in Urban Communities', in B. A. Hanawalt and K. L. Reyerson, eds, *City and Spectacle in Medieval Europe* (Minneapolis, 1994)

McSheffrey, S., *Marriage, Sex and Civic Culture in Late Medieval London* (Philadelphia, 2006)

McVaugh, M., *Medicine before the Plague: Practitioners and their Patients in the Crown of Aragon, 1285–1345* (Cambridge, 2002)

Mead, W. E., *The English Medieval Feast* (London, 1931)

Milne, G., 'Medieval Riverfront Reclamation in London', in G. Milne and B. Hobley, eds, *Waterfront Archaeology in Britain and Northern Europe*, CBA research report 41 (London, 1981)

Minchinton, W., *Life to the City: An Illustrated History of Exeter's Water Supply* (Exeter, 1987)

Mollat, M., *The Poor in the Middle Ages*, trans. A. Goldhammer (New Haven, CT, 1986)

Montford, A., *Health, Sickness, Medicine and the Friars in the Thirteenth and Fourteenth Centuries* (Aldershot, 2004)

Moore, R. I., 'Heresy as a Disease', in W. Lourdaux and V. Verhelst, eds, *The Concept of Heresy in the Middle Ages*, Mediaevalia Louaniensia 1st series 4 (Leuven, 1976)

Mortimer, I., *The Time Traveller's Guide to Medieval England* (London, 2008)

Murray Jones, P., 'Medical Books before the Invention of Printing', in A. Besson, ed., *Thornton's Medical Books, Libraries and Collectors*, 3rd edn (London, 1990)

—— 'Information and Science', in R. Horrox, ed., *Fifteenth-Century Attitudes: Perceptions of Society in Late Medieval England* (Cambridge, 1994)

—— *Medieval Medical Miniatures in Illuminated Manuscripts*, rev. edn (London, 1998)

—— 'Medicine and Science', in L. Hellinga and J. B. Trapp, eds, *The Cambridge History of the Book in Britain*, vol. 3: *1400–1557* (Cambridge, 1999)

Nederman, C. J., 'The Physiological Significance of the Organic Metaphor in John of Salisbury's *Policraticus*', *History of Political Thought* 8 (1987), pp. 211–23

Nevola, F., *Siena: Constructing the Renaissance City* (New Haven, CT, 2007)

Newman, G., *On the History of the Decline and Final Extinction of Leprosy as an Endemic Disease in the British Isles* (London, 1895)

—— *The Rise of Preventative Medicine* (Oxford, 1932)

Nicoud, M., *Les Régimes de santé au moyen âge*, 2 vols (Rome, 2007)

Nightingale, P., *A Medieval Mercantile Community: The Grocers Company and the Politics and Trade of London, 1000–1485* (New Haven, CT, 1995)

—— 'Some New Evidence of Crises and Trends of Mortality in Late Medieval England', *P&P* 187 (2005), pp. 33–68

Nutton, V., 'Continuity or Rediscovery? The City Physician in Classical Antiquity and Medieval Italy', in A. W. Russell, ed., *The Town and State Physician in Europe from the Middle Ages to the Enlightenment* (Wolfenbuttel, 1981)

—— 'Murders and Miracles: Lay Attitudes towards Medicine in Classical Antiquity', in R. Porter, ed., *Patients and Practitioners: Lay Perceptions of Medicine in Pre-Industrial Society* (Cambridge, 1985)

—— 'Did the Greeks Have a Word for It? Contagion and Contagion Theory in Classical Antiquity', in L. I. Conrad and D. Wujastyk, eds, *Contagion: Perspectives from Pre-Modern Societies* (Aldershot, 2000)

—— 'Medical Thoughts on Urban Pollution', in V. M. Hope and E. Marshall, eds, *Death and Disease in the Ancient City* (London, 2000)

O'Boyle, C., 'Surgical Texts and Social Contexts: Physicians and Surgeons in Paris, *c.* 1270 to 1430', in J. Arrizabalaga *et al.*, eds, *Practical Medicine from Salerno to the Black Death* (Cambridge, 1994)

Orme, N., and M. Webster, *The English Hospital, 1070–1570* (New Haven, CT, 1995)

Ormerod, G., *The History of the County Palatine and City of Chester*, vol. 1, 2 parts (London, 1882)

Owen, H., and J. B. Blakeway, *A History of Shrewsbury*, 2 vols (London, 1825)

Owst, G. R., *Literature and Pulpit in Medieval England* (Oxford, 1996)

Page, S., *Magic in Medieval Manuscripts* (London, 2005)

Page, W., ed., *VCH Suffolk*, vol. 2 (London, 1907)

—— ed., *VCH Sussex*, vol. 2 (London, 1907)

—— ed., *VCH Shropshire*, vol. 1 (London, 1908)

—— ed., *VCH Warwickshire*, vol. 2 (London, 1908)

—— ed., *VCH Nottingham*, vol. 2 (London, 1910)

—— ed., *VCH Bedford*, vol. 3 (London, 1912; repr. 1972)

—— ed., *VCH York*, vol. 3 (London, 1913)

—— ed., *VCH Northampton*, vol. 3 (London, 1930)

Pahata, P., and I. Taavitsainen, 'Vernacularisation of Scientific and Medical Writing in its Sociohistorical Context', in I. Taavitsainen and P. Pahata, eds, *Medical and Scientific Writing in Late Medieval English* (Cambridge, 2004)

Palliser, D. M., 'Epidemics in Tudor York', *Northern History* 8 (1973), pp. 45–63

—— 'Urban Decay Revisited', in J. A. F. Thomson, ed., *Towns and Townspeople in the Fifteenth Century* (Gloucester, 1988)

—— 'Civic Mentality and the Government of Tudor York', in J. Barry, ed., *The Tudor and Stuart Town: A Reader in English Urban History, 1530–1688* (London, 1990)

Palliser, D. M., T. R. Slater and E. P. Dennison, 'The Topography of Towns, 600–1300', in D. M. Palliser, ed., *The Cambridge Urban History of Britain*, vol. 1: *600–1540* (Cambridge, 2000)

Palmer, R., 'The Church, Leprosy and Plague in Medieval and Early Modern Europe', *SCH* 19 (1982), pp. 79–99

—— 'In Bad Odour: Smell and its Significance in Medicine from Antiquity to the Seventeenth Century', in W. F. Bynum and R. Porter, eds, *Medicine and the Five Senses* (Cambridge, 1993)

Palmer, R. C., *English Law in the Age of the Black Death, 1348–1381: A Transformation of Governance and Law* (Chapel Hill, NC, 1993)

Park, K., *Doctors and Medicine in Renaissance Florence* (Princeton, NJ, 1985)

Parker, V., *The Making of King's Lynn: Secular Buildings from the Eleventh to the Seventeenth Century*, King's Lynn Archaeological Survey 1 (London, 1971)

Paster, G. K., 'Nervous Tensions: Networks of Blood and Spirit in the Early Modern Body', in D. Hillman and C. Mazzio, eds, *The Body in Parts: Fantasies of Corporeality in Early Modern Europe* (London, 1997)

Pearson, K. L., 'Nutrition and the Early-Medieval Diet', *Speculum* 72 (1997), pp. 1–32

Pelling, M., 'Appearance and Reality: Barber-Surgeons, the Body and Disease', in A. L. Beier and R. Finlay, eds, *London, 1500–1700: The Making of the Metropolis* (London, 1986)

—— *Medical Conflicts in Early Modern London: Patronage, Physicians and Irregular Practitioners, 1550–1640* (Oxford, 2003)

—— 'Health and Sanitation to 1750', in C. Rawcliffe and R. Wilson, eds, *Norwich since 1550* (London, 2004)

Pelner Cosman, M., 'Medieval Medical Malpractice: The *Dicta* and the Dockets', *Bulletin of the New York Academy of Medicine* 49 (1973), pp. 22–47

Pevsner, N., and B. Wilson, *The Buildings of England: Norfolk*, vol. 1, 2nd edn (London, 1997)

Phythian-Adams, C., 'Ceremony and the Citizen: The Communal Year at Coventry, 1450–1550', in P. Clark and P. Slack, eds, *Crisis and Order in English Towns, 1500–1700* (London, 1972)

—— *Desolation of a City: Coventry and the Urban Crisis of the Late Middle Ages* (Cambridge, 1979)

Picherit, J. L. G., *La Métaphore pathologique et therapeutique à la fin du moyen âge* (Tübingen, 1994)

Pickett, J. P., 'A Translation of the "Canutus" Plague Treatise', in L. M. Matheson, ed., *Popular and Practical Science of Medieval England* (East Lansing, MI, 1994)

Platt, C., *Medieval Southampton: The Port and Trading Community, AD 1000–1600* (London, 1973)

—— *The English Medieval Town* (London, 1976)

—— *King Death: The Black Death and its Aftermath in Late-Medieval England* (London, 1996)

Platt, C., and R. Coleman-Smith, *Excavations in Medieval Southampton, 1953–1969*, vol. 1 (Leicester, 1975)

Plummer, C., 'Introduction', in Sir John Fortescue, *The Governance of England* (Oxford, 1875)

Porter, D., *Health, Civilisation and the State* (London, 1999)

Portman, D., *Exeter Houses, 1400–1700* (Exeter, 1966)

Post, J., 'A Fifteenth-Century Customary for the Southwark Stews', *Journal of the Society of Archivists* 5 (1977), pp. 418–28

Pouchelle, M. C., *The Body and Surgery in the Middle Ages*, trans. R. Morris (Oxford, 1990)

Pound, J. F., 'The Social and Trade Structure of Norwich, 1525–1575', *P&P* 34 (1966), pp. 49–69

—— 'Poverty and Public Health in Norwich, 1845–1880', in C. Barringer, ed., *Norwich in the Nineteenth Century* (Norwich, 1984)

Pounds, N., *The Medieval City* (Westport, CT, 2005)

Powell, E., 'Arbitration and the Law in England in the Late Middle Ages', *TRHS*, 5th series 33 (1983), pp. 49–67

Price, R., and M. Ponsford, *St Bartholomew's Hospital, Bristol: The Excavation of a Medieval Hospital*, CBA research report 110 (London, 1998)

Priestley, U., *The Great Market: A Survey of Nine Hundred Years of Norwich Provision Market* (Norwich, 1987)

Pugh, R. B., *Imprisonment in Medieval England* (Cambridge, 1968)

Pullan, B., *Rich and Poor in Renaissance Venice* (Oxford, 1971)

Purvis, J. S., 'Notes from the Diocesan Registry at York', *Yorkshire Archaeological Journal* 30 (1943), pp. 389–403

Quétel, C., *History of Syphilis*, trans. J. Braddock and B. Pike (Oxford, 1990)

Quiney, A., *Town Houses of Medieval Britain* (New Haven, CT, 2003)

Raine, A., *Medieval York* (London, 1955)

Rather, L. J., 'The Six Things Non-Natural: A Note on the Origins and Fate of a Doctrine and a Phrase', *Clio Medica* 3 (1968), pp. 337–47

Rawcliffe, C., 'The Profits of Practice: The Wealth and Status of Medical Men in Later Medieval England', *Social History of Medicine* 1 (1988), pp. 61–78

—— '"That Kindliness Should be Cherished More and Discord Driven Out": The Settlement of Commercial Disputes by Arbitration in Later Medieval England', in J. Kermode, ed., *Enterprise and Individuals in Fifteenth-Century England* (Stroud, 1991)

—— *The Hospitals of Medieval Norwich* (Norwich, 1995)

—— *Medicine and Society in Later Medieval England* (Stroud, 1995)

—— 'Hospital Nurses and their Work', in R. Britnell, ed., *Daily Life in the Late Middle Ages* (Stroud, 1998)

—— *Medicine for the Soul: The Life, Death and Resurrection of a Medieval English Hospital* (Stroud, 1999)

—— '"On the Threshold of Eternity": Care for the Sick in East Anglian Monasteries', in C. Harper-Bill, C. Rawcliffe and R. G. Wilson, eds, *East Anglia's History* (Woodbridge, 2002)

—— 'Passports to Paradise: How English Medieval Hospitals and Almshouses Kept their Archives', *Archives* 27 (2002), pp. 1–22

—— 'Master Surgeons at the Lancastrian Court', in J. Stratford, ed., *The Lancastrian Court* (Donnington, 2003)

—— 'Women, Childbirth and Religion in Later Medieval England', in D. Wood, ed., *Women and Religion in Medieval England* (Oxford, 2003)

—— 'Introduction', in C. Rawcliffe and R. Wilson, eds, *Medieval Norwich* (London, 2004)

—— 'Sickness and Health', in C. Rawcliffe and R. Wilson, eds, *Medieval Norwich* (London, 2004)

—— 'The Earthly and Spiritual Topography of Suburban Hospitals', in K. Giles and C. Dyer, eds, *Town and Country in the Middle Ages: Contrasts, Contacts and Interconnections, 1100–1500* (Leeds, 2005)

—— 'Health and Safety at Work in Late Medieval East Anglia', in C. Harper-Bill, ed., *Medieval East Anglia* (Woodbridge, 2005)

—— *Leprosy in Medieval England* (Woodbridge, 2006)

—— 'A Word from Our Sponsor: Advertising the Patron in the Medieval Hospital', in J. Henderson, P. Horden and A. Pastore, eds, *The Impact of Hospitals, 300–2000* (Oxford, 2007)

—— 'Christ the Physician Walks the Wards: Celestial Therapeutics in the Medieval Hospital', in M. Davies and A. Prescott, eds, *London and the Kingdom: Essays in Honour of Caroline M. Barron* (Donington, 2008)

—— '"Delectable Sightes and Fragrant Smelles": Gardens and Health in Late Medieval and Early Modern England', *Garden History* 36 (2008), pp. 1–21

—— 'Dives Redeemed? The Guild Almshouses of Later Medieval England', *The Fifteenth Century* 8 (2008), pp. 1–27

—— 'A Marginal Occupation? The Medieval Laundress and her Work', *Gender and History* 21 (2009), pp. 147–69

—— 'The Concept of Health in Medieval Society', in S. Cavaciocchi, ed., *Le interazioni fra economia e ambiente biologico nell'Europa preindustriale. Secc. XIII-XVIII* (Florence, 2010)

Rawcliffe, C., and R. Wilson, eds, *Medieval Norwich* (London, 2004)

Reaney, P. H., *The Place-Names of Cambridgeshire and the Isle of Ely* (Cambridge, 1943)

Reddaway, T. F., *The Early History of the Goldsmiths' Company* (London, 1975)

Rexroth, F., *Deviance and Power in Late Medieval London* (Cambridge, 2007)

Reynolds, S., 'Medieval Urban History and the History of Political Thought', *Urban History Yearbook* (1982), pp. 14–23

Richardson, B. W., *Hygeia: A City of Health* (London, 1876)

Rigby, S. H., '"Sore Decay" and "Fair Dwellings": Boston and Urban Decline in the Later Middle Ages', *Midland History* 10 (1985), pp. 47–61

—— 'Urban "Oligarchy" in Late Medieval England', in J. A. F. Thomson, ed., *Towns and Townspeople in the Fifteenth Century* (Gloucester, 1988)

—— *Medieval Grimsby: Growth and Decline* (Hull, 1993)

Rigby, S. H., and E. Ewan, 'Government, Power and Authority, 1300–1540', in D. M. Palliser, ed., *The Cambridge Urban History of Britain*, vol. 1: *600–1540* (Cambridge, 2000)

Risse, G. B., *Mending Bodies, Saving Souls: A History of Hospitals* (New York, 1999)

Roach, J. P. C., ed., *VCH Cambridge and the Isle of Ely*, vol. 3 (London, 1959)

Robbins, R. H., ed., *Historical Poems of the XIVth and XVth Centuries* (New York, 1959)

Roberts, C., and M. Cox, *Health and Disease in Britain* (Stroud, 2003)

Roberts, P., 'Agencies Human and Divine: Fire in French Cities, 1520–1720', in P. Roberts and W. G. Naphy, eds, *Fear in Early Modern Society* (Manchester, 1997)

Robins, F. W., *The Story of Water Supply* (Oxford, 1946)

Roover, R. de, 'The Concept of the Just Price: Theory and Economic Policy', *Journal of Economic History* 18 (1958), pp. 418–38

Rosen, G., *A History of Public Health* (New York, 1958; rev. edn, Baltimore, 1993)

Roskell, J., L. Clark and C. Rawcliffe, eds, *The Commons, 1386–1421*, 4 vols (Stroud, 1992)

Ross, A. S. C., 'The Assize of Bread', *EconHR*, 2nd series 9 (1956), pp. 332–42

Rosser, A. G., 'The Essence of Medieval Urban Communities: The Vill of Westminster, 1200–1500', *TRHS*, 5th series 34 (1984), pp. 91–112

—— *Medieval Westminster, 1200–1540* (Oxford, 1989)

—— 'Going to the Fraternity Feast: Commensality and Social Relations in Later Medieval England', *Journal of British Studies* 30 (1994), pp. 430–46

—— 'Urban Culture and the Church, 1300–1540', in D. M. Palliser, ed., *The Cambridge Urban History of Britain*, vol. 1: *600–1540* (Cambridge, 2000)

Rubin, M., *Charity and Community in Medieval Cambridge* (Cambridge, 1987)

—— 'Development and Change in English Hospitals, 1100–1500', in L. Granshaw and R. Porter, eds, *The Hospital in History* (London, 1990)

—— *Corpus Christi: The Eucharist in Late Medieval Culture* (Cambridge, 1992)

Rushton, N., 'Spatial Aspects of the Almonry Site and the Changing Priorities of Poor Relief at Westminster Abbey, *c.* 1290–1540', *Architectural History* 45 (2002), pp. 66–91

Rutledge, E., 'Immigration and Population Growth in Early Fourteenth-Century Norwich: Evidence from the Tithing Roll', *Urban History Yearbook* 15 (1988), pp. 15–30

—— 'Landlords and Tenants: Housing and the Rented Property Market in Early Fourteenth-Century Norwich', *Urban History* 22 (1995), pp. 1–24

—— 'Economic Life', in C. Rawcliffe and R. Wilson, eds, *Medieval Norwich* (London, 2004)

Rutledge, P., 'Thomas Damet and the Historiography of Great Yarmouth', *NA* 33 (1965), pp. 119–30

——'A Fifteenth-Century Yarmouth Petition', *Great Yarmouth District Archaeological Society* 56 (1976), unpaginated

Sabine, E. L., 'Butchering in Mediaeval London', *Speculum* 8 (1933), pp. 335–53

——'Latrines and Cesspools of Mediaeval London', *Speculum* 9 (1934), pp. 303–21

——'City Cleaning in Mediaeval London', *Speculum* 12 (1937), pp. 19–43

Sagui, S., 'Mid-Level Officials in Fifteenth-Century Norwich', *The Fifteenth Century* 12 (2013), pp. 101–21

Salusbury-Jones, G. T., *Street Life in Medieval England* (Oxford, 1939; repr. 1948)

Salzman, L. F., *Building in England* (Oxford, 1967)

Samuel, M. W., 'The Fifteenth-Century Garner at Leadenhall, London', *Antiquaries Journal* 69 (1989), pp. 119–53

Sandred, K. I., and B. Lindström, *The Place Names of Norfolk*, vol. 1 (Nottingham, 1989)

Saul, A., 'English Towns in the Late Middle Ages: The Case of Yarmouth', *Journal of Medieval History* 8 (1982), pp. 75–88

Saunier, A., *'Le Pauvre malade' dans le cadre hospitalier medieval: France du Nord, vers 1300–1500* (Paris, 1993)

Schleiner, W., 'Infection and Cure through Women: Renaissance Constructions of Syphilis', *Journal of Medieval and Renaissance Studies* 24 (1994), pp. 499–517

Schofield, J., *Medieval London Houses* (New Haven, CT, 1995)

——*London, 1100–1600: The Archaeology of a Capital City* (Sheffield, 2011)

Schofield, J., and G. Stell, 'The Built Environment, 1300–1540', in D. M. Palliser, ed., *The Cambridge Urban History of Britain*, vol. 1: *600–1540* (Cambridge, 2000)

Schofield, J., and A. Vince, *Medieval Towns* (London, 1994)

Scobie, A., 'Slums, Sanitation and Mortality in the Roman World', *Klio* 68 (1986), pp. 399–433

Scully, T., 'The Sickdish in Early French Recipe Collections', in S. Campbell, B. Hall and D. Klausner, eds, *Health, Disease and Healing in Medieval Culture* (New York, 1992)

Seabourne, G., *Royal Regulation of Loans and Sales in Medieval England: Monkish Superstition and Civil Tyranny* (Woodbridge, 2003)

——'Assize Matters: Regulation of the Price of Bread in Medieval London', *Journal of Legal History* 27 (2006), pp. 29–52

Sennett, R., *Flesh and Stone: The Body and the City in Western Civilization* (London, 1994)

Serjeantson, D., and C. M. Woolgar, 'Fish Consumption in Medieval England', in D. Serjeantson, C. M. Woolgar and T. Waldron, eds, *Food in Medieval England: Diet and Nutrition* (Oxford, 2006)

Serjeantson, R. M., and W. R. D. Adkins, eds, *VCH Northampton*, vol. 2 (London, 1906)

Shaw, D., 'The Construction of the Private in Medieval London', *Journal of Medieval and Early Modern Studies* 26 (1996), pp. 447–66

Shaw, D. G., *The Creation of a Community: The City of Wells in the Middle Ages* (Oxford, 1993)

Sheard, S., and H. Power, eds, *Body and City: Histories of Urban Public Health* (Aldershot, 2000)

——'Body and City: Medical and Urban Histories of Public Health', in S. Sheard and H. Power, eds, *Body and City: Histories of Urban Public Health* (Aldershot, 2000)

Shelley, A., *Dragon Hall, King Street, Norwich*, EAA 112 (Norwich, 2005)

Shogimen, T., 'Treating the Body Politic: The Medical Metaphor of Political Rule in Late Medieval Europe and Tokugawa Japan', *The Review of Politics* 70 (2008), pp. 77–104

Shrewsbury, J. F. D., *A History of Bubonic Plague in the British Isles* (Cambridge, 1970)

Siegel, R. E., *Galen on Sense Perception* (Basel, 1970)

Signe Morrison, S., *Excrement in the Late Middle Ages: Sacred Filth and Chaucer's Fecopoetics* (New York, 2008)

Simon, J., *English Sanitary Institutions Reviewed in their Course of Development* (London, 1890)

Singer, D. W., and A. Anderson, *Catalogue of Latin and Vernacular Plague Texts in Great Britain and Eire in Manuscripts Written before the Sixteenth Century* (London, 1950)

Siraisi, N., *Medieval and Early Renaissance Medicine* (Chicago, 1990)

Skelton, R. A., and P. D. A. Harvey, *Local Maps and Plans from Medieval England* (Oxford, 1986)

Slack, P., *The Impact of Plague in Tudor and Stuart England* (London, 1985)

Sloane, B., 'Archaeological Evidence for the Infrastructure of the Medieval City of London', in M. Gläser, ed., *Lübecker Kolloquium zur Stadtarchäologie im Hanseraum IV: Die Infrastruktur* (Lübeck, 2004)

—— *The Black Death in London* (Stroud, 2011)

Smith, A. H., *The Place-Names of Oxfordshire*, vol. 1 (Cambridge, 1953)

Smith, F. F., *A History of Rochester* (London, 1928)

Smith, V., *Clean: A History of Personal Hygiene and Purity* (Oxford, 2007)

Solomon, M., *Fictions of Well-Being: Sickly Readers and Vernacular Medical Writing in Late Medieval and Early Modern Spain* (Philadelphia, 2010)

Somerscales, M. I., 'Lazar Houses in Cornwall', *Journal of the Royal Institution of Cornwall*, n.s. 5 (1965), pp. 61–99

Spooner, Dean, 'The Almshouse Chapel, Hadleigh', *Proceedings of the Suffolk Institute of Archaeology* 7 (1891), pp. 379–80

Statham., M., 'John Baret of Bury', *The Ricardian* 13 (2003), pp. 420–31

Stell, P., *Medical Practice in Medieval York*, Borthwick Paper 90 (York, 1996)

Stevenson, L. G., 'Science Down the Drain', *BHM* 29 (1955), pp. 1–26

Stirland, A., 'The Human Bones', in B. Ayers, ed., *Excavations within the North-East Bailey of Norwich Castle, 1979*, EAA 28 (Norwich, 1985)

—— *Criminals and Paupers: The Graveyard of St Margaret Fyebriggate in Combusto, Norwich*, EAA 129 (Norwich, 2009)

Storey, R. L., 'University and Government, 1430–1500', in J. I. Catto and R. Evans, eds, *The History of the University of Oxford*, vol. 2: *Late Medieval Oxford* (Oxford, 1992)

Strohm, P., *Hochon's Arrow: The Social Imagination of Fourteenth-Century Texts* (Princeton, NJ, 1992)

—— 'Writing and Reading', in R. Horrox and W. M. Ormrod, eds, *A Social History of England, 1200–1500* (Cambridge, 2006)

—— 'Sovereignty and Sewage', in L. H. Cooper and A. Denny-Brown, eds, *Lydgate Matters: Poetry and Material Culture in the Fifteenth Century* (New York, 2007)

Stubbs, W., *The Constitutional History of England*, vol. 3 (Oxford, 1878)

Summerson, H., *Medieval Carlisle: The City and the Borders from the Late Eleventh to the Mid-Sixteenth Century*, 2 vols, Cumberland and Westmorland Antiquarian and Archaeological Society e.s. 25 (Kendal, 1993)

Swanson, H., 'The Illusion of Economic Structure: Craft Guilds in Late Medieval English Towns', *P&P* 121 (1988), pp. 31–48

—— *Medieval Artisans: An Urban Class in Late Medieval England* (Oxford, 1989)

—— 'Artisans in the Urban Economy: The Documentary Evidence from York', in P. Corfield and D. Keene, eds, *Work in Towns, 850–1850* (Leicester, 1990)

Sweetinburgh, S., 'Joining the Sisters: Female Inmates of Late Medieval Hospitals in East Kent', *Archaeologia Cantiana* 202 (2003), pp. 17–40

—— *The Role of the Hospital in Medieval England* (Dublin, 2004)

—— 'Wax, Stone and Iron: Dover's Town Defences in the Late Middle Ages', *Archaeologia Cantiana* 124 (2004), pp. 183–207

—— 'The Hospitals of Medieval Kent', in S. Sweetinburgh, ed., *Later Medieval Kent, 1220–1540* (Woodbridge, 2010)

Taavitsainen, I., 'A Zodiacal Lunary for Medical Professionals', in L. M. Matheson, ed., *Popular and Practical Science of Medieval England* (East Lansing, MI, 1994)

Tachau, K. H., *Vision and Certitude in the Age of Ockham: Optics, Epistemology and the Foundations of Semantics, 1250–1345* (Leiden, 1988)

Talbot, C. H., *Medicine in Medieval England* (London, 1967)

TeBrake, W. H., 'Air Pollution and Fuel Crises in Pre-Industrial London, 1250–1650', *Technology and Culture* 16 (1975), pp. 337–59

Telfer, A., 'Medieval Drainage near Smithfield Market: Excavations at Hosier Lane, EC1', *London Archaeologist* 10.5 (2003), pp. 115–20

Theilmann, J. M., 'The Regulation of Public Health in Late Medieval England', in J. L. Gillespie, ed., *The Age of Richard II* (Stroud, 1997)

Thévenin, E., 'La Léproserie Saint-Ladre de Reims: un espace de festivités', in B. Tabuteau, ed., *Lépreux et sociabilité du moyen âge au temps modernes*, Cahiers du Groupe de Recherche d'Histoire 11 (Rouen, 2000)

Thomas, A. H., 'Notes on the History of the Leadenhall, AD 1195–1488', *London Topographical Record* 13 (1923), pp. 1–22

Thomas, K., *Religion and the Decline of Magic* (Harmondsworth, 1984)

Thomson, D., 'Henry VII and the Uses of Italy: The Savoy Hospital and Henry VII's Posterity', in B. Thompson, ed., *The Reign of Henry VII* (Stamford, 1995)

Thomson, J. A. F., 'Piety and Charity in Late Medieval London', *Journal of Ecclesiastical History* 16 (1965), pp. 178–95

—— *The Early Tudor Church and Society* (London, 1993)

Thorndike, L., 'Sanitation, Baths, and Street Cleaning in the Middle Ages and Renaissance', *Speculum* 3 (1928), pp. 192–203

Thrupp, S. L., *The Merchant Class of Medieval London* (Ann Arbor, MI, 1962)

—— 'The Problem of Replacement Rates in the Late Medieval English Population', *EconHR*, 2nd series 18 (1965–6), pp. 101–19

Tickell, J., *History of the Town and County of Kingston-upon-Hull* (Hull, 1798)

Tierney, B., 'The Decretists and the "Deserving Poor"', *Comparative Studies in Society and History* 1 (1958–9), pp. 360–73

Tillott, P. M., ed., *VCH York: The City of York* (Oxford, 1961)

Tittler, R., 'For the "Re-Edification of Townes": The Rebuilding Statutes of Henry VIII', *Albion* 22 (1990), pp. 591–605

Touati, F. O., *Maladie et société au moyen âge* (Paris, 1998)

Turner, E., 'The Statutes of the Marshes of Pevensey and Romney', *Sussex Archaeological Collections* 18 (1866), pp. 42–53

Vigarello, G., *Concepts of Cleanliness: Changing Attitudes in France since the Middle Ages* (Cambridge, 1988)

Wallace-Hadrill, A., 'Public Honour and Private Shame: The Urban Texture of Pompeii', in T. J. Cornell and K. Lomas, eds, *Urban Society in Roman Italy* (London, 1995)

Walton, M. T., 'Stinking Air, Corrupt Water and the English Sweat', *JHM* 36 (1981), pp. 67–8

—— 'Thomas Forestier and the "false lechys" of London', *JHM* 37 (1982), pp. 71–3

Walton, P., 'Textiles', in J. Blair and N. Ramsay, eds, *English Medieval Industries* (London, 1991)

Warkin, H. R., *Totnes Priory and Town*, 3 vols (Torquay, 1911–17)

Watson, S., 'The Origins of the English Hospital', *TRHS*, 6th series 16 (2006), pp. 75–94

—— 'City as Charter: Charity and the Lordship of English Towns, 1170–1250', in C. Goodson, A. E. Lester and C. Symes, eds, *Cities, Texts and Social Networks: Experiences and Perceptions of Medieval Urban Space* (Aldershot, 2010)

Watts, J., *Henry VI and the Politics of Kingship* (Cambridge, 1996)

Wear, A., 'Making Sense of Health and the Environment in Early Modern England', in A. Wear, ed., *Medicine and Society: Historical Essays* (Cambridge, 1992)

—— *Knowledge and Practice in Early Modern English Medicine, 1550–1680* (Cambridge, 2000)

Webster, C., 'Thomas Linacre and the Foundation of the College of Physicians', in F. Maddison, M. Pelling and C. Webster, eds, *Essays on the Life and Work of Thomas Linacre* (Oxford, 1977)

Weinbaum, M., *The Incorporation of Boroughs* (Manchester, 1937)

Welford, R., *History of Newcastle and Gateshead in the Fourteenth and Fifteenth Centuries* (London, 1884)

—— *History of Newcastle and Gateshead in the Sixteenth Century* (London, 1885)

Wenzel, S., 'Preaching the Seven Deadly Sins', in R. Newhauser, ed., *In the Garden of Evil: The Vices and Culture in the Middle Ages* (Toronto, 2005)

Westholm, G., 'Sanitary Infrastructure in Mediæval Visby', in M. Gläser, ed., *Lübecker Kolloquium zur Stadtarchäologie im Hanseraum IV: Die Infrastruktur* (Lübeck, 2004)

Westlake, H. F., *The Parish Guilds of Medieval England* (London, 1919)

Wheeler, J., 'Stench in Sixteenth-Century Venice', in A. Cowan and J. Steward, eds, *The City and the Senses: Urban Culture since 1500* (Aldershot, 2007)

Williams, G. A., *Medieval London: From Commune to Capital* (London, 1963)

Williams, R., 'The Plague in Cambridge', *Medical History* 1 (1957), pp. 51–64

Winslow, C.-E. A., *The Evolution and Significance of the Modern Public Health Campaign* (New Haven, CT, 1923)

Winter, J., 'The "Agitator of the Metropolis": Charles Cochrane and Early-Victorian Street Reform', *London Journal* 14 (1989), pp. 29–42

Wohl, A. S., *Endangered Lives: Public Health in Victorian Britain* (London, 1983)

Wood, A., '"A Littull Worde ys Tresson": Loyalty, Denunciation and Popular Politics in Tudor England', *Journal of British Studies* 58 (2009), pp. 837–47

Wood, Anthony à, *The History and Antiquities of the University of Oxford*, 2 vols (Oxford, 1792)

Woolgar, C., *The Senses in Late Medieval England* (New Haven, CT, 2006)

Wray, S. K., *Communities and Crisis: Bologna during the Black Death* (Leiden, 2009)

Wright, H. P., *The Story of the 'Domus Dei' of Chichester* (London, 1885)

—— *The Story of the 'Domus Dei' of Stamford* (London, 1890)

Wylie, J. A. H., and L. H. Collier, 'The English Sweating Sickness (*Sudor Anglicus*): A Reappraisal', *JHM* 36 (1981), pp. 425–45

Young, S., *Annals of the Barber-Surgeons of London* (London, 1890)

Ziegler, J., 'Medicine and Immortality in Terrestrial Paradise', in P. Biller and J. Ziegler, eds, *Religion and Medicine in the Middle Ages* (York, 2000)

Ziegler, P., *The Black Death* (Stroud, 1991)

Zimmermann, E. L., 'An Early English Manuscript on Syphilis', *Bulletin of the Institute of the History of Medicine* 5 (1937), pp. 461–82

Zupko, R. E., and R. A. Laures, *Straws in the Wind: Medieval Urban Environmental Law* (Boulder, CO, 1996)

✥ Unpublished Theses and Archaeological Reports

Amor, N., 'The Trade and Industry of Late Medieval Ipswich' (PhD thesis, University of East Anglia, 2009)

Bonfield, C. A., 'The *Regimen Sanitatis* and its Dissemination in England, *c.* 1348–1550' (PhD thesis, University of East Anglia, 2006)

Bowtell, A., 'A Medieval London Hospital: Elsyngspital, 1330–1536' (PhD thesis, Royal Holloway University of London, 2010)

Cullum, P. H., 'Hospitals and Charitable Provision in Medieval Yorkshire, 936–1547' (DPhil thesis, University of York, 1990)

Fay, I. H. H., 'Health and Disease in Medieval and Tudor Norwich' (PhD thesis, University of East Anglia, 2007)

Hawkins, J., 'The Blind in Late Medieval England: Medical, Social and Religious Responses' (PhD thesis, University of East Anglia, 2011)

Juddery, J. Z., and M. J. Stoyle, 'The Aqueducts of Medieval Exeter', Exeter Archaeology report 95.44

Martin, C. A., 'Transport for London, 1250–1550' (PhD thesis, Royal Holloway University of London, 2008)

Nockels Fabbri, C., 'Continuity and Change in Late Medieval Plague Medicine' (PhD thesis, Yale University, 2006)

Palmer, R. J., 'The Control of Plague in Venice and Northern Italy' (PhD thesis, University of Kent at Canterbury, 1978)

Phillips, E. M., 'Charitable Institutions in Norfolk and Suffolk, *c.* 1350–1600' (PhD thesis, University of East Anglia, 2001)

Satchell, A. E. M., 'The Emergence of Leper Houses in Medieval England, 1100–1200' (DPhil thesis, University of Oxford, 1998)

Stoyle, M. J., 'The Underground Aqueduct Passages of Exeter', Exeter Archaeology report 95.45

Wear, R., 'Aspects of Institutional Provision for the Sick Poor in Medieval Ipswich, *c.* 1305–1555' (MA thesis, University of East Anglia, 1997)

❧ Index

This index lists personal names, places and the principal subjects covered in the text. Saints may be found under their first names (e.g. Bridget, Thomas), as also may individuals whose names are toponyms (e.g. Adam of Usk). Numbers in **bold** type denote illustrations.